An Advanced Review of
Speech–Language Pathology

An Advanced Review of Speech–Language Pathology

Preparation for NESPA and Comprehensive Examination

Celeste Roseberry-McKibbin

M. N. Hegde

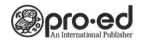

pro·ed
An International Publisher

8700 Shoal Creek Boulevard
Austin, Texas 78757-6897
800/897-3202   Fax 800/397-7633
Order online at http://www.proedinc.com

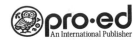

© 2000 by PRO-ED, Inc.
8700 Shoal Creek Boulevard
Austin, Texas 78757-6897
800/897-3202   Fax 800/397-7633
Order online at http://www.proedinc.com

Library of Congress Cataloging-in-Publication Data

Roseberry-McKibbin, Celeste.
    An advanced review of speech–language pathology : preparation for NESPA
and comprehensive examination / Celeste Roseberry-McKibbin, M. N. Hegde.
      p.   cm.
    Includes bibliographical references and index.
    ISBN 0-89079-821-4 (alk. paper)
    1. Speech disorders—Outlines, syllabi, etc. 2. Language disorders—
Outlines, syllabi, etc. 3. Speech therapy Outlines, syllabi, etc.
    4. Audiology—Outlines, syllabi, etc. I. Hegde, M. N. (Mahabalagiri
N.). II. Title.
RC423.R66 1999
616.85'5—dc21   99-24479
                                                CIP

This book is designed in Helvetica and New Century Schoolbook.

Production Director: Alan Grimes
Production Coordinator: Dolly Fisk Jackson
Managing Editor: Chris Olson
Art Director: Thomas Barkley
Designer: Jason Crosier
Print Buyer: Alicia Woods
Preproduction Coordinator: Chris Anne Worsham
Staff Copyeditor: Martin Wilson
Project Editor: Jill Mason
Publishing Assistant: Jason Morris

Printed in the United States of America

2 3 4 5 6 7 8 9 10   03 02 01 00

To our families
Mike and Mark Michael McKibbin
and
Prema and Manu Hegde
with love and gratitude

Contents

CHAPTER 1

Anatomy, Neuroanatomy, and Physiology of the Speech Mechanism

CHAPTER 2

Physiological and Acoustic Phonetics: A Speech Science Foundation

CHAPTER 3

Language Development in Children

CHAPTER 4
Language Disorders in Children

CHAPTER 5
Articulatory-Phonological Development and Disorders in Children

CHAPTER 6
Fluency and Its Disorders

CHAPTER 7
Voice and Its Disorders

CHAPTER 8
Neurologically Based Communicative Disorders and Dysphagia

CHAPTER 9
Communication Disorders in Multicultural Populations

Preface

The idea for this book was born back in 1996. I (Celeste Roseberry-McKibbin) was part of a team that was conducting workshops for speech–language pathologists who needed to pass the National Examination in Speech Pathology and Audiology (NESPA), so that they could become licensed and certified, to accommodate increasingly stringent professional state and federal requirements. These experienced clinicians, who had graduated from school 10–35 years ago, suddenly found themselves faced with the need to quickly learn (or retrieve from memory) a great deal of current information to pass a challenging examination. The task seemed formidable to many of them.

At the same time, M. N. Hegde and I were dealing with many graduate students who were experiencing great stress over the prospect of taking upcoming master's comprehensive examinations as well as the NESPA (usually taken within the same time period). All of these people needed current information covering the entire field of speech–language pathology. Many of them did not have time to go to libraries, check out books, read through each book, and extract the most relevant and up-to-date information that was likely to be asked on the NESPA and on comprehensive examinations in graduate programs. As we reflected upon this situation, an idea was born. Why not write a book that would meet those needs? Why not gather current, relevant material into one book that would help students and practitioners review for examinations that would open (or, sadly, close) career doors to them?

Several years later, this book has come together in one comprehensive package geared toward helping students and practitioners study for and pass the NESPA and comprehensive examinations in graduate programs. But there is also a third purpose for the book. We intend it to be not only a study guide, but also a review for practitioners who want an update of the field for their own professional growth. We have spoken with many practitioners in various professional settings, some of whom are aware that much of their knowledge has become dated but do not have the time or resources to obtain current knowledge in so many areas of an ever-expanding field. Thus, we have also written this book for experienced speech–language pathologists who would like to read current and comprehensive information for their own professional development.

It has been a joy to write a book that is unique in the field of speech–language pathology. No other book is written specifically to meet the needs of students taking comprehensive examinations and the NESPA, experienced practitioners taking the NESPA, and experienced practitioners who are seeking professional growth. When we have discussed the book with students and practitioners, the resounding response has been, "How soon will the book be out? I want to buy it! Please hurry and finish it!" (The last comment has also been heard from our spouses, but that is another story.) It is a great privilege for us to contribute this book to our field, and we hope that it will open doors for those who are seeking further knowledge and opportunities.

The book has unique pedagogical devices to facilitate the learning process. Each chapter has special features to help readers learn and retain the information therein. Each begins with a detailed "Preview Outline" to orient readers to its contents. Next, each chapter section has both a brief introduction and a summary to help readers: (a) become aware of what they will read, (b) read it, and (c) review what they have just read. We believe that repetition is one of the keys to learning and retaining information. At the end of each chapter, "Chapter Highlights" reviews and summarizes the most pertinent information. Readers who are studying for examinations can, soon before the examination, refresh their memories by re-reading section introductions and summaries and chapter highlights.

At the end of each chapter, we also list key terms from the chapter, as well as giving test questions in fill-in-the-blank and multiple-choice formats. The multiple-choice questions are written in a manner similar to that of the questions on the NESPA, to help prepare readers for those questions. Answers to test questions are at the very end of every chapter. For readers who want more information about certain topics within a chapter, we have included a comprehensive list of current references and recommended readings at the end of each chapter. This list will assist readers who want to obtain more information about certain areas.

A unique and key feature of this book is the "Concepts to Consider" questions that are embedded in the body of each chapter. We believe that adults learn best when they can actively interact with information, not just passively read it. To that end, we have written short essay questions to help readers pause, think about, and integrate the information that they have just read. We believe that answering those questions in writing will greatly assist readers in integrating and retaining the information in each chapter.

We would like to acknowledge some very special people who were helpful in the process of writing this book. Floyd and Beverly Roseberry's support and invaluable practical help were greatly appreciated. Dr. James Patton of PRO-ED gave unstinting support and encouragement during the process of completing this book. Thank you so much, Jim. Adriana Peña-Brooks contributed excellent information to the chapters on phonetics, articulatory-phonological disorders, and anatomy and physiology. Her generosity is most appreciated. Dr. Paul Fogle shared pertinent information about swallowing disorders. Dr. Eugene Wiggins gave helpful information about helping prepare test takers for the NESPA. The completion of this book would not have been possible without the continual help of Renee Grover, Christiane Kostecki, and Brittny Johnson, who gave generously of their time to see the book through to the end. Mike McKibbin's patience, love, and support were the foundation for this entire book. It would never have been completed without him.

Again, it is a privilege for us to contribute this work to our field. Thanks to the help and support of many individuals listed above, we are able to offer this book to students and practitioners from all walks of life. It is our hope that it will open doors to those very deserving individuals who have dedicated their lives to serving people with communication disorders.

CHAPTER 1

Anatomy, Neuroanatomy, and Physiology of the Speech Mechanism

PREVIEW OUTLINE

Anatomy and Physiology
Structural Mechanisms and Processes of Speech Production

The process of speech is one most people take for granted. However, speech depends on an intricate and complex system of structures and functions working together to allow human beings to communicate with one another. Respiration, or breathing, supplies the energy for speech. Phonation involves voicing and the structures and processes that create voice. Resonation, the process by which the voice or laryngeal tone is modified by various cavities and structures, is closely tied to articulation, the process of making speech sounds.

RESPIRATION: STRUCTURES AND PROCESSES

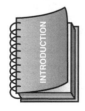

INTRODUCTION

Respiration, the process of breathing, is foundational to speech. The respiratory framework includes the lungs, bronchi, trachea, spinal column, sternum, and ribs. Respiration involves the cycle of inhalation and exhalation; various muscles are necessary for the the completion of that cycle.

Respiration Patterns During Speech Production

■ When we inhale, we bring oxygen to the blood. When we exhale, we get rid of accumulated carbon dioxide. When an excessive amount of carbon dioxide creates a need for oxygen, the *medulla oblongata* in the brain stem fires impulses to the respiratory muscles.

■ *Respiration* is the exchange of gas between an organism and its environment (Seikel, King, & Drumright, 1997). Inhalation (also called inspiration) and exhalation (also called expiration) create the rhythmic cycle of respiration. Inhalation draws air into the lungs, where an exchange of oxygen and carbon dioxide takes place. Through the actions of the diaphragm and other respiratory muscles, we expand the chest cavity and thus the lungs to inhale air.

■ As the lungs expand, the pressure within the lungs is reduced compared to the pressure outside the lungs. The air moves through the open laryngeal valve into the lungs, equalizing the pressure inside and outside the lungs.

■ At that point, muscles contract to reduce the volume of the chest cavity, creating a positive pressure within the lungs. As a result, we exhale. In this manner, the cycle of inhalation and exhalation automatically continues.

■ Respiration provides the air supply needed to set the vocal folds into vibration for speech. Because speech is typically produced on exhalation, the duration of exhalations during speech tends to be longer than the duration of exhalations during silent periods. Longer, louder utterances may require deeper inhalation than usual. Singers often inhale deeply.

■ Compared to quiet breathing, breathing for speech is more consciously monitored and adjusted to meet the demands of speech in various daily situations. These adjustments are continuous and rapid. To make these rapid adjustments, we need to have intact respiratory structures.

Framework of Respiration

■ Respiration is the foundation for speech. As previously stated, respiration involves inhalation and exhalation. Humans generally inhale and then speak on exhaled air. The basic process of inhalation can be summarized as follows (Van Riper & Erickson, 1996):

  – inhale → chest and lungs expand → diaphragm lowers → air flows in through the nose and mouth → air goes down pharynx and between open vocal folds → air continues downward through trachea and bronchial tubes → air reaches final destination of lungs

■ The above process of inhalation, as well as the processes in exhalation and speaking, is complex and requires the support of many structures, including the lungs, bronchi, trachea, spinal column, sternum, and ribs.

Lungs

■ The previously mentioned exchange of gas in respiration is accomplished in the *lungs*. Healthy lungs are soft, spongy, porous, elastic, and pink. They have a rich vascular supply and numerous air sacs.

■ The lungs are located in the thoracic cavity and take up most of the cavity's space. The right lung is shorter and broader and bigger than the left lung because of the liver underneath it, which forces it upward slightly. The lungs are illustrated in Figure 1.1.

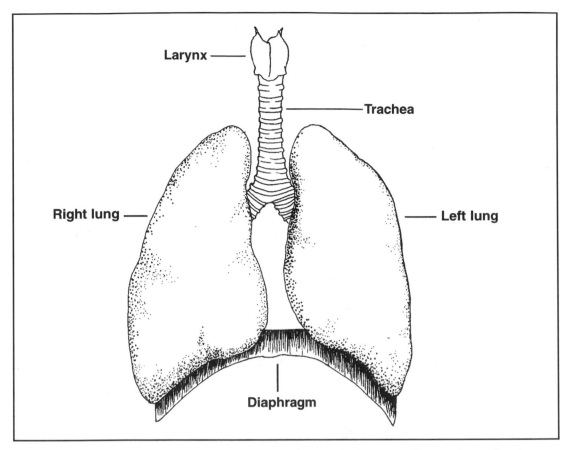

Figure 1.1. The lungs, diaphragm, trachea, and larynx. From *Introduction to Communicative Disorders*, 2nd ed. (p. 67), by M. N. Hegde, 1995, Austin, TX: PRO-ED. Copyright 1995 by PRO-ED, Inc. Reprinted with permission.

Bronchi

■ The *bronchi* are tubes that extend from the lungs upward to the trachea. The bronchi are composed of cartilaginous rings bound together by fibroelastic tissue (Zemlin, 1998).

■ In the lungs, the bronchi subdivide into *bronchioles*. The bronchioles repeatedly divide until they ultimately communicate with *alveolar ducts* that open into tiny air sacs in the lungs. As the bronchi and bronchioles divide, they become less cartilaginous and more muscular in composition.

Trachea

■ As a person inhales, the air goes in through the larynx to the trachea to the lungs, which expand, as previously stated. When a person exhales, the air goes upward again through the *trachea*, a tube formed by approximately 20 rings of cartilage (illustrated in Figure 1.1).

■ These rings of cartilage are incomplete in the back where the trachea comes into direct contact with the esophagus. The first tracheal cartilage is larger than the rest and connects to the inferior or bottom border of the cricoid cartilage.

■ The trachea extends from the larynx, at the level of the sixth cervical vertebra, and the last tracheal ring splits in two or *bifurcates* into the left and right primary bronchi at the level of the fifth thoracic vertebra.

Spinal Column

■ The *spinal column* consists of 32–33 individual vertebrae. These vertebrae are divided into five segments (see Figure 1.2):

- 7 *cervical* vertebrae (C1–C7)

- 12 *thoracic* vertebrae (T1–T12)

- 5 *lumbar* vertebrae (L1–L5)

- 5 *sacral* vertebrae (S1–S5)

- 3–4 *coccygeal* vertebrae (fused together and called the *coccyx*)

■ The thoracic vertebrae provide points of attachment for the ribs. The lumbar vertebrae are large which makes them suitable for weight-bearing functions.

Sternum

■ The *sternum*, also called the *breastbone*, is located on the superior, anterior thoracic wall. The sternum consists of three parts: the manubrium, body, and xiphoid process.

■ The *manubrium* is the uppermost segment of the sternum. The manubrium provides the attachment for the clavicle and the first rib.

■ The corpus or *body* of the sternum is long and narrow. The cartilages of ribs 2 through 7 attach to the body of the sternum.

■ The *xiphoid process* is a small cartilaginous structure at the bottom of the body of the sternum.

Rib Cage

■ The *rib cage*, or *thoracic cage*, is usually called the chest. It consists of 12 pairs of ribs that form a cylindrical structure. The rib cage houses and protects such organs as the heart and lungs. Figure 1.3 shows a schematic of the rib cage.

■ The rib cage is composed of several structures:

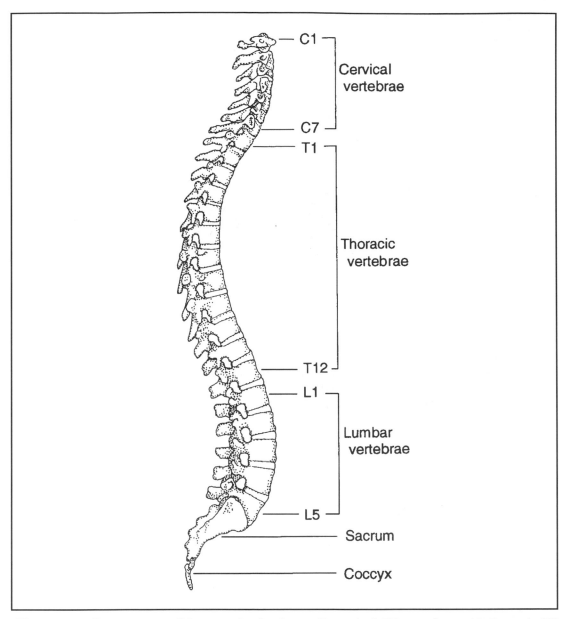

Figure 1.2. Components of the vertebral column: 7 cervical (C) vertebrae, 12 thoracic (T) vertebrae, 5 lumbar (L) vertebrae, 5 fused vertebrae of the sacrum (S), and the coccyx. From *Anatomy and Physiology for Speech, Language, and Hearing* (p. 41), by J. A. Seikel, D. W. King, and D. G. Drumright, 1997, San Diego, CA: Singular Publishing Group, Inc. (401 West A Street, Suite 325, San Diego, CA 92101-7904, 800-521-8545). Copyright 1997 by Singular Publishing Group, Inc. Reprinted with permission.

- sternum in the anterior surface

- 12 thoracic vertebrae in the posterior surface

- 12 pairs of ribs connecting laterally from the vertebrae to their individual *costal cartilages*

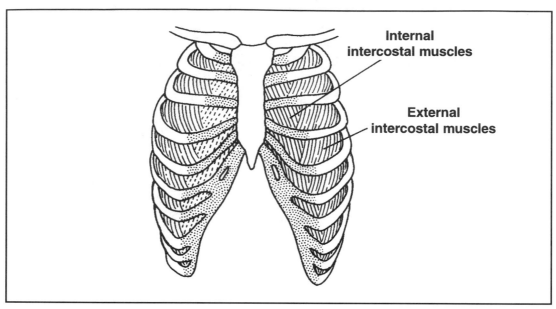

Figure 1.3. Rib cage with the internal and external intercostal muscles. External inter-costals are absent near the sternum, allowing one to see the deeper internal intercostals within that region. On the left rib cage, the fascia covering the internal intercostals has been removed, whereas the fascia remains present and translucent on the right. From *Anatomy and Physiology for Speech, Language, and Hearing* (p. 88), by J. A. Seikel, D. W. King, and D. G. Drumright, 1997, San Diego, CA: Singular Publishing Group, Inc. (401 West A Street, Suite 325, San Diego, CA 92101-7904, 800-521-8545). Copyright 1997 by Singular Publishing Group, Inc. Reprinted with permission.

✎ Concepts To Consider

Briefly describe three structures that are key to adequate respiration. What is the role of each structure?

_____

_____

_____

_____

_____

_____

_____

_____

_____

Muscles of Respiration

Thoracic Muscles of Inspiration

■ The *diaphragm*, illustrated in Figure 1.1, is the floor of the chest cavity. It is a thick, dome-shaped muscle that separates the abdomen from the thorax. The *abdomen* houses structures such as the intestines, liver, and kidneys.

■ Various abdominal muscles are critical in providing support for breathing. Because the lungs rest upon it, the diaphragm plays a major role in breathing.

■ The *intercostal muscles* (illustrated in Figure 1.3) between the ribs are also critical for respiration. The eleven paired *internal intercostals* pull the ribs downward to decrease the diameter of the thoracic cavity for exhalation, and the eleven paired *external intercostals* raise the ribs up and out to increase the diameter of the thoracic cavity for inhalation.

■ Several other muscles also help elevate the rib cage. The *serratus posterior superior, levator costarum brevis, levator costarum longis*, and *external intercostal* muscles are all involved in rib cage elevation.

■ These muscles and their innervations are summarized below (Seikel et al., 1997). (*Note*: The innervations basically arise from the vertebrae and their nerves and branches. For purposes of efficiency, only the vertebrae involved are listed—not the specific vertebral branches and nerves.)

Muscle and Innervation	Function
diaphragm (C3–C5)	distends abdomen, enlarges vertical dimension of thorax, depresses central tendon of diaphragm
serratus posterior superior (C7, T1–T4)	elevates rib cage
levator costarum brevis (T2–T12)	elevates rib cage
levator costarum longis (T2–T12)	elevates rib cage
external intercostal (T2–T11)	elevates rib cage

■ Accessory muscles of the neck are also involved in the process of respiration. Two of the key neck muscles are the sternocleidomastoid and the trapezius.

■ The *sternocleidomastoid* elevates the sternum and thus, indirectly, the rib cage. The *trapezius* controls the head and elongates the neck, and thus also indirectly influences respiration.

■ Muscles of the shoulder and upper arm also act to move the rib cage and increase or decrease its dimensions. These muscles include the *pectoralis major, pectoralis minor, serratus anterior,* and *levator scapulae.*

■ These muscles and their innervations and functions are summarized below (Seikel et al., 1997). (*Note*: The innervations basically arise from the vertebrae and their nerves and branches. For purposes of efficiency, only the vertebrae involved are listed—not the specific vertebral branches and nerves.)

Muscle and Innervation	Function
pectoralis major (C4–T1)	increases transverse dimension of rib cage through elevation of sternum
pectoralis minor (C4–T1)	increases transverse dimension of rib cage
serratus anterior (C5–C7)	elevates ribs 1–9
levator scapulae (C3–C5)	elevates scapula, supports neck
rhomboideus major (C5)	stabilizes shoulder girdle
rhomboideus minor (C5)	stabilizes shoulder girdle
internal intercostal (T2–T11)	depresses ribs 1–11
innermost intercostal (T2–T11)	depresses ribs 1–11
transversus thoracicus (T2–T6)	depresses ribs 2–6

■ Two posterior thoracic muscles are also involved in respiration. The *subcostal muscle* depresses the thorax. The *serratus posterior inferior* muscles, when contracted, pull the rib cage down and thus aid in exhalation.

Abdominal Muscles of Expiration

■ Most muscles involved with breathing assist with inspiration. However, muscle action is also needed for exhalation of air. Muscles of expiration include the *latissimus dorsi, rectus abdominus, transversus abdominus, internal oblique abdominus,* and *quadratus lumborum.*

■ These muscles, their innervations, and their functions are briefly summarized below (Seikel et al., 1997). (*Note*: The innervations basically arise from the vertebrae and their nerves and branches. For purposes of efficiency, only the vertebrae involved are listed—not the specific vertebral branches and nerves.)

Muscle and Innervation	Function
latissimus dorsi (C6–C8)	stabilizes posterior abdominal wall for expiration
rectus abdominus (T7–T12)	flexes vertebral column
transversus abdominus (T7–T12)	compresses abdomen
internal oblique abdominus (T7–T12)	compresses abdomen, flexes and rotates trunk
quadratus lumborum (T12, L1–L4)	supports abdominal compression through bilateral contraction which fixes abdominal walls

Summary

☑ Respiration, the process of breathing involving an exchange of gas between an organism and its environment, is necessary for life itself. It is also the foundation of speech.

☑ The framework of respiration supports the muscles necessary for respiration to take place. These muscles include two primary categories: the thoracic muscles of inspiration, and the abdominal muscles of expiration.

☑ Respiration provides the foundation and energy for phonation.

PHONATION: STRUCTURES AND PROCESSES

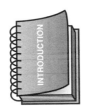

INTRODUCTION

Commonly known as the voice box, the larynx lies at the top of the trachea and houses the vocal folds, which vibrate to produce voice. Optimal laryngeal function and voicing depend upon the integrity of key laryngeal cartilages as well as intrinsic and extrinsic laryngeal muscles. Certain neuroanatomical structures are also critical. These include cortical areas, the cerebellum, and cranial nerves VII and X.

Larynx

▦ During speech, the lungs produce the necessary air for phonation. The air flows upward through the trachea and comes toward the larynx. The *larynx* (called the voice box by laypeople) lies at the top of the trachea in the anterior portion of the neck. It is a valving mechanism, which opens and closes. The major structures of the larynx are shown in Figure 1.4.

▦ The larynx houses the *vocal folds*, which vibrate to produce sound. The vocal folds *adduct* (move toward the midline) and *abduct* (move away from the midline) as they vibrate. When a person is breathing quietly, the vocal folds are abducted.

▦ In addition to producing the sound needed for speech, the larynx has biological functions. These include: (a) closure of the trachea so that food and other substances do not enter the lungs, (b) production of the cough reflex to expel foreign substances that accidentally enter the trachea, and (c) closure of the vocal folds to build subglottic pressure necessary for physical tasks such as excretion and lifting heavy items.

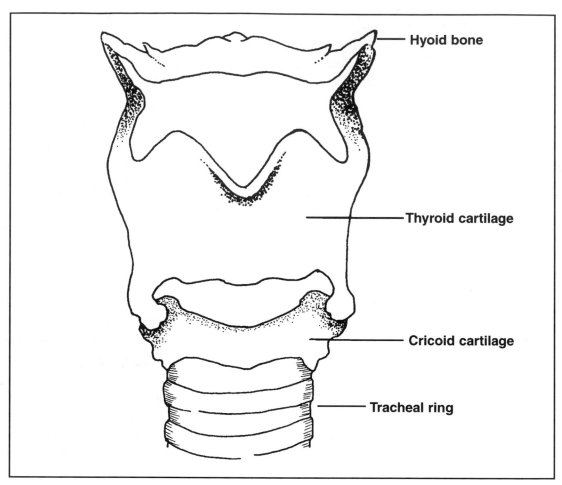

Figure 1.4. Major structures of the larynx. From *Introduction to Communicative Disorders,* 2nd ed. (p. 69), by M. N. Hegde, 1995, Austin, TX: PRO-ED. Copyright 1995 by PRO-ED, Inc. Reprinted with permission.

Laryngeal Structures and Cartilages

■ The larynx is suspended from the U-shaped *hyoid bone*, which floats under the mandible or lower jaw. The muscles of the tongue and various muscles of the mandible, skull, and larynx are attached to the hyoid bone.

■ The *epiglottis*, a protective structure, is a leaf-shaped piece of cartilage medial to the thyroid cartilage and hyoid bone. During swallowing, the epiglottis drops to cover the orifice of the larynx (Seikel et al., 1997). Figure 1.5 illustrates the epiglottis and other key laryngeal structures.

■ Key cartilages of the larynx include the thyroid, cricoid, and arytenoid cartilages. The *thyroid cartilage* forms the anterior and lateral walls of the larynx and protects the larynx.

■ The *cricoid cartilage*, which some view as the uppermost tracheal ring, is linked with the thyroid cartilage and the paired arytenoid cartilages. The cricoid cartilage completely surrounds the trachea.

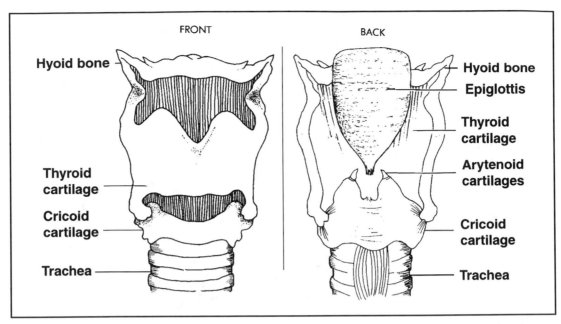

Figure 1.5. A front and back view of key laryngeal structures. From *Introduction to Communicative Disorders,* 2nd ed. (p. 264), by M. N. Hegde, 1995, Austin, TX: PRO-ED. Copyright 1995 by PRO-ED, Inc. Reprinted with permission.

- The *arytenoid cartilages* are small, pyramid-shaped cartilages connected to the cricoid through the *cricoarytenoid joint*, which permits sliding and circular movements.

- The small, cone-shaped *corniculate cartilages* sit on the apex of the arytenoids. The tiny cone-shaped *cuneiform cartilages* are located under the mucous membrane that covers the aryepiglottic folds (defined later).

Intrinsic Laryngeal Muscles

- The *intrinsic laryngeal muscles* are primarily responsible for controlling sound production (Zemlin, 1998). The intrinsic muscles of the larynx are the thyroarytenoids, lateral cricoarytenoids, transverse arytenoids, oblique arytenoids, cricothyroids, and posterior cricoarytenoids.

- The *thyroarytenoids* are attached to the thyroid and arytenoid cartilages. The thyroarytenoid muscles are divided into two muscle masses: the internal thyroarytenoids and the external thyroarytenoids.

- The internal thyroarytenoids are the primary portions of the thyroarytenoid muscle that vibrate and produce sound. Some people also refer to them as the *vocalis muscle, vocal folds,* and *vocal cords.* The vocal folds are illustrated in Figure 1.6.

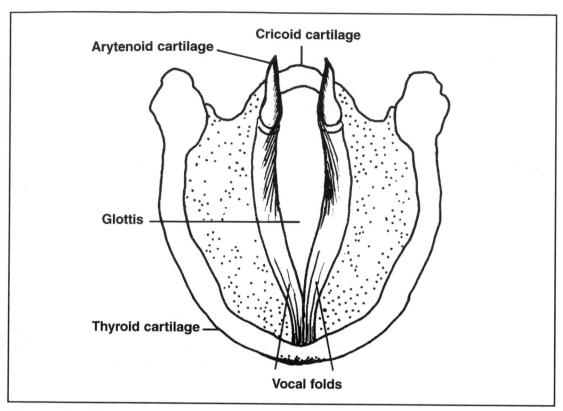

Figure 1.6. The vocal folds and surrounding structures. From *Introduction to Communicative Disorders,* 2nd ed. (p. 70), by M. N. Hegde, 1995, Austin, TX: PRO-ED. Copyright 1995 by PRO-ED, Inc.. Reprinted with permission.

▪ Adductor muscles include the *lateral cricoarytenoids,* transverse arytenoids, and oblique arytenoids. These muscles act to bring the vocal folds together. The lateral cricoarytenoids increase medial compression.

▪ The *cricothyroid muscle* is attached to the cricoid and thyroid cartilages. It lengthens and tenses the vocal folds.

▪ Figure 1.7 illustrates the *posterior cricoarytenoid* muscle and the *oblique* and *transverse arytenoid* muscles. Vocal fold adduction is supported when the oblique and transverse arytenoid muscles contract and pull the arytenoids closer together. Abduction of the vocal folds is accomplished when the posterior cricoarytenoid muscle contracts.

▪ The following lists provide a simple summary of the intrinsic laryngeal muscles, the number of the cranial nerves that innervate them (e.g., "X"), the attachments of each muscle pair, and their functions. (*Note*: Most intrinsic laryngeal muscles are innervated by the recurrent laryngeal nerve branch of cranial nerve X, the vagus nerve. An exception is the cricothyroids, which are innervated by the external branch of the superior laryngeal nerve branch of the vagus.)

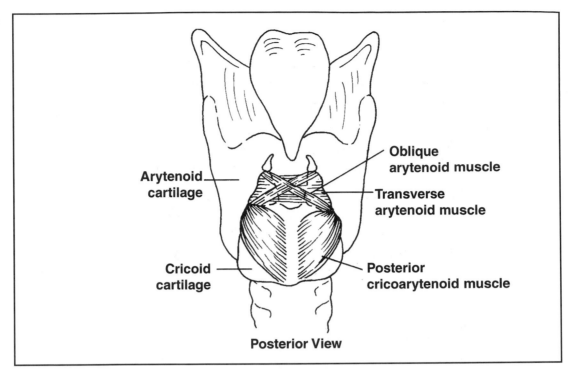

Posterior View

Figure 1.7. Posterior cricoarytenoid muscle and oblique and transverse arytenoid muscles. From *Anatomy and Physiology for Speech, Language, and Hearing* (p. 186), by J. A. Seikel, D. W. King, and D. G. Drumright, 1997, San Diego, CA: Singular Publishing Group, Inc. (401 West A Street, Suite 325, San Diego, CA 92101-7904, 800-521-8545). Copyright 1997 by Singular Publishing Group, Inc. Reprinted with permission.

Muscles and Innervation	Function
thyroarytenoids (X)	internal thyroarytenoids are primary portion of vocal folds that vibrate & produce sound
lateral cricoarytenoids (X)	adducts vocal folds, increases medial compression
transverse arytenoids (X)	adducts vocal folds
oblique arytenoids (X)	pulls apex of arytenoids in a medial direction
cricothyroids (X)	lengthens and tenses vocal folds
posterior cricoarytenoids (X)	abducts vocal folds

■ When the vocal folds are abducted, a small opening is created, which is called the *glottis*. The glottis is not an anatomical structure; it is merely the name of that space.

Extrinsic Laryngeal Muscles

■ The primary function of the *extrinsic laryngeal muscles* is to support the larynx and fix its position (Zemlin, 1998). The extrinsic laryngeal muscles have one attachment to a structure within the larynx and one attachment to a structure outside the larynx. All extrinsic muscles are attached to the hyoid bone and lower or raise the position of the larynx within the neck.

■ The *elevators,* or *suprahyoid muscles,* lie above the hyoid bone. Their primary function is elevation of the larynx. The suprahyoid muscles are the *digastrics, geniohyoids, mylohyoids,* and *stylohyoids, hyoglossus,* and *genioglossus.*

■ The *depressors,* or *infrahyoid muscles,* lie below the hyoid bone. Their primary function is depression of the larynx. The infrahyoid muscles are the *thyrohyoids, omohyoids, sternothyroids,* and *sternohyoids.*

■ The following lists provide a brief summary of the elevators and depressors, their locations, and their functions. Innervation of these muscles is generally provided by branches of cranial nerve V (trigeminal), cranial nerve VII (facial), cranial nerve X (vagus), cranial nerve XII (hypoglossal), and portions of cervical spinal nerves C1–C3. (For more detailed information, see Seikel et al., 1997).

Elevators and Innervation	Depressors and Innervation
digastrics (V, VII)	thyrohyoids (XII, C1)
geniohyoids (XII, C1)	omohyoids (C1–C3)
mylohyoids (V)	sternothyroids (C1–C3)
stylohyoids (VII)	sternohyoids (C1–C3)
hyoglossus (XII)	
genioglossus (XII)	

Vocal Folds

■ The vocal folds have three layers: 1) the *epithelium,* or outer cover, 2) the *lamina propria,* or middle layer (which actually consists of three layers), and 3) the *vocalis muscle,* or body, which provides stability and mass to the vocal fold.

■ There are two other pairs of folds (see Figure 1.8):

  – *Aryepiglottic folds.* The aryepiglottic folds are composed of a ring of connective tissue and muscle extending from the tips of the arytenoids to the larynx. They separate the laryngeal vestibule from the pharynx and help preserve the airway.

  – *Ventricular,* or *false,* vocal folds. The ventricular folds vibrate only at very low fundamental frequencies and usually not during phonation in a normal speaker. The ventricular folds compress during such activities as coughing and lifting heavy items.

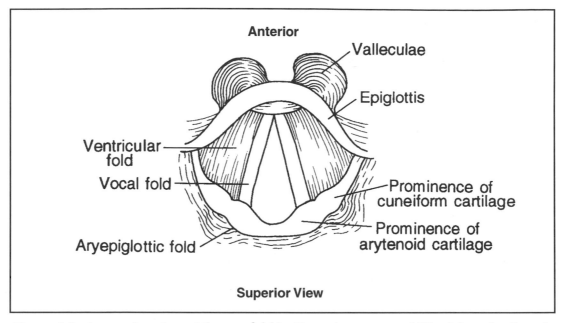

Figure 1.8. A superior view of the vocal folds. From *Anatomy and Physiology for Speech, Language, and Hearing* (p. 172), by J. A. Seikel, D. W. King, and D. G. Drumright, 1997, San Diego, CA: Singular Publishing Group, Inc. (401 West A Street, Suite 325, San Diego, CA 92101-7904, 800-521-8545). Copyright 1997 by Singular Publishing Group, Inc. Reprinted with permission.

Physiology of Phonation

Myoelastic Aerodynamic Theory and Bernoulli Effect

- The *myoelastic aerodynamic theory* states that the vocal folds vibrate because of the forces and pressure of air and the elasticity of the vocal folds.

- The air flowing out of the lungs is temporarily stopped by the closed (or nearly closed) vocal folds. This builds up subglottal air pressure, which eventually blows the vocal folds apart. During this process, the folds are set into vibration as well.

- The air then moves with increased velocity through the glottal opening. As the air moves swiftly through the open, but still somewhat constricted, vocal folds, the pressure between the edges of the vocal folds decreases, and consequently, the folds are sucked together.

- The *Bernoulli effect*, caused by the increased speed of air passing between the vocal folds, is the "sucking" motion of the vocal folds toward one another.

- Once again, the subglottal air pressure builds up and sets the folds in motion. Thus, there is a cycle of opening and closing of the vocal folds; this cycle is repeated more than 100 times per second during vocalization.

✎ Concepts To Consider

Give a brief description of the myoelastic aerodynamic theory and the Bernoulli effect.

_____

_____

_____

_____

_____

_____

_____

Mucosal Wave Action

■ The mucosal wave is critical to vibration of the vocal folds. In *mucosal wave action*, the cover (epithelium and superficial lamina propria, Reinke's space) and the transition (intermediate and deep layers of the lamina propria) over the vocalis muscle slide and produce a wave (Colton & Casper, 1996).

■ This wave travels across the superior surface of the vocal fold about two-thirds of the way to the lateral edge of the fold. Generally, the wave dissipates before reaching the inner surface of the thyroid cartilage. There is no vibration, and thus no phonation, without a mucosal wave.

■ Vocal folds that have been stripped surgically, while being free of overt pathology such as nodules, may be stiff and have difficulty vibrating due to alteration of the normal mucosal wave (Boone & McFarlane, 1994).

Neuroanatomy of the Vocal Mechanism

Cortical Areas

■ The primary cortical areas involved in speech motor control, including phonation, are:

- area 4 (primary motor cortex)

- area 44 (Broca's area)

- areas 3, 1, 2 (somatosensory cortex)

- area 6 (supplementary motor cortex)

Cerebellum

■ The function of the cerebellum is to regulate motor movement. It is critical in the control of speech movement.

■ The cerebellum is key to the coordination of the laryngeal muscles for adequate phonation. It also is involved in other speech systems such as respiration.

Cranial Nerves

■ Cranial nerve VII *(the facial nerve)* innervates the posterior belly of the digastric muscle.

■ *Cranial nerve X* (the vagus nerve) includes the following primary branches, which innervate the larynx:

  – *Superior laryngeal nerve (SLN)*: The superior laryngeal nerve has internal and external branches. The internal branch provides all sensory information to the larynx, and the external branch supplies motor innervation solely to the cricothyroid muscle.

  – *Recurrent laryngeal nerve (RLN)*: The recurrent laryngeal nerve supplies all motor innervation to the interarytenoid, posterior cricoarytenoid, thyroarytenoid, and lateral cricoarytenoid muscles. It supplies all sensory information below the vocal folds.

Summary

☑ Air for speech comes from the lungs, through the trachea, and to the larynx and sets the vocal folds in motion for voicing. Adequate voicing depends upon the integrity of many laryngeal structures.

☑ Key laryngeal structures and cartilages provide protection to the larynx and aid in the process of vocalization.

☑ There are two sets of laryngeal muscles. The intrinsic laryngeal muscles have both their attachments within the larynx. The extrinsic laryngeal muscles have one attachment inside the larynx and one attachment outside the larynx.

☑ The physiology of phonation can be explained by the myoelastic aerodynamic theory and the phenomenon of the Bernoulli effect. Mucosal wave action is critical to vocal fold vibration.

☑ Key neuroanatomical structures involved in vocalization include cortical areas, the cerebellum, and cranial nerves VII (facial nerve) and X (vagus nerve).

RESONATION AND ARTICULATION: STRUCTURES AND PROCESSES

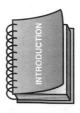

INTRODUCTION

Respiration provides the energy for voicing. As the laryngeal tone travels upward past the larynx, it must be resonated by various structures such as the pharynx, the oral cavity, and the nasal cavity. The resonated tone is then shaped and modified further through articulation, or production of speech sounds. Key structures involved in articulation include the pharynx, the soft palate, the hard palate, the mandible, the teeth, the tongue, the lips, and the cheeks. Functioning of these structures depends in part upon innervation by various cranial nerves.

Fundamentals of Resonation

■ The vocal folds vibrate to produce voice. *Resonation* is the process by which the voice, or laryngeal tone, is modified when some frequency components are dampened and others are enhanced. The resonators that serve to modify laryngeal tone are the pharynx, the nasal cavity, and the oral cavity.

■ The *pharynx*, or throat, is part of the upper airway. It is located superiorly and posteriorly to the larynx. The size and shape of the pharynx are modified by the position of the tongue in the mouth (forward or back) and the vertical positioning of the larynx in the neck (high or low) (Peña-Brooks & Hegde, 1999).

■ The *nasal cavity* has an important role in resonation. Only three sounds in English—/m/, /n/, and /ŋ/—are produced with *nasal resonance*. During the production of those sounds, the soft palate, or velum, is relaxed and lowered, as illustrated in Figure 1.9(A). Thus, there is *coupling* of the nasal and oral cavities; they are not separated from one another.

■ The velum is elevated and retracted for production of all other sounds in English. During production of those sounds, the velum is raised and retracted, or moved back, to make contact with the posterior pharyngeal wall, separating the oral cavity from the nasal cavity, as illustrated in Figure 1.9(B). The cavities are thus *uncoupled*. In this way, the sounds are produced primarily with *oral resonance*.

■ The *oral cavity* is the primary resonating structure for all English sounds, except /m/, /n/, and /ŋ/. The source-filter theory of vowel production provides a widely accepted description of how the oral cavity is capable of producing speech sounds.

■ According to the *source-filter theory*, the vocal tract is visualized as a series of linked tubes: the oral cavity, or mouth; the pharynx; and the nasal cavity (see Figure 1.10). These linked tubes provide the variable resonating cavity that help produce speech (Seikel et al., 1997).

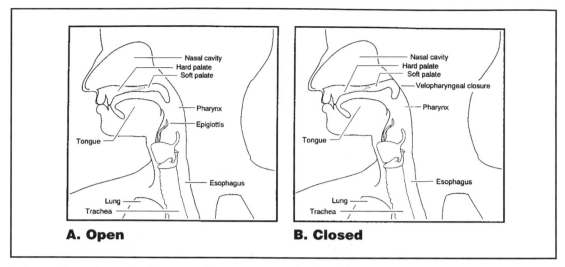

Figure 1.9. The velopharyngeal port, open and closed. From *Manual of Voice Treatment: Pediatrics Through Geriatrics* (p. 72), by M. L. Andrews, 1995, San Diego, CA: Singular Publishing Group, Inc. (401 West A Street, Suite 325, San Diego, CA 92101-7904, 800-521-8545). Copyright 1995 by Singular Publishing Group, Inc. Reprinted with permission.

■ The source-filter theory states that energy from the vibrating vocal folds (the *source*) is modified by the resonance characteristics of the vocal tract (the *filter*) (Kent, 1997).

■ The vocal folds generate a voicing source. This voicing source is routed through the vocal tract, where it is shaped into speech sounds. Those speech sounds may be vowels when the source is phonation, and consonants when the sources include the turbulence of frication or combinations of turbulence and voicing.

■ Changes in the configuration and shape of the articulators (described below) govern the resonance characteristics of the vocal tract. The resonances of the vocal tract determine the sound of each specific vowel. But whether consonants or vowels are produced, in each case the person produces a noise source and passes it through the filter of the oral cavity, which has been specifically configured for production of that sound (Seikel et al., 1997).

■ Structures within the oral cavity are shaped and moved to provide specific resonance for each sound. These structures are key in the process of articulation.

Fundamentals of Articulation

■ Articulation refers to the connection of movable parts or the joining of two elements. In speech, articulation refers to movements of speech structures to produce speech sounds. Articulation may also refer to the act of saying something clearly. In this section, the term *articulation* refers to the movement of

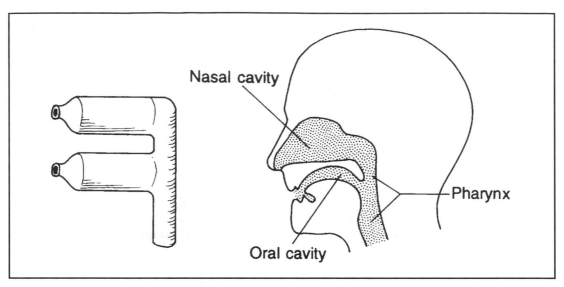

Figure 1.10. Schematic of the pharyngeal, oral, and nasal cavities as a series of linked tubes. From *Anatomy and Physiology for Speech, Language, and Hearing* (p. 258), by J. A. Seikel, D. W. King, and D. G. Drumright, 1997, San Diego, CA: Singular Publishing Group, Inc. (401 West A Street, Suite 325, San Diego, CA 92101-7904, 800-521-8545). Copyright 1997 by Singular Publishing Group, Inc. Reprinted with permission.

joined anatomic parts as well as the production of speech sounds that result from such movements.

■ When a person is speaking, the larynx produces sound. The sound, as stated, travels through the pharynx and the oral cavity (and the nasal cavity for nasal sounds). In the oral cavity, important structures modify the sound into specific sounds for speech. These structures include the pharynx, the soft palate, the hard palate, the mandible, the teeth, the tongue, the lips, and the cheeks.

Pharynx

■ The pharyngeal cavity is divided into three segments, which are illustrated in Figure 1.11:

– the *laryngopharynx*, which begins immediately superior to the larynx and ends at the base of the tongue, is connected to the

– *oropharynx*, which extends up to the soft palate and is connected to the

– *nasopharynx*, which ends where the two nasal cavities begin.

■ The laryngopharynx and the oropharynx add resonance to the sounds produced by the larynx. However, as previously stated, the nasopharynx adds noticeable resonance only to the nasals, /m/, /n/, and /ŋ/.

■ The muscles of the pharynx are summarized in the following lists (Seikel et al., 1997). Most pharyngeal muscles are innervated by cranial nerve X (the vagus nerve) and cranial nerve XI (the accessory nerve) via the pharyngeal

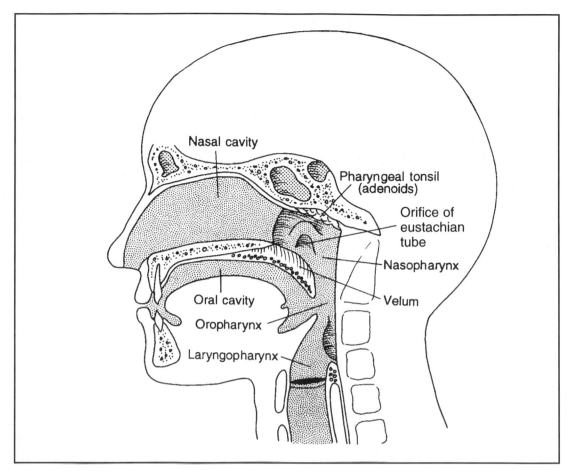

Figure 1.11. The pharyngeal, oral, and nasal cavities. From *Anatomy and Physiology for Speech, Language, and Hearing* (p. 300), by J. A. Seikel, D. W. King, and D. G. Drumright, 1997, San Diego, CA: Singular Publishing Group, Inc. (401 West A Street, Suite 325, San Diego, CA 92101-7904, 800-521-8545). Copyright 1997 by Singular Publishing Group, Inc. Reprinted with permission.

plexus. The *pharyngeal plexus* is formed by the joining of cranial nerves X and XI; it supplies the upper pharyngeal musculature.

Muscle and Innervation	Function
Salpingopharyngeus (X, XI)	elevates lateral pharyngeal wall
Stylopharyngeus (IX)	elevates and opens pharynx
Superior pharyngeal constrictor (X, XI)	constricts pharyngeal diameter, pulls pharyngeal wall forward
Middle pharyngeal constrictor (X, XI)	narrows diameter of pharynx
Inferior pharyngeal constrictor, cricopharyngeus (X, XI)	constricts superior orifice of esophagus
Inferior pharyngeal constrictor, thyropharyngeus (X, XI)	reduces diameter of lower pharynx

Soft Palate

■ The soft palate, also called the *velum*, is a flexible muscular structure at the juncture of the oropharynx and the nasopharynx. It is located in the posterior area of the oral cavity and hangs from the hard palate (roof of the mouth). The *uvula* is the small, cone-shaped structure at the tip of the velum. The soft palate and other major structures of the oral cavity are shown in Figure 1.12.

■ The soft palate is a dynamic structure of muscles that can be elevated or lowered. As previously stated, when the soft palate is lowered, there is coupling of the nasal and oral cavities for nasal sounds or quiet breathing through the nose.

■ When the soft palate is raised and retracted, the muscles of the pharynx also move inward to meet the muscles of the soft palate. With this sphincter-like action, the nasal port is then closed. This action is called *velopharyngeal closure*.

■ If the muscular bulk of the soft palate is inadequate, then the nasal cavity may always remain open to some extent. Speakers with this condition will sound excessively nasal because sound energy passes through the nasal cavities when it should not.

■ The soft palate is composed of a number of muscles (see Figure 1.13). These include the *levator veli palatini*, the *tensor veli palatini*, the *palatoglossus*, and the *palatopharyngeus* muscles. These muscles and their functions and innervations are summarized in the lists below (Seikel et al., 1997). (*Note*: The innervation "X, XI" refers specifically to the pharyngeal plexus, a struc-

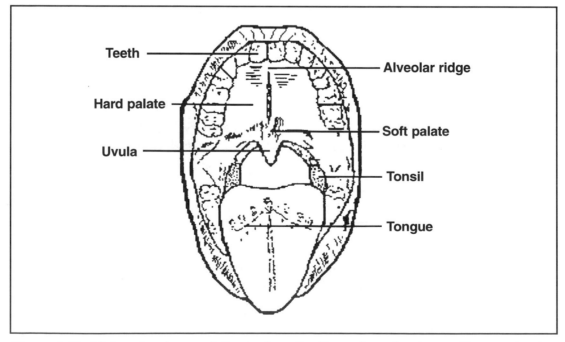

Figure 1.12. Major structures of the oral cavity. From *Introduction to Communicative Disorders,* 2nd ed. (p. 76), by M. N. Hedge, 1995, Austin, TX: PRO-ED. Copyright 1995 by PRO-ED, Inc. Reprinted with permission.

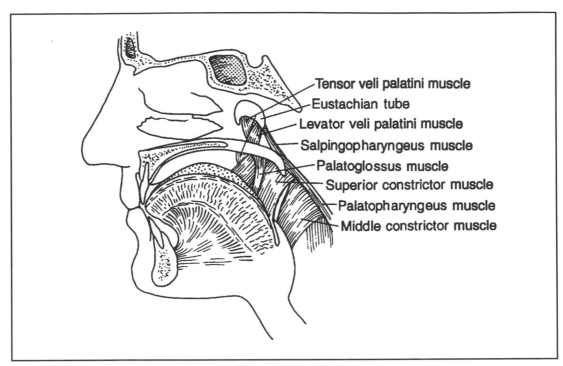

Figure 1.13. Muscles of the pharynx and soft palate. From *Anatomy and Physiology for Speech, Language, and Hearing* (p. 329), by J. A. Seikel, D. W. King, and D. G. Drumright, 1997, San Diego, CA: Singular Publishing Group, Inc. (401 West A Street, Suite 325, San Diego, CA 92101-7904, 800-521-8545). Copyright 1997 by Singular Publishing Group, Inc. Reprinted with permission.

ture arising from cranial nerve X, the vagus nerve, and cranial nerve X1, the spinal accessory nerve.)

Muscle and Innervation	Function
levator veli palatini (X, XI)	primary elevator of velum
tensor veli palatini (V)	tenses velum, dilates Eustachian tube
palatoglossus (X, XI)	elevates and depresses velum
palatopharyngeus (X, XI)	narrows pharyngeal cavity, lowers velum, may assist in elevating larynx

Hard Palate

■ The bony hard palate is the roof of the mouth and the floor of the nose. It is part of the *maxillae*, or paired bones, which are the largest in the face and form the entire upper jaw (Zemlin, 1998). The maxillae are also referred to as the maxillary bone. The hard palate is illustrated in Figure 1.14.

■ The front portion of the maxillary bone is called the *premaxilla*. The premaxilla houses the four upper front teeth known as the incisors.

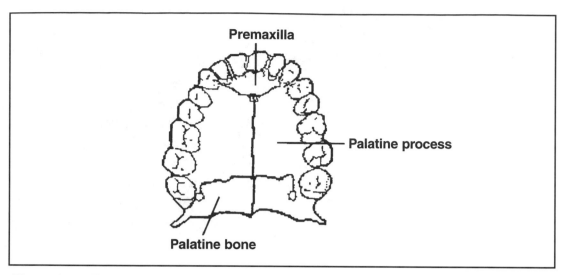

Figure 1.14. Hard palate and surrounding structures. From *Introduction to Communicative Disorders*, 2nd ed. (p. 77), by M. N. Hegde, 1995, Austin, TX: PRO-ED. Copyright 1995 by PRO-ED, Inc. Reprinted with permission.

- The portion of the maxillary bone that forms most of the hard palate is called the *palatine process*. The palatine process consists of two pieces of bone that grow and fuse at the midline during the fetal stage.

- The outer edges of the maxillary bone are called the *alveolar process*, which houses the molar, bicuspid, and cuspid teeth.

- Due to genetic and toxic environmental reasons, the premaxilla may fail to fuse with the maxillary bone. Also, the palatine process may fail to fuse at midline. These failures cause clefts of the palate.

- Posteriorly, the maxillary bone joins with the *palatine bone* (different from the palatine process, which is part of the maxillary bone). The soft palate attaches to the palatine bone.

Mandible

- Also known as the lower jaw, the mandible is an important facial bone. It houses the lower teeth and forms the floor of the mouth. The mandible is formed by the fusion of two bones in the midpoint of the chin, but it is considered to be one bone in adults.

- The *alveolar arch* is the part of the mandible that houses the teeth. The two arches of the mandible are hinged to the skull with a set of muscles and tendons. The mandible is attached to the temporal bone of the skull by a joint called the *temporomandibular joint*.

- The muscles of the mandible serve two major functions: 1) opening and closing the mouth, and 2) chewing food. Although its major task is to chew food, the mandible is important for speech because it houses the lower teeth, serves as a framework for the tongue and lower lip, and is an integral part of the oral cavity.

■ The muscles of the mandible can be categorized as either elevators or depressors (Seikel et al., 1997). They arise from branches of cranial nerves V (trigeminal nerve), VII (facial nerve), and XII (hypoglossal nerve); the geniohyoid also rises from the C1 spinal nerve. These muscles are summarized below.

Elevators and Innervation	Function
masseter (V)	elevates mandible
temporalis (V)	elevates mandible, draws mandible back if protruded
medial (internal) pterygoid (V)	elevates mandible
lateral (external) pterygoid (V)	protrudes mandible
Depressors and Innervation	
anterior belly of digastric (V)	depresses mandible in conjunction with posterior belly of digastric; pulls hyoid forward
posterior belly of digastric (VII)	depresses mandible in conjuction with anterior belly of digastric; pulls hyoid back
geniohyoid (XII, C1)	depresses mandible
mylohyoid (V)	depresses mandible

Teeth

■ The lower dental arch is part of the mandible, and the upper dental arch is part of the maxillary bone. The major function of the teeth is *mastication* (chewing), but the teeth also aid in production of some speech sounds. For example, the labiodental sounds /f/ and /v/ require the lower lip to come in contact with the upper teeth. Thus, the teeth are considered articulators.

■ Teeth, illustrated in Figure 1.15, are called by different names (e.g., molars, bicuspids) depending upon their location in the mouth. *Deciduous teeth* are temporary teeth that appear in a baby, usually around 6–9 months of age. Babies normally have 20 deciduous teeth, 10 in each arch. Of the 10, 4 are incisors, 2 are canine, and 4 are molar.

■ Adults have 32 teeth, 16 in each arch; of the 16 teeth, 4 are incisors, 2 are canine, 4 are premolar, and 6 are molar. The deciduous dental arch does not have premolars or the third molar.

■ *Occlusion* refers to the way the two dental arches come together when a person "bites down." Occlusion is normal if 1) the upper and lower dental arches meet each other in a symmetrical manner, and 2) if the individual teeth in the two arches are properly aligned.

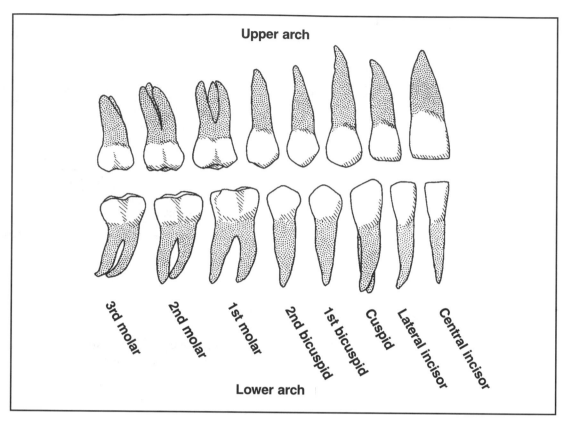

Figure 1.15. Types of teeth. From *Anatomy and Physiology for Speech, Language, and Hearing* (p. 294), by J. A. Seikel, D. W. King, and D. G. Drumright, 1997, San Diego, CA: Singular Publishing Group, Inc. (401 West A Street, Suite 325, San Diego, CA 92101-7904, 800-521-8545). Copyright 1997 by Singular Publishing Group, Inc. Reprinted with permission.

■ *Malocclusions* include deviations in the positioning of individual teeth and the shape and relationship of the upper and lower dental arches. Types of malocclusions are further described in Chapter 5.

✎ Concepts To Consider

List three pharyngeal muscles, three soft palate muscles, and three mandibular muscles that are key in the process of articulation.

_____

_____

_____

_____

_____

_____

Tongue

- The tongue plays an important role in eating and in speech production. The taste buds of the tongue help people taste their food, and the muscles of the tongue help it to move food around in the oral cavity for efficient mastication and swallowing. Movements of the tongue are critical to articulation.

- For example, tongue movement is necessary to produce /k/, /ŋ/, and many other sounds. The tongue can constrict the air passage and thus create the friction needed for sounds such as /ʃ/.

- Anatomically, the tongue is divided into four parts: tip, blade, dorsum, and root (see Figure 1.16):

  - The *tip* is the thinnest and most flexible part of the tongue, and it plays an important role in articulation.

  - The *blade* is a small region adjacent to the tip; in a resting position, the blade is the portion of the tongue that lies just inferior to the alveolar ridge.

  - The *dorsum* is the larger area of the tongue that lies in contact with both the hard and soft palates.

  - The *root* is contained in the very back of the tongue.

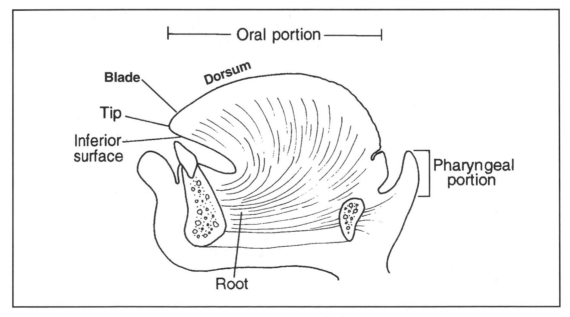

Figure 1.16. Major areas of the tongue. From *Anatomy and Physiology for Speech, Language, and Hearing* (p. 311), by J. A. Seikel, D. W. King, and D. G. Drumright, 1997, San Diego, CA: Singular Publishing Group, Inc. (401 West A Street, Suite 325, San Diego, CA 92101-7904, 800-521-8545). Copyright 1997 by Singular Publishing Group, Inc. Reprinted with permission.

■ The *lingual frenulum* (or *frenum*) connects the mandible with the inferior portion of the tongue. This band of tissue may stabilize the tongue during movement (Seikel et al., 1997).

■ There are two sets of important tongue muscles: intrinsic and extrinsic muscles. Upon contraction, these muscles perform important functions in articulation. The tongue muscles are innervated by cranial nerve XII, the hypoglossal nerve.

■ The genioglossus muscle forms the bulk of the tongue and allows it to move freely. Figure 1.17 illustrates the genioglossus and related muscles.

Intrinsic Tongue Muscles and Innervation	Function
superior longitudinal muscle (XII)	shortens tongue, turns tip upward, assists in turning lateral margins upward
inferior longitudinal muscle (XII)	shortens tongue, pulls tip downward, assists in retraction
transverse muscles (XII)	narrow and elongate tongue
vertical muscles (XII)	flatten the tongue

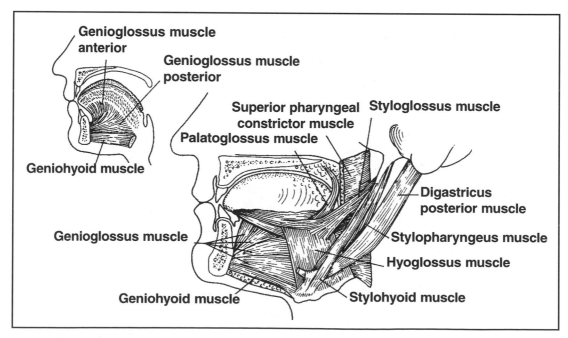

Figure 1.17. The genioglossus and related muscles. From *Anatomy and Physiology for Speech, Language, and Hearing* (p. 317), by J .A. Seikel, D. W. King, and D. G. Drumright, 1997, San Diego, CA: Singular Publishing Group, Inc. (401 West A Street, Suite 325, San Diego, CA 92101-7904, 800-521-8545). Copyright 1997 by Singular Publishing Group, Inc. Reprinted with permission.

Extrinsic Tongue Muscles and Innervation	Function
genioglossus (XII)	forms bulk of tongue; is able to retract tongue, draw tongue downward, draw entire tongue anteriorly to protrude tip or press tip against alveolar ridges and teeth
styloglossus (XII)	draws tongue up and back, may draw sides of tongue upward to help make dorsum concave
hyoglossus (XII)	retracts and depresses tongue
chondroglossus (XII)	depresses the tongue

Face: Lips and Cheeks

■ Several important bones of the face have already been discussed. There are major facial muscles, involving the lips and cheeks, that are important for articulation (see Figure 1.18). These muscles assist in production of various sounds, especially the labial sounds /m/, /b/, and /p/.

■ The primary muscle of the lips is the *orbicularis oris* muscle. The cheeks are primarily comprised of the *buccinator* muscle, a large flat muscle whose inner surface is covered with mucous membrane.

■ Most of the facial muscles are innervated by either the *buccal branches* or the *mandibular marginal branch* of cranial nerve VII, the facial nerve. These muscles are summarized in the following lists (Seikel et al., 1997).

Muscle and Innervation	Function
mentalis (VII)	pulls lower lip out, wrinkles and elevates chin
platysma (VII)	depresses mandible
risorius (VII)	retracts lips at corners
buccinator (VII)	constricts oropharynx; moves food onto grinding surfaces of molars
depressor labii inferioris (VII)	pulls lip down and out to dilate orifice
depressor anguli oris (triangularis) (VII)	helps to press lower and upper lips together; depresses corners of mouth
zygomatic minor (VII)	elevates upper lip
zygomatic major (VII)	retracts and elevates angle of mouth
orbicularis oris inferioris & superioris (VII)	pull lips together, seal lips, serve as point of insertion for other muscles, interact with other muscles to produce facial expressions
levator anguli oris (VII)	draws corner of mouth upward and toward medial
levator labii superioris (VII)	elevates upper lip
levator labii superioris alaeque nasi (VII)	elevates upper lip

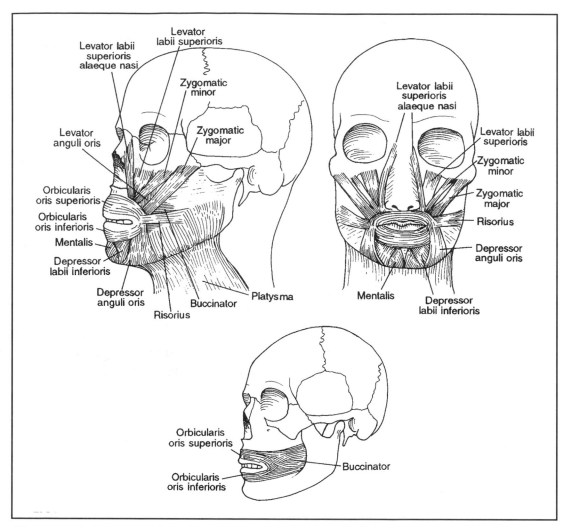

Figure 1.18. Muscles of the face. From *Anatomy and Physiology for Speech, Language, and Hearing* (p. 308), by J. A. Seikel, D. W. King, and D. G. Drumright, 1997, San Diego, CA: Singular Publishing Group, Inc. (401 West A Street, Suite 325, San Diego, CA 92101-7904, 800-521-8545). Copyright 1997 by Singular Publishing Group, Inc. Reprinted with permission.

Summary

☑ Tones generated by the larynx travel upward and are resonated by the pharynx, oral cavity, and nasal cavity. This process of resonation is explained by the source-filter theory.

☑ Articulation refers to the movement of speech structures to produce sounds. It depends upon the integrity of the following structures: the pharynx, soft palate, hard palate, mandible, teeth, tongue, lips, and cheeks.

☑ Cranial nerves mostly involved with innervating the muscles involved in articulation include cranial nerve V (trigeminal), VII (facial), X (vagus), XI (spinal accessory), and XII (hypoglossal).

Neuroanatomy and Neurophysiology
The Nervous System

Neurology is the study of neurological disorders and diseases and their diagnosis and treatment. *Neuroanatomy* is a branch of neurology concerned with the study of *structures* of the nervous system. *Neurophysiology*, another branch of neurology, is concerned with the study of the *function* of the nervous system.

In this section, we discuss basic neuroanatomy and neurophysiology of speech, language, and hearing. It is assumed that the reader has taken coursework in these areas, and thus this section provides only a basic "refresher" of some foundational ideas.

This section covers neurons and neural transmission. It discusses basic facts about the workings of the peripheral and autonomic nervous systems, including information about the cranial nerves. The central nervous system is then described according to its general parameters: the brain stem, reticular activating system, diencephalon, basal ganglia, cerebellum, cerebrum, pyramidal system, extrapyramidal system, connecting fibers in the brain, cerebral ventricles, protective layers of the brain, and cerebral blood supply. (*Note*: The extrapyramidal system is not technically a part of the central nervous system; however, it is closely related to the central nervous system and is thus discussed in this section.)

NEURONS AND NEURAL TRANSMISSION

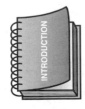

INTRODUCTION

The nervous system comprises of billions of specialized cells that function interconnectedly. Neurons are the most important of these cells. Sensory or afferent neurons carry sensory impulses toward the brain, while motor or efferent nerves transmit impulses away from the brain. Nerves may be organized into systems.

Anatomy and Physiology of Nerve Cells

■ The central nervous system is made up of different types of cells. *Glial cells* or *neuroglia* include *Schwann cells* and *oliodendroglia*, which are related to myelin production, and *microglia,* which act as scavengers to remove dead cells and other waste (Freed, 1999).

- ■ *Neurons* are the most important type of nerve cells. There are billions of neurons which receive information from other neurons, process that information, and then transmit the information to still other neurons (Bhatnagar & Andy, 1995).

- ■ The neuron or nerve cell has two parts: (1) nerve fibers, and (2) the soma, or cell body, which contains the nucleus. Figure 1.19 shows a typical nerve cell.

- ■ The core of the cell body is called the *nucleus.* The cell body is covered with a membrane. The axons and dendrites are projections of the cell body and specialize in receiving and conducting stimuli.

- ■ *Dendrites* are short fibers that extend from the cell body. They receive neural impulses generated from the axons of other cells, and they transmit those impulses to the cell body.

- ■ Each cell has a single *axon*, which is wrapped in a myelin sheath (defined later). Axons are longer fibers than dendrites and have *terminal,* or *end, buttons* at the tip. The end button of one neuron either makes close contact with or actually touches the dendrite of another neuron. Axons send out impulses generated within the neuron; these impulses are sent away from the cell body to other neurons.

- ■ Neurons communicate with each other through junctions called *synapses.* An axon branches out into several smaller fibers, which form terminals. These terminals connect to a synapse, although this neural junction includes a small gap or space. Thus, a synapse consists of the terminal button of one neuron, the receptive site of another neuron, and the synaptic cleft or space between the two (Peña-Brooks & Hegde, 1999).

- ■ *Neural transmission* is a chemical process of information exchange at the level of the synapse. A *neurotransmitter,* a chemical contained within the terminal buttons, helps make contact between two cells by diffusing itself across the synaptic space.

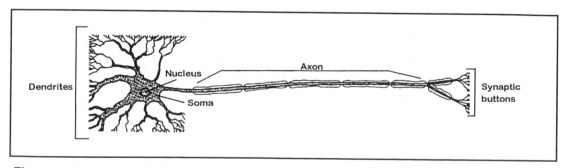

Figure 1.19. A typical neuron. From *A Coursebook on Aphasia and Other Neurogenic Language Disorders*, 2nd ed. (p. 17), by M. N. Hegde, 1998, San Diego, CA: Singular Publishing Group, Inc. (401 West A Street, Suite 325, San Diego, CA 92101-7904, 800-521-8545). Copyright 1998 by Singular Publishing Group, Inc. Reprinted with permission.

■ Such diffused neurotransmitters become bound to receptors in the postsynaptic membrane. The diffused neurotransmitter may cause the inhibition or excitation of the next neuron. *Dopamine* and *acetylcholine* are two important neurotransmitters in the motor system.

■ Neurons have certain specialized functions. There are three basic types of neurons: motor neurons, sensory neurons, and interneurons.

✎ Concepts To Consider

Describe neurons in terms of their key parts and their function in the human body.

_____

_____

_____

_____

_____

_____

_____

_____

_____

_____

■ *Sensory neurons*, also called *afferent neurons*, carry sensory impulses from the peripheral sense organs *toward* the brain. *Motor neurons*, also called *efferent neurons*, transmit impulses *away* from the central nervous system. Motor neurons cause glandular secretions or muscle contractions (movement).

■ *Interneurons*, the most common type of neuron in the nervous system, link neurons with other neurons. Because they form connections with other neurons, interneurons play an important role in controlling movement (Freed, 1999).

■ Many axons, especially the larger axons of the central nervous system and those in the peripheral nervous system, have a white insulating sheath called *myelin* around them. Schwann cells and oliodendroglia provide the myelin sheath around the axon. The myelin has breaks at the junction between the cells to facilitate the impulse transfer.

■ Neurons are arranged in the form of fibers. A *nervous system*, on the other hand, is an organization of nerves according to specific spatial, structural, and functional principles. The peripheral, autonomic, and central nervous systems are often collectively referred to as the nervous system. In the next sections, each of these systems is explained.

Summary

☑ Neurons, the central building blocks of the nervous system, are composed of a cell body, dendrites, and an axon.

☑ Some of these nerves have myelin sheaths around them. Various types of nerves transmit impulses to and from the central nervous system.

THE PERIPHERAL AND AUTONOMIC NERVOUS SYSTEMS

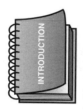

INTRODUCTION

The peripheral nervous system, a collection of nerves outside the spinal column and skull, carries sensory and motor impulses back and forth from the brain to various parts of the body. The 12 pairs of cranial nerves are part of the peripheral nervous system; some of these are critical to language, speech, and hearing. The 31 pairs of spinal nerves are indirectly involved with speech because they control automatic functions such as breathing. Part of the peripheral nervous system is the autonomic nervous system, with its sympathetic and parasympathetic branches, which may have an indirect effect upon speech in certain situations.

Peripheral Nervous System

Basic Principles

■ The *peripheral nervous system* (PNS) is a collection of nerves that are outside the skull and spinal column. These nerves carry *sensory* impulses originating in the peripheral sense organs to the brain, and *motor* impulses originating in the brain to the glands and muscles of the body.

■ The PNS contains three types of nerves: the spinal, the cranial, and the peripheral autonomic nerves. There are 12 pairs of cranial nerves and 31 pairs of spinal nerves. Of the three types of nerves, the cranial nerves are the most directly involved in speech, language, and hearing.

Cranial Nerves

■ The cranial nerves emerge from the brain stem and are attached to the base of the brain. They are part of the lower motor neuron system of the cortico-bulbar tract of the pyramidal system (discussed later in more detail). The cranial nerves exit through *foramina*, or holes, in the base of the skull. They exit at different levels of the brain stem and the top portion of the spinal cord.

■ Consequently, the cranial nerves are numbered according to the vertical order in which they exit from the skull. They go out to connect to various sense organs and muscles of the neck and head. Table 1.1 lists the cranial nerves and their numbers and basic functions. Some students remember the cranial nerves by the following mnemonic: On old Olympus' towering top, a fin and German viewed some hops.

■ *Sensory nerves* are those cranial nerves carrying sensory information from a sense organ (e.g., the nose) to the brain. *Motor* (movement-related) *nerves* carry impulses from the brain to the muscles that make those muscles move. Several cranial nerves are *mixed nerves* because they carry both sensory and motor impulses.

■ There are 12 pairs of cranial nerves. The first two cranial nerves are related to the cerebral cortex. Cranial nerves III–XII originate from the brain stem and innervate the muscles of the pharynx, tongue, larynx, head, neck, and face (Bhatnagar & Andy, 1995). Figure 1.20 illustrates an inferior view of the brain showing cranial nerves as well as other cerebral structures (described later).

TABLE 1.1

Cranial Nerves

Nerve No.	Name	Function
I	Olfactory	Sense of smell (sensory)
II	Optic	Vision (motor)
III	Oculomotor	Eye movement (motor)
IV	Trochlear	Eye movement (motor)
V	Trigeminal	Face (sensory); jaw (motor)
VI	Abducens	Eye movement (motor)
VII	Facial	Tongue (sensory); face (motor)
VIII	Vestibular acoustic	Hearing and balance (sensory)
IX	Glossopharyngeal	Tongue and pharynx (sensory); pharynx only (motor)
X	Vagus	Larynx, respiratory, cardiac, and gastrointestinal systems (sensory and motor)
XI	Accessory	Shoulder, arm, and throat movements (motor)
XII	Hypoglossal	Mostly tongue movements (motor)

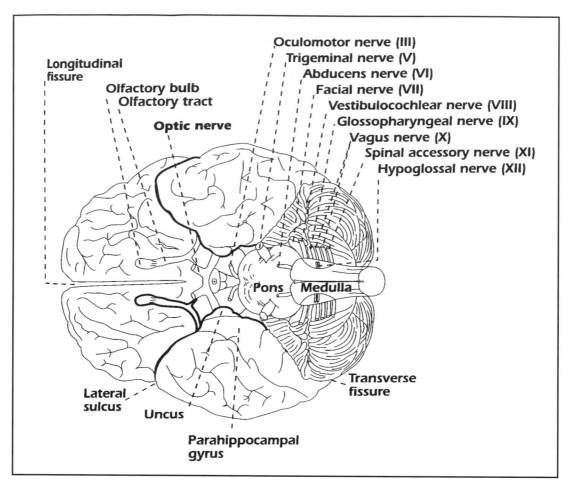

Figure 1.20. Inferior view of the brain showing cranial nerves and other cerebral structures. From *Neuroscience of Communication* (p. 79), by D. B. Webster, 1995, San Diego, CA: Singular Publishing Group, Inc. (401 West A Street, Suite 325, San Diego, CA 92101-7904, 800-521-8545). Copyright 1995 by Singular Publishing Group, Inc. Reprinted with permission.

▣ Cranial nerves I, II, III, IV, and VI are not concerned with speech, language, or hearing:

- *Cranial nerve I (the olfactory nerve)* is a sensory nerve originating in the nasal cavity. It is involved with smell.

- *Cranial nerve II (the optic nerve)* is a sensory nerve originating in the retina of the eye.

- *Cranial nerve III (the oculomotor nerve)* and *cranial nerve IV (the trochlear nerve)* are motor nerves that originate in the midbrain area and innervate muscles corresponding to eye movement.

- *Cranial nerve VI (the abducens nerve)* is a motor nerve that controls eye movement.

■ Cranial nerves V and VII–XII are involved with speech, language, and hearing and, as such, are described in more detail below.

■ *Cranial nerve V, the trigeminal nerve*, is a mixed (both motor and sensory) nerve (see Figure 1.21).

　　— Its *sensory fibers* are composed of three branches: opthalmic, maxillary, and mandibular branches. The opthalmic nerve has sensory branches to the nose, eyes, and forehead. The maxillary branch has sensory branches to the upper lip, maxilla, upper cheek area, upper teeth, maxillary sinus, and palate. The mandibular branch has sensory branches to the mandible, lower teeth, lower lip, tongue, part of the cheek, and part of the external ear.

　　— The *motor fibers* of cranial nerve V innervate various jaw muscles, including the temporalis, lateral and medial pterygoids, masseter, tensor veli palatini, tensor tympani, mylohyoid, and anterior belly of the digastric muscle.

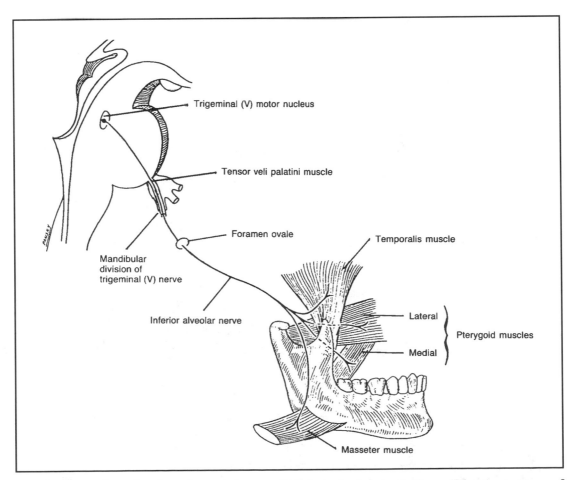

Figure 1.21. Distribution of cranial nerve V (trigeminal nerve). From "Neuroanatomy of Speech" (p. 125), by J. G. Kennedy and D. P. Kuehn, 1989, in *Neural Bases of Speech, Hearing, and Language,* by D. P. Kuehn, M. L. Lemme, and J. M. Baumgartner (Eds.), Austin, TX: PRO-ED. Copyright 1989 by PRO-ED, Inc. Reprinted with permission.

– Damage to cranial nerve V may result in an inability to close the mouth, difficulty in chewing, and *trigeminal neuralgia* (sharp pain in the facial area) (Newman & Ramadan, 1998; Zemlin, 1998).

■ *Cranial nerve VII, the facial nerve,* is also a mixed nerve (see Figure 1.22).

– The *sensory fibers* of the facial nerve are responsible for taste sensations on the anterior two-thirds of the tongue.

– The *motor fibers* of the facial nerve have branches (Figure 1.22) that innervate muscles important to facial expression and speech. These muscles include the buccinator, zygomatic, orbicularis oris, orbicularis oculi, platysma, stapedius, stylohyoid, frontalis, procerus, nasalis, depressor labii inferioris, depressor anguli oris, auricular muscles, various labial muscles, and the posterior belly of the digastric muscle.

– A person with damage to the facial nerve often has a masklike appearance with minimal or no facial expression.

■ *Cranial nerve VIII, the vestibular acoustic (or vestibulocochlear) nerve,* is a sensory nerve for balance and hearing. It has two branches (described further in Chapter 10).

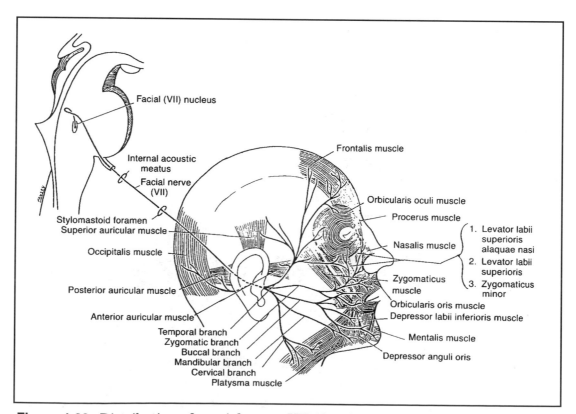

Figure 1.22. Distribution of cranial nerve VII (facial nerve). From "Neuroanatomy of Speech" (p. 126), by J. G. Kennedy and D. P. Kuehn, 1989, in *Neural Bases of Speech, Hearing, and Language,* by D. P. Kuehn, M. L. Lemme, and J. M. Baumgartner (Eds.), Austin, TX: PRO-ED. Copyright 1989 by PRO-ED, Inc.. Reprinted with permission.

- The *vestibular branch* is primarily responsible for the maintenance of equilibrium or balance.

- The *acoustic branch* transmits sensory information from the cochlea of the inner ear to the primary auditory cortex of the brain, where it is interpreted.

- Damage to the vestibular acoustic nerve results in a hearing loss, problems with balance, or both.

■ *Cranial nerve IX, the glossopharyngeal nerve*, is a mixed nerve. It has sensory, motor, and autonomic components.

- The *sensory* component of the glossopharyngeal nerve assists in processing taste sensations from the posterior third of the tongue. This component also provides general sensation for the tympanic cavity, ear canal, eustachian tube, faucial pillars, tonsils, soft palate, and pharynx.

- The *motor* fibers of the glossopharyngeal nerve innervate the stylopharyngeus, a muscle that raises and dilates the pharynx.

- Experts differ on whether the motor fibers of the glossopharyngeal nerve also innervate the superior pharyngeal constrictor (Newman & Ramadan, 1998; Seikel et al., 1997). According to Zemlin (1998), the glossopharyngeal nerve, along with fibers of the vagus nerve (X), supplies motor fibers to the *pharyngeal plexus*, which innervates the upper pharyngeal constrictor muscles.

- Lesions of the glossopharyngeal nerve may create difficulty in swallowing, unilateral loss of the gag reflex, and loss of taste and sensation from the posterior third of the tongue.

■ *Cranial nerve X, the vagus nerve*, is a mixed nerve containing motor, sensory, and autonomic fibers (see Figure 1.23). It is called a wandering ("vagus") nerve because it extends into the chest and the stomach.

- The *motor* fibers of the vagus nerve supply the digestive system, heart, and lungs.

- The *sensory* fibers convey information from the digestive system, heart, trachea, pharynx, and larynx.

- The *recurrent laryngeal nerve* (RLN), a branch of the vagus nerve, regulates the intrinsic muscles of the larynx, excluding the cricothyroid, which is supplied by the superior laryngeal nerve branch. The RLN can be damaged during thyroid surgery, resulting in total or partial paralysis of the vocal folds.

- The *pharyngeal branch* of the vagus nerve supplies the pharyngeal constrictors. It also supplies all the muscles of the velum except the tensor tympani, which is innervated by the trigeminal nerve.

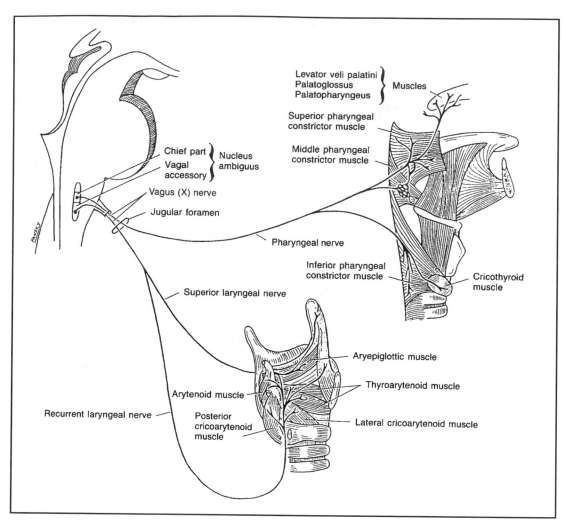

Figure 1.23. Distribution of cranial nerve X (vagus nerve). From "Neuroanatomy of Speech" (p. 123), by J. G. Kennedy and D. P. Kuehn, 1989, in *Neural Bases of Speech, Hearing, and Language*, by D. P. Kuehn, M. L. Lemme, and J. M. Baumgartner (Eds.), Austin, TX: PRO-ED. Copyright 1989 by PRO-ED, Inc. Reprinted with permission.

- Damage to the vagus nerve includes a variety of possible sequelae such as difficulty swallowing, paralysis of the velum, and voice problems if the RLN is damaged.

■ *Cranial nerve XI, the spinal accessory nerve*, is a motor nerve (see Figure 1.24). It is both a cranial and spinal nerve because of its cranial and spinal origin.

- The spinal root supplies the trapezius and sternocleidomastoid muscles, which assist in head and shoulder movements.

- In concert with the vagus nerve, the cranial fibers of the accessory nerve innervate the uvula and levator veli palatini muscles of the soft palate.

- Lesions of the spinal accessory nerve may result in neck weakness, paralysis of the sternocleidomastoid, and consequent inability to turn

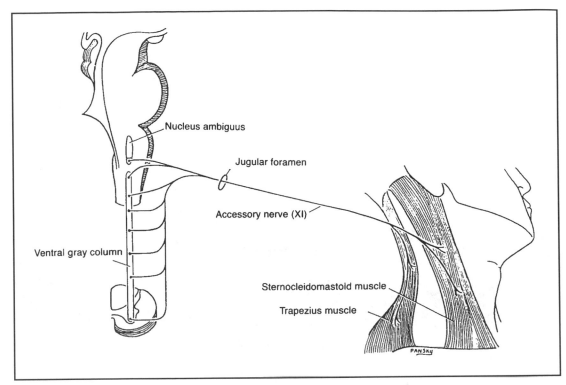

Figure 1.24. Distribution of cranial nerve XI (spinal accessory nerve). From "Neuroanatomy of Speech" (p. 132), by J. G. Kennedy and D. P. Kuehn, 1989, in *Neural Bases of Speech, Hearing, and Language,* by D. P. Kuehn, M. L. Lemme, and J. M. Baumgartner (Eds.), Austin, TX: PRO-ED. Copyright 1989 by PRO-ED, Inc. Reprinted with permission.

the head, as well as an inability to shrug the shoulders or raise the arm above shoulder level (Zemlin, 1998).

■ *Cranial nerve XII, the hypoglossal nerve,* is a motor nerve that runs under the tongue (see Figure 1.25).

- – This nerve supplies three extrinsic tongue muscles: the styloglossus, hyoglossus, and genioglossus.

- – The hypoglossal nerve also supplies all the intrinsic muscles of the tongue.

- – Lesions to the hypoglossal nerve can result in tongue paralysis, diminished intelligibility, and possible swallowing problems.

Spinal Nerves

■ The spinal nerves of the PNS are closely related to the autonomic nervous system. Together, they control various bodily activities that are executed with little conscious effort or knowledge.

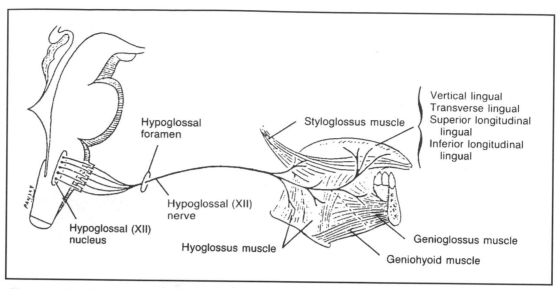

Figure 1.25. Distribution of cranial nerve XII (hypoglossal nerve). From "Neuroanatomy of Speech" (p. 126), by J. G. Kennedy and D. P. Kuehn, 1989, in *Neural Bases of Speech, Hearing, and Language,* by D. P. Kuehn, M. L. Lemme, and J. M. Baumgartner (Eds.), Austin, TX: PRO-ED. Copyright 1989 by PRO-ED, Inc. Reprinted with permission.

- The spinal nerves can be motor, sensory, or mixed. They transmit motor information from the central nervous system, or CNS, to the muscles, and carry sensory information from peripheral receptors to the CNS.

- Not all the spinal nerves are directly involved with speech production. However, some nerves contribute to speech through innervation of the respiratory musculature. For example, the internal and external intercostals are innervated by the thoracic spinal nerves. The diaphragm is innervated by the motor branches of the C3–C5 spinal nerves (Peña-Brooks & Hegde, 1999).

- There are 31 pairs of spinal nerves. These nerves are attached to the spinal cord through two roots: one is efferent and ventral (toward the front) and the other is afferent and dorsal (toward the back).

- The 31 pairs of spinal nerves are divided into segments. They are named after the region of the spinal cord to which they are attached (cervical, thoracic, lumbar, sacral, and coccygeal; see Figure 1.26):

C1–C8	=	8 pairs of cervical spinal nerves
T1–T12	=	12 pairs of thoracic spinal nerves
L1–L5	=	5 pairs of lumbar spinal nerves
S1–S5	=	5 pairs of sacral spinal nerves
C1	=	1 pair of coccygeal spinal nerves

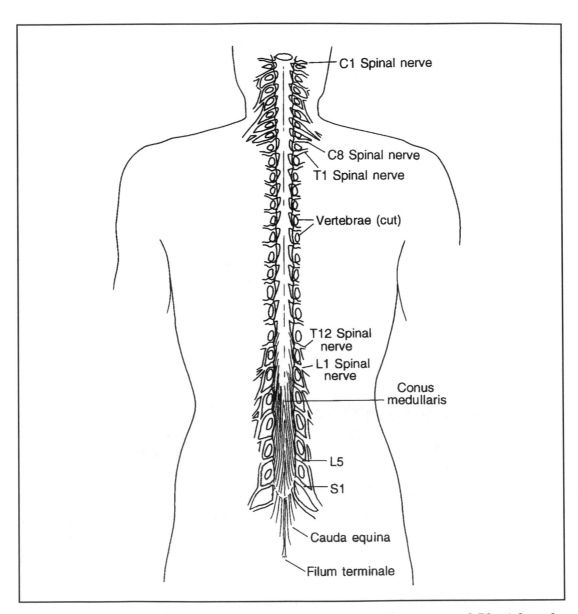

Figure 1.26. The spinal cord and emerging nerves. From *Anatomy and Physiology for Speech, Language, and Hearing* (p. 395), by J. A. Seikel, D. W. King, and D. G. Drumright, 1997, San Diego, CA: Singular Publishing Group, Inc. (401 West A Street, Suite 325, San Diego, CA 92101-7904, 800-521-8545). Copyright 1997 by Singular Publishing Group, Inc. Reprinted with permission.

■ There are several other important spinal cord structures. One is the *conus medullaris*, where the spinal cord ends at the L1 vertebra level. The lowermost nerves are described as the *cauda equina* (horse's tail), which is beneath the *filum terminale,* where there are no spinal cord segments (Seikel et al., 1997).

✎ Concepts To Consider

Compare the cranial nerves and the spinal nerves. What is the role of each type of nerve in speech and language?

_____

_____

_____

_____

_____

_____

_____

_____

Autonomic Nervous System

■ The *autonomic nervous system* (ANS) is generally viewed as part of the peripheral nervous system (Zemlin, 1998). Here, it is artificially presented separately for purposes of simplifying the following information.

■ The ANS controls and regulates the internal environment of our bodies; for example, heartbeat is controlled by the ANS. The heartbeat is controlled through the sympathetic and parasympathetic divisions of the ANS, which supply the body's smooth muscles and various glands that secrete hormones.

■ The *sympathetic* branch of the ANS mobilizes the body for "fight or flight" situations. Activation of the sympathetic branch accelerates the heart rate, dilates the pupils, raises the blood pressure, and increases the blood flow to the peripheral body structures (e.g., the legs, which run from danger). Humans feel emotionally aroused when the sympathetic branch of the ANS is activated.

■ The *parasympathetic* branch of the ANS helps bring the body back to a state of relaxation. After the body has mobilized for highly charged situations, the parasympathetic branch lowers blood pressure, slows the heart rate, increases activity within the stomach, and generally relaxes the body. Humans feel relaxed and calm during activation of the parasympathetic branch of the ANS.

■ The ANS does not have a direct effect upon speech, language, or hearing. However, the emotionally relaxed and aroused states created by ANS actions may have some effect on various parameters of communication.

■ For example, people who stutter may become more dysfluent when the sympathetic branch is aroused. In another example, people who habitually speak too quickly and loudly with consequent trauma to the vocal folds might benefit from the feelings of relaxation provided from activation of the parasympathetic branch.

Summary

☑ The most important part of the peripheral nervous system in relationship to communication is the cranial nerves. Cranial nerves V, VII, VIII, IX, X, XI, and XII are the cranial nerves most directly connected with speech, language, and hearing.

☑ The spinal nerves of the peripheral nervous system control automatic functions such as breathing.

☑ The sympathetic and parasympathetic branches of the autonomic nervous system have an indirect effect on speech when they cause speakers to feel emotionally relaxed or aroused.

The Nervous System

Peripheral Nervous System	Central Nervous System
Cranial Nerves	Spinal cord
Spinal Nerves	Brain
Autonomic Nervous System	
• sympathetic branch	
• parasympathetic branch	

THE CENTRAL NERVOUS SYSTEM

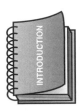

INTRODUCTION

The central nervous system is composed of the spinal cord and the brain. Key structures of the brain include the brain stem, the reticular activating system, the diencephalon, the basal ganglia, the cerebellum, and the cerebrum. Other key structures and systems include the pyramidal and extrapyramidal systems, connecting fibers within the brain, the cerebral ventricles, the protective layers of the brain, and structures that provide the cerebral blood supply. (As noted earlier, the extrapyramidal system is technically not part of the CNS but is included here as it is highly related and interconnected to CNS structures.)

Basic Principles

■ The brain gathers information about the environment from the PNS and then sends impulses that lead to actions. The peripheral systems and organs send and receive a variety of kinds of information and possibly demand directions for action.

■ The brain acts as a "central station," which coordinates this activity, integrates information, and issues commands.

■ The central nervous system is composed of the brain and the spinal cord, as depicted in Figure 1.27. The CNS acts as a *motor command center* for planning, originating, and carrying out the transmission of messages (Van Riper & Erickson, 1996).

■ The CNS is enclosed within the vertebral column and the cranial structure. The spinal cord is an elongated structure within the spinal canal of the vertebral columns.

■ Pairs of spinal nerves branch out on either side of the vertebral column and reach most parts of the body. The upper portion of the spinal cord is continuous with the lower portion of the brain.

■ The brain is the most important structure in the body for language, speech, and hearing. It is housed in and protected by the cranial cavity of the skull.

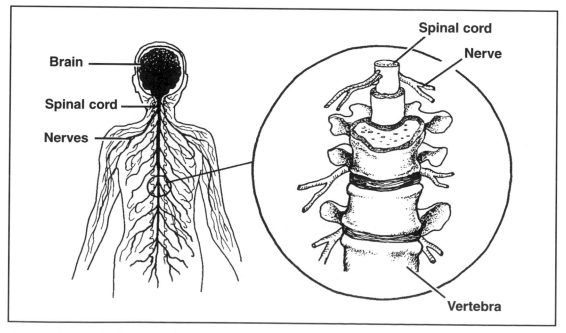

Figure 1.27. The brain and spinal cord. From *Introduction to Communicative Disorders*, 2nd ed. (p. 92), by M. N. Hegde, 1995, Austin, TX: PRO-ED. Copyright 1995 by PRO-ED, Inc. Reprinted with permission.

The *skull* is not a single structure but rather is made up of separate pieces of bone that eventually become a unified structure.

■ Because the brain is so much more related to speech and language than the spinal cord, the rest of this section is devoted to a description of the structures and processes of the brain. Information about the spinal cord is integrated as necessary.

The Brain Stem

■ The *brain stem* is said to be the oldest part of the brain. It connects the spinal cord with the brain via the diencephalon. It also serves as a bridge between the cerebellum and all other CNS structures, including the spinal cord, the thalamus, the basal ganglia, and the cerebrum.

■ Internally, the brain stem consists of *longitudinal fiber tracts, cranial nerve nuclei,* and the *reticular formation.* Outwardly, one sees the key structures of the brain stem as illustrated in Figure 1.28: the midbrain, the pons, and the medulla.

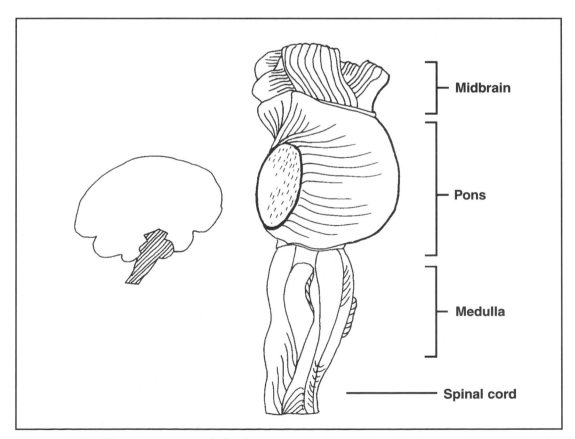

Figure 1.28. The structures of the brain stem. From *Introduction to Communicative Disorders*, 2nd ed. (p. 93), by M. N. Hegde, 1995, Austin, TX: PRO-ED. Copyright 1995 by PRO-ED, Inc. Reprinted with permission.

Midbrain

■ The *midbrain*, also called the *mesencephalon*, is a narrow structure that lies superior to the pons and inferior to the diencephalon. The midbrain's *superior peduncles* help connect the brain stem and the cerebellum. The *substantia nigra* (described later) runs the vertical length of the midbrain at the level of the peduncles.

■ The midbrain contains structures that control many motor and sensory functions, including postural reflexes, visual reflexes, eye movements, and coordination of vestibular-generated eye and head movements.

■ The midbrain contains the cranial nerve nuclei for the trochlear (IV) and oculomotor (III) nerves. These nerves are not involved in speech production.

Pons

■ The *pons*, also called the *metencephalon*, is a roundish, bulging structure that bridges the two halves of the cerebellum. It is located directly inferior to the midbrain.

■ The pons and the midbrain together serve as a connection point between the cerebellum and various cerebral structures through the *inferior* and *middle peduncles*. The pons transmits information relative to movement from the cerebral hemispheres to the cerebellum.

■ The pons contains many descending motor fibers and is involved with hearing and balance. It also houses the nuclei for the trigeminal (V) and facial (VII) nerves, which are important for speech production.

Medulla

■ The *medulla*, also called the *myelencephalon*, is inferior to the midbrain and the pons. It is the uppermost portion of the spinal cord, which enters the cranial cavity through the *foramen magnum* at the base of the skull.

■ The medulla contains all the fibers that originate in the cerebellum and cerebrum and move downward to form the spinal cord. It includes several centers that control vital, automatic bodily functions such as breathing, digestion, heart rate, and blood pressure.

■ The medulla is very important for speech production because it contains descending fibers that transmit motor information to several cranial nerve nuclei.

■ Cranial nerves whose nuclei are housed within the medulla include the vestibulocochlear (VIII), vagus (X), glossopharyngeal (IX), accessory (XI), and hypoglossal (XII) nerves.

▦ The medulla contains nerve fibers that carry commands from the motor center of the brain to various muscles. These fibers are called *pyramidal tracts*. The pyramidal tracts, described in more detail later, control many movements and supply some of the muscles that are involved in speech.

▦ At the level of the medulla, many of the pyramidal tracts from the left and right sides of the brains *decussate* or cross over to the other side. Thus, the right side of the body is primarily controlled by the left side of the brain and vice versa.

Reticular Activating System

▦ The *reticular activating system* (RAS) is a structure within the midbrain, brain stem, and upper portion of the spinal cord. It integrates motor impulses flowing out of the brain with sensory impulses flowing into it.

▦ The RAS thus plays a role in the execution of motor activity. It sends diffuse impulses to various regions of the cortex and alerts the cortex to incoming impulses.

▦ The RAS is the primary mechanism of attention and consciousness. It is important in controlling sleep-wake cycles. It plays a critical role in states of consciousness, in whether a person is asleep, drowsy, alert, or very excited. Generally, the RAS can be viewed as the part of the CNS that responds to incoming information by affecting the state of a person's alertness and consciousness (Webster, 1995).

Diencephalon

▦ The *diencephalon* lies above the midbrain and between the brain stem and the cerebral hemispheres. (*Note*: Some experts, such as Zemlin [1998] consider the diencephalon to be part of the brain stem.)

▦ The diencephalon contains the *third ventricle*, a tall and narrow space filled with cerebrospinal fluid. The diencephalon also contains the thalamus and the hypothalamus.

▦ The *thalamus* is the largest structure in the diencephalon. It regulates the sensory information that flows into the brain and relays sensory impulses to various portions of the cerebral cortex.

▦ The thalamus also receives information about motor impulses from the cerebellum and the basal ganglia and relays this information to motor areas of the cerebral cortex.

▦ The thalamus is critical in maintenance of consciousness and alertness. The exact role of the thalamus in speech and language is unclear.

- The *hypothalamus*, which lies inferior to the thalamus, helps integrate the actions of the ANS. The hypothalamus also controls emotions.

Basal Ganglia

- The *basal ganglia*, illustrated in Figure 1.29, are structures deep within the brain that are located near the thalamus and lateral ventricles. They are primarily composed of gray matter.

- The basal ganglia are a highly complex system of neural pathways that have connections with many subcortical and cortical areas. The basal ganglia receive input primarily from the frontal lobe and relay information back to the higher centers of the brain via the thalamus.

- Experts differ on the exact structure of the basal ganglia, but most agree that they consist of at least three nuclear masses: the globus pallidus, the putamen, and the caudate nucleus. *Corpus striatum* is the collective term for these structures (Love & Webb, 1996).

- The basal ganglia are part of the extrapyramidal system. The *extrapyramidal system* helps regulate and modify cortically initiated motor movements, including speech. The *substantia nigra*, which is functionally related to (but not a part of) the basal ganglia, is an important part of the extrapyramidal system (Peña-Brooks & Hegde, 1999).

- The extrapyramidal system, described in more detail later, is considered an indirect activation system because motor movements are not directly controlled in the basal ganglia. The extrapyramidal system primarily affects motor movements by communicating with the cerebral cortex via other subcortical structures such as the thalamus.

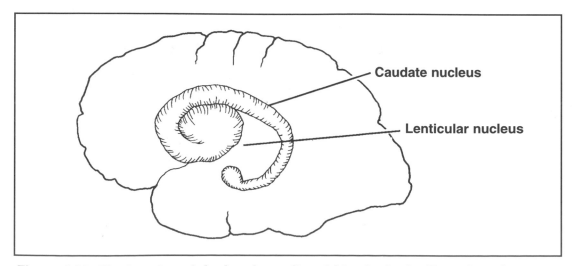

Figure 1.29. The location of the basal ganglia within the brain. From *Introduction to Communicative Disorders*, 2nd ed. (p. 94), by M. N. Hegde, 1995, Austin, TX: PRO-ED. Copyright 1995 by PRO-ED, Inc. Reprinted with permission.

■ Lesions in the basal ganglia can result in unusual body postures, dysarthria (described in Chapter 8), changes in body tone, and involuntary and uncontrolled movements (dyskinesias) that interfere with a person's voluntary attempts to walk, speak, or do many other activities (Freed, 1999).

✎ Concepts To Consider

Describe one way that the brain stem, the RAS, and the basal ganglia are involved in speech and language functioning.

_____

_____

_____

_____

_____

_____

_____

_____

_____

The Cerebellum

■ The cerebellum, illustrated in Figure 1.30, lies just below the cerebrum and behind the brain stem. Also called the "little brain," the cerebellum has two hemispheres (which are different from the cerebral hemispheres).

■ Three primary fiber bundles serve as connections between the brain stem and cerebellum. These are the *superior, middle*, and *inferior cerebellar peduncles,* which connect with the midbrain, the pons, and the medulla, respectively. All efferent and afferent fibers going to and from the cerebellum pass through these peduncles.

■ Afferent fibers originate from the motor cortex, temporal lobes, cranial nerve VIII, spinal cord, and brain stem. They travel through the middle and inferior cerebellar peduncles and mediate almost all sensorimotor information to the cerebellum.

■ Efferent fibers travel through the superior cerebellar peduncle. These fibers transmit cerebellar outputs to the brain stem and then to the thalamus, motor cortex, and spinal cord.

■ The cerebellum is not a primary motor integration or initiation center. It receives neural impulses from other brain centers and helps coordinate and

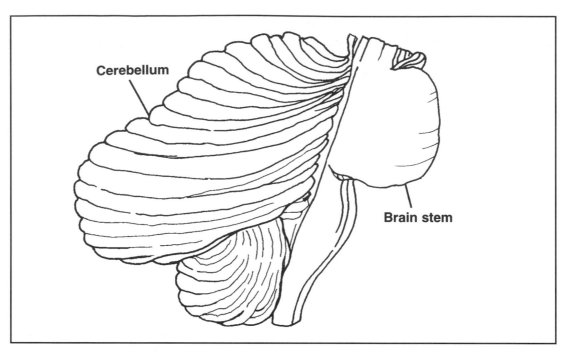

Figure 1.30. The cerebellum. From *Introduction to Communicative Disorders*, 2nd ed. (p. 95), by M. N. Hegde, 1995, Austin, TX: PRO-ED. Copyright 1995 by PRO-ED, Inc. Reprinted with permission.

regulate those impulses. Therefore, it acts as a "modulator" of neuronal activity through its efferent and afferent circuits.

■ The cerebellum regulates equilibrium (balance), body posture, and coordinated fine-motor movements. Because these movements are necessary for rapid speech, cerebellar intactness is very important to speech production.

■ Damage to the cerebellum results in a neurological disorder called *ataxia*, found in some people with cerebral palsy and in people who have suffered cerebellar damage. These people are likely to show abnormal gait, disturbed balance, and a speech disorder called *ataxic dysarthria* (described in Chapter 8). Damage to the cerebellum also creates other problems described in Chapter 8.

The Cerebrum

Basic Facts

■ The cerebrum, or *cerebral cortex* (terms are used interchangeably here), is the biggest and most important CNS structure for language, speech, and hearing. It is a complex structure of intricate neural connections that contains approximately 10–15 billion neurons and weighs about 3 pounds.

■ The brain is often referred to as gray matter because the cerebrum has gray cells on top. This differs from the spinal cord and the brain stem, which have gray cells inside.

■ The cortex includes the topmost portion of the brain but is actually arranged in six layers. Each layer consists of a different type of cell.

■ The surface of the cerebrum appears wrinkled because it is folded to accommodate as much tissue as possible in a small space. Billions of neural cells are packed into this structure and folded into ridges and valleys.

■ A *gyrus* is a ridge on the cortex, and the cortex has many gyri (plural). A shallow valley is a *sulcus*, and there are many sulci on the surface of the brain. Deeper valleys are called *fissures*, and there are fewer fissures than sulci. The fissures are the boundaries of the broad divisions of the cerebrum.

■ The *longitudinal fissure* courses along the middle of the brain from front to back, and divides the cerebrum into the left and right hemispheres. The *fissure of Rolando*, or *central sulcus*, is a major fissure, which runs laterally, downward, and forward and arbitrarily divides the anterior from the posterior half of the brain.

■ The *Sylvian fissure*, or *lateral cerebral fissure* (sulcus), starts at the inferior portion of the frontal lobe at the base of the brain and moves laterally and upward. The areas of the brain surrounding the Sylvian fissure are especially critical in language, speech, and hearing.

■ There are four lobes in the right hemisphere and four lobes in the left hemisphere of the cerebrum. The names of these lobes are based on the cranial bones with which they are in contact, not on function. The four lobes each have their own function, but they work interconnectedly. These cortical lobes are the frontal, parietal, occipital, and temporal lobes. They are illustrated in Figure 1.31.

Frontal Lobe

■ The frontal lobe is located on the anterior portion of the cerebrum in front of the central fissure and above the lateral fissure. It makes up approximately one-third of the surface area of the cerebrum.

■ Intact frontal lobe functioning is critical to the deliberate formation of plans and intentions that dictate a person's conscious behavior. People with damage to the frontal lobe thus have difficulty carrying out consciously organized activity (Luria, 1973).

■ The frontal lobe contains areas that are especially critical to speech production. These include the primary motor cortex containing the precentral gyrus, a supplementary motor cortex, and Broca's area. The major areas pertinent to speech, language, and hearing are illustrated in Figure 1.32.

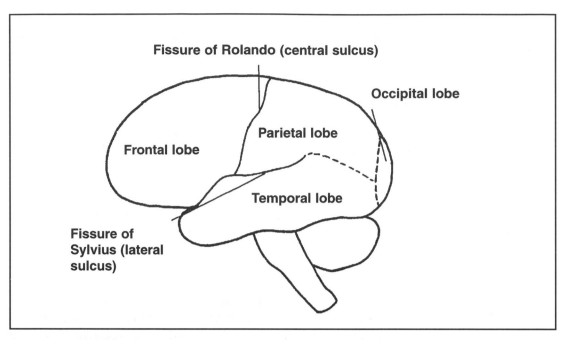

Figure 1.31. The lobes of the cerebral cortex. From *Introduction to Communicative Disorders*, 2nd ed. (p. 96), by M. N. Hegde, 1995, Austin, TX: PRO-ED. Copyright 1995 by PRO-ED, Inc. Reprinted with permission.

▧ The *primary motor cortex*, or *motor strip*, is located on the *precentral gyrus*, a large ridge that lies anterior to the central sulcus. This area controls voluntary movements of skeletal muscles on the opposite side of the body. This demonstrates the neurological principle of *contralateral motor control*, which means that each cerebral hemisphere controls the opposite side of the body.

▧ All muscles of the body, including those for speech production, are connected to the primary motor cortex through descending motor nerve cells. Figure 1.33 shows regions of the motor cortex that govern motor activation of specific body regions.

▧ It has been found that when specific areas of the primary motor cortex are stimulated, corresponding motor responses (e.g., movement of the hand or lip) occur. There is a large area representing the larynx, jaw, tongue, and lips; this suggests the importance of cortical control of structures involved in speech.

▧ The motor strip controls muscle movements through an aforementioned neural pathway called the pyramidal system. The motor impulses are modified by the extrapyramidal system with its indirect and complex relay stations (Hegde, 1998).

▧ The *supplementary motor cortex* of the frontal lobe is believed to be involved in the motor planning of speech. It also plays a secondary role in regulating muscle movements.

▧ An important motor speech center is *Broca's area*, which is named after the 19th-century French anthropologist and neurosurgeon who "discovered" it during a brain autopsy of a patient with aphasia.

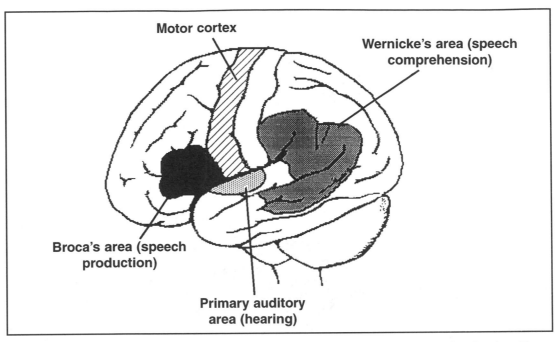

Figure 1.32. The major speech, language, and hearing areas of the brain. From *Introduction to Communicative Disorders*, 2nd ed. (p. 97), by M. N. Hegde, 1995, Austin, TX: PRO-ED. Copyright 1995 by PRO-ED, Inc. Reprinted with permission.

■ Broca's area is located in the third convolution of the left cerebral hemisphere. It is anterior to the portion of the primary motor cortex that controls lip, tongue, jaw, and laryngeal movements.

■ Broca's area is also called the motor speech area because it controls motor movements involved in speech production. An intact Broca's area is important for production of well-articulated, fluent speech (Love & Webb, 1996). Lesions in Broca's area cause motor speech problems, which are further described in Chapter 8.

Parietal Lobe

■ The parietal lobe is located on the upper sides of the cerebrum behind the frontal lobe and is considered to be the primary somatic sensory area. It integrates contralateral *somesthetic* sensations such as pressure, pain, temperature, and touch.

■ The *postcentral gyrus*, also called the *sensory cortex* or *sensory strip*, lies just behind the central sulcus. It is the primary sensory area that integrates and controls somesthetic sensory impulses.

■ Two specific areas of the parietal lobe are important for speech and language. These are the areas including and surrounding the supramarginal gyrus and the angular gyrus.

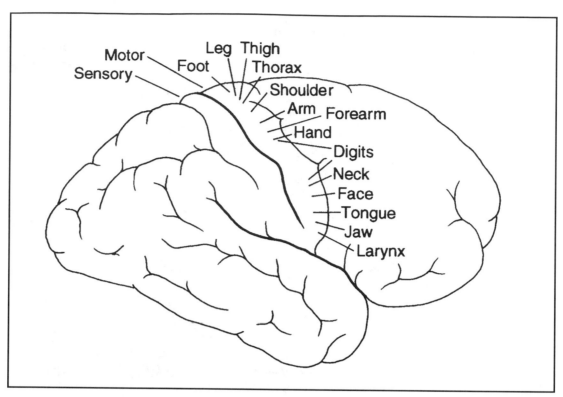

Figure 1.33. The right hemisphere, showing regions of the motor cortex that govern motor activation of specific body regions. From *Anatomy and Physiology for Speech, Language, and Hearing* (p. 456), by J. A. Seikel, D. W. King, and D. G. Drumright, 1997, San Diego, CA: Singular Publishing Group, Inc. (401 West A Street, Suite 325, San Diego, CA 92101-7904, 800-521-8545). Copyright 1997 by Singular Publishing Group, Inc. Reprinted with permission.

■ The *supramarginal gyrus* lies superior to the lateral fissure in the inferior portion of the parietal lobe. Its posterior portion curves around the lateral fissure. Damage to the supramarginal gyrus can cause conduction aphasia (described in Chapter 8) and agraphia, a writing disorder.

■ The *angular gyrus* lies posterior to the supramarginal gyrus. Damage to this area can cause writing, reading, and naming difficulties and, in some cases, transcortical sensory aphasia (described in Chapter 8).

Occipital Lobe

■ The occipital lobe lies behind the parietal lobe at the lower posterior portion of the head, just above the cerebellum. It is not very relevant to speech and hearing because it is primarily concerned with vision.

■ The major structure of the occipital lobe is the *primary visual cortex*. The remainder of the occipital lobe is composed of association visual cortices (Webster, 1995).

Temporal Lobe

- The temporal lobe is the lowest one-third of the cerebrum (see Figure 1.34). It lies inferior to the frontal and parietal lobes and in front of the occipital lobe. There are three major gyri in the temporal lobe: the *superior temporal gyrus*, the *middle temporal gyrus*, and the *lower temporal gyrus*.

- The temporal lobe contains two general areas that are critical to adequate hearing and speech. The first critical area is the *primary auditory cortex*, located on the superior temporal gyrus.

- The second critical area, the *auditory association area*, lies posterior to the primary auditory cortex. *Heschl's gyri* is a term sometimes used in reference to the transverse convolutions that make up the auditory association cortex and the primary auditory cortex (Kuehn, Lemme, & Baumgartner, 1989).

- The primary auditory cortex receives sound stimuli from the acoustic nerve (cranial nerve VIII) bilaterally. The auditory association area then synthesizes that information so that it can be recognized as whole units.

- In the dominant hemisphere (left hemisphere for most people), the auditory association area generally analyzes speech sounds so that the person recognizes words and sentences. In the nondominant hemisphere (right hemisphere for most people), the auditory association area generally analyzes nonverbal sound stimuli like environmental noises and music.

- The second critical area within the temporal lobe is *Wernicke's area*, named for Carl Wernicke, a famous neurologist. Wernicke's area is the posterior two-thirds of the superior temporal gyrus in the left hemisphere. It is close to the intersection of the parietal, occipital, and temporal lobes.

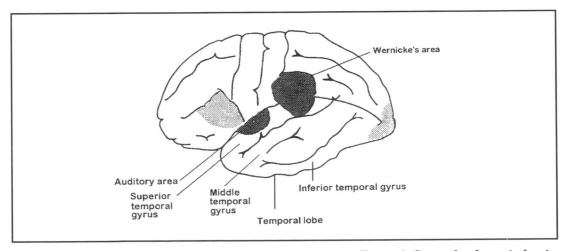

Figure 1.34. The temporal lobe and its primary areas. From *A Coursebook on Aphasia and Other Neurogenic Language Disorders*, 2nd ed. (p. 34), by M. N. Hegde, 1998, San Diego, CA: Singular Publishing Group, Inc. (401 West A Street, Suite 325, San Diego, CA 92101-7904, 800-521-8545). Copyright 1998 by Singular Publishing Group, Inc. Reprinted with permission.

- Wernicke's area is critical to the comprehension of spoken and written language. It is connected to Broca's area through the arcuate fasciculus (described later in this chapter).

- A lesion in the posterior portion of the superior temporal gyrus causes *Wernicke's aphasia* (described in Chapter 8), in which the patient demonstrates fluent, meaningless speech and significant language comprehension problems.

✎ Concepts To Consider

List and briefly describe two important speech- and language-related structures in the frontal lobe and the temporal lobe.

_____

_____

_____

_____

_____

_____

_____

_____

_____

Pyramidal System

Basic Facts

- The *pyramidal system*, as previously stated, is the direct motor activation pathway that is primarily responsible for facilitating voluntary muscle movement (including speech).

- The nerve fiber tract of the pyramidal system comes from the cerebral cortex to the spinal cord and brain stem to ultimately supply the muscles of the head, neck, and limbs. Voluntary movements needed to produce speech are initiated in the primary motor cortex.

- The pyramidal system is composed of the corticobulbar and the corticospinal tracts. Because tracts are bundles of nerve fibers coursing through the CNS, one can imagine the pyramidal system and its two tracts as a group of myelinated nerve fibers carrying crucial neural impulses (Peña-Brooks & Hegde, 1999).

■ The projection fibers of both the corticospinal and the corticobulbar tracts originate in the cerebral cortex, and the tracts are part of one unified system. However, these tracts are often discussed separately, if somewhat artificially, for purposes of simplification.

Corticospinal Tract

■ The *corticospinal tract* (see Figure 1.35) has nerve fibers that descend from the motor cortex of each hemisphere through the internal capsule. These fibers continue to course vertically through the midbrain and the pons. At the level of the medulla, approximately 85–80% of the fibers decussate.

■ The decussated fibers of the corticospinal tract synapse in the anterior horn (motor gray matter) of the spinal cord and communicate with the spinal nerves at different levels. Finally, the spinal nerves exit through the *vertebrae foramina* along the spinal column to innervate the muscles of the limbs and trunk.

■ Because of the decussation of fibers at the medullary level, the right side of the body is generally controlled by nerve fibers that originate in the left cerebral cortex, and vice versa. Many stroke patients, for example, have had left-hemisphere strokes and have consequent weakness on the right side of the body.

Corticobulbar Tract

■ The *corticobulbar tract* is critical to speech production. The fibers of this tract control all the voluntary movements of the speech muscles (except the respiratory muscles).

■ As stated, the fibers of the corticobulbar tract originate in the cerebral cortex—primarily the motor cortex. They course downward vertically through the internal capsule and run along with the corticospinal tract fibers.

■ A difference is that the corticobulbar tract fibers terminate in the brain stem at the motor nuclei of cranial nerves III–XII (see Figure 1.36). These fibers then decussate at the level of the brain stem where they terminate. For example, the fibers that terminate at the motor nuclei of the trigeminal nerve decussate in the pons. The fibers that terminate at the motor nuclei of the facial nerve decussate in the medulla (Peña-Brooks & Hegde, 1999).

■ The cranial nerves involved in speech exit the skull via small foramina and innervate the muscles of the larynx, pharynx, soft palate, tongue, face, and lips. This innervation allows the muscles to function for production of speech.

■ For practical clinical purposes, the corticospinal and corticobulbar tracts are further subdivided into lower and upper motor neurons. This division is

(text continues on page 66)

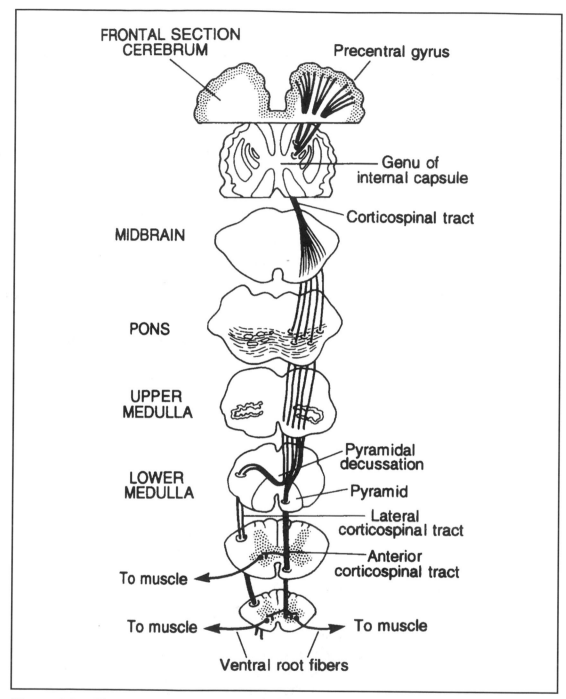

Figure 1.35. The corticospinal pathway as traced from the cerebral cortex to the spinal cord. From *Anatomy and Physiology for Speech, Language, and Hearing* (p. 407), by J. A. Seikel, D. W. King, and D. G. Drumright, 1997, San Diego, CA: Singular Publishing Group, Inc. (401 West A Street, Suite 325, San Diego, CA 92101-7904, 800-521-8545). Copyright 1997 by Singular Publishing Group, Inc. Reprinted with permission.

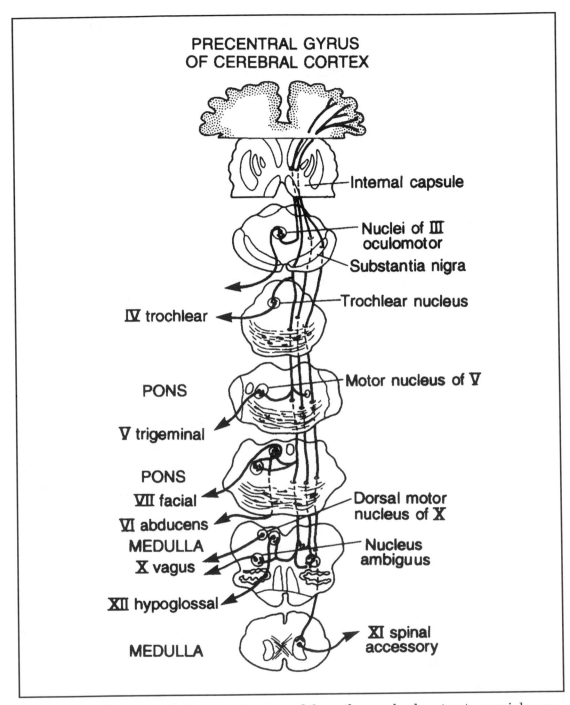

Figure 1.36. The corticobulbar tract as traced from the cerebral cortex to cranial nerve nuclei. From *Anatomy and Physiology for Speech, Language, and Hearing* (p. 410), by J. A. Seikel, D. W. King, and D. G. Drumright, 1997, San Diego, CA: Singular Publishing Group, Inc. (401 West A Street, Suite 325, San Diego, CA 92101-7904, 800-521-8545). Copyright 1997 by Singular Publishing Group, Inc. Reprinted with permission.

clinically helpful in classifying the symptoms associated with lower versus upper motor neuron damage.

■ *Lower motor neurons* are the motor neurons in the spinal and cranial nerves. They include nerve fibers that exit the neuraxis (spinal cord or brain) and communicate with the peripheral (cranial and spinal) nerves for innervation of muscles.

■ Thus, lower motor neurons are part of the peripheral nervous system and as such are the final route by which centrally mediated neural impulses are communicated to peripheral muscles. Lower motor neuron activity eventually results in muscular movement.

■ *Upper motor neurons* are the motor fibers within the central nervous system. Upper motor neurons can be thought of as all the descending motor fibers that course through the central nervous system. As such, upper motor neurons include the pathways of both the pyramidal and the extrapyramidal systems.

Extrapyramidal System

■ A general distinction between the pyramidal and the extrapyramidal systems is that the pyramidal system is responsible for carrying the impulses that control voluntary, fine-motor movements. The *extrapyramidal system* transmits impulses that control the postural support needed by those fine-motor movements (Freed, 1999).

■ The extrapyramidal system ("extra" referring to the motor tracts that are not part of the pyramidal system) is important in motor speech production. It is composed of different subcortical nuclei including the red nucleus, the substantia nigra, the subthalamus, the basal ganglia, and the pathways that connect these structures to one another.

■ Whereas the pyramidal system has a direct connection with lower motor neurons, the extrapyramidal system is considered a more indirect activation system, which interacts with various motor systems in the nervous system.

■ The neuronal activity of the extrapyramidal system begins in the cerebral cortex and ultimately influences lower motor neurons. The extrapyramidal system helps maintain posture and tone and helps regulate the movement that results from lower motor neuron activity.

■ Damage to the extrapyramidal system creates motor disturbances that fall under the rubric of "involuntary movement disorders." Patients may show unusual movement patterns of various muscles (including facial muscles) and bizarre postures.

Connecting Fibers in the Brain

■ The structures of the brain are connected with one another through specialized bundles of nerve fibers. These connecting fibers keep information flowing throughout the brain. This alerts various brain structures about sensory stimuli that have been received and actions that are planned and performed.

■ Connecting fibers differ in length. Adjacent areas are connected by shorter fibers; distant areas are connected by longer fibers called *fasciculi* (singular = fasciculus).

■ *Intrahemispheric fibers* allow areas within each hemisphere to communicate with each other. *Interhemispheric fibers* permit communication between hemispheres and are composed mostly of myelinated axonal fibers, or white matter. Interhemispheric fibers form the medullary center of the brain. Depending upon the nature of their connections, the nerve fibers of the medullary center are divided into three types.

■ The three types of connecting fibers are (Bhatnagar & Andy, 1995):

 – projection fibers
 – association fibers
 – commissural fibers

Projection Fibers

■ *Projection fibers* create connections between the cortex and subcortical structures like the cerebellum, basal ganglia, brain stem, and spinal cord.

■ Some fibers transmit motor information to the glands and muscles. Other fibers carry sensory information to the brain. The *internal capsule* contains the concentrated and compact projection fibers near the brain stem.

■ The motor projection fibers originate primarily in the premotor and primary motor areas in the frontal lobe. They form the upper motor neuron system of the pyramidal tract, which is the direct activation pathway for voluntary motor movements.

■ As projection fibers move upward toward the upper regions of the brain, they fan out in a structure called the *corona radiata*. Through the corona radiata, information is transmitted to other portions of the brain.

■ Afferent projection fibers relay sensory information (such as smell) from the peripheral sense organs (e.g., the nose) to the brain. Efferent projection fibers come together in the internal capsule and pass through the thalamus and basal ganglia. These efferent fibers relay motor commands to glands and muscles.

Association Fibers

■ *Association fibers* may be long or short; whatever their length, they connect areas within a hemisphere. Association fibers assist in maintaining communication between the structures in a hemisphere.

■ The most important of the association fibers is the bundle of *superior longitudinal fibers*, also called *arcuate fasciculus*, which lies just below the surface of the cortex. The arcuate fasciculus arches backward from the lower part of the frontal lobe to the posterior superior part of the temporal lobe.

■ The arcuate fasciculus connects Broca's area with Wernicke's area. It is important for verbal memory, language acquisition, and meaningful language production.

Commissural Fibers

■ The left and right hemispheres are divided by the medial longitudinal fissure. The *commissural fibers* are interhemispheric connectors; they run horizontally and connect the corresponding areas of the two hemispheres.

■ The most important of the commissural fibers, the *corpus callosum*, is a thick, broad band of myelinated fibers that connects the two hemispheres at their base (see Figure 1.37).

■ Damage to the corpus callosum disconnects the two hemispheres, resulting in *disconnection syndromes* characterized by problems in naming, reading, movement, and other functions.

The Cerebral Ventricles

■ The term *cerebral ventricles* refers to a system of cavities deep within the brain. These interconnected cavities are filled with *cerebrospinal fluid*.

■ This fluid is produced by the *choroid plexus*, which is composed of vascular membranous materials. The cerebrospinal fluid circulates throughout the nervous system and nourishes the neural tissues, removes waste products, cushions the brain, and regulates intracranial pressure (Hegde, 1998).

■ There are four cerebral ventricles. The largest of the four ventricles are the two *lateral ventricles* (one in each hemisphere). Located immediately inferior to the corpus callosum, the lateral ventricles are C-shaped and course through the lobes of the cortex.

■ The *third ventricle* is behind the lateral ventricles at the top of the brain stem. It looks like a broad disk and is connected with the lateral ventricles by the *foramen of Munro*.

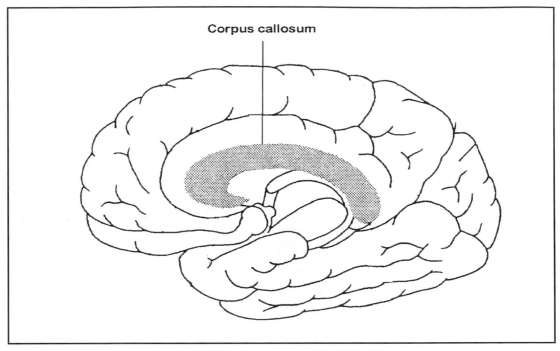

Corpus callosum

Figure 1.37. The corpus callosum. From *A Coursebook on Aphasia and Other Neurogenic Language Disorders*, 2nd ed. (p. 27), by M. N. Hegde, 1998, San Diego, CA: Singular Publishing Group, Inc. (401 West A Street, Suite 325, San Diego, CA 92101-7904, 800-521-8545). Copyright 1998 by Singular Publishing Group, Inc. Reprinted with permission.

■ The *fourth ventricle* is located between the cerebellum and the pons. This ventricle is continuous with the central canal of the spinal cord below and the *cerebral aqueduct* above. The cerebral aqueduct connects the fourth and the third ventricles.

Protective Layers of the Brain

■ The spinal cord of the CNS is protected by the vertebral column. The brain is protected by three structures: a layer of skin, skull bones, and layers of tissue called the meninges.

■ The *meninges* contain three layers of membranes that cover the brain and spinal cord (see Figure 1.38):

 - The *dura mater* ("tough mother") is the thick, tough, outermost membrane whose one side adheres to the skull and whose other side adheres to the arachnoid.

 - The *arachnoid* ("spider web") is the semitransparent, thin, vascular, delicate, and weblike middle membrane; cerebrospinal fluid fills the subarachnoid space between the arachnoid and the pia mater.

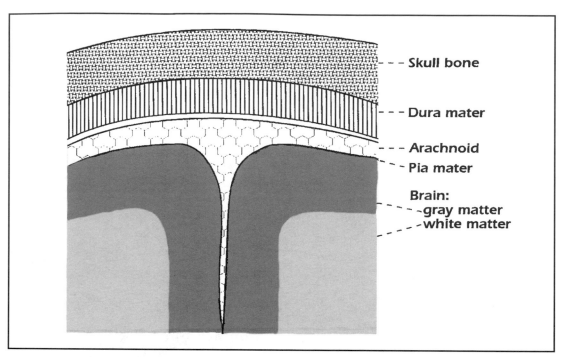

Figure 1.38. The relationship of the meninges to the brain and skull. The pia mater and part of the arachnoid extend into every groove of the brain. The dura mater, however, does not. From *Neuroscience of Communication* (p. 61), by D. B. Webster, 1995, San Diego, CA: Singular Publishing Group, Inc. (401 West A Street, Suite 325, San Diego, CA 92101-7904, 800-521-8545). Copyright 1995 by Singular Publishing Group, Inc. Reprinted with permission.

— The *pia mater* ("tender mother") is the delicate, thin, transparent membrane that adheres to the brain surface and closely follows its gyri and sulci; many blood vessels penetrate the pia mater to enter the brain.

✎ Concepts To Consider

Describe and compare the pyramidal and extrapyramidal systems. What are the implications for speech and language of lesions in these systems?

_____

_____

_____

_____

_____

_____

_____

Cerebral Blood Supply

■ The brain makes up approximately 2% of the body's weight; however, it consumes 25% of the body's oxygen and requires 20% of the body's blood.

■ The wonderfully complex and intricate brain is a highly vulnerable structure. If its blood supply is interrupted, consciousness may be lost within 10 seconds, electrical activity ceases after 20 seconds, and the brain is permanently damaged within 4 to 6 minutes.

■ The blood supplies oxygen and other nutrients required by the brain. The major structures that supply blood to the brain are the aorta, the vertebral arteries, the carotid arteries, and the circle of Willis.

Aorta

■ The *aorta* is the main artery of the heart. It carries blood from the left ventricle to all parts of the body except the lungs.

■ Just above the heart, the aortic arch divides into four branches. These branches are the two carotid arteries and the two subclavian arteries. Figure 1.39 illustrates the major vascular supply of the cerebral cortex.

Vertebral Arteries

■ The right and left *vertebral arteries* branch out from the two subclavian arteries that emerge from the aortic arch. The subclavian arteries supply primarily the upper extremities.

■ The vertebral arteries enter the skull and then branch out to supply the spinal cord and many organs of the body. As they move up to the lower level of the pons, the two vertebral arteries join to form the *basilar artery*.

■ As the basilar artery moves toward the upper portion of the pons, it divides again into two *posterior cerebral arteries*. These arteries supply the lateral and lower portions of the temporal lobes and the lateral and middle portions of the occipital lobes.

■ Several other branches of the basilar artery, such as the anterior, posterior, superior, and inferior cerebellar arteries, supply other structures such as the inner ear, cerebellum, and pons.

Carotid Arteries

■ As the left and right *carotid arteries* (one on each side of the neck) enter the neck, they each branch out into an internal carotid artery and an external

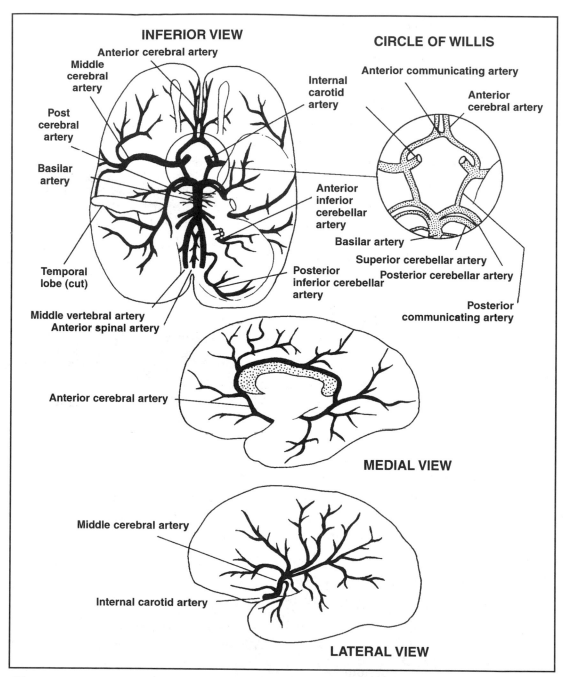

Figure 1.39. The major vascular supply of the cerebral cortex. From *Anatomy and Physiology for Speech, Language, and Hearing* (p. 469), by J. A. Seikel, D. W. King, and D. G. Drumright, 1997, San Diego, CA: Singular Publishing Group, Inc. (401 West A Street, Suite 325, San Diego, CA 92101-7904, 800-521-8545). Copyright 1997 by Singular Publishing Group, Inc. Reprinted with permission.

carotid artery. The arteries enter the brain through the base of the skull and go through the dura mater and subarachnoid space.

- The *external carotid artery* moves toward the face and branches into smaller arteries. It supplies blood to the muscles of the mouth, nose, forehead, and face.

- The *internal carotid artery* is the major supplier of blood to the brain. This artery branches into several smaller blood vessels that supply different parts of the brain. Two key branches of the internal carotid artery are the middle cerebral artery and the anterior cerebral artery.

- The *middle cerebral artery* is the biggest branch of the internal carotid artery, and it supplies the entire lateral surface of the cortex, including the major regions of the frontal lobe.

- The middle cerebral artery supplies blood to major areas involved with motor and sensory functions and language, speech, and hearing functions.

- The areas supplied by the middle cerebral artery include the motor cortex in the precentral gyrus, Broca's area, the primary auditory cortex, Wernicke's area, the supramarginal gyrus, the angular gyrus, and the somatosensory cortex.

- Damage to the middle cerebral artery may result in strokes, aphasia, reading and writing deficits, contralateral hemiplegia, and an impaired sense of pain, temperature, touch, and position.

- The *anterior cerebral artery* supplies primarily the middle portion of the parietal and frontal lobes. It also supplies blood to the corpus callosum and basal ganglia. Branches of the anterior cerebral artery join with the posterior cerebral artery in the posterior medial areas of the brain.

- Damage to the anterior cerebral artery can cause cognitive deficits such as impaired judgment, concentration, and reasoning. Damage can also cause paralysis of the feet and legs.

Circle of Willis

- The *circle of Willis* (*circulus arteriosus*) is formed at the base of the brain where the two carotid and the two vertebral arteries join. The circle is completed by the anterior and posterior communicating arteries. The posterior cerebral, anterior cerebral, and middle cerebral arteries branch out from the circle of Willis.

- The circle of Willis provides a common blood supply to various cerebral branches. If an artery is blocked above the circle, brain damage will occur because the brain has no alternate source of blood. If an artery is blocked below the circle of Willis, however, brain damage may be minimal because alternate channels of blood flow may be maintained.

Summary

☑ The central nervous system, composed of the brain and the spinal cord, is a complex and intricate system that depends upon the intact functioning of and interconnections between many structures.

☑ These structures include the brain stem, the reticular activating system, the diencephalon, the basal ganglia, the cerebellum, and the cerebrum with its frontal, parietal, occipital, and temporal lobes.

☑ The pyramidal and extrapyramidal systems are concerned with movement. Projection, association, and commissural fibers connect key brain structures.

☑ Other critical components of the brain include the cerebral ventricles, meninges, and various arteries that supply blood to the brain and its structures.

CHAPTER HIGHLIGHTS

▶ Respiration, or breathing, consists of a rhythmic cycle of inhalation and exhalation. Respiration provides the energy for voicing and ultimately for speech. The process of respiration relies upon the integrity of many structures. These include the lungs, bronchi, trachea, spinal column, sternum, rib cage, and muscles of inspiration and expiration.

▶ Voice is usually produced as exhaled air comes from the lungs through the trachea to the larynx. The larynx houses the vocal folds, which vibrate to produce voice. Optimal voicing relies upon key laryngeal cartilages and structures as well as the functioning of the intrinsic and extrinsic laryngeal muscles. The myoelastic aerodynamic theory helps explain the physiology of phonation. Cranial nerves VII (facial nerve) and X (vagus nerve) are key in the phonation process.

▶ The vocal folds vibrate to produce voice, and the voice travels upward to be modified or resonated by the pharynx and the oral and nasal cavities. English sounds have primarily oral or nasal resonance. The source-filter theory explains how speech sounds are ultimately produced through modification of the oral cavity and adjacent structures.

▶ Articulation for speech involves movements that produce particular sounds. Key structures for articulation in the oral cavity include the pharynx, soft palate, hard palate, mandible, teeth, tongue, lips, and cheeks. Cranial nerves primarily responsible for innervation of articulatory structures include V (trigeminal nerve), VII (facial nerve), IX (glossopharyngeal nerve), X (vagus nerve), XI (spinal accessory nerve), and XII (hypoglossal nerve).

(continues)

▶ The nervous system, composed of neurons and other specialized cells, can be divided into two basic parts: the peripheral and central nervous systems. The peripheral nervous system is composed of the spinal nerves and the cranial nerves. Cranial nerves most critical to speech, language, and hearing include trigeminal nerve V, facial nerve VII, vestibulocochlear nerve VIII, glossopharyngeal nerve IX, vagus nerve X, spinal accessory nerve XI, and hypoglossal nerve XII.

▶ The central nervous system is composed of the brain and the spinal cord. The brain contains many structures, including the brain stem, reticular activating system, diencephalon, basal ganglia, cerebellum, and cerebrum. The brain stem, composed of the midbrain, pons, and medulla, connects the spinal cord with the brain via the diencephalon.

▶ The cerebellum helps coordinate and regulate neural impulses going to and from the brain. It regulates equilibrium, body posture, and coordinated fine-motor movements. An intact cerebellum is critical to speech production, and people with cerebellar damage may show ataxia and dysarthria.

▶ The cerebrum, or cerebral cortex, has four lobes: the occipital, frontal, parietal, and temporal lobes. The occipital lobe is primarily concerned with vision. The frontal lobe contains motor areas, such as Broca's area, that are critical to speech production. The parietal lobe, which integrates sensations such as pain, temperature, and touch, contains the angular gyrus and the supramarginal gyrus, which are critical to speech. The temporal lobe contains the key structures of the primary auditory cortex, the auditory association area, and Wernicke's area.

▶ The pyramidal and extrapyramidal systems are involved in motor movement. The pyramidal system, consisting of the corticospinal and corticobulbar tracts, is primarily responsible for facilitating voluntary movements of muscles, including speech muscles. The extrapyramidal system is a more indirect activation system, which helps maintain posture and tone as well as regulating movement.

▶ Important connecting fibers in the brain include projection fibers, association fibers, and commissural fibers. The corpus callosum, a critical commissural fiber, connects the two hemispheres. Other important brain structures include the cerebral ventricles, meninges, and structures that supply blood to the brain.

▶ Add your own chapter highlights here:

_____

_____

_____

_____

KEY TERMS

abdomen
abduct
adduct
afferent neuron
alveolar arch
alveolar ducts
alveolar process
angular gyrus
anterior belly of
  digastric
anterior cerebral artery
aorta
arachnoid
arcuate fasciculus
articulation
aryepiglottic folds
arytenoid cartilages
association fibers
ataxia
ataxic dysarthria
auditory association
  area
autonomic nervous
  system
axon
basal ganglia
basilar artery
Bernoulli effect
blade (of tongue)
body (of sternum)
brain
brain stem
Broca's area
bronchi
bronchioles
buccinator
carotid arteries
caudate nucleus
central nervous system
central sulcus
cerebellar peduncles
  (superior, middle,
  inferior)
cerebellum
cerebral cortex
cerebral ventricles
cerebrospinal fluid

cerebrum
cervical vertebrae
chondroglossus
choroid plexus
circle of Willis
coccygeal vertebrae
commissural fibers
contralateral motor
  control
corniculate cartilages
corona radiata
corpus callosum
corpus striatum
cortex
corticobulbar tract
corticospinal tract
costal cartilages
cranial nerves
cranial nerve I
  (olfactory)
cranial nerve II (optic)
cranial nerve III
  (oculomotor)
cranial nerve IV
  (trochlear)
cranial nerve V
  (trigeminal)
cranial nerve VI
  (abducens)
cranial nerve VII (facial)
cranial nerve VIII
  (vestibular acoustic or
  vestibulocochlear)
cranial nerve IX
  (glossopharyngeal)
cranial nerve X (vagus)
cranial nerve XI (spinal
  accessory)
cranial nerve XII
  (hypoglossal)
cricoarytenoid joint
cricoid cartilage
cricothyroids
cuneiform cartilages
deciduous teeth
dendrite
depressor anguli oris

(triangularis)
depressor labii inferioris
depressors
diaphragm
diencephalon
digastrics
disconnection syndrome
dorsum (of tongue)
dura mater
efferent neuron
elevators
epiglottis
eustachian tube
external carotid artery
external intercostals
extrapyramidal system
extrinsic laryngeal mus-
  cles
fasciculi
fissure
fissure of Rolando
foramen magnum
foramen of Munro
foramina
fourth ventricle
frontal lobe
ganglion
genioglossus
geniohyoids
globus pallidus
glottis
gyrus
hard palate
Heschl's gyri
hyoglossus
hyoid bone
hypothalamus
inferior longitudinal
  muscle
inferior peduncle
inferior pharyngeal
  constrictor, crico-
  pharyngeus
inferior pharyngeal
  constrictor, thyro-
  pharyngeus
infrahyoid muscles

innermost intercostals
interarytenoid muscles
intercostal muscles
interhemispheric fibers
internal capsule
internal carotid artery
internal intercostals
internal oblique
   abdominus
interneuron
intrahemispheric fibers
intrinsic laryngeal
   muscles
laryngopharynx
larynx
lateral cerebral fissure
lateral cricoarytenoid
   muscles
lateral ventricles
latissimus dorsi
levator anguli oris
levator costarum brevis
levator costarum longis
levator labii superioris
levator labii superioris
   alaeque nasi
levator scapulae
levator veli palatini
lingual frenulum
   (frenum)
longitudinal fissure
lower motor neurons
lower temporal gyrus
lumbar vertebrae
lungs
malocclusion
mandible
manubrium
masseter
mastication
maxillae
medial (internal)
   pterygoid
medulla
medulla oblongata
meninges
mentalis muscle
mesencephalon
metencephalon
midbrain

middle cerebral artery
middle peduncle
middle pharyngeal
   constrictor
middle temporal gyrus
mixed nerves
motor nerves
motor neuron
mucosal wave action
myelin
myelencephalon
mylohyoids
myoelastic aerodynamic
   theory
nasopharynx
nervous system
neural transmission
neurotransmitter
nucleus
oblique arytenoids
occipital lobe
occlusion
omohyoids
orbicularis oris
orbicularis oris inferioris
   and superioris
oropharynx
palatine bone
palatine process
palatoglossus muscle
palatopharyngeus
   muscle
parasympathetic
   (branch of autonomic
   nervous system)
parietal lobe
pectoralis major
pectoralis minor
peripheral nervous
   system
pharyngeal branch (of
   vagus nerve)
pharyngeal plexus
pharynx
pia mater
platysma
pons
postcentral gyrus
posterior belly of
   digastric

posterior cerebral
   arteries
posterior cricoarytenoids
precentral gyrus
premaxilla
primary auditory cortex
primary motor cortex
   (motor strip)
primary visual cortex
projection fibers
putamen
pyramidal system
pyramidal tracts
quadratus lumborum
rectus abdominus
recurrent laryngeal
   nerve
resonation
respiration
reticular activating
   system
rhomboideus major
rhomboideus minor
rib cage
risorius muscle
root (of tongue)
sacral vertebrae
salpingopharyngeus
sensory cortex (strip)
sensory nerves
sensory neuron
serratus anterior
serratus posterior
   inferior
serratus posterior
   superior
skull
soft palate
source-filter theory
spinal column
spinal cord
sternocleidomastoid
sternohyoids
sternothyroids
sternum
styloglossus
stylohyoids
stylopharyngeus
subcostal muscle
substantia nigra

sulcus (sulci)
superior laryngeal nerve
superior longitudinal fibers
superior longitudinal muscle
superior peduncles
superior pharyngeal constrictor
superior temporal gyrus
supplementary motor cortex
suprahyoid muscles
supramarginal gyrus
Sylvian fissure
sympathetic (branch of autonomic nervous system)
synapse

temporal lobe
temporalis
temporomandibular joint
tensor veli palatini
terminal (end) knob
thalamus
third ventricle
thoracic vertebrae
thyroarytenoids
thyrohyoids
thyroid cartilage
tip (of tongue)
tongue
trachea
transverse arytenoids
transverse (tongue) muscles
transversus abdominus

transversus thoracicus
trapezius
trigeminal neuralgia
upper motor neurons
uvula
velopharyngeal closure
velum
ventricular (false) vocal folds
vertebrae foramina
vertebral arteries
vertical (tongue) muscles
vocal folds (or vocal cords)
vocalis muscles
Wernicke's area
xiphoid process
zygomatic major
zygomatic minor

STUDY AND REVIEW QUESTIONS

Fill in the Blank

1. Respiration relies upon muscles of inspiration and expiration. A key muscle is the _diaphragm_, a thick, dome-shaped muscle that separates the abdomen from the thorax. The _internal intercostal_ muscles pull the ribs downward to decrease the diameter of the thoracic cavity for exhalation, and the _external intercostal_ raise the ribs up and out to increase the diameter of the thoracic cavity for inhalation.

2. Most pharyngeal muscles are innervated by cranial nerves _X_ and _XI_, which join to form the _pharyngeal plexus_, which supplies the upper pharyngeal musculature.

3. The primary muscle of the lips is the _orbicularis oris_ muscle; the cheeks are primarily composed of the _buccinator_ muscle.

4. _neurons_, the most important type of cells in the nervous system, are composed of three parts: _cell body_, _axon_, and _dendrite_. _afferent_ neurons carry sensory information from the peripheral sense organs toward the brain, and _efferent_ neurons transmit impulses away from the brain.

5. The three sections of the brain stem are the _midbrain_, _pons_, and _medulla_. An important adjacent structure is the _diencephalon_, which lies between the brain stem and the cerebral hemispheres and contains the _hypothalamus_, which controls emotions, and the _thalamus_, which relays sensory impulses to various portions of the cerebral cortex.

6. The _basal_ _ganglia_, which lie deep within the brain, contain the corpus striatum, which is composed of three nuclear masses: the _globus pallidus_, _caudate nucleus_, and _putamen_.

7. The _cerebellum_ is a structure that regulates equilibrium, body posture, and coordinated fine-motor movements. People with damage to this structure may have a neurological disorder called _ataxia_.

8. The _middle_ _cerebral_ artery is the largest branch of the internal carotid artery, supplying the entire lateral surface of the cortex. The _anterior_ _cerebral_ artery supplies blood to the corpus callosum and the basal ganglia.

9. _Lower_ motor neurons are the motor neurons in the spinal and cranial nerves and are part of the PNS. _Upper_ motor neurons are the motor fibers within the CNS.

10. The _internal_ _capsule_ contains concentrated and compact projection fibers near the brain stem, while the _corona_ _radiata_ is a fanlike structure of projection fibers in the upper regions of the brain.

Multiple Choice

11. The cranial nerve that innervates the larynx and also innervates the levator veli palatini, palatoglossus, and palatopharyngeus muscles is:

   A. cranial nerve X, the vagus nerve.
   B. cranial nerve V, the trigeminal nerve.
   C. cranial nerve XI, the spinal accessory nerve.
   D. cranial nerve VII, the facial nerve.
   E. cranial nerve XII, the hypoglossal nerve.

12. Muscles that contribute to velopharyngeal closure through tensing and/or elevating the velum are the:

   A. tensor veli palatini, levator veli palatini, and salpingopharyngeus.
   B. stylopharyngeus, salpingopharyngeus, and levator veli palatini.

C. levator veli palatini, genioglossus, and salpingopharyngeus.

D. palatoglossus, tensor veli palatini, and levator veli palatini.

E. tensor veli palatini and levator veli palatini.

13. The structure at the inferior portion of the tongue that connects the tongue with the mandible is called the:

   A. dorsum.
   B. root.
   C. blade.
   D. tip.
   E. lingual frenum.

14. When a person is producing voiced and voiceless /th/, the muscle that is most involved is the:

   A. palatopharyngeus.
   B. sternocleidomastoid.
   C. genioglossus.
   D. styloglossus.
   E. buccinator.

15. When a person is adducting and abducting the vocal folds, which muscles from the list below are the most involved with that process?

   I. thyroarytenoids
   II. digastrics
   III. lateral cricoarytenoids
   VI. transverse arytenoids
   V. sternothyroids

   A. I, III, V   C. I, IV, V   E. II, III, IV, V
   B. II, III, IV   D. I, III, IV

16. The cerebral hemispheres are connected by:

   A. projection fibers.
   B. association fibers.
   C. commissural fibers.
   D. cerebrocortical fibers.
   E. extrapyramidal fibers.

17. The central nervous system's primary mechanism of attention, alertness, and consciousness, which is also related to sleep-wake cycles, is the:

   A. diencephalon.
   B. mesencephalon.

C. reticular activating system.

D. corticobulbar tract.

E. circle of Willis.

18. The primary motor cortex in the frontal lobe is located on the:

A. precentral gyrus.

B. homunculus.

C. supramarginal gyrus.

D. angular gyrus.

E. middle temporal gyrus.

19. Which one of the following is FALSE?

A. Wernicke's area in the temporal lobe is critical to the comprehension of spoken language.

B. Wernicke's area is connected to Broca's area in the frontal lobe through the arcuate fasciculus.

C. The occipital lobe contains the primary visual cortex.

D. The angular gyrus in the occipital lobe is important for interpretation of somesthetic sensations such as pain, touch, and temperature.

E. The pyramidal system consists of the corticospinal and corticobulbar tracts.

20. Which of the following are TRUE?

   I. The cerebral ventricles are interconnected cavities filled with fluid produced by the dura mater.

   II. The meninges of the brain consist of the dura mater, the pia mater, and the arachnoid.

   III. The basilar artery eventually divides into the two posterior cerebral arteries.

   IV. The external carotid artery is the major supplier of blood to the brain.

   V. The circle of Willis is formed at the base of the brain where the two carotid and two vertebral arteries join.

A. II, III, IV, V   C. I, III, IV   E. II, III, V

B. All of the above   D. II, IV, V

REFERENCES AND RECOMMENDED READINGS

Andrews, M. L. (1995). *Manual of voice treatment: Pediatrics through geriatrics*. San Diego, CA: Singular Publishing Group.

Bhatnagar, S. C., & Andy, O. J. (1995). *Neuroscience for the study of communicative disorders*. Baltimore, MD: Williams & Wilkins.

Boone, D. R., & McFarlane, S. C. (1994). *The voice and voice therapy* (5th ed.). Englewood Cliffs, NJ: Prentice-Hall.

Colton, R., & Casper, J. K. (1996). *Understanding voice problems: A physiological perspective for diagnosis and treatment* (2nd ed.). Baltimore, MD: Williams & Wilkins.

Freed, D. B. (1999). *Motor speech disorders: Diagnosis and treatment*. San Diego: Singular Publishing Group.

Hegde, M. N. (1995). *Introduction to communicative disorders* (2nd ed.). Austin, TX: PRO-ED.

Hegde, M. N. (1998). *A coursebook on aphasia and other neurogenic language disorders* (2nd ed.). San Diego, CA: Singular Publishing Group.

Kent, R. (1997). *The speech sciences*. San Diego, CA: Singular Publishing Group.

Kuehn, D. P., Lemme, M. L., & Baumgartner, J. M. (Eds.). (1989). *Neural bases of speech, hearing, and language*. Austin, TX: PRO-ED.

Love, R. J., & Webb, W. G. (1996). *Neurology for the speech–language pathologist* (3rd ed.). Boston: Butterworth-Heinemann.

Luria, A. R. (1973). *The working brain: An introduction to neuropsychology*. New York: Basic Books.

Newman, D., & Ramadan, N. (1998). Neurologic disorders: An orientation and overview. In A. F. Johnson & B. H. Jacobson (Eds.), *Medical speech–language pathology: A practitioner's guide* (pp. 211–242). New York: Thieme.

Peña-Brooks, A., & Hegde, M. N. (1999). *Articulatory and phonological disorders in children: A dual level text*. Austin, TX: PRO-ED.

Seikel, J. A., King, D. W., & Drumright, D. G. (1997). *Anatomy and physiology for speech, language, and hearing*. San Diego, CA: Singular Publishing Group.

Van Riper, C., & Erickson, R. L. (1996). *Speech correction: An introduction to speech pathology and audiology* (9th ed.). Needham Heights, MA: Allyn & Bacon.

Webster, D. B. (1995). *Neuroscience of communication*. San Diego, CA: Singular Publishing Group.

Zemlin, W. R. (1998). *Speech and hearing science: Anatomy and physiology* (4th ed.). Needham Heights, MA: Allyn & Bacon.

ANSWERS TO STUDY AND REVIEW QUESTIONS

1. Diaphragm, internal intercostals, external intercostals

2. X, XI, pharyngeal plexus

3. Orbicularis oris, buccinator

4. Cell body, dendrites, axon; afferent, efferent

5. Midbrain, pons, medulla; diencephalon, hypothalamus, thalamus

6. Basal ganglia, globus pallidus, caudate nucleus, putamen

7. Cerebellum, ataxia

8. Middle cerebral, anterior cerebral

9. Lower, upper

10. Internal capsule, corona radiata

11. A. The cranial nerve that innervates the larynx and also innervates the levator veli palatini, palatoglossus, and palatopharyngeus muscles is cranial nerve X, the vagus nerve.

12. D. Muscles that contribute to velopharyngeal closure through tensing and/or elevating the velum are: the palatoglossus, tensor veli palatini, and levator veli palatini.

13. E. The structure at the inferior portion of the tongue that connects the tongue with the mandible is called the lingual frenum.

14. C. When a person is producing voiced and voiceless /th/, the muscle that is most involved is the genioglossus.

15. D. When a person is adducting and abducting the vocal folds, the muscles most involved with this process are the thyroarytenoids, lateral cricoarytenoids, and transverse arytenoids.

16. C. The cerebral hemispheres are connected by the commissural fibers.

17. C. The central nervous system's primary mechanism of attention, alertness, and consciousness, which is also related to sleep-wake cycles, is the reticular activating system.

18. A. The primary motor cortex in the frontal lobe is located on the precentral gyrus.

19. D. The angular gyrus is in the parietal lobe.

20. E. The meninges of the brain consist of the dura mater, the pia mater, and the arachnoid; the basilar artery eventually divides into the two posterior cerebral arteries; and the circle of Willis is formed at the base of the brain where the two carotid and two vertebral arteries join.

CHAPTER 2

Physiological and Acoustic Phonetics: A Speech Science Foundation

PREVIEW OUTLINE

CHAPTER INTRODUCTION

Sounds can be very broadly categorized into two key areas: production and perception. The *production* of sounds is generally concerned with articulatory physiology; that is, how sounds are produced. The *perception* of sounds is generally concerned with the relationship between sound production and the acoustic signal of speech. *Phonetics*, the study of speech sounds, is the science concerned with the production and perception of speech sounds in terms of their articulatory and physical characteristics (Nicolosi, Harryman, & Kresheck, 1996; Yavas, 1998). Because much research effort in the speech sciences relates to issues in phonetics, phonetics is a central aspect of speech science (Kent, 1997). Thus, in this chapter, we integrate information in phonetics and speech science through describing *physiological phonetics*, which focuses on speech sound production, and *acoustic phonetics*, which focuses on the acoustic properties of sound waves that result when sounds are produced. Our discussion focuses on the production and perception of Standard American English.

BASIC PRINCIPLES AND DEFINITIONS: A FOUNDATION

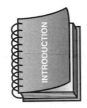

Every language exists as a system with organized components. Phonetics, the study of speech sounds, organizes these sounds into systematic categories according to their perception and production. Speakers of any language need adequate respiration, phonation, resonation, and articulation to produce sounds for speech.

Definitions

■ *Language* is a code or system of symbols used to express concepts formed through exposure and experience (Bloom & Lahey, 1978). *Speech* is the sensorimotor production of that code, and *phonology* is the scientific study of the sound systems and patterns used to create the words of a language.

■ *Phonemes* are the smallest units of sound that can affect meaning. For example, *man* and *fan* mean different things because of the different initial phonemes /m/ and /f/. Phonemes are families of sounds; the listener perceives members of a family as belonging to the same phoneme. Phonemes are represented by other families or categories of sounds called allophones (Lowe, 1994).

■ *Allophones* are variations of phonemes. Allophones do not change word meanings, and listeners do not perceive them as different from one another. The individual sound /r/ is a phoneme, but it sounds slightly different when it is produced differently by different speakers in different contexts.

■ For instance, the /r/ in *green* would be produced with more tongue retraction than the /r/ in *red*, which would be produced slightly more toward the front of the mouth. A speaker from New York would produce /r/ differently than a speaker from California. These different productions are allophonic variations of the /r/ phoneme.

■ The term *phonemic* refers to the abstract system of sounds; for example, the idealized and abstract description of /s/ is phonemic. Slash marks indicate phonemic representation of a sound, or a general and abstract class of sounds.

■ The term *phonetic* refers to concrete productions of specific sounds. Phonetic productions are enclosed in square brackets [ ], indicating specific sound productions by given speakers.

■ The term *phonetics* is derived from the word *phone*. A phone may or may not be a speech sound; the word refers generically to any sound that can be produced by the vocal tract (Edwards, 1997). Usually, a phone is considered a single speech sound. Phonetics is the study of speech sounds.

■ Researchers have divided the area of phonetics into different categories. A synthesis of these categories follows (Edwards, 1997; Kent, 1998; Nicolosi et al., 1996; Yavas, 1998):

– *Acoustic phonetics* examines the relationship between articulation and the acoustic signal of speech. The focus is upon the acoustic properties of sound waves (e.g., periodicity and aperiodicity).

– *Auditory phonetics* is the study of hearing, perception, and the brain's processing of speech.

– *Articulatory* or *physiological phonetics* focuses on speech sound production; emphasis is on how the articulators produce individual sounds.

– *Applied phonetics* focuses on the practical application of research in articulatory, perceptual, acoustic, and experimental phonetics.

– *Experimental phonetics* involves the use of objective laboratory techniques to scientifically analyze speech sounds.

– *Descriptive phonetics* refers to the study and explanation of the unique sound properties of various dialects and languages.

Anatomy and Physiology: A Brief Review

■ To produce sounds intelligibly, the speaker needs adequate respiration, phonation, articulation, and resonation. These processes work together synergistically.

Respiration

■ The respiratory system consists of the lungs, diaphragm, rib cage, airway, and many other structures.

■ Inhalation and exhalation are necessary components of breathing for speech. They create the rhythmic cycle of respiration. The process of respiration supplies the air necessary for speech production.

Phonation

■ As air travels upward from the lungs and through the airway, it reaches the vocal folds housed within the larynx.

■ Vocal fold vibrations create phonation, which is necessary for all voiced sounds (described in more detail later). Sounds cannot be properly voiced without adequate phonation.

Resonation

■ The air continues to travel upward past the level of the vocal folds and enters cavities above the larynx. In these nasal, pharyngeal, and oral cavities, the air is modified. Resonance is the modification of sound by structures or cavities through which the sound passes.

■ Resonating bodies do not produce sound; rather, they modify sound produced by another source (e.g., the vocal folds).

Articulation

■ Articulation refers to the production of speech sounds.

■ The articulators, or primary structures involved in the process of articulation, are: lips, mandible, pharynx, velum, hard palate, tongue, and teeth.

Summary

☑ Every language has a system of sounds that are used to create words in that language. Phonetics is the study of speech sounds.

☑ When speakers produce speech sounds, they need adequate respiration, phonation, resonation, and articulation.

☑ Phonetics can be divided into six specific categories; in this chapter, we focus on physiological and acoustic phonetics.

PHONETIC TRANSCRIPTION

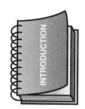

INTRODUCTION

All languages share the challenge of how to best record the sounds of the language as spoken by its people. Many languages of the world have written symbols for the sounds of the language. A problem for many languages, including English, is that the same sound can be written, or spelled, many different ways. To deal with this problem and to provide clarity, the International Phonetic Alphabet was developed. In this section, we describe this alphabet and its broad and narrow symbols.

The International Phonetic Alphabet

■ As stated above, the International Phonetic Alphabet (IPA) was developed to deal with the challenges of *orthographic symbols*, or written representations of sounds. Different orthographic symbols can be used to denote the same sound. For example, the letters *ough* are pronounced differently in the words *through, tough, bough, trough*, and *though*.

■ Developed in 1888, the IPA is used internationally today. It was most recently revised in 1989. The IPA provides a set of phonetic symbols that represents sounds accurately and consistently.

✎ Concepts To Consider

What is the IPA? Why was it developed?

_____

_____

_____

_____

_____

_____

_____

_____

_____

Broad Phonetic Transcription

■ When professionals use IPA symbols to transcribe words or sounds, they use _phonemic transcriptions_ which are indicated by enclosing phonemes between slash marks, as /s/. These transcriptions are phonemic because variations in phoneme production are not depicted.

■ In _phonetic transcription_, allophones are indicated by placing them in brackets, as [s].

■ Table 2.1 lists and gives examples of the consonant and vowel symbols in the IPA. These symbols fall into three basic categories: consonants, vowels, and diphthongs.

Narrow Phonetic Transcription

■ Professionals use narrow phonetic transcription to record more detail about how a speaker produces a sound. Narrow phonetic transcription is especially important when clinicians are assessing speakers with challenges such as a cleft palate, a severe phonological disorder, and hearing loss.

■ _Diacritical markers_ are special symbols used in narrow phonetic transcription. Table 2.2 shows the most widely used diacritical markers in the profession of speech pathology.

Summary

☑ The International Phonetic Alphabet is an internationally recognized system of representing speech sounds consistently and accurately.

☑ Speech–language pathologists can transcribe speech using broad phonetic symbols and narrow phonetic symbols. Narrow phonetic symbols give increased detail about how individual speakers produce sounds.

TABLE 2.1

The International Phonetic Alphabet (IPA)

IPA Symbol	Examples	IPA Symbol	Examples
/p/	pot	/ʃ/	shine
/b/	bat	/ʒ/	vision
/m/	mat	/θ/	thin
/n/	net	/ð/	then
/ŋ/	sing	/tʃ/	chin
/d/	dime	/dʒ/	Jane
/t/	time	/v/	van
/g/	gum	/w/	wine
/k/	Kim	/l/	lean
/f/	fun	/j/	yawn
/s/	sun	/h/	hen
/z/	Zen	/r/	run
/ɑ/	fall	/ɛ/	bet
/æ/	fat	/e/	late
/ɔ/	fought	/o/	overcoat
/ə/	atop	/ʊ/	put
/ʌ/	upset	/u/	boot
/ɪ/	infect	/ɝ/	shirt
/i/	eat	/ɚ/	later
/eɪ/	main		
/aɪ/	lime		
/oʊ/	dome		
/aʊ/	how		
/ɔɪ/	boy		
/ɪʊ/	fuse		

Note. From *Introduction to Communicative Disorders,* 2nd ed. (p. 113), by M. N. Hegde, 1995, Austin, TX: PRO-ED. Copyright 1995 by PRO-ED, Inc. Reprinted with permission.

PRODUCTION OF SEGMENTALS: CONSONANTS AND VOWELS

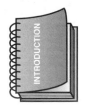

Speech sounds can be broadly classified into two categories: consonants and vowels. Consonants and vowels are often described by their role in the production and perception of syllables. In speech–language pathology, it is useful to further divide consonants and vowels into categories or classification systems. The two most widely used classification systems are: (a) the distinctive feature approach, and (b) the place-voice-manner approach. (*Note:* Some of this information is also contained in Chapter 5, on articulatory and phonological disorders. In this chapter, the information is more detailed.)

TABLE 2.2

Diacritic Markers

[ː] *full lengthening.* This mark, when placed to the right of a phoneme, indicates that the duration of the phoneme has been increased considerably (almost doubled); e.g., /ɛg/ becomes /ɛːg/.

[·] *half lengthening.* This mark, when placed to the right of a phoneme, indicates that the duration of the phoneme has been somewhat increased (not as much as for full lengthening); e.g., /tɔk/ becomes [tɔ·k].

[~] *nasalization.* This mark, when placed above a phoneme, indicates that the phoneme, usually nonnasal, has become nasalized; e.g., /tɔp/ becomes [tɔ̃p].

[̥] *devoicing.* This mark, when placed below a phoneme, indicates that the phoneme, usually voiced, has become devoiced; e.g., /beɪbɪ/ becomes [b̥eɪb̥ɪ].

[̬] *voicing.* This mark, when placed below a phoneme, indicates that the phoneme, usually voiceless, has become voiced; e.g., /sup/ becomes [s̬up].

[ʰ] or [ʻ] *aspiration.* This mark, when placed at the top right side of a phoneme, indicates that the phoneme, usually unaspirated, becomes aspirated; e.g., /tek/ becomes [tekʻ].

[ʼ] *unaspiration.* In American English, this mark, placed at the top left side of phoneme /p, t, k/ in the word-initial position, indicates that the phonemes, usually aspirated, become unaspirated; e.g., /pɑt/ becomes [ʼpɑt].

[̫] *labialization.* This mark, placed directly below the phoneme, indicates that the phoneme, usually nonlabial, becomes labialized; e.g., /nouz/ becomes [n̫ouz].

[̼] *nonlabialization.* This mark, placed directly below the phoneme, indicates that the phoneme, usually labial, becomes nonlabial; e.g., /wɪθ] becomes [w̼ɪθ].

[̪] *dentalization.* This mark, placed directly below the phoneme, indicates that the phoneme, usually not linguadental, is produced at the linguadental place of articulation; e.g., /tɪtʃ/ becomes [t̪ɪt̪ʃ].

[̇] *palatalization.* This mark, placed directly above the phoneme, indicates that the phoneme, usually nonpalatal, becomes palatalized; e.g., /zu/ becomes [żu].

[ ] *closing of vowel.* This mark, placed directly below the vowel phoneme, indicates that the phoneme is produced with greater closing than normally required for its production; e.g., /edʒ/ becomes [e̝dʒ].

[ ] *opening of vowel.* This mark, when placed directly below the vowel phoneme, indicates that the phoneme is produced with greater opening than normally required for its production; e.g., /ˈeɪnˌdʒəl/ becomes [ˈe̞ɪnˌdʒəl].

[˔] *tongue raising.* This mark, when placed to the right of the vowel phoneme, indicates that the phoneme is produced with more than usual tongue raising; e.g., /ðe/ becomes [ðe˔].

[˕] *tongue lowering.* This mark, when placed to the right of the vowel phoneme, indicates that the phoneme is produced with more than usual tongue lowering; e.g., /blu/ becomes [blu˕].

[+] or [˧] *tongue advancement.* This mark, when placed to the right of the vowel phoneme, indicates that the phoneme is produced with more than usual tongue advancement; e.g., /tu/ becomes [tu+].

[−] or [˗] *tongue retraction.* This mark, when placed to the right of the vowel phoneme, indicates that the phoneme is produced with more than usual tongue retraction; e.g., /tʃik/ becomes [tʃi−k].

[ ] *lip rounding.* This mark, when placed at the top right side of the vowel phoneme, indicates that the phoneme is produced with more than usual lip rounding; e.g., /ʃit/ becomes [ʃiᵓt].

[ ] *lip spreading.* This mark, when placed at the top right side of the vowel phoneme, indicates that the phoneme is produced with more than usual lip spreading; e.g., /sun/ becomes [suᶜn].

[-] *vowel centralization.* This mark, when placed across the vowel phoneme, indicates that the phoneme, usually noncentral, becomes centralized; e.g., /it/ becomes [ɨt].

[ ] *consonant syllabification.* In American English, this mark is placed below the consonants /m, n, ŋ, l/ when these consonants perform the function of the nucleus in a syllable; e.g., /bɑtəl/ becomes [bɑtl̩].

Note. From *Phonetics: Principles and Practices*, 2nd ed. (pp. 227–229), by S. Singh & K. S. Singh, 1982, Austin, TX: PRO-ED. Copyright 1982 by PRO-ED, Inc. Reprinted with permission of the authors.

Consonant and Vowel Functions: The Syllable as a Unit

- Consonants and vowels may be defined by their role in speech production of syllables. The *syllable* is defined as the smallest phonetic unit.

- Yavas (1998) describes syllables as motor units comprised of three parts:

    1. *onset*, or the initial consonant or consonant cluster of the syllable, created by release of the syllable pulse through articulatory movements or action of the chest muscles;

    2. *nucleus*, or a vowel or dipthong in the middle of the syllable, created by vowel-shaping movements of the vocal tract; and

    3. *coda*, the consonant at the end of the syllable, created by arrest of the syllable pulse through articulatory movements, action of the chest muscles, or both.

- Thus, vowels form the nucleus of syllables; consonants release and arrest syllables. Vowels may also stand alone to form syllables. For example, utterances such as "ah," "oh," and "I" are vowels and may stand alone. Consonants may not stand alone; they function only with vowels. Table 2.3 illustrates basic comparisons between vowels and consonants; these comparisons will be described in more detail later.

- Vowels may also be termed *syllabics* because they carry syllables. A few consonants have a syllabic nature in that they also can form the nucleus of a syllable (Creaghead, Newman, & Secord, 1989). These syllabic consonants are /l/, /n/, and /m/. The diacritic marker / ̩/ is used to indicate the syllabic nature of these consonants. Examples follow:

TABLE 2.3

Comparisons of Vowels and Consonants

Vowels	Consonants
Always voiced	May be voiced or voiceless
May stand alone	Always combined with vowel
Velum always elevated	Velum elevated or lowered
Vocal tract open	Vocal tract modified or constricted
Airflow continuous	Airflow modified or stopped
May be described by: • distinctive features • tongue and lip position • tension vs. laxness	May be described by: • distinctive features • place-voice-manner

/m̩/: love 'em, leave 'em

/n̩/: button, more 'n' more

/l̩/: bottle, middle

■ Syllables may be open or closed. *Open syllables* end in vowels; *my, hey*, and *ski* are open syllables. *Closed syllables* end in consonants; *cook, lip,* and *hiss* are closed syllables.

■ *Syllabification* is the skill involved in identifying the number of syllables in words. Speakers using syllabification would know, for example, that *categorize* has four syllables whereas *dog* has one syllable.

Classification Systems

Distinctive Feature Approach

■ The distinctive feature approach to classification was created by linguists to describe the languages of the world. These linguists believed that each phoneme was a collection of independent features. A distinctive feature is a unique characteristic of a phoneme that distinguishes one phoneme from another (Chomsky & Halle, 1968; Jakobson, Fant, & Halle, 1952).

■ Each phoneme (consonant or vowel) is described according to a cluster of features that are either present or absent in that phoneme. The binary system of plus or minus a feature is a hallmark of the distinctive feature approach.

■ If a feature is present, a phoneme is given a plus (+) for that feature. If a feature is absent, a phoneme is given a minus (−) for that feature. For example, according to the distinctive feature classification system, /s/ would be described as follows: −vocalic, +consonantal, +anterior, +coronal, +continuant, −high, −low, −back, −nasal, +strident, −vocalic.

■ Although phonemes may share certain features, each phoneme has a unique set of features that distinguishes it from all the other phonemes. Table 2.4 lists each phoneme according to the distinctive feature model.

Place-Voice-Manner Approach

■ The place-voice-manner approach to classification categorizes consonants in terms of three parameters: place, voice, and manner of production. *Place of articulation* refers to the location of the sound's production, indicating the primary articulators that shape the sounds. For example, /p/ is termed a "bilabial" because it is produced by putting the lips together.

■ *Voicing* refers to vocal fold vibration during production of sounds. *Voiced* sounds are those produced while the vocal folds are vibrating. *Voiceless* sounds are those produced while the vocal folds are not vibrating. The /p/ is a voiceless sound.

TABLE 2.4

The Chomsky-Halle Distinctive Features of English Consonants

	w	f	v	θ	ð	t	d	s	z	n	l	ʃ	ʒ	j	r	tʃ	dʒ	k	g	ŋ	h	p
Voiced	+	−	+	−	+	−	+	−	+	+	+	−	+	+	+	−	+	−	+	+	−	−
Consonantal	−	+	+	+	+	+	+	+	+	+	+	+	+	−	+	+	+	+	+	+	−	+
Anterior	+	+	+	+	+	+	+	+	+	+	+	−	−	−	−	−	−	−	−	−	−	+
Coronal	−	−	−	+	+	+	+	+	+	+	+	+	+	−	+	+	+	−	−	−	−	−
Continuant	+	+	+	+	+	−	−	+	+	−	+	+	+	+	+	−	−	−	−	−	+	−
High	−	−	−	−	−	−	−	−	−	−	−	+	+	+	−	+	+	+	+	+	−	−
Low	−	−	−	−	−	−	−	−	−	−	−	−	−	−	−	−	−	−	−	−	+	−
Back	−	−	−	−	−	−	−	−	−	−	−	−	−	−	−	−	−	+	+	+	−	−
Nasal	−	−	−	−	−	−	−	−	−	+	−	−	−	−	−	−	−	−	−	+	−	−
Strident	−	+	+	−	−	−	−	+	+	−	−	+	+	−	−	+	+	−	−	−	−	−
Vocalic	−	−	−	−	−	−	−	−	−	−	+	−	−	−	+	−	−	−	−	−	−	−

Note. From *Introduction to Communicative Disorders*, 2nd ed. (p. 120), by M. N. Hegde, 1995, Austin, TX: PRO-ED. Copyright 1995 by PRO-ED, Inc. Reprinted with permission.

 Manner of articulation refers to the degree or type of constriction of the vocal tract during consonant production. For example, /p/ is termed a "stop" because it is produced by putting the lips together and completely stopping the air-flow. Table 2.5 illustrates how English consonants may be classified according to the place-voice-manner approach.

✎ Concepts To Consider

Compare and contrast the distinctive feature and place-voice-manner approaches to categorizing phonemes.

_____

_____

_____

_____

_____

_____

_____

TABLE 2.5

Manner of Production

Place of Articulation	Nasals	Stops	Fricatives	Affricates	Liquids	Glides	Laterals
Bilabial	ⓜ	pⓑ				ⓦ	
Labiodental			fⓥ				
Linguadental			θⓓ̶				
Lingua-alveolar	ⓝ	tⓓ	sⓩ		Ⓘ		Ⓘ
Linguapalatal			ʃ③	tʃ ⓓ̶ʒ	ⓡ	ⓙ	
Linguavelar	ⓝ̇	kⓖ					
Glottal			h				

Note. Voiced sounds are circled. Place-Voice-Manner Classification of English Consonants. From *Introduction to Communicative Disorders*, 2nd ed. (p. 117), by M. N. Hegde, 1995, Austin, TX: PRO-ED. Copyright 1995 by PRO-ED, Inc. Reprinted with permission.

Consonants

Basic Principles

■ Consonants are speech sounds produced by movements of articulatory muscles. These movements modify the airstream in some manner through interrupting it, stopping it, and/or creating a narrow opening through which it must pass. Consonants may be voiced or voiceless.

■ Consonants may be described according to distinctive features and their place, voice, and manner of production. In this section, we describe these parameters and provide a summary of them for each consonant either singly or as a member of a cognate pair (defined later).

Distinctive Feature Approach

When a person produces /ə/, the tongue is neutral and at rest. For production of many consonants, the tongue moves to a different position. In the distinctive feature system, many sounds are described according to where and how the tongue moves away from the neutral resting position /ə/. The following descriptions are summarized from Peña-Brooks and Hegde (1999); Kent (1997); Creaghead et al. (1989); Yavas (1998); and Borden, Harris, and Raphael (1994):

■ *Vocalic* sounds include all vowels and the consonants /r/ and /l/. They have little constriction and are associated with spontaneous voicing.

■ *Consonantal* sounds include /m/, /b/, /p/, /ŋ/, /g/, /k/, /dʒ/, /tʃ/, /ʒ/, /ʃ/, /r/, /l/, /n/, /s/, /z/, /d/, /t/, /ð/, /θ/, /v/, /f/. These sounds have marked constriction along the midline region of the vocal tract.

■ *Lateral* sound includes /l/ only. The /l/ is produced by placing the front of the tongue against the alveolar ridge (midline closure) and lowering the midsection of the tongue bilaterally (lateral opening).

■ *Voiced* sounds include /m/, /n/, /ŋ/, /b/, /g/, /l/, /r/, /z/, /d/, /v/, /w/, /dʒ/, /j/, /ʒ/, /ð/. When these sounds are produced, the vocal folds vibrate.

■ *Back* sound includes (+) back consonants /k/, /g/, /ŋ/. These sounds are produced with the tongue retracted from the neutral *schwa* position.

■ *Low* sounds include only (+) low /h/. The tongue is lowered from the neutral schwa position.

■ *Continuant* sounds include /h/, /r/, /l/, /s/, /z/, /f/, /v/, /w/, /j/, /ʒ/, /ʃ/, /ð/, /θ/. These sounds are produced with an incomplete point of constriction. Because of this, the airflow is not entirely stopped at any time and these sounds may be produced continuously until the person runs out of breath.

■ *Nasal* sounds include /m/, /n/, /ŋ/. These sounds are produced by lowering the velum so that there is coupling of the oral and nasal cavities and sounds are resonated in the oral cavity.

■ *Anterior* sounds include /m/, /p/, /b/, /l/, /n/, /s/, /z/, /t/, /d/, /v/, /f/, /w/, /ð/, /θ/. These sounds are produced with a point of constriction located more anteriorly than that of /ʃ/. The production of /ʃ/ defines the boundary between anterior and nonanterior sounds.

■ *Coronal* sounds include /r/, /l/, /n/, /s/, /z/, /t/, /d/, /dʒ/, /tʃ/, /ʒ/, /ʃ/, /ð/, /θ/. These sounds are produced with the tongue blade raised above the neutral schwa position.

■ *Round* sounds include /r/ and /w/. These sounds are produced with the lips protruded or rounded.

■ *Tense* sounds include /l/, /s/, /f/, /k/, /t/, /p/, /ʃ/, /ð/, /θ/, /dʒ/, /tʃ/. All these consonants are voiceless except /dʒ/ and /l/. These sounds are produced with a relatively greater degree of contraction or muscle tension at the root of the tongue.

■ *High* sounds include (+) high consonants /k/, /g/, /ŋ/, /ʃ/, /ʒ/, /j/, /tʃ/, /dʒ/. These sounds are produced with the tongue elevated above the neutral /ə/ position.

■ *Strident* sounds include /tʃ/, /dʒ/, /ʒ/, /ʃ/, /s/, /z/, /f/, /v/. These sounds are produced by forcing the airstream through a small, constricted opening. The result is strident or intense noise.

■ *Sonorant* sounds include /n/, /m/, /ŋ/, /l/, /r/, /w/, /j/. These sounds are produced by allowing the airstream to pass relatively uninterrupted through the nasal or oral cavity. There is no stoppage or point of constriction.

■ *Interrupted* sounds include /tʃ/, /dʒ/, /t/, /d/, /k/, /g/, /p/, /b/. These sounds may be thought of as the opposites of sonorants because the interrupted sounds are produced by complete blockage of the airstream at the point of constriction.

Although the above list comprises the primary distinctive feature categories used by speech–language pathologists, there are other categories of distinctive features that have some clinical utility (Bleile, 1996; Ohde & Sharf, 1992; Peña-Brooks & Hegde, 1999; Shriberg & Kent, 1995; Yavas, 1998). These categories are:

- *Syllabics* include liquids /r/, /l/ and nasals /m/, /n/, /ŋ/. All vowels are syllabics, and most consonants are not. Syllabics serve as the nucleus for a syllable.

- *Obstruents*, which include affricates /tʃ/, /dʒ/; fricatives /f/, /v/, /ð/, /θ/, /s/, /z/, /h/, /ʃ/, /ʒ/; and stops /p/, /b/, /t/, /d/, /k/, /g/, are made with a notable amount of air obstruction in the vocal tract. Obstruents are made with a narrow constriction or complete closure of the oral cavity so a friction noise is produced or the airstream is stopped completely.

- *Sibilants* include affricates /tʃ/ and /dʒ/ and fricatives /s/, /z/, /ʃ/, /ʒ/. Sibilants are high-frequency sounds that have longer duration and more stridency than most other consonants.

- *Approximants* include glides /w/ and /j/ and liquids /r/ and /l/. Approximants are named thus because of the approximating nature of the contact between the two articulators that help form them. The degree of contact is *approximate*, not nearly as firm or closed as it is for fricatives, affricates, and stops.

- *Rhotic* is a term sometimes used to describe /r/ and its allophonic variations.

Place-Voice-Manner Approach

Consonants can be described according to place-voice-manner of production as well as distinctive features. The following descriptions are summarized from Peña-Brooks & Hegde (1999), Kent (1997), Creaghead et al. (1989), Yavas (1998), and Borden et al. (1994).

Place of Articulation

- *Linguavelars* (also called velars) are produced when the dorsum of the tongue contacts the velum. Linguavelars are /g/, /j/, /ŋ/.

- *Linguapalatals* are produced when the tongue blade is pressed against the hard palate to form the point of constriction just posterior to the alveolar ridge. Linguapalatals are /j/, /r/, /dʒ/, /tʃ/, /ʒ/, and /ʃ/.

- *Lingua-alveolars* are produced by contact of the tip of tongue with the alveolar ridge. Lingua-alveolars are /s/, /z/, /n/, /l/, /t/, and /d/.

- *Linguadentals*, also called *interdentals*, are produced by protuding the tongue tip slightly between the cutting edge of the lower and upper front teeth, forming a narrow constriction. Airflow is directed through this constriction, and contact between the tongue and teeth is light. The sounds /θ/ and /ð/ are linguadental.

■ *Bilabials* are produced by mutual contact of the upper and lower lips. Bilabials are /w/, /m/, /p/, /b/.

■ *Labiodentals* are produced by placing the lower edge of the upper central incisors on the upper portion of the lower lip. A narrow point of constriction is formed from this light contact of the incisors and lip. The sounds /f/ and /v/ are labiodentals.

■ *Glottals* are produced at the level of the glottis. The vocal folds are open, and the air passes through them. The only glottal in American English is /h/.

Voicing

■ The characteristic of voicing refers to whether the vocal folds are vibrating when a consonant is produced. Sounds such as /r/, /g/, and /z/ are *voiced*. Sounds such as /k/, /t/, and /s/ are *voiceless*.

■ *Cognate pairs* are those sounds that are identical in every way except voicing. Place and manner of production are the same, but the feature of voicing is different. For example, /p-b/ and /k-g/ are cognate pairs.

Manner of Articulation

■ The following information about manner of articulation is summarized from Peña-Brooks & Hegde (1999), Kent (1997), Creaghead et al. (1989), Yavas (1998), and Borden et al. (1994). All sounds in each manner-of-articulation category are described according to place, voice, and manner of articulation as well as distinctive features. Though redundant, this brief description is intended to help the reader quickly remember key attributes of each consonant.

Nasals: /m/, /n/, /ŋ/

■ Nasals are produced by lowering the velum to keep the velopharyngeal port open. The open velopharyngeal port allows the sound produced by the vibrating vocal folds to pass through the nasal cavity.

■ The vocal tract is lengthened, and there is an overall increase in the area for resonance. Thus, the resonance characteristic is changed by low-frequency components being added to the sounds.

/m/: place = bilabial

voice = voiced

manner = nasal

distinctive features = +voiced, +consonantal, +anterior, +nasal

/n/: place = lingua-alveolar

voice = voiced

manner = nasal

distinctive features = +voiced, +consonantal, +anterior, +coronal, +nasal

/ŋ/: place = linguavelar

voice = voiced

manner = nasal

distinctive features = +voiced, +consonantal, +high, +back, +nasal

Fricatives: /h/, /ʒ/, /ʃ/, /s/, /z/, /ð/, /θ/, /f/, /v/

■ Fricatives derive their name from the friction, the hissing-type quality that results from the continuous forcing of air through a narrow constriction.

■ The constrictions in the vocal tract generate aperiodic noise as the airflow passes through them. The constrictions must be narrow enough and the airflow strong enough to create a turbulent airflow. This turbulent airflow creates noisy random vibrations, or frication. Two closely approximating articulators form the constriction through which a continuous airstream must pass. Firm velopharyngeal closure is necessary.

/h/: place = glottal

voice = voiceless

manner = fricative

distinctive features = +continuant, +low

/ʒ-ʃ/: place = linguapalatal

voice = /ʒ/ voiced, /ʃ/ voiceless

manner = fricative

distinctive features = +consonantal, +coronal, +continuant, +high, +strident

/s-z/: place = lingua-alveolar

voice = /s/ voiceless, /z/ voiced

manner = fricative

distinctive features = +consonantal, +anterior, +coronal, +continuant, +strident

/ð-θ/: place = lingua-dental

    voice = /ð/ voiced, /θ/ voiceless

    manner = fricative

    distinctive features = +consonantal, +coronal, +anterior, +continuant

/f-v/: place = labiodental

    voice = /f/ voiceless, /v/ voiced

    manner = fricative

    distinctive features = +consonantal, +anterior, +continuant, +strident

Affricates: /tʃ/, /dʒ/

- The affricates /tʃ/ and /dʒ/ have both a fricative and a stop component. These sounds begin as stops and are released as fricatives. The speaker makes alveolar closure for /d/ or /t/; when the closure is released, the tongue is retracted and shaped for production of /tʃ/ or /dʒ/.

- Usually, the lips are slightly rounded as the fricative portion of the affricate sound is produced.

    /tʃ-dʒ/: place = lingua-alveolar

        voice = /tʃ/ voiceless, /dʒ/ voiced

        manner = affricate

        distinctive features = +consonantal, +coronal, +strident

Stops: /p/, /b/, /t/, /d/, /k/, /g/

- The stops are produced by complete constriction or closure of the vocal tract at some point so the airflow is totally stopped. Stops are formed at three basic places: *alveolar* (closure between the tip of the tongue and the alveolar ridge), *velar* (closure between the tongue blade and roof of the mouth), and *labial* (closure of the lips) (Kent, 1997).

- When the airflow is stopped, pressure builds up behind the point of contact; when the built-up air is released, there is a short audible burst of noise. Because of this, stops may also be called *stop-plosives*.

    /p-b/: place = bilabial

        voice = /p/ voiceless, /b/ voiced

        manner = stop

        distinctive features = +consonantal, +anterior

/t-d/: place = lingua-alveolar

voice = /t/ voiceless, /d/ voiced

manner = stop

distinctive features = +consonantal, +anterior, +coronal

/k-g/: place = lingua-velar

voice = /k/ voiceless, /g/ voiced

manner = stop

distinctive features = +consonantal, +high, +back

Glides: /w/, /j/

■ The glides, also called *semivowels* and *sonorants*, are produced by a quick transition of the articulators as they move from a partially constricted state to a more open state for the vowels that follow them. The term *onglide* is used to describe this movement (Edwards, 1997). In comparison to stops, fricatives, and affricates, glides are formed by a relatively transitory and unrestricted point of constriction.

/w/: place = bilabial

voice = voiced

manner = glide

distinctive features = +anterior, +continuant

/j/: place = labiodental

voice = voiced

manner = glide

distinctive features = +continuant, +high

Liquids: /r/, /l/

■ The liquids are produced with the least oral cavity restriction of all the consonants. The vocal tract is obstructed only slightly more than for vowels.

■ The /r/ is also called a *rhotic*. and is commonly produced in two ways. One way is as a *retroflex*, made with the tongue tip retracted and approximating the hard palate; a second way is as a *bunched* /r/, where the dorsum of the tongue is "bunched" or retracted and elevated toward the hard palate.

■ The /l/ is also called a *lateral* because when the /l/ is produced, the midsection portion of the tongue is relaxed and open, and thus air is directed through the sides of the tongue.

/r/: place = lingua-palatal

    voice = voiced

    manner = liquid

    distinctive features = +consonantal, +coronal, +continuant, +vocalic

/l/: place = lingua-alveolar

    voice = voiced

    manner = liquid

    distinctive features = +consonantal, +anterior, +coronal, +continuant, +vocalic

Concepts To Consider

Describe /m/ and /s/ in terms of place-voice-manner of articulation and distinctive features.

_____

_____

_____

_____

_____

_____

_____

_____

_____

Consonant Clusters

- While many consonants are produced alone or adjacent to vowels, others are produced adjacent to other consonants. These *consonant clusters*, also known as *blends*, may occur in the initial, medial, or final position of words.

- Most consonant clusters in American English consist of two consonants. However, some three-consonant clusters occur. Examples of two-consonant clusters are: *mosquito*, *bless*, *silk*. An example of a three-consonant cluster is *burst*.

Vowels

Basic Principles

■ Unlike consonants, which are mostly produced with some constriction of the vocal tract, vowels are produced with an open vocal tract. The vocal tract is open from the vocal folds to the lips, with no points of constriction.

■ Because all vowels are voiced, the sound source for vowels is the vocal folds. Resonance patterns for the vowels are shaped by the vocal tract. The distinctive resonance features for each vowel sound are produced by changing the size and shape of the oral cavity.

Distinctive Feature Approach

Like consonants, vowels can be described according to their distinctive features. The following descriptions are summarized from Peña-Brooks & Hegde (1999), Kent (1997), Creaghead et al. (1989), Yavas (1998), and Borden et al. (1994):

■ *Vocalics* include all vowels. These sounds are produced without a marked constriction in the vocal tract.

■ *Sonorants* include all vowels. Sonorants are produced by an airstream that passes unconstricted through the oral or nasal cavity.

■ *Voiced* vowels include all vowels. All vowels are produced with vocal fold vibration.

■ *Rounded* vowels are /o/, /u/, /ʊ/, and /ɔ/. These sounds are produced with the lips protruded or rounded.

■ *Tense* vowels are /e/, /i/, /ʌ/, /ɝ/, /o/, and /u/. These sounds are produced with muscle contraction or tension at the root of the tongue.

■ *Front* vowels include /ɪ/, /i/, /e/, /ɛ/, and /æ/. The tongue is in a position anterior to the neutral schwa position.

■ *Back* vowels are /a/, /ɔ/, /o/, /ʊ/, and /u/. These sounds are made with the tongue retracted from the neutral schwa position.

■ *High* vowels include /i/, /ɪ/, /ʊ/, and /u/. These sounds are made with the tongue elevated above the neutral schwa position.

■ *Low* vowels include /æ/ and /a/. These vowels are made with the tongue lowered from the neutral schwa position.

■ *Rhotic* refers to sounds made with an /r/ coloring. These sounds include the mid-central vowels /ɚ/ and /ɝ/.

Vowel Position Characteristics

■ While it is helpful to describe vowels according to their distinctive features, it is also useful to describe vowel production from a position of physiologic rest—that is, what amount of mandibular, tongue, and lip movement away from physiologic rest is necessary for production of each vowel? Figure 2.1 demonstrates the tongue positions with which vowels are typically produced.

■ Using this paradigm, vowels can be characterized according to four dimensions:

– *lip position*, which causes vowels to be categorized as *rounded* or *unrounded*. For rounded vowels, the lips are protruded. For unrounded vowels, the lips are in a neutral or slightly retracted position.

– *tense/lax qualities*. Tense vowels have longer duration and are produced with increased tension, while lax vowels are of shorter duration and are produced with less muscular tension.

– *tongue height*, which causes vowels to be categorized as *high, mid*, or *low* in terms of production within the oral cavity.

– *tongue forwardness* or *retraction*, which causes vowels to be categorized as front, central, or back in terms of production within the oral cavity.

– In the following section, vowels are described according to these dimensions. Key words containing each vowel serve as examples.

Front Vowels: /ɪ, i, e, ɛ, æ/.

■ *High* front vowels /ɪ/ and /i/

/i/: tense, unround; tongue is in a high and forward position. Key words: *heat, meeting, see.*

/ɪ/: lax, unround; tongue is slightly lower and more posterior than for /i/. Key words: *bit, sick, tin.*

■ *Mid* front vowels /e/ and /ɛ/

/e/: tense, unround; as compared to production of /ɪ/, /e/ involves keeping the tongue lower and slightly more retracted. Key words: *make, later, fate.*

/ɛ/: lax, unround; the /ɛ/ vowel is produced slightly lower than /e/. Key words: *let, ten, sent.*

■ *Low* front vowel /æ/

/æ/: lax, unround; one of the lowest vowels in English, /æ/ is produced with the tongue lower and more retracted than required for production of /ɛ/. Key words: *tan, matter, sat.*

Central Vowels: /ɝ/, /ɚ/, /ə/, /ʌ/.

■ The place of production varies for each of the central vowels, also called mid-central vowels.

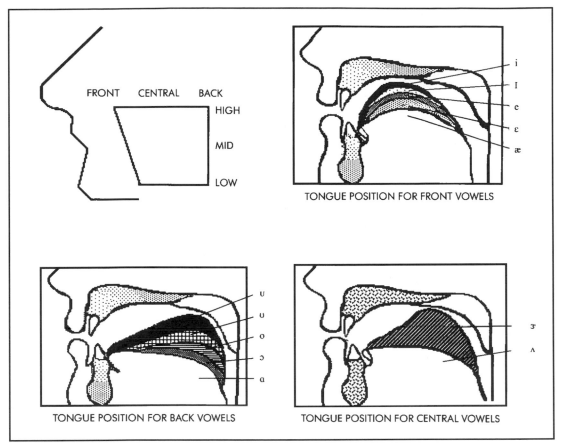

Figure 2.1. The vowel chart. From *Introduction to Communicative Disorders,* 2nd ed. (p. 116), by M. N. Hegde, 1995, Austin, TX: PRO-ED. Copyright 1995 by PRO-ED, Inc. Reprinted with permission.

■ /ɝ/ and /ɚ/

/ɝ /: tense, half-round, retroflexed; the tongue blade is bunched and elevated toward the hard palate. The tongue is retracted toward /o/, and tongue height is approximately equivalent to /ɪ/ and /e/. The /ɝ/ is transcribed to represent /r/ production in syllables receiving primary stress (e.g., *certain*). Key words: *curtain, hurt, dirty*.

/ɚ/: lax, half-round, and retroflexed. The /ɚ/, called *schwar*, is produced in the same manner as /ɝ/. However, schwar is transcribed to represent /r/ production in unstressed syllables such as that in *butter*. Key words: *letter, color, ladder*.

■ /ə/ and /ʌ/

/ə/: lax, unround; the tongue blade is lowered in relation to /ɝ/. The unstressed /ə/ occurs in unstressed syllables such as <u>a</u>bove. Key words: <u>a</u>ttempt, <u>a</u>head, pizz<u>a</u>.

/ʌ/: lax, unround; the /ʌ/ vowel is produced in a manner similar to that for /ə/, but the tongue is slightly more retracted toward /a/. The /ʌ/ occurs in stressed syllables. Key words: m<u>o</u>ney, fl<u>oo</u>d, <u>u</u>p.

Back Vowels: /u/, /ʊ/, /o/, /ɔ/, /a/.

■ *High* back vowels /u/ and /ʊ/

/u/: tense, round; the tongue is in the highest, most retracted position when a speaker is producing /u/. Key words: *spoon, fruit, bruise*.

/ʊ/: lax, round; the /ʊ/ vowel is produced in a slightly lower and more forward manner than /u/. Key words: *took, put, foot*.

■ *Mid* back vowels /o/ and /ɔ/

/ɔ/: lax, round; the /ɔ/ vowel is produced a little lower than /u/. Key words: *fought, caught, shawl*.

/o/: tense, round; in comparison to /u/, /o/ is produced slightly lower in the oral cavity. Key words: *coat, lower, soapy*.

■ *Low* back vowel /a/

/a/: lax, unround; the /a/ vowel is produced with the lowest, most retracted tongue position of all the vowels. Key words: *calm, pocket, father*.

Diphthongs

■ Diphthongs are produced as a slow gliding movement from one vowel (the *onglide*) to the adjacent vowel (the *offglide*) (Kent, 1997). For example, in the diphthong /aɪ/, /a/ is the onglide vowel, and /ɪ/ is the offglide vowel. Diphthongs contain both an initial and a final segment.

■ Diphthongs are represented phonetically by digraph symbols that highlight the initial and final segments (Peña-Brooks & Hegde, 1999). The diphthongs are:

- /aɪ / (e.g., m*igh*t, sk*y*, T*y*ler)

- /aʊ/ (e.g., cl*ou*d, h*ow*)

- /ɔɪ/ (e.g., h*oi*st, t*oy*)

- /eɪ/ (e.g., w*eigh*, h*ay*)

■ *Phonemic* diphthongs /aɪ/, /ɔɪ/, and /aʊ/ cannot be reduced to pure vowels without changing word meaning. For example, /tɑɪp/ and /tɑp/ represent two different meanings. *Nonphonemic* diphthongs /oʊ/ and /eɪ/ do not change word meanings. For example, the listener perceives /soʊp/ and /sop/ as the same words.

Summary

- ☑ Consonants and vowels may be defined by their role in the production of syllables, the smallest phonetic unit.

- ☑ Two classification systems frequently used to describe consonants and vowels are distinctive features in place-voice-manner of articulation.

- ☑ Vowels may also be described according to lip position, tense-lax qualities, and tongue height and position within the oral cavity.

THE EFFECTS OF CONTEXT IN SPEECH SOUND PRODUCTION

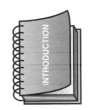

INTRODUCTION

The sounds of a language may be produced in isolation. Typically, however, they are produced within a context of some kind. Within this context, sounds are influenced by one another in running speech. Sounds as parts of words and ultimately conversational speech are also influenced by suprasegmental parameters, which add variety and expression to speech.

Dynamics of Speech Production

- In most cases, sounds are produced as part of connected speech. Sounds may influence each other in three ways: through adaptation, through assimilation, and through coarticulation.

- Phonetic *adaptations* comprise two types of variations according to preceding and following sounds: (a) variations in the way the articulators move, and (b) the extent to which vocal tract configurations change shape (Creaghead et al., 1989).

- For example, the /m/ in *meek* is produced with more lip retraction than the /m/ in *moo*, which is produced with slight lip protrusion. The adjacent vowels influence the production of /m/.

- In *assimilation*, speech sounds are modified due to the influence of adjacent sounds. Modifications are so extensive that there are perceptible changes in sounds. For example, in the phrase "great zoo," the /z/ in *zoo* is devoiced because of the voiceless /t/ in the preceding word.

■ *Coarticulation* refers to the influence of one phoneme upon another phoneme in production or perception. In coarticulation, two different articulators move simultaneously to produce two different speech sounds. Coarticulation creates both adaptation and assimilation.

Suprasegmentals

■ Suprasegmentals, also referred to as features of *prosody*, add meaning, variety, and color to running speech. They involve larger units than individual units or segmentals do, such as syllables, words, phrases, and sentences.

■ Suprasegmentals are affected by a number of variables. These include a person's cultural and linguistic background, emotional state, gender, and age. The most commonly described suprasegmentals or prosodic features that affect speech production are length, stress, rate, pitch, volume, and juncture.

✎ Concepts To Consider

What is meant by the term *suprasegmentals*? List two suprasegmentals that impact speech production.

_____

_____

_____

_____

_____

_____

_____

_____

■ *Length* of vowels and consonants is related to syllable perception and production. If syllables have long vowels, they will tend to have short consonants. If syllables have short vowels, they will tend to have long consonants.

■ *Stress* is an important characteristic of syllables, for it can change meanings of words. Stressed syllables are often called syllables containing *primary stress*, while unstressed syllables are referred to as those with *secondary* or *weak* stress.

■ Stressed and unstressed syllables differ in four ways relative to each other:

Stressed Syllable	Unstressed Syllable
loud	soft
greater length	shorter length
higher in pitch	lower in pitch
greater muscular effort	less muscular effort

■ Syllable stress is especially important in differentiating noun and verb pairs that have identical sounds. The words *object, permit, insult*, and *import* become nouns or verbs depending upon which syllables are stressed (Yavas, 1998).

■ *Rate* of speech refers to the speed with which a person speaks. When people are speaking rapidly, they tend to reduce duration of vowels and to produce consonants with less articulatory effort. Rate reflects the phonetic duration of both sound and silence and may be impacted by the speaker's emotion (Nicolosi et al., 1996).

■ *Pitch* is the *perception* of the frequency with which the vocal folds vibrate, while frequency is a *physical property* of the actual sound waves. Pitch is determined by mass, tension, and elasticity of the vocal folds. In English, pitch can be used to indicate different meanings of spoken units. For example, "We are having fun reading this book" can be a statement if the pitch falls at the end. A rising pitch at the end of this statement turns it into a question.

■ *Volume* is the *perception* of a speaker's intensity of speech. This perception is related to amplitude, a *physical property* of the actual sound waves. A speaker's loudness may be influenced by many variables, including the amount of background noise in the situation, the speaker's feelings at the moment, and the speaker's or listener's ability to hear.

■ *Juncture*, also called vocal punctuation, is a combination of suprasegmentals such as intonation and pausing, which mark special distinctions or grammatical divisions in speech. These distinctions affect the meaning of an utterance. For example, one would say "<u>What</u> did you eat?" differently than one would say "What, did you <u>eat</u>?" Or, one might use juncture to make distinctions between similar-sounding words like *night rate* and *nitrate*, or *I scream* and *ice cream* (Kent, 1998).

Summary

☑ Speech sounds are generally produced within a context where they are influenced by one another.

☑ Suprasegmentals such as juncture, pitch, and stress add meaning and variety to speech as part of human interaction.

SPEECH SCIENCE: PHYSIOLOGICAL PHONETICS, ACOUSTIC PHONETICS, AND SPEECH PERCEPTION

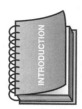

Acoustics is the study of sound as a physical phenomenon. Sound is an audible vibration or disturbance in the air that creates sound waves. These waves, which are disturbances of molecules, may be periodic or aperiodic. Vibratory motion can be characterized according to two properties: intensity and frequency.

Acoustics: Basic Definitions

▓ *Acoustics,* a branch of physics, is the study of the physical properties of sound and how sound is generated and propagated.

▓ *Psychoacoustics* is a study of how humans respond to sound as a physical phenomenon; it is a branch of both psychology and acoustics.

▓ *Sound* may be defined both physically and psychologically (perceptually). Physically defined, sound is the result of vibration or disturbance in the air. Psychologically defined, sound is *audible* vibration or disturbance in the air. *Sound waves* are movements of particles in a medium containing expansions and contractions of molecules.

▓ *Compression,* or *condensation,* is a phase of sound in which the vibratory movements of an object (e.g., the tines of a tuning fork) increase the density of air molecules because the molecules are compressed or condensed; it is the opposite of rarefaction (see below).

▓ *Rarefaction* is the thinning of air molecules when the vibrating object returns to equilibrium; it is the opposite of condensation.

▓ *Simple harmonic motion* refers to the back-and-forth movement of particles when the movement is symmetrical and periodic; it is also known as a sine wave.

▓ *Sinusoidal motion* or *wave* is a wave with horizontal and vertical symmetry because it contains one peak or crest and one valley or trough; a sinusoidal wave contains a single frequency; it is a result of simple harmonic motion.

▓ *Aperiodic waves* are those that do not repeat themselves at regular intervals; their vibratory patterns are random and difficult to predict from one time interval to the next. *Periodic waves* are sound waves that repeat themselves at regular intervals.

■ *Amplitude* is one of two characteristics of vibratory motion and is the magnitude and direction of displacement. In acoustics, it is the strength or magnitude of a sound signal; the greater the amplitude, the louder the sound signal.

■ *Intensity* is the quality of sound that creates the sensation of loudness; physically, intensity is the amount of energy transmitted per second over an area of one square meter; it is measured in terms of watt per square meter; it is also expressed in decibels.

■ *Bel* is a logarithmic unit of measure of sound intensity; it is a basic and relative reference measure; it helps express the wide range of sound intensities to which the human ear is sensitive by means of a compressed, logarithmic scale. *Decibel* (dB) is a measure of sound intensity; it equals one-tenth of a bel.

■ *csg system* is a metric system of measuring length in centimeters (cm), time in seconds (sec), and mass in grams (g); it can be contrasted with the MKS system. The *MKS system* is a metric system of measuring length in meters (m), mass in kilograms (kg), and time in seconds.

■ *Dyne* is a measure of force in the cgs metric system; 1 dyne is the force required to accelerate a mass of 1 gram from a velocity of 0 cm per second to a velocity of 1 cm per second in 1 second.

■ *Density* is the amount of mass per unit volume. Density of matter that serves as a medium for sound affects sound transmission.

■ *Displacement* is change in position; air molecules are said to be displaced because of the vibratory action of an object. *Oscillation* refers to the to-and-fro movement of the air molecules because of a vibrating object.

■ *Force* is a vector quantity that tends to produce an acceleration of a body in the direction of its application; it is also defined as the product of mass and acceleration. Force is measured in terms of Nt (newton); 1 newton equals the force required to accelerate a mass of 1 kg from a velocity of 0 m (meter) per second to a velocity of 1 m per sec in 1 sec.

■ *Elasticity* is a property that makes it possible for matter (that helps transmit sound) to recover its form and volume when subjected to distortion; all matter is subjected to distortion when force is applied to it.

■ *Velocity* is a change in position of, for example, air molecules when an object is set to vibration. Velocity is measured in terms of the distance an object moves per the time and the direction it takes as it moves.

■ *Frequency* is one of the two characteristics of vibratory motion and is the rate of vibratory motion that is measured in terms of the number of cycles completed per second or, more recently, in terms of hertz (Hz). *Hertz* is the unit of measure for frequency; it is the same as the cycle per second; 1 cycle per sec is 1 Hz.

■ *Natural frequency* is the frequency with which a source of sound normally vibrates. It is determined by the source's mass and stiffness. *Mass* is the quantity of matter, and is not to be confused with *weight*, which is gravitational force exerted on mass. The mass of a medium of sound affects its transmission. Increased mass results in decreased frequency, and increased stiffness results in increased frequency.

■ *Formant frequency* is a frequency region with concentrated acoustic energy; it is the center frequency of a *formant*, which is a resonance. *Fundamental frequency* is the lowest frequency of a periodic wave; it is the first harmonic.

✎ Concepts To Consider

Define the terms *sound* and *acoustics*.

_____

_____

_____

_____

_____

_____

_____

_____

■ An *octave* is an indication of interval between two frequencies. The intervals always maintain a ratio of 1:2; thus, each octave doubles a particular frequency (e.g., 200 Hz is one octave above 100 Hz, and 2,000 Hz is one octave above 1,000 Hz).

■ *Impedance* is acoustic, mechanical, or electrical resistance to motion or sound transmission.

■ *Newton's laws of motion* explain motion and its characteristics. Basically, sound involves motion; the law of inertia states that all bodies remain at rest or in a state of uniform motion unless another force acts in opposition. In other words, a body in motion tends to remain in motion and a body at rest tends to stay at rest. The law of reaction forces states that every force is associated with a reaction force of opposite direction.

■ *Pressure* is the amount of force per unit area. Force is measured either as dynes or as newtons and is important in understanding the amount of force sound waves exert on the eardrum.

■ *Reflection* refers to the phenomenon of sound waves traveling back after hitting an obstacle with no change in the speed of propagation. *Refraction* is the bending of the sound wave due to change in its speed of propagation; this happens, for example, when sound waves move from one medium (e.g., air) to another (e.g., water).

■ *Resonance* is the modification of sound by other sources; in speech acoustics, resonance refers to modification of the laryngeal tone predominantly by the nasal and oral cavities.

■ A *transmitting medium* is any matter that carries or transmits sound; air, liquids, and solids can all transmit sound; *mass* and *elasticity* of transmitting media affect sound (see the next section).

Summary

☑ Acoustics, the study of sound, defines sound as an audible vibration or disturbance in the air that creates sound waves. These waves may be periodic or aperiodic.

☑ Vibratory motion can be characterized according to intensity and frequency. Intensity is measured in decibels, and frequency is measured in Hertz.

☑ Sound may be resonated for speech by the nasal and oral cavities.

INTRODUCTION TO THE STUDY OF SOUND

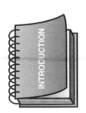 Sound is the result of vibrations of an elastic object. Physically, sound is a compressional wave; psychologically, it is a compressional wave that produces a sensation. Sound exists both as a physical phenomenon and as a sensory experience (Borden et al., 1994; Kent, 1997; Speaks, 1996). It is perceived in terms of pitch and loudness.

Sound Wave Generation and Propagation

■ Sound or vibration propagation needs a medium. Air, liquid, or gas can serve as such a medium. The two main properties of the medium that affect the transmission of sound are the mass (density) and the elasticity.

■ More massive objects (sound media) require greater force to set them into vibratory motion because of their higher inertia. Vibratory motion is possible partly because of the elasticity of objects.

■ For example, the tines of a tuning fork can be set into a to-and-fro motion by striking them because of their elasticity. Elastic objects get distorted when a force is applied to them and in due course recover their original form or position. As they change these, they create waves of molecular disturbances (vibratory motion).

■ Vibrations repeat themselves in *cycles* or *Hertz*. The number of times a cycle of vibration repeats itself within a second is the frequency of vibration. When a tone contains a single frequency, it is called a *pure tone*.

■ *Simple harmonic motion* results in a tone of single frequency that repeats itself. Simple harmonic motion also is called *sinusoidal motion*. A graphical representation of a sinusoidal motion is called a *sine wave*.

■ A *complex tone* is created when two or more sounds of differing frequencies are added. The vibrations that make up a complex tone may be *periodic* or *aperiodic*. When waves repeat themselves at regular and predictable intervals, they are said to be periodic. When the vibratory patterns are random and the next pattern cannot be predicted from the previous pattern, they are said to be aperiodic. Although it is not always the case, periodic waves are equated with noise.

■ It is important to realize that sound waves only imply motion; there is no physical movement of matter. What moves (actually, gets transferred) is energy. Sound is propagated because of the to-and-fro movements of molecules. During these movements, there is a time when the molecules are pressed together (*compression*) and a time when they move apart (*rarefaction*). Thus, only the molecules swing back and forth to create a wave of disturbance the human ear may detect as sound.

■ The amount of molecular displacement per unit of time is measured in terms of *velocity*. A change in velocity is described as *acceleration* or *deceleration*. Acceleration also is related to direction of movement; when direction changes, velocity also changes.

■ Vibratory motion has two important but independent characteristics that create distinctly different auditory sensation: frequency and amplitude.

Frequency and Pitch

■ *Frequency* is a measure of the number of cycles per second or Hz. A single cycle (or 1 Hz) consists of one instance of compression and one instance of rarefaction within a second.

■ A related measure is called a *period* (T), which is the amount of time needed to complete a cycle. The frequency of vibration is a function of the properties of the vibrating object. For instance, the frequency of vibration of a tuning fork is determined by its metallic density and length. The air molecules vibrate at the same rate as the vibrating object (Speaks, 1996).

■ The medium that transmits the sound does not affect the frequency of sound. However, it does affect the speed of sound. A more dense medium will retard the speed of sound transmission more than a less dense medium, which will propagate sound faster.

■ However, a more elastic medium (even if it is more dense) will propagate sound faster than a less elastic (even if it is less dense) medium. Therefore, steel, which is more dense but also more elastic than air, will transmit sound faster than air, which is less dense but also much less elastic than steel.

■ Variations in the frequency of vibration create variations in sensation we call pitch. Thus, *pitch* is a sensory (perceptual) experience related to changes in frequency, a physical event. A sound of higher frequency is perceived as a sound of higher pitch than a sound of lower frequency.

■ The human ear is not sensitive to all frequencies of sound that exist. The normal ear of a young adult can respond to 20 Hz to 20,000 Hz. The human ear is more sensitive to changes in lower frequencies (below 1,000 Hz) than in higher frequencies.

Amplitude and Loudness

■ Amplitude, the second important characteristic of vibratory motion, is a measure of the *magnitude* (intensity, strength) of the sound signal. In most cases, a measure of amplitude refers to sound pressure.

■ Measured in dynes or newtons, sound pressure is the amount of force per unit area. Amplitude is the extent of molecular displacement; the greater the degree of molecular displacement, the higher the amplitude or intensity of sound.

■ While amplitude, intensity, magnitude, and strength of a sound signal are physical concepts, loudness is a sensory concept. *Loudness* is a sensation related to physical amplitude or intensity of the sound. The higher the amplitude of a sound, the greater the perceived loudness of that sound.

■ The human ear is sensitive to a wide range of sound intensity, perhaps 10 trillion units of intensity on a linear scale. Measuring this wide range presents a cumbersome problem; therefore, a logarithmic scale is used to express the intensity range to which the human ear is sensitive. On this scale, the ear is sensitive to 130 units called *decibels* (dB). As mentioned earler, a decibel is one-tenth of a *bel*, a unit of measure named after Alexander Graham Bell.

🖉 Concepts To Consider

Distinguish between the concepts of frequency and amplitude as physical phenomena. Relate them to their corresponding psychological or perceptual experiences.

_____

_____

_____

_____

_____

_____

_____

_____

_____

_____

Sound Pressure Level and Hearing Level

- Instead of describing intensity, one can measure the pressure of sound. Therefore, intensity of a sound is expressed in terms of decibels at a certain *sound pressure level* (dB SPL). Sound pressure is the square root of *power*, which is measured in *watts*. The pressure itself is measured in terms of *pascals* (pa).

- Sound should reach a certain minimum intensity to stimulate the human auditory system. This minimum level is called the *hearing level* (HL). Sounds of different frequencies need to reach different minimum levels before they stimulate the human ear.

- For example, sounds of 1,000 to 4,000 Hz can stimulate the auditory system at lower intensities than those at other frequencies. This differential sensitivity of the ear to different frequencies creates problems in the measurement of hearing and hearing loss. This problem has been solved by arbitrarily setting the minimum sound pressure level required to stimulate the auditory system at zero for all frequencies. This minimum level is known as the 0 dB hearing level.

- Loudness or intensity of speech also is measured in terms of dB SPL. Intensity of normal conversational speech varies between 50 and 70 dB SPL. Very intense sounds exceed 100 dB SPL and may induce pain.

Summary

☑ Sound, the result of vibrations of an elastic object, exists both as a physical phenomenon and as a sensory experience.

☑ Physically, sound is a compressional wave; psychologically, it is a compressional wave that produces a sensation.

☑ The frequency of sound is measured by the number of cycles per second or Hz. The intensity of sound is expressed in units called decibels.

CHAPTER HIGHLIGHTS

▶ Phonetics is the study of speech sounds. The key categories of phonetics include acoustic, articulatory/physiological, auditory, applied, experimental, and descriptive phonetics. This chapter focuses on acoustic and articulatory/physiological phonetics.

▶ Because a sound can be represented visually in many different ways, the International Phonetic Alphabet or IPA was developed. The IPA is a set of internationally used phonetic symbols of vowels and consonants. Phonetic transcription of sounds can be broad, reflecting only vowels and consonants, or narrow, reflecting more detail about an individual speaker's sound production.

▶ Speech sounds can be broadly classified as consonants or vowels, which are described by their role in the production and perception of syllables. Syllables are motor units comprised of an onset, a nucleus, and a coda.

▶ Speech sounds can be more narrowly classified according to two major approaches. The distinctive feature approach describes each phoneme according to a cluster of features that are either present (+) or absent (–) in that phoneme. The place-voice-manner approach describes consonants according to place and manner of articulation as well as voicing.

▶ Sounds, or phonemes, are usually produced within the context of conversational speech. Within that context, sounds influence each other through adaptation, assimilation, and coarticulation. Running speech is given variety and meaning through suprasegmentals such as length of sounds, stress, rate of speech, pitch, loudness, and juncture.

▶ Acoustics, a branch of physics, is the study of sound as a physical phenomenon. Psychoacoustics is the study of how humans respond to sound as a physical phenomenon. Physically, sound is a compressional wave; psychologically, it is a compressional wave that produces a sensation. Sound exists both as a physical phenomenon and as a sensory experience.

(continues)

▶ Sound is the result of vibrations of an elastic object. It is propagated through waves of disturbances in molecules. A vibrating object is the source of sound, and media such as air, gas, water, and metal can transmit sound. Mass (density) and elasticity are two main properties of the medium that affect the transmission of sound.

▶ Vibrations repeat themselves (in frequencies, cycles, or Hertz). Pure tones contain a single frequency and are the result of simple harmonic motion, also known as a sine wave or sinusoidal motion. Complex tones are a combination of two or more sounds of differing frequencies.

▶ Pitch is a sensory (perceptual) experience related to physical changes in frequency. The normal ear of a young adult can respond to frequencies within the range of 20 Hz to 20,000 Hz. Loudness is a sensation related to physical amplitude or intensity of sound. Amplitude is measured in dynes or newtons. Intensity is often expressed in terms of decibels at a certain sound pressure level. A decibel is one-tenth of a bel, a basic unit of measure.

▶ The minimum intensity of sound needed to stimulate the human auditory system, called the hearing level, differs for different frequencies. However, on all audiometers, the minimum required to stimulate the human ear is arbitrarily set at 0 dB for all frequencies. The intensity of normal conversational speech varies between 50 and 70 dB SPL.

▶ Add your own chapter highlights here:

_____

_____

_____

_____

KEY TERMS

acoustic phonetics
acoustics
adaptation
affricates
allophones
amplitude
anterior
aperiodic waves
applied phonetics
approximants
articulatory/physiological phonetics
assimilation
auditory phonetics
back (sounds)
bel
bilabials
coarticulation
coda
cognate pairs
compression or condensation
consonant cluster (blend)
consonantal
continuant
coronal
csg system
decibel
density
descriptive phonetics
diphthong
displacement
distinctive feature approach
dyne
elasticity
experimental phonetics
force
formant frequency
frequency
fricatives

front (sounds)
fundamental frequency
glides
glottals
Hertz
high (sounds)
impedance
intensity
International Phonetic Alphabet
interrupted (sounds)
juncture
labiodentals
language
lateral
length (of vowels)
lingua-alveolars
linguadentals (interdentals)
linguapalatals
linguavelars
liquid
loudness
low (sounds)
mass
MKS system
nasal
natural frequency
Newton's laws of motion
nucleus
obstruents
octave
offglide
onglide
onset
orthographic symbols
oscillation
periodic waves
phone
phonemes
phonemic
phonemic transcription

phonetic
phonetic transcription
phonetics
phonology
pitch
place-voice-manner approach
pressure
primary stress
psychoacoustics
rarefaction
rate
reflection
refraction
resonance
retroflex
rhotic
round (sounds)
secondary (weak) stress
semivowels
sibilants
simple harmonic motion
sinusoidal motion
sonorants
sound
sound waves
speech
stops
stop-plosives
stress
stridents
suprasegmental
syllabics
syllabification
syllable
tense (sounds)
transmitting medium
velocity
vocalic
voiced
voiceless

STUDY AND REVIEW QUESTIONS

Fill in the Blank

1. _acoustic_ phonetics examines the relationship between articulation and the acoustic signal of speech, whereas _articulatory/phonoroq__ phonetics focuses on speech sound production.

2. In the distinctive feature approach to describing consonants, the term _Sibilant_ refers to affricates and fricatives, which are high-frequency sounds that have longer duration and more stridency than most other consonants. The term _Obstruent_ refers to sounds produced by allowing the airstream to pass relatively uninterrupted through the oral or nasal cavity.

3. In the place-voice-manner approach to describing consonants, _linguavelar_ are those consonants produced when the dorsum of the tongue contacts the velum, while _bilabials_ are those consonants produced by mutual contact of the upper and lower lips.

4. In the distinctive feature approach, _rhotic_ is a term used to refer to sounds made with an /r/ coloring.

5. _Phonemic_ diphthongs /aɪ/, /ɔɪ/, and /aʊ/ cannot be reduced to pure vowels without changing word meaning, while _nonphonemic_ diphthongs /oʊ/ and /eɪ/ do not change word meaning.

6. Stressed syllables are often called syllables that contain _primary_ stress, while unstressed syllables are referred to those with _secondary_ or _weak_ stress.

7. _Compression - condensation_ is a phase of sound in which the vibratory movements of an object increase the density of air molecules.

8. _refraction_ is the bending of the sound wave due to a change in its speed of propagation; this happens, for example, when sound waves move from one medium (e.g., air) to another (e.g., water).

9. Simple _harmonic_ motion refers to the back-and-forth movement of particles when the movement is _symmetrical_ and _periodic_.

10. Pressure is the amount of _force_ per square unit area; it is measured either as _dynes_ or as _newtons_.

Multiple Choice

11. The "typical" speaker of Standard American English would produce the word "emancipation" as:

    A. /ɪmansʌpeʃʌʌ/

    B. /imansʌpeɪʃən/

    C. /imænsəpeɪʃən/

    D. /ɪmʌnsʌpeʃʌʌ/

    E. /ɪmænsʌpɛʃən/

12. The /r/ and /l/ sounds may both be categorized as:

    A. rhotics

    B. glides

    C. laterals

    D. liquids

    E. retroflexes

13. A semivowel that can be categorized as a voiced bilabial glide that is +anterior and +continuant is the:

    A. /j/

    B. /w/

    C. /ʃ/

    D. /r/

    E. /h/

14. The term *coarticulation* refers to:

    A. speech sounds being modified due to the influence of adjacent sounds to the point that there are perceptible changes in sounds.

    B. the extent to which vocal tract configurations change shape during the production of consonants and vowels in running speech.

    C. vocal punctuation, or a combination of suprasegmentals such as intonation and pausing.

    D. the influence of various syllables upon one another when a client recites a phonetically balanced list of words.

E. the influence of one phoneme upon another in production and perception wherein two different articulators move simultaneously to produce two different speech sounds.

15. Broad phonemic transcription involves:

    A. the use of IPA symbols to transcribe phonemes by enclosing them within slash marks (e.g., /f/).

    B. the use of diacritical markers to transcribe phonemes by enclosing them within slash marks (e.g., /f/).

    C. the transcription of allophones by placing them within brackets (e.g., [f]).

    D. the transcription of allophones by the use of diacritical markers.

    E. the use of orthographic symbols to transcribe phonemes by enclosing them within slash marks (e.g., /r/).

16. If a speaker said, "I just love 'em and leave 'em," the phrase "leave 'em" could be transcribed as:

    A. [liv um]

    B. [lev] [em]

    C. /liv uhm/

    D. /liv m̩/

    E. /lev m/

17. The two properties of a medium that affect sound transmission are:

    A. amplitude and intensity.

    B. mass and elasticity.

    C. compression and rarefaction.

    D. pressure and force.

    E. elasticity and compression.

18. A sinusoidal wave is a sound wave:

    A. with horizontal and vertical symmetry.

    B. with one peak and one valley.

    C. with a single frequency.

    D. that is a result of simple harmonic motion.

    E. all of the above.

19. A natural frequency is a frequency:

    I. with which a source of sound vibrates naturally.

    II. that is affected by the mass and stiffness of the vibrating body.

    III. that is the center frequency of a formant.

    IV. that is the first harmonic.

    V. that is the lowest frequency of a periodic wave.

    A. I, II   C. I, IV, V   E. All of the above

    B. I, III, V   D. II, III

20. An octave is:

    A. the amount of molecular displacement per unit of time.

    B. the amount of time between cycles.

    C. an indication of interval between two frequencies.

    D. a measure of the magnitude (intensity, strength) of the sound signal.

    E. the unit of measure for frequency; it is the same as the cycle per second.

REFERENCES AND RECOMMENDED READINGS

Bleile, K. M. (1996). *Articulation and phonological disorders: A book of exercises* (2nd ed.). San Diego, CA: Singular Publishing Group.

Bloom, L., & Lahey, M. (1978). *Language development and disorders*. New York: Macmillan.

Borden, G. J., Harris, K. S., & Raphael, L. J. (1994). *Speech science primer: Physiology, acoustics, and perception of speech* (3rd ed.). Baltimore, MD: Williams & Wilkins.

Chomsky, N., & Halle, M. (1968). *The sound pattern of English*. New York: Harper & Row.

Creaghead, N. A., Newman, P. W., & Secord, W. A. (1989). *Assessment and remediation of articulatory and phonological disorders* (2nd ed.). Columbus, OH: Merrill Publishing Company.

Edwards, H. T. (1997). *Applied phonetics: The sounds of American English* (2nd ed.). San Diego: Singular Publishing Group.

Jakobson, R., Fant, G., & Halle, M. (1952). *Preliminaries to speech analysis* (2nd ed). Cambridge, MA: MIT Press.

Kent, R. (1997). *The speech sciences*. San Diego, CA: Singular Publishing Group.

Kent, R. (1998). Normal aspects of articulation. In J. E. Bernthal & N. W. Bankson, *Articulation and phonological disorders* (4th ed.). Needham Heights, MA: Allyn & Bacon.

Lowe, R. J. (1994). *Phonology: Assessment and intervention applications in speech pathology*. Baltimore, MD: Williams & Wilkins.

Nicolosi, L., Harryman, E., & Kresheck, J. (1996). *Terminology of communication disorders: Speech–language-hearing* (4th ed.). Baltimore, MD: Williams & Wilkins.

Ohde, R. N., & Sharf, D. J. (1992). *Phonetic analysis of normal and abnormal speech*. New York: Merrill.

Peña-Brooks, A., & Hegde, M. N. (1999). *Articulatory and phonological disorders in children: A dual level text*. Austin, TX: PRO-ED.

Shriberg, L. D., & Kent, R. D. (1995). *Clinical phonetics* (2nd ed.). Boston: Allyn & Bacon.

Speaks, C. E. (1996). *Introduction to sound* (2nd ed.). San Diego, CA: Singular Publishing Group.

Yavas, M. (1998). *Phonology: Development and disorders*. San Diego, CA: Singular Publishing Group.

ANSWERS TO STUDY AND REVIEW QUESTIONS

1. Acoustic, articulatory/physiological

2. Sibilant, obstruent

3. Linguavelars, bilabials

4. Rhotic

5. Phonemic, nonphonemic /oʊ/, /eɪ/

6. Primary, secondary, weak

7. Compression (condensation)

8. Refraction

9. Harmonic, symmetrical, periodic

10. Force, dynes, newtons

11. C.

12. D. The /r/ and /l/ sounds may both be categorized as liquids.

13. B. The /w/ sound is a semivowel that can be categorized as a voiced bilabial glide that is +anterior and +continuant.

14. E. Coarticulation is specifically defined as the influence of one phoneme upon another in production and perception wherein two different articulators move simultaneously to produce two different speech sounds.

15. A. Broad phonemic transcription involves use of IPA symbols to transcribe phonemes by enclosing them within slash marks.

16. D. If a speaker said, "I just love 'em and leave 'em," the phrase "leave 'em" could be transcribed as /liv m̩/.

17. B. The two properties of a medium that affect sound transmission are mass and elasticity.

18. E. A sinusoidal wave is a sound wave with horizontal and vertical symmetry. It contains one peak or crest and one valley or trough. It contains a single frequency and is a result of simple harmonic motion.

19. A. A natural frequency is a frequency with which a source of sound vibrates naturally and that is affected by the mass and stiffness of the vibrating body.

20. C. An octave is an indication of interval between two frequencies.

PREVIEW OUTLINE

CHAPTER INTRODUCTION

It is language that makes people so efficient at communication. It is language that provides people with a mechanism for social interaction and communication with one another. As societies have become more complex, organized, and interrelated, effective communication has gained in importance. Language and communication are now crucial for even mundane occupational success or survival as vocations have become more sophisticated and interrelated.

A *language* can be defined as a form of social behavior shaped and maintained by a verbal community. It can also be viewed as a system of symbols used to represent concepts that are formed through exposure and experience (Bloom & Lahey, 1978). In order to understand what constitutes language disorders in children, it is necessary to first understand normal language development. In this chapter, we discuss: (a) basic definitions of language, (b) normal language development milestones, and (c) theories of language development.

TERMS AND DEFINITIONS

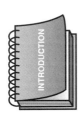

There are various approaches to the study of language. The behavioral approach, which will be described in a later section, views language as verbal behavior. The linguistic approach describes different components of language.

Linguistics is the study of language, its structure, and the rules that govern its structure. Linguists, specialists in linguistics, have traditionally described several components of language. These include morphology, syntax, semantics, pragmatics, and phonology. Phonology is described in Chapter 5.

Morphology

■ Morphology is the study of *word structure*. It describes how words are formed out of more basic elements of language called morphemes.

■ A *morpheme* is the smallest meaningful unit of a language. Morphemes are considered minimal because if they were subdivided any further, they would become meaningless (McLaughlin, 1998). Each morpheme is different from the others because each signals a distinct meaning. Morphemes are used to form words.

■ *Base, root,* or *free* morphemes are words that have meaning, cannot be broken down into smaller parts, and can have other morphemes added to them. Examples of free morphemes are: *ocean, establish, book, color, connect,* and *hinge.* These words mean something, can stand by themselves, and cannot be broken down into smaller units.

■ These words can have other morphemes added to them. *Bound* or *grammatic morphemes,* which cannot convey meaning by themselves, must be joined with free morphemes in order to have meaning.

■ In the following examples, the free morphemes are underlined; the bound morphemes are in capital letters:

<u>ocean</u>S   <u>establish</u>MENT   DIS<u>connect</u>   <u>color</u>FUL   UN<u>hinge</u>

■ Common bound or grammatic morphemes include the following:

   – ing, the present progressive (cook*ing,* writ*ing*)
   – s, the regular plural morpheme (cat*s,* basket*s*)
   – s, the possessive inflection (man*'s,* lady*'s*)
   – ed, the regular past tense (comb*ed,* wash*ed*)

■ Bound morphemes can be divided into the subcategories of prefixes and suffixes. A *prefix* is added at the beginning of a base morpheme; a *suffix* is added at the end of a base morpheme. For example:

Whole Word	Prefix	Base Word	Suffix
prearranged	pre	arrange	ed
disestablishment	dis	establish	ment
misunderstanding	mis	understand	ing

■ *Allomorphs* are variations of morphemes; they do not alter the original meaning of the morpheme. For example, the plural morpheme can be denoted by the following allomorphs (with their sounds in parentheses): box*es* (ez), leav*es* (z), cat*s* (s).

■ Morphemes are a means of modifying word structures to change meaning. The morphology of a given language describes the rules of such modifications. It describes what kinds of morphemic combinations are permissible in a given language.

■ Speakers arrange morphemes so that they can change the meaning of a sentence. For example, one can change "He cook*s* a meal" to "He cook*ed* a meal." By adding the past-tense *-ed* morpheme and omitting the third-person singular *-s,* the speaker changes sentence meaning.

■ Sentence meaning is also conveyed by the order of words in a sentence. This order is dictated by the rules of syntax.

Syntax

■ Syntax and morphology constitute the two major categories of language structure. Whereas morphology is the study of word structure, syntax is the study of sentence structure. The basic meaning of the word *syntax* is to join, to put together.

■ In the study of language, syntax involves (McLaughlin, 1998):

   – the arrangement of words to form meaningful sentences

   – word order and overall structure of a sentence

   – a collection of rules that specify the ways and order in which words may be combined to form sentences in a particular language

■ The syntactic rules of languages differ from one another. For example, in English, one might use the phrase "the new car." In Spanish, one might say *"el carro nuevo"* ("the car new"). All languages are creative, and speakers can generate an infinite variety of structures.

■ These structures, however, are governed by rules of syntax. Normal speakers of a language do not produce structures with random and meaningless word order. For example, an English speaker could say, "He said he was going to come but didn't." Due to syntactic rules, a speaker could not say, "He going to was said he didn't but come."

■ Sentences can be classified according to their functions. For example:

   – *passive* sentences, in which the subject receives the action of the verb ("The puppy was petted by Mike.")

   – *active* sentences, in which the subject performs the actions of the verb ("Mike petted the puppy.")

   – *interrogatives* or questions ("Did you see that gorgeous sunset?")

   – *declaratives*, which make statements ("The sunset was gorgeous.")

   – *imperatives*, which state commands ("Shut the door.")

   – *exclamatory* sentences, which express strong feeling ("I never said that!")

■ As they mature in syntactic development, children begin to use *compound* and *complex* sentences, which can be defined as follows:

   – A *compound sentence* contains two or more *independent clauses* joined by a comma and a conjunction or by a semicolon. There are no subordinate clauses in a compound sentence. A *clause* contains a subject and a predicate. An *independent* or *main clause* has a subject and predicate and can stand alone. For example:

The officer waved his hands,	and	the cars stopped.
(independent clause)	*(conjunction)*	*(independent clause)*

The bird sang in the tree;	later it flew away.
(independent clause + semicolon)	*(independent clause)*

- A *complex sentence* contains one independent clause and one or more *dependent or subordinate clauses*. A dependent or subordinate clause has a subject and predicate but cannot stand alone. For example:

I will be at the station	if it doesn't rain.
(independent clause)	*(dependent clause)*
You can have the lollipop	after you take a bath.
(independent clause)	*(dependent clause)*

■ Languages have different syntactic structures. In English, the basic syntactic structure is subject + verb + object. This structure, usually called the *kernel sentence*, can also be called the *phrase structure* or *base structure*.

Concepts To Consider

Briefly define the terms *morphology* and *syntax*. What do these terms mean?

_____

_____

_____

_____

_____

_____

Semantics

■ Semantics is the study of *meaning* in a language. The semantic component is the meaning conveyed by words, phrases, and sentences.

■ Semantics involves a person's *vocabulary* or lexicon. Vocabulary development depends heavily upon environmental exposure as well as the individual capacity each child brings to the learning situation.

- Important aspects of vocabulary development include knowledge of:

  - antonyms or opposites (e.g., *big–little*)

  - synonyms or words that mean similar things (e.g., *attractive–pretty*; *clear–transparent*)

  - multiple meanings of words (e.g., *rock, pound*)

  - humor (e.g., riddles, puns, jokes)

  - figurative language, including

    —metaphors (*He's drowning in money.*)

    —idioms (*It's raining cats and dogs*; *She kicked the bucket.*)

    —proverbs (*Don't put all your eggs in one basket.*)

  - deictic words, or words whose referents change depending on who is speaking (e.g., *this, here, that, come, go*)

- *Semantic categories* are used to sort words. Examples of a few of these categories are *recurrence* (concept of *more*), *rejection* (*no*), and *causality* (*cause and effect*). A child using recurrence might say, "More milk"; if that child didn't want any more, she might show rejection by saying, "No milk."

- Most words in a child's first 50 spoken words refer to things that the child can act upon (e.g., toys, objects). Young children may use *overextension* (e.g., all round items are balls) or *underextension* (only an Oreo is a cookie).

- Semantics can be viewed as relating word knowledge and world knowledge. *World knowledge* involves a person's autobiographical and experiential memory and understanding of particular events. *Word knowlege* is primarily verbal and contains word and symbol definitions.

- A child's word knowledge depends heavily upon his or her world knowledge. For example, an urban child who has never visited a zoo or been exposed to books about a zoo (world knowledge) might have difficulty understanding and using the word *zoo* (word knowledge).

- An important concept emphasized today in semantics is called *quick incidental learning* or *fast mapping*. This refers to children's ability to learn a new word on the basis of just a few exposures to it (Reed, 1994). Normal children use fast mapping to rapidly expand their vocabularies.

- Another important semantic aspect of children's language development is developing the ability to categorize words. For example, children must learn that *tiger, lion, dog, cat, pig*, and *horse* fall under the category of *animals*.

- The use of categories helps bring order to the child's experiences. The child who successfully categorizes does not need to treat each experience as a totally new one (Reed, 1994). New experiences may be "filed" under preexisting categories, or under mental constructs of the child that allow him or her to group similar items together.

Pragmatics

▨ Pragmatics is the study of rules that govern the use of language in social situations. In pragmatics, one focuses on use of language in context. Pragmatics places greater emphasis on *functions*, or uses of language, than on structure.

▨ *Functions of language* (described in more detail later) include:

- *labeling* (naming something; e.g., a child is playing with a puppy and says "tail")

- *protesting* (objecting to something; e.g., "Don't do that!")

- *commenting* (describing or identifying objects; e.g., "That's a cookie.")

▨ One can view pragmatics as the dimension of language that considers the *context* of the utterance (i.e., the situation, the listener-speaker relationship) and the *function* of the utterance (i.e., its purpose or goal).

▨ Language context involves:

- where the utterance takes place

- to whom the utterance is directed

- what and who are present at the time

▨ Important functions of utterances include:

- providing listeners with adequate information without redundancy

- making the sequence of statements coherent and logical

- taking turns with other speakers

- maintaining a topic

- repairing communication breakdowns

▨ Children with effective pragmatic skills display adequate *cohesion*, or the ability to order and organize utterances in a message so that they build logically on one another (Reed, 1994).

▨ As they get older, children with effective pragmatic skills distinguish between and appropriately use *direct* and *indirect speech acts*. For example, as a direct speech act, a child could say, "Bring me the ball." As an indirect speech act, the child could say, "Will you bring me the ball?" Indirect speech acts are used to convey politeness.

▨ Pragmatic skills involve the appropriate knowledge and use of discourse. *Discourse* refers to how utterances are related to one another; it has to do with the connected flow of language. Discourse can involve a monologue, a dialogue between two people, or even conversational exchange in a small group. When people talk with one another, they are engaging in discourse.

■ *Narratives* are a form of discourse in which the speaker tells a story. The speaker talks about a logical sequence of events. This sequence can involve an actual episode from the speaker's life, such as a trip he or she took; or it can involve a story about an event (such as a fairy tale or movie) that did not happen to the speaker directly.

■ Pragmatics is heavily influenced by culture. For example, in Japanese culture, the use of indirect speech acts is believed to convey speaker sophistication and sensitivity. In American culture, people who use many indirect speech acts may be viewed as weak, unassertive, and unsure of themselves.

■ Pragmatic skills are increasingly recognized today as important for social, academic, and vocational success. Effective pragmatic skills enable speakers to relate successfully to others within their linguistic and cultural milieu.

Summary

☑ The linguistic approach analyzes language according to five components: morphology, syntax, semantics, pragmatics, and phonology. In this section, we have discussed the first four components.

☑ Morphology involves the study of word structure. Syntax includes rules for word order and rules for combining words into sentences.

☑ Semantics involves word meanings. A child's semantic skills refer to his vocabulary skills, which are influenced by word and world knowledge.

☑ Pragmatics refers to the social skills of language—how, where, when, and with whom language is used.

NORMAL LANGUAGE DEVELOPMENT: DEVELOPMENTAL MILESTONES

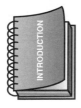

INTRODUCTION

The development of language rests upon several major variables which interact with one another. First, the individual child brings innate characteristics to the situation. Such characteristics may include, for example, a high IQ or a limited attention span. Second, the child's environment plays a major role in language development. The more stimulating the environment, the better and faster children will develop language skills. Language development also depends on cultural expectations. In some cultures, children are to be seen and not heard; those children may develop good visual skills, but their verbal skills may not develop at a rate expected by mainstream American clinicians.

(continues)

In this section, we describe language development milestones that represent a range of expectations for when children may develop certain language structures. These milestones depend heavily on the child's linguistic and cultural background; various cultures differ in their expectations for children's language development. This section focuses on semantic, syntactic, morphological, and pragmatic development as consistent with general mainstream American social expectations. Chapter 5 has detailed information regarding phonological development.

Birth to 1 Year

The following developmental milestones are observed in normally developing children from birth to one year of age.

Birth to 3 Months

The child:

- displays startle response to loud sound.

- visually tracks, or moves eyes, to source of sound.

- attends to and turns head toward voice; turns toward sound source.

- smiles reflexively.

- quiets when picked up.

- ceases activity or coos back when person talks (by 2 months).

4–6 Months

The child:

- responds by raising arms when mother says, "Come here," and reaches toward child (by 6 months).

- moves or looks toward family members when they are named (e.g., "Where's Daddy?").

- explores the vocal mechanism through vocal play such as growling, squealing, yelling, making "raspberries" (bilabial trills).

- begins to produce adult-like vowels.

- begins marginal babbling; produces double syllables (e.g., "baba"), puts lips together for /m/.

7–9 Months

The child:

- looks at some common objects when their names are spoken.

- comprehends "no."

- begins to use some gestural language; plays pat-a-cake, peek-a-boo; shakes head for "no."

- uses wide variety of sound combinations.

- uses inflected vocal play, intonation patterns.

- imitates intonation and speech sounds of others (by 9 months).

- begins variegated babbling—e.g., "mabamaba" (at approximately 9 months).

- uncovers hidden toy (beginning of object permanence).

10–12 Months

The child:

- understands up to 10 words, such as *no, bye-bye, pat-a-cake, hot*; understands one simple direction like "sit down," especially when command is accompanied by gesture.

- begins to relate symbol and object; uses first true word.

- gives block, toy, or object upon request.

- understands and follows simple directions regarding body action.

- looks in correct place for hidden toys (object permanence).

- turns head instantly to own name.

- gestures and/or vocalizes to indicate wants and needs.

- jabbers loudly; uses wide variety of sounds and intonations; varies pitch when vocalizing.

- uses all consonant and vowel sounds in vocal play.

Pragmatics

As infants develop pragmatics skills, they typically go through the following stages:

- uses *perlocutionary behavior,* in which child's "signals" have an effect on the listener or observer but lack communicative intent. For example, if a child smiles reflexively, an observer may smile back or laugh, even though the child didn't intend to express pleasure or joy.

■ at 9–10 months, uses *illocutionary behavior*—signals to carry out some socially organized action such as pointing and laughing; uses intentional communicaton.

■ at approximately 12 months, enters *locutionary* stage—begins to use words.

■ establishes *joint reference*, or the ability to focus attention on an event or object as directed by another person. (Caretakers begin by establishing eye contact in the early months; later, they point to or name objects that both they and the child can focus on.)

1–2 Years

The following developmental milestones are observed in normally developing children between 1 and 2 years of age.

Syntax

■ The child uses one-word sentences, and is in the *holophrastic* single-word phase—one word represents a complex idea. For example, "Up" might mean "Please pick me up because I don't want to sit here playing with the dog anymore." Average MLU (mean length of utterance) 1.0–2.0.

■ The child uses sentence-like words; communicates relationships by using one word plus vocal and bodily cues. The sentence-like word can have several basic functions:

- The emphatic or imperative statement: e.g., "Car!" (child telling you to look at a car)

- The question: e.g., "Car?" (child asking if that's a car)

- The declarative statement: e.g., "Car." (child saying it's a car and not something else)

■ At approximately 18 months, some children begin to put two words together.

■ The child may use three- or four-word responses at 2 years.

■ Approximately 51% of the child's utterances consist of nouns.

Semantics

■ As mentioned, the child uses *holophrastic* speech—1 word is used to communicate a variety of meanings. The child uses 3–20 words and uses gestures. Around 18 months, the child produces 10–50 words.

■ The child shows understanding of some words and simple commands; understands "no." Around 18 months, child understands about 200 words.

- The child's most frequent lexical categories are nominals (e.g., *ball, Mommy*) and verbs (e.g., *drink, run*).

- The child uses *semantic relations*, or utterances that reflect meaning based on relationships between different words (e.g., cause-effect relationships). The child begins with one-word utterances and gradually progresses to two-word utterances (see Table 3.1 and Table 3.2).

- The child also exhibits the following during this period:

  - Uses overextensions. For example, all tall men are "Daddy."

  - Answers the question "What's this?" Responds to yes/no questions by nodding or shaking head.

  - Says "All gone" (emerging negation).

  - Follows one-step commands or simple directions accompanied by gestures (e.g., "Give Mommy the spoon.").

  - Follows directions using one or two spatial concepts such as *in* or *on* (19–24 months).

  - Points to one to five body parts on command; points to recognized objects (emerging nomination).

  - Listens to simple stories; especially likes to hear stories repeated (19–24 months).

  - Asks for "more."

  - Refers to self with pronoun and name ("Me Johnny") (19–24 months).

  - Verbalizes immediate experiences (e.g., "Bath hot!").

  - Begins to use some verbs and adjectives.

Pragmatics

- *Presuppositions* emerge. Between 1 and 2 years of age, the child uses expressions that have shared meaning for the listener and speaker.

- The child begins to understand some rules of dialogue, e.g., "When someone talks, you need to listen." The child is able to take the role of both speaker and listener.

- The child uses nonverbal as well as verbal communication to signal intent. Halliday (1975) considered the listener's responses in describing the following seven functions of communicative intent that develop between 9 and 18 months of age:

  - *Imaginative.* Children pretend or do play-acting; they use language to create an environment; there is a communicative function ("Let's pretend"; child may vocalize to herself while playing with dolls).

TABLE 3.1

Relations Expressed by Single-Word Utterances

Before children reach the two-word utterance stage, they typically use single words to express themselves. The relations expressed by single words are as follows:

Relation	Definition	Example
Attribution	An adjective; a property or characteristic of an event, person, or object	*Big* doggy *Clean* dolly Face *dirty*
Action	Child requests or labels an action; indicates movement relationships between objects and people	*Open* box Kitty *run* *Close* door
Locative action	Child refers to a change in an object's location	*There* doggy Ball *up*
Existence	Child is attending to item or object present in the immediate environment, especially a novel one	What's *that*? *This* kitty
Nonexistence or disappearance	An action or object is expected to be present but is not; something was present but disappeared	*All gone* juice *Bye bye* Mom *No* doggy
Denial	Child denies a statement or previous utterance (e.g., in response to a parent saying "Is this a kitty?")	*No* kitty
Rejection	Child does not want something to happen; child refuses an object or action	*No* bath *No* beans
Recurrence	An event happens again; an object reappears or replaces another	*More* cookie *Another* doggie
Possession	Child identifies something as belonging to him or her, or to another person	*His* block Doll *mine*

Note. Adapted from *An Introduction to Children with Language Disorders*, 2nd ed., by V. A. Reed, 1994, New York: Macmillan College Publishing Company.

- *Heuristic.* Children attempt to have their environment and events in their environment explained to them; they organize and investigate the environment ("Tell me why." "What that?")

- *Regulatory.* Children attempt to control the behavior of others ("Do as I tell you to do.").

- *Personal.* Children express own feelings and attitudes (e.g., child says "yummy" as she licks a lollipop); self-awareness.

- *Informative.* Children can tell someone something, communicate experiences ("I have something to tell you.").

- *Instrumental.* Children attempt to get assistance, material things from others ("I want ball.").

- *Interactional.* Children initiate interactions with others ("Hi, Daddy.").

TABLE 3.2

Semantic Relations Expressed by Two-Word Utterances

Semantic Relation	Structure	Example
Notice	Hi + noun	Hi doggy
Nomination	Demonstrative + noun	That chair
Instrumental	Verb + noun	Cut [with scissors]
Conjunction	Noun + noun	Knife spoon
Recurrence	More + noun	More juice
Action-object	Verb + noun	Pet kitty
Action-indirect object	Verb + noun	Give [to] Mommy
Agent-action	Noun (agent) + verb	Doggy bark
Agent-object	Noun (agent) + noun	Baby [drink] juice
Possessor-possession	Noun (possessor) + noun	Mommy sock
Attribute-entity	Adjective/attributive + noun	Red ball
Entity + locative	Noun + locative	Juice [in] glass
Action + locative	Verb + noun	Jump [on] bed

■ Dore (1975) focused on the 12–24 month period in which children use early words to signal communicative intent, focusing more on children's intentions and less on listeners' reactions:

- Practicing (language)

- Protesting ("no" and resisting)

- Greeting ("Hi, Grandma" as Grandma comes in door)

- Calling/addressing ("Mommy")

- Requesting action (says "juice" to get juice)

- Requesting an answer ("Cow?")

- Labeling (points out and names "hair," "eyes," etc. of a doll)

- Repeating/imitating (overhears and repeats the word "cat")

- Answering (adult: "What's this?" child: "bottle")

2–3 Years

The following developmental milestones are observed in normally developing children between 2 and 3 years of age.

Syntax

The child:

■ uses word combinations, has beginning phrase and sentence structure.

■ has an average MLU of 2.0–4.0; at 36 months, sentences often average 3–4 words.

■ combines 3–4 words in subject-verb-object format; e.g., "Daddy throw ball."

■ uses telegraphic speech; word order is often object-verb (e.g., "doggy sit"), verb-object (e.g., "push Barbie"), subject-verb. Most sentences are incomplete.

■ asks wh-questions (e.g., "What's that?" "When go home?"), yes-no questions.

■ expresses negation by adding "no" or "not" in front of verbs—e.g., "Me not do it," or "He no bite."

Semantics

■ Comprehension usually precedes production. At 30 months, the child comprehends up to 2,400 words.

■ At 36 months, the child comprehends up to 3,600 words.

■ Expressive vocabulary is 200–600 words; average is 425 words at 30 months.

■ Meanings seem to be learned in sequence: objects, events, actions, adjectives, adverbs, spatial concepts, temporal (time) concepts.

■ First pronouns used are self-referents such as *I, me.*

The child:

– answers simple "wh" questions (e.g., "What runs?"); generally understands questions; begins asking wh-questions of adults (30 months).

– can identify simple body parts.

– carries out one- and two-part commands such as "Pick up the sock and give it to Mommy."

– understands plurals.

– can give simple account of experiences and tell understandable stories (36 months).

Morphology

The child's use of bound morphemes expands greatly between 2 and 3 years of age. The child:

- develops inflections such as *-ing,* spatial prepositions *in* and *on,* plurals, possessives, articles, and pronouns (see Table 3.3).

- develops simple, irregular past tense—e.g., *went.*

- develops copular *were.*

- develops *is* plus adjective—e.g., "That is pretty."

- develops regular past-tense verbs—e.g., *walked.*

- overregularizes past-tense inflections—e.g., *goed, throwed, falled.*

- overgeneralizes plural morphemes—e.g., *feets, mouses.*

- uses some memorized contractions, such as *don't, can't, it's, that's.*

Pragmatics

- The child's utterances, although occasionally egocentric, generally have a communicative intent.

- The child demonstrates rapid topic shifts; a 3-year-old can sustain topic of conversation only about 20% of the time.

- Communication includes criticism, commands, requests, threats, questions, and answers.

- Interpersonal communication expands; the child learns to adopt a role to express his own opinions and personality.

3–4 Years

The following developmental milestones are observed in normally developing children between 3 and 4 years of age.

Syntax

The child:

- learns set of clause-connecting devices: coordination (e.g., "and"), subordination (e.g., "because"), and uses these in sentences.

- begins using complex verb phrases—e.g., "I should have been able to do it."

- begins using modal verbs (e.g., *could, should, would*).

- begins using *tag questions*—e.g., "You want to go, *don't you?*"

- begins using *embedded* forms, which rearrange or add elements within sentences—e.g., "The man *who came to dinner* stayed a week."

TABLE 3.3

Average Order of Acquisition of 14 Grammatic Morphemes in Three Children

	Morphemes	Examples	Average MLU	Stage	Age of Mastery (months)
1	Present progressive -ing	Mom com*ing* Dog bark*ing*	2.25	II	19–28
2/3	Prepositions in, on	Toy *in* box Book *on* table	2.25	II	27–30
4	Regular plural inflection -s	My crayon*s* Dog bone*s*	2.25	II	24–33
5	Irregular past-tense verbs	*Came, ran sat, broke*	2.75	III	25–46
6	Possessive -s	Daddy'*s* hat Baby'*s* bottle	2.75	III	26–40
7	Uncontractible copula	Here *it is* There *I am*	2.75	III	27–39
8	Articles	I want *a* cookie Give me *the* ball	3.50	IV	28–46
9	Past-tense regular -ed	Mom pour*ed* juice I color*ed* pictures	3.50	IV	26–48
10	Regular third-person -s	Daddy cook*s* Kitty meow*s*	3.50	IV	26–46
11	Irregular third person	*Does, has*	4.00	V	28–50
12	Uncontractible auxiliary	She *was* working	4.00	V	29–48
13	Contractible copula	He *is* nice or He'*s* nice	4.00	V	29–49
14	Contractible auxiliary	Mom *is* coming or Mom'*s* coming	4.00	V	30–50

Note. Adapted from *A First Language: Early Stages,* by R. Brown, 1973, Cambridge, MA: Harvard University Press.

- begins using passive voice—e.g., "She's been bitten by a dog."

- uses mostly complete sentences; at 48 months, sentences average 5–5 1/2 words per utterance. MLU is approximately 3.0–5.0.

- uses mostly nouns, verbs, and personal pronouns.

- acquires do-insertions and ability to make transformations—e.g., "Does the kitty run around?"

- uses negation in speech—e.g., "Timmy can't swim."

- begins using complex and compound sentences—e.g., "I can sing and dance." Seven percent of sentences are compound or complex.

Semantics

The child:

- comprehends up to 4,200 words (by 42 months; at 48 months, comprehends up to 5,600 words).

- uses 800–1500 words expressively.

- asks how, why, and when questions.

- understands some common opposites—e.g., *day–night, little–big, fast–slow.*

- knows full name, name of street, several nursery rhymes.

- labels most things in the environment.

- relates experiences and tells about activities in sequential order.

- can recite a poem from memory or sing a song (by 48 months).

- answers appropriately questions such as "Which is the boy?" "Where is the dress?" "What toys do you have?" (by 42 months).

- can complete opposite analogies such as "Daddy is a man; Mommy is a _____ ." (by 48 months).

- understands most preschool children's stories (by 48 months).

- uses pronouns *you, they, us,* and *them,* as well as others such *I, me.*

- understands concepts such as heavy–light, empty–full, more–less, around, in front of–in back of, next to, big–little, hard–soft, rough–smooth (by 42 months).

- understands agent-action—e.g., "Tell me what flies, swims, bites," etc.

- supplies last word of sentence—e.g., "The apple is on the _____." (closure).

- appropriately answers "what if" questions—e.g., "What would you do if you fell down?" (by 43–48 months).

Morphology

The child:

- uses irregular plural forms—e.g., *children.*

- uses third-person singular, present tense—e.g., "he runs."

- consistently uses simple (regular) past and present progressives (e.g., *is running*) and negatives (e.g., *not*).

- uses inflection to convert adjective to causative—e.g., *sharp, sharpen.*

- uses simple (regular) plural forms correctly—e.g., *boys, houses, lights.*

- begins to use *is* at beginning of questions.
- uses contracted forms of modals—e.g., *can't, won't.*
- uses *and* as a conjunction.
- uses *is, are,* and *am* in sentences.
- uses possessive markers consistently—e.g., *the boy's clothes* (by 43–48 months).
- begins to use reflexive pronoun *myself* (by 43–48 months).
- begins to use conjunction *because* (by 43–48 months).

Pragmatics (adapted from Shulman, 1983)

The child:

- can maintain conversation without losing track of topic.
- begins to modify speech to age of listener—e.g., uses simplified language with a younger child.
- begins to produce indirectives—e.g., "Are the cookies done?" meaning "I want a cookie."
- uses requesting (e.g., yes–no questions, wh-questions).
- responds with structures such as *yes, no, because*; expresses agreement or denial (e.g., "That's not really her dress"), compliance or refusal (e.g., "I won't take a bath!").
- uses conversational devices:
    - boundary markers such as *hi, bye* (indicate beginning, end of communication)
    - calls such as "Hey, Mommy!"
    - accompaniments such as "Here you are"
    - politeness markers such as *please, thanks*
- uses communicative functions:
    - role-playing, fantasies
    - protests/objections such as "Don't touch that!"
    - jokes such as "I threw the juice in the ceiling!"
    - game markers such as "You have to catch me!"
    - claims such as "I'm first!"
    - warnings such as "Look out or you'll fall!"
    - teases such as "You can't have this!"

✎ Concepts To Consider

Briefly describe the syntactic development of a normally developing child between 3 and 4 years of age. What forms is the child using at this stage?

_____

_____

_____

_____

_____

_____

_____

4–5 Years

The following developmental milestones are observed in normaly developing children between 4 and 5 years of age.

Syntax

The child:

■ averages 6–6.5 words per sentence (by 5 years); has an average MLU of 4.5–7.0.

■ speaks in complete sentences.

■ uses complex sentences; interprets complex sentences correctly. By 4 1/2, only about 8% of sentences are incomplete.

■ uses future tense, e.g., "She will go to the store."

■ uses _if, so_ in sentences.

■ begins to use passive voice (some children)—e.g., "The cat was fed by the man."

Semantics

The child:

■ uses concrete meanings and words, but responds to some abstract ideas appropriately.

- has an expressive range of approximately 1,500–2,000 words.

- comprehends about 5,600 words at 48 months; by 54 months, comprehends approximately 6,500 words; by 60 months, comprehends up to 9,600 words.

- can name items in a category—e.g., food, animals. Able to point to categorical item (e.g., fruit).

- uses most pronouns, including possessives (e.g., *mine, his, her*).

- uses *why* and *how.*

- understands time concepts such as *early in the morning, tomorrow, after.*

- uses *what do, does, did* in questions.

- answers simple "when" questions like "When do you sleep?" (55–60 months).

- responds appropriately to "how often, how long" questions (55–60 months).

- asks meaning of words.

- tells long stories accurately.

- can give whole name (first, middle, last).

- begins to understand right and left (5 years).

- can define 10 common words (4½ years).

- shows objects by use and function (e.g., if directed, "Show me what tells time," "Show me which one gives us milk").

- identifies past and future verbs ("Show me the man who kicked the ball," "Who will kick the ball?").

- demands explanations with frequent use of *why.*

Morphology

The child:

- uses comparatives—e.g., *bigger, nicer, taller.*

- uses *could, would* in sentences.

- uses irregular plurals (e.g., *mice, teeth*) fairly consistently.

Pragmatics

The child:

- modifies speech as a function of listener age (beginning at 4 years).

- begins to judge grammatical correctness and appropriateness of sentences.

- can maintain topic over successive utterances.

- uses egocentric monologue about a third of the time (this monologue does not communicate information to the listener).

- uses indirect speech acts, softens speech—e.g., "I think that goes in there" rather than "Put that in there."

- begins to tell jokes and riddles (around 5 years).

5–6 Years

The following developmental milestones are observed in normally developing children between 5 and 6 years of age.

Syntax

The child:

- has an average MLU of 6.0–8.0.

- uses present, past, and future tenses consistently.

- uses conjunctions to string words together (e.g., "A bear and a wolf and a fox").

- asks "how" questions.

- uses auxiliary *have* correctly at times.

- uses "if" sentences—e.g., "If I had a cookie, I'd eat it."

- increases understanding and use of complex sentences; decreases grammatical errors as sentences and vocabulary become more sophisticated.

- comprehends verb tenses in the passive voice (e.g., "The bus was hit by the car," "The cat was fed by the man").

- uses a language form that approximates the adult model.

Semantics

The child:

- knows spatial relations and prepositions such as *on top, behind, far, near.*

- can distinguish *alike, same, different.*

- distinguishes right and left in self, not in others.

- knows complete address.

- knows most common opposites—e.g., *hard–soft, fat–thin, high–low;* understands "opposite of"—e.g., "What's the opposite of cold?"

- defines objects by use, composition (e.g., "Napkins are made of paper; you wipe your mouth with them").
- tells long stories; retells tales of past and present events.
- comprehends 13,000–15,000 words (by age 6).
- can answer "What happens if . . . ?" questions.
- understands concepts such as yesterday–tomorrow, more–less, some–many, several–few, most–least, before–after, now–later.
- can state similarities and differences of objects.
- can name position of objects: first, second, third.
- can name days of week in order.
- comprehends *first, last*.
- knows functions of body parts.

Morphology

The child:

- knows passive forms of main verbs.
- knows indefinite pronouns—*any, anything, anybody, every, both, few, many, each*, and others.
- uses irregular plurals with general consistency.
- uses possessives and negatives consistently.
- uses all pronouns consistently.
- uses superlative *-est* (e.g., *smartest*).
- begins to use adverbial word endings (e.g., *-ly*).

Pragmatics

The child:

- understands humor, surprise.
- corrects potential errors by modifying the message.
- can recognize a socially offensive message and reword it in polite form.
- modifies speech according to listener's needs.
- begins to use and understand formal levels of address (e.g., *Mr, Mrs.*).
- gains greater facility with indirect requests (e.g., "I would like a sticker" instead of "Gimme a sticker").

- can differentiate 80% of the time between polite and impolite utterances.

- uses expressions such as "thank you" and "I'm sorry."

- often asks permission to use objects belonging to others.

- contributes to adult conversation.

6–7 Years

The following developmental milestones are observed in normally developing children between 6 and 7 years of age.

Syntax

The child:

- uses *if* and *so*.

- uses reflexive pronouns (e.g., *himself, myself*).

- begins to use perfect tense forms (e.g., *have, had*).

- has full use of passive voice.

- has an average MLU of 7.3 words.

- uses embedding more frequently (e.g., "The girl *who bought the dress* went to the party.").

Semantics

The child:

- comprehends 20,000–26,000 words.

- understands seasons of the year and knows what you do in each.

- forms letters left to right (reversals and inversions are common).

- prints alphabet and numerals from previously printed model.

- recites the alphabet sequentially, names capital letters, matches lower to upper case letters.

- rote counts to 100.

- tells time related to specific daily schedule.

Morphology

The child:

- uses most morphological markers fairly consistently.
- uses irregular comparatives (*good, better, best*) more correctly.
- continues to improve in correct use of irregular past tense and plurals.
- begins to produce *gerunds* (a noun form produced by adding *-ing* to a verb infinitive, e.g., *fish, fishing*).
- acquires use of *derivational morphemes*, in which verbs are changed into nouns (e.g., *catch* becomes *catcher*).

Pragmatics

The child:

- becomes aware of mistakes in other people's speech.
- is apt to use slang and mild profanity.

7–8 Years

The following developmental milestones are observed in normally developing children between 7 and 8 years of age.

Syntax

The child:

- has an MLU of approximately 7.0–9.0
- uses predominantly complex sentence forms

Semantics

The child:

- interprets jokes and riddles literally.
- anticipates story endings.
- uses some figurative language.
- uses details in description.
- creates conversation suggested by a picture.
- enjoys telling stories and anecdotes.
- retells a story, keeping main ideas in correct sequence.

Morphology

The child:

■ uses most irregular verb forms, though with some mistakes in irregular past tense.

■ uses superlatives (*biggest, prettiest*).

■ uses adverbs regularly.

Pragmatics

The child:

■ initiates, maintains conversation in small groups.

■ is able to role-play, to take the listener's point of view.

■ determines and uses appropriate discourse codes and styles—e.g., informal with friends, formal with adults.

■ uses nonlinguistic and nonverbal behaviors—posture, gestures—appropriately.

■ takes more care in communicating with unfamiliar people; announces topic shifts.

■ can sustain a topic through a number of conversational turns, but topics tend to be concrete (by 8 years; after age 11, discussions involving abstract topics can be sustained).

Summary

☑ Children develop language based on their innate characteristics, the environment they are exposed to, and the expectations of their particular cultures.

☑ The development of syntactic, semantic, morphological, and pragmatic skills depends in large part on those factors. Each child develops at his or her own rate, and variation among children is to be expected.

THEORIES OF LANGUAGE DEVELOPMENT

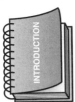

Theory drives practice. The way clinicians conduct assessment and treatment depends greatly on their theoretical viewpoints. Some clinicians are eclectic in their approach; that is, they blend aspects of several different theories to achieve what they see as a balanced approach to language assessment and treatment. Other clinicians depend primarily on and operate from one theory.

In this section, we describe five major theories of language development: nativist, cognitive, behavioral, information-processing, and social interactionism. These theories differ in describing how language is developed and in their implications for (a) areas that clinicians should target in assessment and intervention, and (b) what procedures should be used to facilitate language learning.

Nativist Theory

■ The nativist theory, an influential theory of syntax proposed by Noam Chomsky in the 1950s, has had a significant impact on linguistics and on speech–language pathology.

■ Chomsky stated that syntactic structures are the essence of language and that language is a product of the unique human mind. He said that there are universal rules of grammar that apply to all languages.

■ The nativist theory states that children are born with a *language acquisition device* (LAD). The LAD is assumed to be a specialized language processor that is a physiological part of the brain (Bohannon & Bonvillian, 1997). The LAD knows about languages in general, because it contains the universal rules of language.

■ The child's environment provides information about the unique rules of the language the child is exposed to. The LAD then integrates the universal rules and the unique rules of that language and thus helps the child learn language in a relatively short period of time.

■ Nativists believe that children are born with an innate capacity to learn language and that because the basic knowledge necessary to acquire language is already present at birth, language is not learned through environmental stimulation, reinforcement, or teaching.

■ Chomsky described language *competence* and language *performance*. Competence, the knowledge of the rules of universal grammar, is innate. Thus, the child learns language relatively independently of the environment. Performance, the actual production of language, is imperfect because of such factors as fatigue and distraction.

■ Chomsky introduced the ideas of *surface* structure and *deep* structure. Surface structure is the actual arrangement of words in a syntactic order. It is the phrase or sentence that one hears. Underlying this surface structure is the abstract deep structure, which primarily contains the rules of sentence formation.

■ Chomsky stated that surface and deep structures are related through grammatic transformations. A *transformation* is an operation that relates the deep and surface structures and yields different forms of sentences.

■ A transformation can further be viewed as a process by which one arranges and rearranges words to change sentences. Grammatic transformations involve deleting, adding, substituting, and rearranging words to change meaning. Consider the following examples:

- The boy kicked the ball.

- Who kicked the ball? (a question transformation)

- Did the boy kick the ball? (another question transformation)

- The ball was not kicked by the boy. (a negative transformation)

- The ball was kicked by the boy. (a passive transformation)

■ Each of these examples involves a transformation of adding, deleting, substituting, or rearranging words to form a different kind of sentence. These transformations account for the creative nature of language.

■ Because Chomsky believed that such creative transformation of sentence forms is the essence of language, his theory is often called the *transformational generative theory of grammar*. According to Chomsky, with knowledge of the rules of grammar and the use of transformations, speakers can generate an endless variety of sentences.

■ A revision of Chomsky's theory was proposed in the early 1980s. The *government binding theory* attempts to describe the way the mind represents language. Government binding theory tries to account for the great diversity in human languages and to explain more about children's development of grammar on the basis of limited input (Owens, 1996).

■ The nativist theory and its variants lead to few specific implications for assessment and treatment of children who have language disorders. However, Chomskyan theorists do believe that in therapy, it is necessary to focus heavily on syntax in selecting treatment goals.

■ Reinforcement, however, is unnecessary. Because language knowledge is innate, reinforcing a child for talking would be tantamount to reinforcing a child for walking. Manipulating the child's environment, as the behaviorist does, is unlikely to be successful, according to this theory.

Cognitive Theory

■ Described as a variant of the nativist theory, the cognitive theory emphasizes *cognition*, or knowledge and mental processes such as attention, memory, and auditory and visual perception. Cognitivists focus on the child's regulation of learning and on internal aspects of behavior (Klein & Moses, 1999).

■ According to cognitive theory, language acquisition is made possible by cognition and general intellectual processes. Language is only one expression of a more general set of cognitive activities, and proper development of the cognitive system is a necessary precursor of linguistic expression (Bohannon & Bonvillian, 1997).

■ Thus, a child must first acquire concepts before producing words. For example, a child who does not know about a dog or a triangle is not likely to say those words.

■ Proponents of the *strong cognition hypothesis* believe in cognitive precursors to language. They state that there are cognitive abilities that are essential prerequisites to language skills. Without these prerequisite cognitive abilities, language skills will not be optimally developed. Language development is dependent on cognitive development.

■ Piaget, a supporter of the strong cognition hypothesis, described four stages of cognitive development that children must go through (see Table 3.4). He believed that children successively acquire the necessary cognitive operations that, in turn, lead to higher levels of language development. Children must master the features of one stage in order to progress to the next (McLaughlin, 1998).

■ Children pass through each cognitive stage in the *order* given but may show variation in the *rate* at which they progress through the stages.

■ Although researchers have not proven that there is a causal relationship between cognitive and language skills, it has been observed that certain language skills develop at about the same time as certain cognitive skills. For example, children's use of "all gone" (a disappearance phrase) is associated with the emerging understanding of object permanence.

■ The *weak cognition hypothesis* states that while cognition accounts for some of a child's language abilities, it cannot account for all of them; some aspects of language do not develop directly as a result of underlying cognitive skills (Reed, 1994).

■ Cognitive theorists believe that while nonlinguistic, cognitive precursors are innate, language is not. Thus, because they believe that language is neither innate (nativist view) nor learned (behaviorist view), they view language as emerging as a result of cognitive growth.

TABLE 3.4
Piaget's Stages of Cognitive Development

Sensorimotor (0–2 years)

Usually divided into six substages; children gain increased control over their environments:

- Child displays reflexive vocal and sensorimotor behavior
- Child engages in symbolic play (e.g., using a tissue for a doll's blanket; using a block to represent a car)
- Child coordinates hand-eye and hand-mouth movements
- Child begins to search for objects
- Child starts causing objects to move
- Child imitates sounds; babbling
- Object permanence occurs; child looks for an item that is out of sight
- Around 12 months, first word appears
- Child uses words for people or things that are not in present environment
- Child demonstrates means-ends behavior (e.g., pulling a string to get a toy)

Preoperational (2–7 years)

Frequently divided into two stages: preconceptual (2–4 years) and intuitive (4–7 years):

- Child is egocentric; has difficulty taking perspective of others
- Child overextends word meanings (all men are "Daddy")
- Child underextends word meanings (only the family pet, Rover, is a "dog")
- Child demonstrates concreteness of thought
- Child displays lack of conservation (e.g., lack of ability to see that a ball of clay can be rolled into a snake shape and still be the same clay)
- Child has difficulty with classification skills

Concrete Operations (7–11 years)

- Child is less egocentric, has increasing ability to see others' points of view
- Child aquires conservation skills
- Child employs logical causality
- Child uses effective classification skills

Formal Operations (more than 11 years)

- Child displays lack of egocentricity, ability to see others' point of view
- Child displays ability to think and speak in the abstract
- Child can use inductive and deductive thought processes
- Child can use verbal reasoning and make "if...then" statements
- Child is able to use hypothetical reasoning

Note. Adapted from *An Introduction to Children with Language Disorders,* 2nd ed., by V. Reed, 1994, New York: Macmillan.

■ Thus, a clinical implication of the cognitive theory is that clinicians must assess cognitive precursors to language and facilitate the development of those precursors before working on language itself (Van Kleeck & Richardson, 1989). Language will not improve until cognitive precursors are developed.

Behavioral Theory

■ The behavioral theory does not explain the acquisition of language, because language often is described by linguists and others as a mental system. Behavioral psychologist B. F. Skinner did not describe language as a mental or cognitive system, because he considered that such a view would preclude an experimental study of language.

■ Skinner's (1957) system of behavioral analysis explains the acquisition of *verbal behavior*. Verbal behavior is considered to be a form of social behavior maintained by the actions of a verbal community. Verbal behaviors are acquired under appropriate conditions of stimulation, response, and reinforcement.

■ Behavioral scientists suggest that learning, not innate mechanisms, plays a major role in the acquisition of verbal behaviors. They do not believe, as nativists do, that a child has an innate knowledge of the universal rules of grammar. Behaviorists focus on the *measurable* and *observable* aspects of language behavior and emphasize performance over competence (Bohannon & Bonvillian, 1997).

■ To behaviorists, the events in the child's *environment* are important (McLaughlin, 1998; Klein & Moses, 1999). Children learn only the language they are exposed to; severe social deprivation results in language deprivation as well.

■ Verbal behavior is characteristically produced under social stimulation. An audience is necessary; the audience, or person(s) interacting with the speaker, sets the stage for speech. Put differently, verbal behavior is a form of social behavior shaped and maintained by the members of a verbal community.

■ Practically all forms of verbal behaviors can be increased or decreased experimentally. Social reinforcement, for example, can increase babbling, word and phrase responses, and the production of grammatic features.

■ Thus, behaviorists question the nativist assumption that the environment offers little assistance to the child in acquiring language. In treatment, behaviorists teach verbal behavior to children by modeling correct responses and reinforcing children's correct productions.

■ Verbal behavior is broken down into cause-effect (functional) units, not structures of language. These *functional units* include:

- *Mands.* Derived from related traditional terms such as *demands* and *commands,* mands involve requests (McLaughlin, 1998). In some cases, a physiological need such as thirst or hunger stimulates speech ("Do you have something to eat?"). Needs of this sort cause various kinds of requests, commands, and demands. These mands are caused by states of motivation and are reinforced by food and other biologically satisfying events.

- *Tacts.* Sometimes physical objects and events stimulate speaking; verbal responses to this kind of stimulation are called tacts. A tact is a group of verbal responses that describe and comment on the things and events around us. For example, a child is using a tact when she says, "This car is big and red." Tacts are reinforced socially; a smile, a nod of approval, and similar statements by a listener may all reinforce a tact.

- *Echoics.* Echoics are imitative verbal responses whose stimuli are the speech of another person. Reinforcement for an echoic is based on a close resemblance betwen the stimulus and the response. Thus, a clinician will model target responses, which a child imitates. The clinician reinforces only when the child's imitations at least approximate the clinician's modeled response.

- Clinicians who conduct language treatment according to principles of the behavioral theory believe that one can teach language by targeting any observable behavior and manipulating the elements of a stimulus, a response, and some type of reinforcement.

- In treatment, the clinician selects specific target responses, creates appropriate antecedent events, and reinforces correct responses (Fey, 1986). There is a clearly established criterion for success (e.g., 8 out of 10 responses produced accurately).

- For example, a clinician teaching a child to use plural *-s* might create a game using toy cars. If the clinician points to the cars and asks, "What are these?" and the child says, "Cars," the clinician might respond with "Good job!"

Concepts To Consider

Compare and contrast the nativist and behavioral theories. What are the main points of difference between the two?

_____

_____

_____

_____

_____

_____

_____

_____

_____

_____

_____

Information-Processing Theory

- Proponents of the information-processing theory are mostly concerned with cognitive *functioning*, not cognitive structures or concepts—in other words, with *how* language is learned.

- Information-processing theorists view the human information-processing system as a mechanism which encodes stimuli from the environment, operates on interpretations of those stimuli, stores the results in memory, and permits retrieval of previously stored information (Nelson, 1998).

- Of primary concern are the steps involved in handling or processing incoming and outgoing information. Included in these steps are organization, memory, transfer, attention, and discrimination. Long- and short-term memory are especially important (Owens, 1996).

- In the area of language, auditory processing has received more attention than visual processing. The role of auditory processing in language learning has continued to be highly controversial. Yet, many speech–language pathologists provide treatment for "auditory-processing problems," believing that such treatment will result in enhanced language skills.

- Foundational to adequate auditory processing is normal auditory sensitivity. When normal auditory sensitivity is established, some clinicians address components of auditory processing in their treatment programs (Mokhemar, 1999; Reed, 1994):

  - *Auditory discrimination.* These skills enable children to identify differences between sound stimuli. Popular available tests ask children, for example, "Listen: cat–bat. Are these words the same or different?" The validity of these tests has been questioned by many professionals. Although the role of auditory discrimination in language development is heavily debated, researchers have found that language-impaired children have poorer auditory discrimination skills than their normally developing peers.

- *Auditory attention.* This is the ability to ignore irrelevant acoustic stimuli and focus on important information. Children with poor auditory attention have difficulty filtering relevant and irrelevant stimuli. Without appropriate auditory attention, children focus equally on all incoming stimuli, thus experiencing sensory overload. Optimal language learning cannot take place under such conditions; children cannot sort out and attend to the important aspects of speech.

- *Auditory memory.* This refers to the ability to mentally store speech stimuli, or remember what one has heard. Many clinicians and researchers have found that language-impaired children have difficulty with auditory memory. Yet research suggests that while auditory memory may be a factor that exists *concomitantly with* language impairment, there is insufficient evidence to demonstrate that auditory memory problems are a *cause of* language impairment.

- *Auditory rate.* This refers to children's ability to process acoustic stimuli that are presented at different rates or speeds. Much research has suggested that language-impaired children have difficulty processing incoming stimuli presented at rapid rates and that if the rate of incoming information is slowed down, language-impaired children can process it better.

- *Auditory sequencing.* This is the ability to identify the temporal order in which auditory stimuli occur. Although the role of auditory sequencing in language development has been debated, it has been found that children with language disorders do more poorly on auditory-sequencing tasks than children who are developing normally.

■ Many researchers would argue that at this time there is insufficient evidence to support the idea that speech–language pathologists should target auditory-processing skills as a part of language therapy. Because auditory-processing skills have not been conclusively demonstrated to be causally related to language impairment, many believe that addressing these skills as part of treatment is a waste of time.

■ However, recent research with small numbers of language-impaired children has shown that directly targeting auditory-processing skills leads to direct improvement in language skills (Miller, Merzenich, Saunders, Jenkins, & Tallal, 1997; Tallal et al., 1996). More research, with larger numbers of subjects, needs to be conducted in this area.

■ Information-processing models as a whole have been criticized because they speculate about processes that are inaccessible and nonobservable (Klein & Moses, 1999; McLaughlin, 1998). It is difficult to quantify and measure the phenomenon of "information processing."

Social Interactionism Theory

■ The social interactionism theory does not focus on innate linguistic competence (nativism) or specific reinforcement principles (behaviorism). Rather, this theory stipulates that the structure of human language has possibly arisen from language's social-communicative function in human relations (Bohannon & Bonvillian, 1997).

■ Proponents of social interactionism emphasize language *function*, not *structure*. They give credence to the situations in which social interactions occur, believing that interactions vary depending on the situation (Nelson, 1998).

■ Social interactionists believe that language develops because people are motivated to interact socially with other people around them. For example, infants seek out human faces and respond to them (Bruner, 1968; cited in Nelson, 1998). Thus, the environment and its inherent social experiences are crucial to the emergence of language (Bohannon & Bonvillian, 1997).

■ Proponents of social interactionism believe that the *child*, as well as his or her caretakers and the environment, plays an active role in language acquisition.

■ Lev Vygotsky, a Russian psychologist, believed that language is a tool for social interaction. He saw language as being intrinsically linked with the social-interactive context.

■ According to Vygotsky, language knowledge is acquired through social interaction with more competent and experienced members of the child's culture (Van Kleeck & Richardson, 1989). Vygotsky emphasized the importance of verbal guidance and adult modeling (Klein & Moses, 1999).

■ Vygotsky stated that a child's conversational partners, including the parents, are significant contributors to the language acquisition process. They contribute by *scaffolding*, or by supplying the necessary communicative structure that allows the child to communicate despite limited communication skills.

■ Unlike Piaget, who believed that cognitive development preceded language development, Vygotsky thought that children first learned language in interpersonal interactions and then used that language to structure thought.

■ Vygotsky further believed that as children's language develops, they increasingly use language internally to structure their actions and direct their thoughts. For example, small children playing house by themselves may be observed talking to themselves as they play. Eventually, as they mature, children use language silently internally to mediate thought.

■ Social interactionism theorists believe that language, both oral and written, continues to develop across the span of a person's life. Adolescents, for example, continue to refine their skills in figurative language and pragmatics as they mature. Adults who change jobs or vocations must learn the vocabulary relevant to their new station in life.

■ Clinicians whose practice is driven by social interactionist theory focus on children's *motivation* for communication. In other words, treatment sessions are built around increasing children's motivation to communicate.

■ To motivate children to use language, clinicians supply external situations and contexts, both verbal and nonverbal, that encourage the child to use language to meet his or her needs. For example, a clinician might withhold an attractive bottle of bubbles until the child says, "I want bubbles."

Summary

☑ The nativist, cognitive, behavioral, information-processing, and social interactionism theories have been briefly described. Although other models of language development certainly exist, these five theories have done much to influence research and practice.

☑ Most speech–language pathologists, rather than allowing their practice to be driven by a single theory, incorporate aspects of all five theories to allow an eclectic blend to serve as a foundation for optimal assessment and treatment of language-impaired children.

CHAPTER HIGHLIGHTS

▶ Language is a form of social behavior that is shaped and maintained by a verbal community. Language can also be defined as a system of symbols used to represent concepts that are formed through exposure and experience.

▶ Linguists have traditionally described several components of language: morphology (the study of word structure), syntax (rules specifying how words may be combined to form meaningful sentences), semantics (the study of meaning), and pragmatics (the study of rules that govern language use in various social situations). (Phonology, frequently studied under the aegis of language, is defined and discussed in Chapter 5).

▶ Language development in children depends on several factors: the innate characteristics the individual child brings to the situation (e.g., a high IQ, a limited attention span); the child's environment; and cultural expectations.

(continues)

▶ There are language developmental milestones that clinicians can use to guide their expectations about language characteristics of children at certain chronological ages. However, a great deal of individual variability exists among children, and developmental milestones can serve only as a *general* guide and frame of reference.

▶ Theories of language development provide the foundational underpinnings for assessment and treatment of children with language problems. Key theories that have impacted clinical practice include the nativist theory (Chomsky), the cognitive theory (Piaget), the behavioral theory (Skinner), the information-processing theory, and the social interactionism theory (Vygotsky).

▶ According to the nativist theory, proposed by Chomsky, children are born with a language acquisition device that contains the universal rules of language. Chomsky has described the concepts of deep and surface structures as well as the concepts of language competence and language performance.

▶ Proponents of the cognitive theory state that cognition and intellectual processes make language acquisition possible. Piaget, a supporter of the strong cognition hypothesis, stated that children pass through four overlapping developmental cognitive stages: the sensorimotor, preoperational, concrete operations, and formal operations stages.

▶ The behavioral theory was proposed by Skinner, who explained language acquisition as the development of verbal behavior. He suggested that learning, not an innate and unmeasurable mechanism such as the language acquisition device, plays a major role in language development. He emphasized the importance of the environment in language learning.

▶ The information-processing theory focuses on *how* language is learned; that is, on what types of cognitive functioning are necessary for language learning. A strong emphasis of this theory is auditory processing, comprised of the components of auditory discrimination, attention, memory, rate, and sequencing.

▶ Proponents of the social interactionism theory, influenced by Vygotsky, emphasize language function over language structure. Social interactionists believe that language develops as a function of social interaction between a child and his environment (including significant others in that environment). Motivation is key in using language.

▶ Add your own chapter highlights here:

_____

_____

_____

_____

KEY TERMS

auditory attention
auditory discrimination
auditory memory
auditory rate
auditory sequencing
base morpheme
behavioral theory
bound morpheme
clause
cohesion
competence
complex sentence
compound sentence
declarative
deep structure
dependent clause
discourse
echoic
embedding
exclamatory
fast mapping
free morpheme
government binding
   theory
grammatic morpheme

illocutionary
imperative
independent clause
information-processing
   theory
interrogative
joint reference
kernel sentence
language
language acquisition
   device
linguistics
linguists
locutionary
main clause
mand
morpheme
morphology
narrative
nativist theory
overextension
passive
performance
perlocutionary
pragmatics

prefix
presupposition
quick incidental learning
root morpheme
semantic relations
semantics
social interactionism
   theory
strong cognition
   hypothesis
subordinate clause
suffix
surface structure
syntax
tact
transformation
transformational
   generative theory of
   grammar
underextension
verbal behavior
weak cognition
   hypothesis

STUDY AND REVIEW QUESTIONS

Fill in the Blank

1. A(n) _morpheme_ is the smallest meaningful unit of a language;
   a(n) _allomorph_ is a variation that does not alter the
   original meaning of the morpheme.

2. Proponents of the information-processing theory describe auditory
   attention, or the ability to ignore irrelevant acoustic stimuli and
   focus on important information; these proponents also describe auditory
   sequencing, or the ability to identify the temporal order in
   which auditory stimuli occur.

3. The _nativist_ theory was an influential theory of syntax proposed by _Chomsky_; a revision of this theory came in
   the early 1980s and was called the _gov't binding_ theory.

4. The ___behaviorist___ theory, proposed by ___Skinner___, viewed language as verbal behavior or a form of social behavior maintained by the actions of a verbal community.

5. A ___compound___ sentence has two or more independent clauses joined by a comma and a conjunction or joined by a semicolon; a ___complex___ sentence contains one independent clause and one or more dependent or subordinate clauses.

6. The stage in which a child uses one word to communicate a variety of meanings is called the ___holophrastic___ stage.

7. A child who labels all round items as cookies is using ___overextension___, while a child who thinks that only the family pet Phydeaux is a dog is using ___underextension___.

8. In English, the basic syntactic structure is the subject-verb-object sequence. Usually called the ___kernel sentence___, this can also be called the ___phrase___ structure or the ___base___ structure.

9. The form of discourse in which the speaker tells a story about a logical sequence of events is called a(n) ___narrative___.

10. Signals issued by a child that have an effect on the listener but lack communicative intent are called ___perlocutionary___ behaviors. At 9–10 months, normally developing children begin using ___illocutionary___ behaviors, or signals to carry out some socially organized action; there is intentional communication. At about 12 months of age, the child enters the ___locutionary___ stage as she or he begins to use words.

Multiple Choice

11. A child says "red crayon." This is an example of which type of semantic relations?

   A. attribute + entity

   B. action + locative

   C. agent + action

   D. attribute + locative

   E. possession + attribute

12. A child using *recurrence* would say:

    A. "Face dirty."

    B. "All gone juice."

    C. "More cookie."

    D. "Doll mine."

    E. "Close door."

13. An example of a sentence using an *embedded form* would be:

    A. I saw the squirrel climbing the tree.

    B. The girl ate a cookie, three crackers, and some fruit.

    C. Mom and Dad are going to the store to buy some groceries.

    D. Because he was on time, they were happy with him.

    E. The boy who got a haircut looks nice.

14. Which one of the following does NOT occur between 8 and 10 months of age in the normally developing child?

    A. comprehension of *no*

    B. using the phrase *all gone* to express emerging negation

    C. using variegated babbling (e.g., "madamada")

    D. uncovering a hidden toy (beginning of object permanence)

    E. use of gestural language such as shaking head no, playing peek-a-boo

15. Which of the following statements is/are true with regard to Brown's morphemes?

    A. Children may vary in terms of the *rate* with which they develop the morphemes, but children usually develop them in the same *sequence*.

    B. One of the last morphemes to develop, in Stage V, is uncontractible copula (e.g., "There *it is*").

    C. The first morpheme to develop is present progressive *-ing* (e.g., "Dad cook*ing*").

    D. A, B

    E. A, C

16. A clinician assesses a 7-year-old girl who has difficulties in the area of *discourse*. Treatment goals would most likely involve which one of the following?

    A. increasing mean length of utterance and sentence complexity

    B. increasing accurate use of morphological structures

    C. expanding vocabulary to be more commensurate with age level

    D. increasing ability to converse appropriately with peers over a range of topics

    E. increasing ability to comprehend and use metaphors and idioms

17. Pragmatic skills involve:

    A. understanding words with multiple meanings (e.g., *rock*)

    B. use of narratives, a form of discourse in which a speaker tells a story

    C. use of appropriate cohesion, or the logical order and organization of utterances in a message

    D. B, C

    E. A, B, C

18. You are conducting a language sample with a 5-year-old who says, "Him no eat cookies." This is an example of:

    A. 4 words, 5 morphemes, personal pronoun + negative + verb + plural noun

    B. 4 words, 6 morphemes, modal + negative + verb + auxiliary

    C. 4 words, 4 morphemes, personal pronoun + copula + negative + noun

    D. 4 words, 5 morphemes, negative + personal pronoun + copula

    E. 4 words, 5 morphemes, personal pronoun + auxiliary + negative + plural noun

19. Which one of the following Piagetian stages, which includes object permanence, corresponds with the emergence of a normally developing child's first word?

    A. preoperational

    B. formal operations

    C. sensorimotor

    D. concrete operations

    E. none of the above

20. Halliday described seven functions of communicative intent that develop between 9 and 18 months of age. Which of the following is an example of the *heuristic* function?

    A. "Yummy" (said by a child eating a cookie)

    B. "Why airplane fly?"

    C. "I want juice."

    D. "Hi, Grandpa."

    E. "I go store."

REFERENCES AND RECOMMENDED READINGS

Berko Gleason, J. (1997). *The development of language* (4th ed.). Needham Heights, MA: Allyn & Bacon.

Bloom, L., & Lahey, M. (1978). *Language development and disorders*. New York: Macmillan.

Bohannon, J. N., & Bonvillian, J. D. (1997). Theoretical approaches to language acquisition. In J. Berko Gleason, *The development of language* (4th ed.) (pp. 259–316). Needham Heights, MA: Allyn & Bacon.

Brown, R. (1973). *A first language: Early stages*. Cambridge, MA: Harvard University Press.

Bruner, J. (1968). *Processes of cognitive growth: Infancy* (Vol. III, Heinz Werner Lecture Series). Worcester, MA: Clark University Press.

Dore, J. (1975). Holophrase, speech acts, and language universals. *Journal of Child Language, 2,* 21–40.

Fey, M. E. (1986). *Language intervention in young children*. Boston: Little, Brown.

Halliday, M. (1975). *Learning how to mean: Explorations in the development of language*. London: Edward Arnold.

Johnson, B. A. (1996). *Language disorders in children: An introductory clinical perspective*. Albany, NY: Delmar Publishers.

Klein, H. B., & Moses, N. (1999). *Intervention planning for children with communication disorders: A guide for clinical practicum and professional practice* (2nd ed.). Needham Heights, MA: Allyn & Bacon.

McLaughlin, S. (1998). *Introduction to language development*. San Diego, CA: Singular Publishing Group.

Miller, S., Merzenich, M. M., Saunders, G., Jenkins, W. M., & Tallal, P. (1997). Improvements in language abilities with training of children with both attentional and language impairments. *Society for Neuroscience, 23,* 490–492.

Mokhemar, M. A. (1999). *The central auditory processing kit*. East Moline, IL: Linguisystems, Inc.

Nelson, N. W. (1998). *Childhood language disorders in context: Infancy through adolescence* (2nd ed.). Needham Heights, MA: Allyn & Bacon.

Owens, R. E. (1996). *Language development: An introduction* (4th ed.). Needham Heights, MA: Allyn & Bacon.

Paul, R. (1995). *Language disorders from infancy through adolescence: Assessment and intervention*. St. Louis, MO: Mosby-Year Book.

Reed, V. A. (1994). *An introduction to children with language disorders* (2nd ed.). New York: Macmillan College Publishing Company.

Shulman, B. (1983). *Pragmatic development chart*. San Francisco: Word-Making Productions.

Skinner, B. F. (1957). *Verbal behavior*. Norwalk, CT: Appleton-Century-Crofts.

Tallal, P., Miller, S. L., Bedi, G., Byma, G., Wang, X., Nagarajan, S. S., Schreiner, C., Jenkins, W. M., & Merzenich, M. M. (1996). Language comprehension in language-learning impaired children improved with acoustically modified speech. *Science, 271,* 77–84.

Van Kleeck, A., & Richardson, A. (1989). Language delay in the child. In J. L. Northern (Ed.), *Study guide for handbook of speech–language pathology and audiology* (pp. 170–177). Philadelphia, PA: B.C. Decker.

ANSWERS TO STUDY AND REVIEW QUESTIONS

1. Morpheme, allomorph

2. Attention, sequencing

3. Nativist, Chomsky, government binding

4. Behavioral, Skinner

5. Compound, complex

6. Holophrastic

7. Overextension, underextension

8. Kernel sentence, phrase, base

9. Narrative

10. Perlocutionary, illocutionary, locutionary

11. A. When a child says "red crayon," this is an example of attribute + entity.

12. C. A child using recurrence would say "*more* cookie."

13. E. Embedding refers to adding or rearranging elements within sentences; in this example, the phrase "who got a haircut" makes the sentence one that uses an embedded form.

14. B. Most children use "all gone" to express emerging negation between 1 and 2 years of age.

15. E. Children tend to develop Brown's morphemes in the same sequence, but the rate of acquisition may vary. The *-ing* morpheme is the first to develop, and the uncontractible copula develops in Stage III.

16. D. Discourse involves how utterances are related, and has to do with the connected flow of language between speakers.

17. D. Pragmatic skills involve the ability to use narratives and to use appropriate cohesion.

18. A. If you are conducting a language sample with a 5-year-old and the child says, "Him no eat cookies," this is an example of 4 words, 5 morphemes, personal pronoun + negative + verb + plural noun.

19. C. Children usually use their first word at 10–14 months of age, which corresponds to the sensorimotor cognitive development stage.

20. B. The heuristic function involves children attempting to have events in their environment explained to them ("Tell me why").

CHAPTER 4

Language Disorders in Children

PREVIEW OUTLINE

As stated in the previous chapter, *language* may be defined as a form of social behavior shaped and maintained by a verbal community. It may also be viewed as a system of symbols used to represent concepts that are formed through exposure and experience (Bloom & Lahey, 1978). Children with disorders of language have a disruption within this system. They are not able to interact, within their families, communities, or cultures, in a manner consistent with that of their peers or with societal expectations. Children with language disorders find themselves at a disadvantage throughout their lives as they attempt to go to school, interact within various realms of society, and eventually find productive and fulfilling vocations.

Language problems are caused by or associated with a number of factors. Experts have proposed many paradigms or models from which to view these problems, their causes, and associated factors. In this chapter we discuss three broad categories of children with language problems: (a) children with *language-learning disabilities* or *specific language impairment*, (b) children with *language problems associated with physical and sensory disabilities in specific categories* such as mental retardation, autism, and acquired brain injury, and (c) children who have language difficulties related to a combination of *physical and social-environmental factors* such as poverty, neglect or abuse, alcohol or drug exposure in utero, and attention-deficit disorder. We then discuss assessment and treatment principles and procedures that can be used when serving children with language problems.

CHILDREN WITH LANGUAGE-LEARNING DISABILITIES

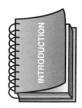

INTRODUCTION

Limited language skills are described by many terms: language delay, language disorder, specific language impairment, and language problem. Some children, who are normal in most respects yet manifest language problems, are described as having a *language-learning disability* (LLD). Children with LLD have certain characteristics that distinguish them from other populations.

Characteristics of Children with Language-Learning Disabilities

General Characteristics

■ Children with LLD manifest an impairment specific to language. This impairment is not demonstrated secondary to other developmental disabilities (Casby, 1997).

■ LLD children have no known etiology or associated condition such as a sensory-motor problem, mental retardation, or significant neurological impairment. LLD children may have deficiencies in certain cognitive functions, although general intelligence is within the normal range.

■ The sequence of language development in LLD children is the same as that seen in normally developing children. However, problems may be seen with various components of language.

■ LLD children display varied profiles. Some may have great difficulty in syntax, with relatively normal pragmatic performance and moderate difficulty with the semantic component of language, for example. LLD children represent a widely varied and heterogeneous group.

■ There are two major explanations of LLD. The first is that of *underlying deficits*. In this view, LLD is due to deficits in cognitive, auditory, perceptual, and intellectual functions that underlie language.

■ The second explanation is that LLD reflects the normal variation in linguistic skills, that LLD children are at the lower end of the normal continuum of language skills. Just as some people have poor math or musical skills, some people have poor linguistic skills (Leonard, 1991).

Specific Characteristics

■ Children with LLD often have articulatory and phonological problems. They may have poor speech intelligibility and may exhibit *phonological processes* (simplification rules such as final consonant deletion) longer than normal children.

■ LLD children may manifest less complex syllable structure; for example, they may use more consonant-vowel (CV) combinations than same-age peers who are using CVCV combinations. LLD children may also have fewer consonants in their phonetic repertoire.

■ Recent research has indicated that young LLD children with phonological problems are at risk for later problems with reading and spelling.

▓ LLD children are often late in starting to talk. They have a slow rate of word acquisition, especially between 18 and 24 months of age, when normal children show a great vocabulary spurt.

▓ LLD children often have *word-finding* or *word-retrieval problems*, in which they are unable to retrieve specific words appropriate to the situation. These word-finding problems may result in dysfluencies such as pauses and interjections or fillers (*um, you know*). Word-finding problems may also result in use of vague or general words (*this, that, thing*) instead of specific referents.

▓ Learning abstract or figurative words is often hard for LLD children. They frequently use concrete, not abstract words, to express themselves. For example, a child with LLD might say "I'm mad" instead of "I feel frustrated with this situation."

▓ The majority of LLD children have marked morphological problems. Experts believe that these problems may be due to:

  – *perceptual problems*; children do not perceive morphological features as well as they do other features, because those features are produced with less stress and lower intensity;

  – *syntactic problems*; the syntactic complexity involved in sentence comprehension and production may have a negative impact on morphology.

▓ Morphological problems include omissions of:

  – regular and irregular plural morphemes

  – possessive morphemes

  – present progressive *-ing*

  – third-person singular

  – articles (*a, an, the*)

  – auxiliary and copula verbs

  – regular and irregular past-tense inflections

▓ LLD children may also show confusion with the following structures:

  – singular and plural forms of words

  – plural and singular forms of auxiliary and copula verbs (*are, is*)

  – subject case markings (*him, he,* or *her, she*)

  – regular and irregular forms of plural and past-tense morphemes

▓ LLD children frequently have shorter utterances than normally developing children. Their MLU is shorter than that of normal peers.

▓ LLD children use transformations and complex and compound sentences less frequently or not at all; simple, declarative sentences may predominate.

■ The speech of some LLD young children is *telegraphic*. Instead of saying "The cat is eating her food," the child might say, "Cat eat food." The child preserves the meaning of the utterance while omitting the smaller grammatical elements.

■ Understanding or comprehending complex sentences is difficult for many LLD children. This especially presents problems in the classroom setting, where LLD students spend much of their time in large groups of normally developing children who understand complex teacher talk.

■ Pragmatic skills of LLD children vary greatly. Fey (1986) described two conversational components that can be seen, in different combinations, in LLD children:

  – *assertiveness*—the ability to initiate conversation or take a conversational turn when none has been solicited by the partner

  – *responsiveness*—how responsive the child is to the conversational partner

■ Many LLD children are passive—that is, unassertive and unresponsive—in communicative interactions. Other LLD children are assertive yet unresponsive; they initiate conversations but are unaware of and unresponsive to their partners' needs.

■ LLD children may have difficulty with the following aspects of pragmatics:

  – turn taking

  – topic maintenance

  – appropriate conversational repair strategies

  – discourse and narrative skills

■ LLD children's narratives are less complete, contain fewer utterances, and show more communication breakdowns than those of normally developing children.

Summary

☑ Children with LLD manifest an impairment specific to language. This impairment is not due to known etiological factors or associated conditions such as sensory-motor problems or mental retardation.

☑ Children with LLD generally show specific difficulties in all aspects of language skills: syntax, morphology, phonology, semantics, and pragmatics.

☑ However, there is great heterogeneity in the LLD population, with children manifesting different profiles of problems with various language components.

CHILDREN WITH LANGUAGE PROBLEMS ASSOCIATED WITH PHYSICAL AND SENSORY DISABILITIES

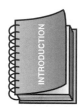

INTRODUCTION

Some children are born with conditions such as mental retardation or autism. While it cannot be said that these conditions *cause* language problems, it is known that language problems *coexist* with these conditions. In addition, children who experience brain injury usually have coexisting language and cognitive problems as a result.

Mental Retardation

■ Children with mental retardation (MR), also known as children who are "developmentally delayed," are a diverse group. Some are affected by inherited genetic syndromes such as Down syndrome; others are affected by environmentally induced genetic abnormalities. Consequently, children with MR show a variety of communicative problems.

■ The severity of these problems varies with the extent of the retardation. The greater the extent of the retardation, the more severe the communicative problems. The language of children with MR is deficient in phonologic, morphologic, semantic, syntactic, and pragmatic components.

■ Most experts agree that the language of children with MR is *delayed* rather than deviant. That is, children with MR show language skills that are commensurate with those of younger normally developing children; they follow the same *sequence* of language development as those children. However, profoundly retarded children may show *echolalia* (parrotlike repetition of what others say).

■ Some children with MR have concomitant problems, such as:

　— distractibility and a short attention span

　— congenital microcephaly ("small head")

　— difficulties with gross- and fine-motor skills

　— physical structural deficits such as a cleft palate

■ Cognitively, children with MR tend to have depressed skills. These children are very concrete and have difficulty with abstract concepts. This is thought to affect language skills, particularly semantic skills.

- Children with MR have semantic difficulties in that they frequently have smaller, more concrete vocabularies than normally developing children. There may be a gap between comprehension and expression skills, comprehension being superior to expression.

- Morphologic skills are especially poor in most children with MR. Due to the abstract nature of bound morphemes especially, many children with MR use telegraphic speech. Such children tend to omit bound morphemes and *function words*, or the small words that help make up sentences (e.g., instead of saying "The man is going to the store," children with MR might say, "Man go store.")

- The syntax of children with MR is reduced both expressively and receptively. They master syntactic constructions as normally developing children do but at a slower pace. They frequently use short and simple syntactic structures and have difficulty understanding long and complex sentences.

- Pragmatically, children with MR may be passive in interacting with others. Or, because of their reduced communication skills, they may be physically aggressive and communicate physically rather than verbally.

- Because many children with MR may have other problems (e.g., medical, gross motor), it is usually necessary to utilize a multidisciplinary approach to assessment and treatment.

✏ Concepts To Consider

Many parents believe that LLD and MR are the same thing and think that if their child is diagnosed as LLD, then their child has mental retardation. Describe how you would explain to a parent the differences between LLD and MR.

_____

_____

_____

_____

_____

_____

_____

_____

Autism

■ Leo Kanner (1943), a child psychiatrist, originally described *autism* as a profound emotional disorder of childhood. It was believed for many years that autism was a form of child psychosis. Currently, most experts support genetic or neurophysiological theories of autism, including hypotheses that cortical and/or subcortical dysfunction is involved.

■ Nowadays, the phenomenon is described as autism spectrum disorder. The term *autism spectrum disorder* implies that autism exists on a continuum of severity. For example, the term *pervasive developmental delay* is used to describe a child who demonstrates a basic impairment in communication and relating to others but does not meet all the formal criteria for autism. In this section, the term *autism* is used for purposes of consistency.

■ Characteristics of children with autism include:

- a lack of responsiveness to and awareness of other people

- a preference for solitude and objects rather than people

- a lack of interest in nonverbal and verbal communication

- stereotypic body movements such as rocking

- insistence on routines; strong dislike of change

- a dislike of being touched or held

- self-injurious behaviors such as head banging (in some children)

- unusual talent in some areas such as arithmetic

■ Specific language problems associated with autism include:

- inadequate or lack of response to speech

- lack of interest in human voices and a better response to environmental noises; a fascination with mechanical noises

- slow acquisition of speech sound production and language in general

- disinterest in interaction with others

- use of language in a meaningless, stereotypic manner including echolalia

- perseveration on certain words or phrases

- faster learning of concrete than abstract words, including more ready learning of words that refer to objects as opposed to emotions

- lack of generalization of word meanings

- lack of understanding of the relationships between words

- pronoun reversal (use of *you* for *I* and *I* for *you*; referring to self as *she, him,* or *her*)

- use of short, simple sentences; occasional use of incorrect word order

- omission of grammatic features such as plural inflections, conjunctions

- pragmatic problems such as lack of eye contact and lack of topic maintenance; reduced initiation or lack of assertiveness

- difficulty establishing joint reference

■ Children with autism may have associated problems, such as:

- motor deficits

- central auditory problems

- mental retardation

- evidence of brain injury, especially damage to the left cerebral hemisphere

- abnormal electrical activity of the brain

- seizures

- hearing loss

- hypo- or hypersensitivity to touch

■ Because many children with autism have one or more of these associated problems, it is frequently necessary to utilize a multidisciplinary team approach to assessment and intervention.

■ Treatment for autism has emphasized social skills training. Systematic and prolonged language training has resulted in meaningful communication patterns in many children. Behavioral management techniques, when combined with behavioral language training, have been shown to be effective. If the autism is severe, the use of alternative, augmentative communication devices may be warranted.

Brain Injury

Children can have brain injury due to various causes. Brain-injured children can be classified into various subgroups depending on the injury's cause and sequelae. Two major subgroups of brain-injured children include those who sustain injury due to head trauma (with resulting traumatic brain injury), and those who have cerebral palsy.

Traumatic Brain Injury (TBI)

■ TBI in children is cerebral damage due to external physical force. The injury is not congenital, nor is it a result of a neurological disease. A *focal injury* is restricted to one area of the brain; *diffuse injury* involves multiple areas because damage is widespread.

■ TBI in children is most frequently caused by vehicular and sports-related accidents, falls, physical abuse, assaults, and gunshot wounds.

■ A multidisciplinary team approach to assessment and treatment is always necessary. Medical personnel may be especially involved.

■ Immediate effects of TBI include:

- coma or loss of consciousness

- confusion and post-traumatic amnesia (memory loss)

- abnormal behaviors including possible aggression, anxiety, irritability, hyperactivity, lethargy, and withdrawal

- motor dysfunctions including tremors, rigidity, spasticity, ataxia, and apraxia

■ Cognitive and language problems can be associated with TBI. Some of these may be observed only initially and then may resolve; others may be long term:

- comprehension problems, especially of sentences

- word-retrieval problems leading to reduced fluency

- syntactic problems, including limited MLU, fewer utterances, and difficulty expressing and understanding long, complex sentences

- reading and writing problems; poor academic performance

- pragmatic problems such as difficulty with turn taking and topic maintenance (often related to poor inhibition and lack of self-monitoring)

- difficulty with attention and focus

- memory problems

- inability to recognize one's own difficulties

- reduced speed of information processing

- difficulties with reasoning and organization

■ Children with TBI have unique needs. Frequently, their problems may persist over time. A problem in the schools for children with TBI is that traditional, standardized language tests are often not sensitive to the special problems manifested by these children (Ylvisaker, 1995).

■ Children with TBI need to be assessed regularly in natural settings to determine how they are functioning in those settings. Such children should be served through a comprehensive team approach that helps them integrate back into school and society.

Cerebral Palsy

■ *Cerebral palsy* (CP) is a disorder of early childhood in which the immature nervous system is affected. This results in muscular incoordination and associated problems.

■ Associated problems may include orthopedic abnormalities, seizures, feeding difficulties, hearing loss, perceptual disturbances, and intellectual deficits. However, not all children with CP have all these problems.

■ CP is not a progressive disease. It generally occurs for the following reasons:

  – *prenatal brain injury* due to maternal rubella, mumps, accidents, or other factors

  – *perinatal brain injury* due to difficulties in the birth process such as prolonged labor, prematurity, breech delivery

  – *postnatal brain injury* due to anoxia, accidents, infections, and diseases such as scarlet fever and meningitis

■ Children with CP can manifest paralysis of various body parts. These can be categorized as follows:

  – *hemiplegia* (one side of the body, the right or left, is paralyzed)

  – *paraplegia* (only the legs and lower trunk are paralyzed)

  – *monoplegia* (only one limb or a part thereof is paralyzed)

  – *diplegia* (either the two legs or the two arms are paralyzed)

  – *quadriplegia* (all four limbs are paralyzed)

■ Although many types of CP have been described, most professionals categorize CP into three major types:

  – *ataxic CP*, which involves disturbed balance, awkward gait, and uncoordinated movements (due to cerebellar damage)

  – *athetoid CP*, which is characterized by slow, writhing, involuntary movements (due to damage to the indirect motor pathways, especially the basal ganglia)

  – *spastic CP*, which involves increased spasticity (increased tone, rigidity of the muscles) as well as stiff, abrupt, jerky, slow movements (due to damage to the motor cortex or direct motor pathways)

■ Speech and language problems associated with CP depend heavily on the type of CP and the presence of associated problems such as mental retardation. Some children with CP have normal language skills, while others have severe language problems.

■ Treatment for children with CP should involve a multidisciplinary team approach and the use of alternative, augmentative methods of communication if necessary.

Summary

☑ Children who have physical and sensory disabilities such as mental retardation, autism, and brain injury manifest unique language characteristics that tend to coexist with the disabilities.

☑ Children whose disabilities are severe may require the use of augmentative, alternative communication devices.

☑ A comprehensive team approach to assessment and treatment is necessary for children whose language problems co-occur with physical and sensory disabilities.

CHILDREN WITH LANGUAGE PROBLEMS RELATED TO PHYSICAL AND SOCIAL-ENVIRONMENTAL FACTORS

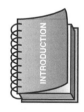

INTRODUCTION

Some children manifest language difficulties that are related to a combination of physical and social-environmental factors such as poverty, neglect or abuse, alcohol or drug exposure in utero, and attention-deficit disorders. Researchers and clinicians today are seeing increasing numbers of children who have a wide variety of language problems that coexist with these factors.

Language Problems Related to Poverty

■ There is no demonstrable causal or even correlational relationship between poverty and language-learning difficulties. Professionals should be careful never to equate poverty with dysfunction. Many children from low-income backgrounds have excellent language skills because they have had good stimulation in the home.

■ Other children, however, show problems in language development and learning. Research shows that while not directly causing language problems, limited access to health care and low educational levels of caretakers tend to affect the language skills of children from low-income homes (Roseberry-McKibbin & Brice, 1998).

▢ Socioeconomic status is more critical to language development than ethnic background. The factor most highly related to socioeconomic status is the mother's educational level (Battle & Anderson, 1998).

▢ Limited access to health care can affect language skills because:

— children who are often sick and do not get adequate medical treatment miss much school, thus limiting academic and language exposure;

— children who come to school sick have difficulty concentrating and learning;

— children who do not have access to medical care frequently have untreated ear infections;

— mothers of low-income children often get inadequate prenatal care, which affects the development of the fetus's central nervous system;

— mothers who get inadequate prenatal care tend to have premature and/or low-birthweight babies; prematurity and low birth weight are associated with language and cognition problems.

▢ Research has documented a strong correlation between education and income levels. Studies show that long-term welfare dependency is strongly associated with lack of a high school diploma and low literacy levels (Friedlander & Martinson, 1996). This may affect the language development of children from low-income homes because some caretakers who have had limited educational opportunities may not :

— provide adequate oral language stimulation for their children

— provide opportunities for literacy

— have the economic means to expose their children to a variety of enriching experiences (e.g., trips to zoos, museums)

— have the economic means to purchase toys and books that stimulate language development

▢ Children from backgrounds of poverty show wide variation in their language skills. Some of these children have excellent language skills. Others show such deficits as the following:

— difficulty in reading and writing;

— difficulty referencing time and temporal concepts due to a lack of routine and structure in the home;

— lack of familiarity with "school-type" tasks such as reciting the alphabet, singing rhyming songs, reading books;

    – delayed vocabulary skills due to lack of language stimulation and lack of exposure to a variety of experiences;

    – delayed morphosyntactic skills;

    – less verbal elaboration and overall verbalization.

Language Problems Related to Neglect or Abuse

- Statistics indicate that increasing numbers of children come from backgrounds in which they experience neglect, abuse, or both (NA). NA can be found across all socioeconomic levels and ethnic groups.

- The effect of NA on language depends greatly upon the *extent* and *severity* of the NA. A child who regularly undergoes severe physical, emotional, or verbal abuse, or all of these, will have more severe language problems than the child who experiences neglect without abuse.

- While it is difficult to make generalizations about this heterogeneous group of children, certain trends have emerged characterizing the effect of NA on language development and skills.

- Among mother-child pairs in which abuse has been identified, mothers have been observed to be less likely to engage in reciprocal interactions with their infants. In addition, some of these mothers have been found to punish normal exploration and risk-taking that accompany development (Nelson, 1998).

- Children who undergo abuse tend to have *expressive language delays*. Some of these children are hit or yelled at when they speak; thus, they speak less and therefore do not develop oral language optimally.

- Children who experience NA are frequently deprived of adequate language stimulation related to *isolation*. Physical or social isolation or both reduces the human contacts needed to acquire language optimally. Children's opportunities for hearing and practicing a variety of language structures are reduced. Thus, expressive and receptive language skills are underdeveloped.

- Research has shown a relationship between communicative disorders (particularly those associated with physical anomalies and disabilities) and NA. Parents of children with special needs tend to become frustrated more easily than parents of normally developing children. Frustration creates stress, which can lead to NA.

- To best serve children who experience NA, speech–language pathologists may serve on multidisciplinary teams that address the emotional and physical as well as the language needs presented by these children.

✎ Concepts To Consider

List two language problems (per area) one might find in children who (a) have autism, (b) have experienced TBI, (c) have cerebral palsy, (d) are from low-income backgrounds, or (e) have experienced neglect and/or abuse.

_____

_____

_____

_____

_____

_____

_____

_____

Language Problems Related to Parental Drug and Alcohol Use

■ Speech–language pathologists are participating on multidisciplinary teams to serve increasing numbers of children who have language problems related to maternal alcohol consumption and/or drug use during pregnancy. Children who have been prenatally exposed to drugs, alcohol, or both present a wide variety of problems depending on the extent, pattern, and type of exposure to such substances.

■ Recent research has shown that *paternal* alcohol consumption, drug use, smoking, or exposure to environmental toxins can also negatively affect fetal development. Sperm can be damaged by cigarette smoke, marijuana, and alcohol. Men exposed to those teratogens have a greater chance of fathering babies with abnormalities like hydrocephalus, Bell's palsy (paralysis of cranial nerve VII), and mouth cysts.

■ *Fetal alcohol syndrome* (FAS) is a pattern of mental, physical, and behavioral defects that develop in infants born to some women who drink heavily during the pregnancy. FAS is the leading cause of mental retardation in the Western world.

■ FAS causes direct language problems and creates difficulties in areas associated with language development. Problems associated with FAS include:

  – pre- and post-natal growth problems; abnormally low birth weight and length; small head size (microcephaly);

- central nervous system dysfunction: delayed motor development, mild-profound mental retardation or learning disabilities;

- abnormal craniofacial (skull and face) features;

- malformations of major organ systems, especially of the heart; the child may have a small trachea and kidney problems;

- behavior problems, including hyperactivity and attention-deficit disorder;

- poor play and social skills, including poor organizational responses to environmental stimuli;

- learning and academic problems; poor reading, writing;

- speech problems such as articulation delay; may have cleft palate or oral-motor coordination problems;

- swallowing problems, including impaired sucking reflex at birth;

- language delays;

- cognitive problems—reasoning, memory, learning;

- auditory processing problems;

- hearing problems—conductive and sensorineural losses.

■ *Fetal alcohol effects* (FAE) are signs in babies (e.g., mild physical and cognitive deficits) that have been linked to the mother's drinking during pregnancy. Babies with FAE do not meet the diagnostic criteria for FAS.

■ Children who are prenatally exposed to drugs also have difficulties in language and related skills. Some of these difficulties include the following:

- in motor/neurological development

  • poor visual tracking

  • blanking out, staring spells, bizarre eye movements

  • gross- and fine-motor problems

  • tremors; increased startling

  • decreased awareness of body in space

- in affective/behavioral development

  • emotional lability; mood swings from apathy to aggressiveness

  • depressed affect, decreased laughter

  • great difficulty with transitions and changes

  • refusal to comply with simple commands; testing of limits

  • inability to self-regulate, modify own behavior

- in social attachment, development

  - decreased use of eye contact, gestures to initiate social interaction

  - separation anxiety

  - indiscriminate attachment to new people

  - aggressiveness with peers

  - decreased responsiveness to praise, rewards

- in cognitive skills

  - poor on-task attention

  - increased distractibility to extraneous sounds, movements

  - impulsivity; poor use of trial-and-error strategies

  - difficulty with immediate, short-term, and long-term memory

- in language development

  - fewer spontaneous vocalizations from infancy

  - delayed language acquisition

  - decreased use of words, gestures to communicate wants and needs

  - word-finding problems

  - prolonged infantile articulatory-phonological disorders

  - difficulty following directions

  - difficulty answering wh-questions

  - difficulty understanding opposites, uses for objects

- Children prenatally exposed to drugs and alcohol may have language problems that are not readily detected by standardized language measures. Thus, such children may be denied services in the public schools because they do not fit a recognized category such as *learning disabled* or *mentally retarded*.

- Early intervention is critical with drug- and alcohol-exposed children. These children appear to especially benefit from structure and routine. Caregivers need to be involved as much as possible in treatment efforts.

Language Problems Related to Attention-Deficit Disorder

- Speech–language pathologists are seeing increasing numbers of students with language problems related to *attention-deficit disorder* (ADD). The nature of this relationship is not clear, but many students with ADD also manifest language problems, auditory-processing problems, or both. Thus, speech–language pathologists are increasingly involved on multidisciplinary teams that identify and serve students with ADD.

- Students with ADD are at risk because they frequently experience academic and behavior problems. In some cases, language and auditory-processing difficulties contribute to those problems. It is important for clinicians to provide intervention in cases where these factors are present.

- Students with ADD are described as having chronic difficulties in the areas of impulsivity, attention, and overactivity to a degree inappropriate to their age and developmental level. They are more likely to receive lower grades in academic subjects, and over half of children with ADD will fail at least one grade by adolescence (Westby & Cutler, 1994).

- Behavioral characteristics of ADD students include:

  - frequent fidgeting with hands or feet or squirming in seats
  - difficulty remaining seated when required to do so
  - high distractibility by extraneous stimuli
  - difficulty sustaining attention in tasks or activities
  - difficulty waiting turns in games or group situations
  - frequent loss of things necessary for tasks or activities at school or at home
  - frequent participation in physically dangerous activities without considering the possible consequences

- Research and clinical experience indicate that students with ADD tend to manifest the greatest amount of difficulty in auditory processing and social interaction skills. Specifically, ADD students (England, 1994; Westby & Cutler, 1994):

  - often blurt out answers to questions before the questions have been completed;
  - have difficulty following through on instructions;
  - often do not seem to be listening;
  - often talk excessively;
  - often interrupt or intrude on others;
  - use non sequiturs during discourse;
  - have poor turn-taking skills
  - frequently manifest false starts because they change their minds while structuring a response;
  - use an excessive number of fillers and pauses because verbal expression occurs with minimal preplanning;
  - have difficulty describing things in an organized, coherent manner— have general difficulty with expressive language organization;

- do not tell stories or use narrative skills effectively due to disorganization and impulsivity of thought;

- have difficulty with social entry (limited knowledge of how to successfully initiate or join ongoing interactions);

- experience problems with verbal reciprocity, tend to be less talkative and responsive when others initiate interactions;

- use inappropriate register; for example, use the same interactive style with adults and peers;

- do not perceive or act appropriately upon interlocutors' nonverbal cues;

- do not use comprehension monitoring strategies; for example, do not request a repetition of information when they experience a comprehension breakdown.

■ Speech–language pathologists must become actively involved in interdisciplinary, collaborative teams that create effective service delivery models for students with ADD. Goals of treatment may include work on auditory-processing skills, pragmatics, and expressive language organization.

Summary

☑ Increasing numbers of children have language problems related to physical and social-environmental factors such as poverty, neglect or abuse, alcohol or drug exposure in utero, and attention-deficit disorders.

☑ Speech–language pathologists are increasingly serving on multidisciplinary teams that address the comprehensive profile of needs presented by these children.

ASSESSMENT PRINCIPLES AND PROCEDURES

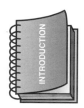

INTRODUCTION

Language assessment is a process of observation and measurement of a child's language behaviors to determine (a) whether a clinically significant problem exists, (b) the nature and extent of the problem, and (c) the course of action that must be taken to help the child. In this section, we discuss common underlying procedures and principles that can be applied to children of any age, use of standardized and nonstandardized forms of assessment, and specific recommendations for preschool children, elementary-aged children, and adolescents.

Language Assessment: General Principles and Procedures

■ Whatever the age of the child being assessed, clinicians typically follow a set of common procedures that serve as the foundation for the assessment (Hegde, 1996a):

  – obtain results of visual and/or audiological evaluations;

  – obtain any available relevant medical data that might be important;

  – obtain psychological data, including the results of cognitive functioning and intelligence testing; and

  – for elementary-aged and adolescent students:

    • obtain assessment data on educational achievement that might suggest learning disabilities

    • obtain samples of the student's writing from his or her teachers

    • examine classroom textbooks to select words, phrases, and sentences that could be included in the assessment

■ Language assessment generally falls into three broad categories: screening, standardized assessment, and nonstandardized or informal assessment.

Screening

■ Screening refers to the process of quickly obtaining a general overview of a child's language skills.

■ Most clinicians use screening initially to decide whether further assessment is necessary. Screening usually indicates one of two things: (a) there is not a clinically significant language problem, and no further assessment needs to be completed, or (b) there is a possible language problem and further assessment is needed.

■ Many clinicians use informal measures to screen language. These are often constructed by individual clinicians and consist of simple activities such as conversational samples that quickly sample children's expressive and receptive language skills. Published screening tests are also available.

Standardized Assessment

■ Standardized tests provide clinicians with a quantitative means of comparing the child's performance to the performance of large groups of children in a similar age category (Johnson, 1996).

■ Standardized tests are preferred by many clinicians because they yield quantitative, psychometrically based measures such as language age, percentile rank, and standard deviation. Federal or state laws may require the use of these quantitative measures for placement of a child into special education services within the public school system (Klein & Moses, 1999).

■ When using standardized tests, clinicians must consider *subject sampling*. All standardized tests sample subjects, and few or no tests sample all segments of the population. Therefore, many tests are not applicable across all population groups. This is especially true of culturally and linguistically diverse populations because of their underrepresentation in the normative samples.

■ It is important to avoid using a test whose normative sample does not include subjects who represent the child being tested. Clinicians must consider all relevant variables: socioeconomic class, urban or rural environment, and ethnocultural and linguistic background (Roseberry-McKibbin, 1995).

■ Standardized tests, even when they sample subjects adequately, tend to sample behaviors inadequately. For example, a behavior tested, such as use of a regular plural, is tested only in one or two contexts. This is inadequate sampling. Clinicians must follow-up standardized tests with extended, informal sampling of behaviors targeted on items a child has missed on a standardized test.

■ Clinicians must avoid using a standardized test as the sole measure for making clinical judgments about a child's language skills and the presence of a language-learning disability. Standardized tests should be supplemented with language samples and other informal measures.

Nonstandardized, Informal Assessment

■ Although widespread use of standardized language tests continues in the United States, many researchers and clinicians are increasingly turning to informal, nonstandardized measures of language. There are several reasons for this.

■ One major reason is that the use of standardized tests is often biased and inappropriate with the increasing number of linguistically and culturally diverse students in the United States.

■ Another reason is that many standardized tests do not reflect children's day-to-day lives and functional communication skills and needs. Some professionals view standardized tests as artificial measures of formal, noncontextual language that is not reflective of children's language interaction in daily life. Thus, clinicians are increasingly using several current major alternatives to standardized tests.

Individualized Assessment

- *Client-specific procedures* are a preferred alternative to standardized tests. Client-specific procedures form a valid basis for developing client-specific treatments. These procedures utilize the evocation of language samples over time, using culturally appropriate client-specific materials instead of standard stimuli.

- *Baselines* can be used as *extended measurements*. Baselines are measures of target behaviors in the absence of planned treatment. Clinicians can establish baselines of communicative behaviors targeted for treatment. Because they are extended and repeated, baselines provide more reliable assessment data than tests and other procedures.

Authentic Assessment

- *Dynamic assessment*, a form of authentic assessment, looks at learner modifiability, or a child's ability to learn when provided with instruction. It often takes place in a test-teach-retest paradigm, in which the child is tested, taught new material, and then retested to see how well and quickly he or she learned the material. A major advantage of dynamic assessment is that a child is not penalized for a lack of experiences assumed by many standardized tests (Roseberry-McKibbin, 1995).

- *Portfolio assessment*, another form of authentic assessment that is popular in many public schools, involves collecting samples of a child's work or performance over a period of time and observing the growth that occurs when instruction is provided.

Social Assessment Methods (Gallagher, 1991)

- *Peer assessment*. Peers can be interviewed as to their perceptions of the child as an interlocutor, classmate, and/or friend.

- *Teacher and parent assessment*. Interviews and rating instruments can be filled out by teachers and parents indicating their perceptions of the student's language skills.

- *Self-assessment*. The student can fill out a rating scale, complete an interview, or use a combination of these to assess his or her own language skills and language needs.

Language Sampling

- Language sampling is a measure of language vital to a diagnosis of language disorders in children. This is a procedure of recording a student's language under relatively normal conditions, which usually involve conversation.

■ The clinician's main task in obtaining a language sample is to stimulate the child to speak as freely and naturally as possible. This can be accomplished through the use of a variety of toys, books, stories, pictures, and games. Other conversation partners, such as peers and family members, may interact with the child.

■ Clinicians need to remember that a single language sample is not sufficient; additional samples must be obtained. Brief language samples should be recorded subsequent to the first sample.

■ Clinicians may informally analyze a language sample or use a number of published protocols that are available. These include *Language Assessment, Remediation, and Screening Procedure* (LARSP; Crystal, Fletcher, & Garman, 1976); *Developmental Sentence Scoring* (Lee, 1974); and *Language Sampling, Analysis, and Training Procedure* (LSAT; Tyack & Gottsleben, 1974).

■ Some language sampling programs are available on computer; these include *Computerized Profiling* (Long & Fey, 1993); *Lingquest 1* (Mordecai & Palin, 1982); and *Systematic Analysis of Language Transcripts* (SALT; Miller & Chapman, 1983).

■ Many clinicians use a language sample to obtain a measure of a child's *mean length of utterance* (MLU), which is usually calculated in morphemes through the following method:

$$MLU = \frac{\text{number of morphemes}}{\text{number of utterances}}$$

■ Clinicians can analyze not only the child's MLU, but also the presence or absence of Brown's 14 grammatical morphemes (see Chapter 3, Table 3.3).

■ Language samples can also be analyzed through a *type-token ratio* (TTR), which is calculated as follows:

$$TTR = \frac{\text{number of different words in sample}}{\text{total number of words in sample}}$$

■ TTR represents the variety of different words the child uses expressively. To calculate TTR as shown above, the clinician first counts all the words in the sample (even if they're repeated). These words become the denominator. The clinician then counts each different word in the sample—for example, if "dog" occurs 10 times, the clinician counts it only once. The number of different words the child uses becomes the numerator. For children 3–8 years of age, the TTR is typically 1:2, or .5. In other words, the total number of words spoken by the child during the language sample is usually about twice the number of different words in the sample (Johnson, 1996).

✎ Concepts To Consider

Briefly compare and contrast standardized, formal language assessment and non-standardized, informal language assessment. In what situations would you want to use each type of assessment?

_____

_____

_____

_____

_____

_____

_____

Assessment of Infants and Toddlers

■ The assessment and treatment of infants and toddlers has taken on increasing visibility in past years. There are several reasons for this. First, laws such as P.L. 99-457 have provided incentives at the state and federal levels for speech–language pathologists to identify and treat infants and toddlers with established risk of language disorders or who experience conditions that put them at risk for developing language disorders.

■ Second, due to advances in medical science, many more medically fragile pre-term infants are surviving; these infants often have needs in multiple areas such as speech and language, motor skills, and others. The assessment of infants and toddlers holds special challenges for clinicians, who must account for risk factors as well as overt language problems.

Risk Factors for Language Disorders in Infants and Toddlers

■ As mentioned, infants and toddlers may fall into one of two categories: those with an _established risk_ of developing language disorders, and those who experience conditions that put them _at risk_ of developing language disorders.

■ Factors involving an _established risk_ of developing language disorders are mostly biological or disease related. These factors include (Rossetti, 1996):

- congenital malformations (e.g., cleft palate, spina bifida)

- genetic syndromes (e.g., Down syndrome)

- atypical developmental disorders (e.g., autism)

- sensory disorders (e.g., hearing loss, visual impairment)

- neurologic disorders (e.g., cerebral palsy, muscular dystrophy)

- metabolic disorders (e.g., Tay-Sachs disease, pituitary diseases)

- chronic illnesses (e.g., diabetes, cystic fibrosis)

- severe infectious diseases (e.g., HIV, encephalitis)

- severe toxic exposure (e.g., lead poisoning, fetal alcohol syndrome)

■ Conditions that place children *at risk* for developing language disorders include environmental factors, genetic background, and some disease-related conditions (Rossetti, 1996):

- serious prenatal and natal complications, including low birth weight (<1,500 g), child being small for gestation age (<10th percentile), and anoxia;

- early signs of behavior disorders (e.g., irritability, withdrawal);

- child's tendency toward frequent and unusual accidents;

- chronic middle ear infections (otitis media);

- family history of predisposing genetic or medical conditions;

- chronic or severe physical illness, mental illness, or mental retardation in the primary caregiver or one or both parents;

- serious questions raised by a professional, a parent, or a caregiver about the child's development;

- chronically dysfunctional interaction between members of the family;

- caregiver or parental substance abuse; caregiver or parental history of abuse;

- parental education below ninth grade, parental unemployment, or chronic welfare dependency;

- isolation of the child or separation of the child from the primary caretaker or parent;

- unstable or dangerous living conditions (e.g., homelessness);

- lack of health insurance; poor family health care; inadequate prenatal care.

Prelinguistic Behavioral Deficiencies

■ Although language problems in infants and toddlers may be caused by or associated with many factors, such as those listed above, some infants who later exhibit LLD may not show primary impairment. Several characteristics distinguish such infants:

- difficulty establishing eye contact, mutual gaze, and joint reference;

- communication of needs through greater use of gestures and vocalizations than words and phrases; frequent delays in onset of first word and onset of two-word combinations;

- reduced amount of babbling, fewer consonants during babbling, and less complex babbling.

General Assessment Guidelines and Procedures

■ Make a family-centered communication assessment of infants and toddlers in both home and clinic settings (Hegde, 1996a).

■ Begin assessment as early as possible and repeat assessments throughout the childhood period. Assess the family constellation, family resources, family strengths and limitations, and family communication patterns.

■ Work on a team with other professionals. Make interdisciplinary decisions regarding assessment materials and methods and how assessment results will be used.

■ Conduct interviews and gather an extensive case history, including maternal health during pregnancy, circumstances of the birth, and early development patterns of the infant (e.g., fine and gross motor, speech and language).

■ Take into consideration the cultural practices in family communication patterns, child rearing, caretaker-child interactions, and accepted roles for children in adult-child interactions.

Specific Assessment Guidelines and Procedures

■ With infants and toddlers (depending upon the age), clinicians generally need to assess language-related areas such as hearing and infant readiness for communication as well as language comprehension, verbal communication, infant-caregiver interaction, and play activities.

Language-Related Areas

■ Assess the infant's attentional and physiological state (including alertness, drowsiness, light or deep sleep states, eye opening, crying, toleration of handling, etc.).

■ Assess the infant's readiness for communication (e.g., whether the baby shows reciprocal interaction with the environment).

■ If necessary, refer the infant to an audiologist.

Language Comprehension and Verbal Communication

- ▓ Use language development milestones (see Chapter 3) to assess the presence or absence of verbal communication behaviors as well as language comprehension skills. This can be done through direct observation, parent report, or both.

Infant-Caregiver Interaction

- ▓ Use instruments such as the *Mother-Infant Play Interaction Scale* by Walker and Thompson (1982) and the *Observation of Communication Interaction* by Klein and Briggs (1986). These instruments offer suggestions for observing the baby and the mother or another caregiver, preferably in the home setting or in a natural interactive clinical situation. These instruments help assess:

  - the infant's mood and affect, responsiveness or lack thereof;

  - how the caregiver modifies the interaction when the infant gives negative cues (e.g., when the infant is tired of peek-a-boo and averts her gaze, the caregiver changes activities);

  - how the caregiver visually focuses on the baby (e.g., the caregiver holds or places the infant at his or her eye level and maintains eye contact);

  - how the caregiver stimulates and handles the baby (holding, rocking, cuddling, stroking);

  - how the caregiver expresses his or her affection for the baby (smiling and laughing, for example).

Play Activities

- ▓ Observe the child engaged in play with one or several other children. Observe the child's pattern of interaction during play and evaluate whether the child:

  - exhibits aggressive or uncooperative behaviors

  - does not share toys

  - talks little during play

  - passively watches others play

  - plays cooperatively with other children

  - engages in isolated or parallel play

  - engages in constructive activities with or alongside other children

  - engages in pretend play and role playing

Published Assessment Instruments

Few standardized instruments are available to use in the assessment of children under 3 years of age. Most instruments for children age 3 and under are developmental scales that help structure clinicians' and/or parents' observations of the child to take note of the presence or absence of behaviors of interest. Clinicians can also use the developmental milestones list in Chapter 3 to structure individualized assessments for infants and toddlers. Clinicians can consider using the published instruments listed in Table 4.1.

TABLE 4.1

Commonly Used Published Assessment Instruments for Infants and Toddlers

Assessment Instrument	Description
Preschool Language Scale–3 (I. Zimmerman, V. Steiner, & R. Pond)	Used to assess expressive and receptive language in infants and children through 6-11 years
Birth to 3 Developmental Scale (T.S. Bangs & S. Dodson)	Used to assess developmental delays in multiple areas
Early Language Milestone Scale (2nd ed.) (J. Coplan)	Used to assess speech and language development in children from birth through 3 years
Bayley Scales of Infant Mental Development–Revised (N. Bayley)	Used to assess cognitive, psychomotor, social, visual, and auditory skills in infants
Sequenced Inventory of Communication Development –Revised (D. Hedrick, E. Prather, & A. Tobin)	Used to assess nonverbal and verbal communication in infants and children through 4 years
Receptive-Expressive Emergent Language Test–2 (K. Bzoch & R. League)	Used to interview parents and gain a multidimensional analysis of emergent language in children from birth through 3 years
Battelle Developmental Inventory (J. Newbord, J. Stock, L. Wnek, J. Guidubaldi, & J. Svinicki)	Used to assess the following skills in infants: memory, discrimination, perceptual, conceptual, motor, adaptive, and communication
Rossetti Infant-Toddler Language Scale (L. Rossetti)	Used to assess interaction and communication patterns in infants and toddlers
Communication and Symbolic Behavior Scales (A.M. Wetherby & B. Prizant)	Used to assess nonverbal and verbal communication patterns in infants and children through 6 years
Assessment of Preterm Infant Behavior (H. Als, B. Lester, E. Tronick, & T. Brazelton)	Used with infants in NICU (neonatal intensive care unit); assesses attentional and physiological states
Vineland Adaptive Behavior Scale (S. Sparrow, D. Balla, & D. Cicchetti)	Used to assess daily living, socialization, and motor skills as well as receptive and expressive language in infants and toddlers
Preschool Language Assessment Instrument (M. Blank, S.A. Rose, & L.J. Berlin)	Used from ages 3–0 to 5–11 to assess ability to integrate vocabulary and language structure knowledge to solve problems and follow directions (also available in Spanish)

Assessment of Preschool and Elementary-Aged Children

■ Language problems often become apparent during the elementary school years. They are frequently brought to the surface by reading and writing deficiencies that cause academic problems and even failure. It is when children experience academic difficulties that they are usually referred for speech–language assessment. In ideal circumstances, language problems would be noted and dealt with when children are in preschool.

Description of Language Disorders in Preschool and Elementary-Aged Children

Language problems of preschool and elementary-aged children can be associated with a variety of factors such as language-learning disability, mental retardation, environmental factors, and others. Characteristics of such children with language problems can include the following:

■ *Difficulty in comprehending spoken language.* This includes problems with comprehending syntactically longer and more complex productions as well as difficulty comprehending meaning of complex words, phrases, sentences, and abstract terms.

■ *Slow or delayed language onset.* This can include delayed babbling, slower vocabulary growth rate, delayed acquisition of vocabulary, slowness in combining words into phrases and sentences, and overall slower acquisition of language milestones.

■ *Limited amount of language output or expressive language.* This includes generally limited verbal repertoire, lack of complex or longer word productions, limited amount of vocabulary produced and comprehended, and lack of abstract words in the child's repertoire.

■ *Problematic syntactic skills.* This includes use of shorter instead of longer sentences, simpler instead of more complex sentences, single words or phrases in place of sentences, and a limited variety of syntactic structures.

■ *Problematic pragmatic skills.* This includes difficulty with initiating and maintaining conversations, turn taking, using conversational repair strategies, maintaining eye contact, and narrative skills.

■ *Problematic learning of grammatic morphemes.* This includes difficulty with comparatives and superlatives (e.g., *small, smaller, smallest*), omission of bound morphemes (e.g., past tense-*ed*, plural-*s*), and incorrect use of learned grammatic morphemes, including overgeneralizations (e.g., *womans/women, goed/went*) past the appropriate developmental point.

General Assessment Guidelines and Procedures

■ Begin by screening language to determine if a more detailed assessment is needed; do this through brief language sampling or through formal screening measures such as those listed in Table 4.2.

■ Obtain a case history.

■ Use social assessment methodologies; conduct interviews as appropriate and necessary. Obtain information from parents, teachers, and peers about the child's communication patterns.

■ Evaluate semantic, syntactic, morphologic, and pragmatic aspects of expressive and receptive oral language.

■ Evaluate reading and writing skills if relevant, and relate communication skills to academic demands and performance if relevant.

■ Assess the family constellation and communication patterns. Consider factors related to bilingualism, second-language acquisition, and use of a social dialect if relevant.

■ Suggest treatment targets based on the findings generated by use of these assessment procedures.

Specific Assessment Guidelines and Procedures

Obtain an extended speech and language sample for a typical analysis of language functions. Language samples can be collected on different days with different interlocutors (e.g., peers, teachers, family members) over a period of time in order to obtain the most representative sample of the child's language.

TABLE 4.2
Commonly Used Standardized Screening Measures

Assessment Instrument	Description
Denver Developmental Screening Test II (W.K. Frankenburg & Associates)	Used from age 2 weeks to 6 years to assess motor, language, and personal-social development
The Communication Screen (N. Striffler & S. Willig)	Used from age 2-10 to 5-9 to assess auditory comprehension and vocabulary skills
Preschool Language Screening Test (E. Hannah & J. Gardner)	Used from age 3 to 5-6 to assess motor, visual, and auditory perceptual concepts
Bankson Language Screening Test–2 (N.W. Bankson)	Used from age 4 to 7 to screen syntactic, semantic, and morphologic skills and visual and auditory perception
Fluharty Preschool Speech and Language Screening Test–3 (N. B. Fluharty)	Used from age 2 to 6 to screen basic language skills

- Language samples can be analyzed and a description given of the child's skills in the areas of semantics, morphology, syntax, and pragmatics. Language comprehension can also be analyzed.

- To assess *syntactic skills*, calculate the child's mean length of utterance (MLU), as well as the complexity of his or her utterances. Evaluate the child's use of:

  - verb phrases (e.g., *he is swimming, that is red*)

  - noun phrases (e.g., *my books, big dress, that crayon*)

  - prepositional phrases (e.g., *the crayons in the box*)

  - sentence types such as simple, declarative, compound, complex, active, questions, negatives, and requests

- To assess *morphologic skills*:

  - use appropriate pictures to assess a child's production of regular and irregular plural nouns as well as present progressive -*ing* (e.g., "What are these things? What is the boy doing?")

  - assess production of comparatives and superlatives by showing three pictures and saying things like, "This man is big; this man is even _____, and this man is the very ____.")

  - evoke the possessive morpheme by showing pictures and asking questions such as "whose hat is this?"

  - evoke the production of the third-person singular by asking such questions as "What flies?" and "Who cooks?" after showing pictures of a bird flying and a man cooking

  - assess production of adjectives by showing pictures and asking the child to complete such sentences as "This boy is..." (short); "This car is..." (green); and so forth

  - evoke past-tense constructions by telling a story, through pictures, and then asking the child to use the pictures to retell the story

- To assess *semantic skills*:

  - ask parents to list words the child uses, especially if the child only produces a few words

  - ask parents to describe the types and number of words the child uses at home

  - have the child name and describe pictures, toys, and objects as you show them

  - have a child tell a story depicted pictorially (e.g., using a book or cards)

  - tell the child a short story and then have the child retell the story to you

- note phenomena such as unusual word usage, over- and underextensions of words, signs of misunderstanding words, and the use of general terms (e.g., *this, that, thing*) for more specific ones

■ To assess *pragmatic skills*, observe the following parameters:

- eye contact and other nonverbal behaviors

- narrative skills

- topic initiation and maintenance

- turn-taking skills

- conversational repair—is the child able to ask questions when messages are not clear, and to respond effectively to listener requests for clarification?

■ To assess *language comprehension:*

- note inappropriate or irrelevant responses that indicate lack of comprehension

- note the complexity level at which comprehension breaks down (e.g., comprehension of phrases or sentences but not paragraphs)

- give specific commands that gradually increase in length and complexity (e.g., "Point to the blue square," "Point to the small blue square," "Point to the blue square and the green triangle," "Point to the big blue square and the small green triangle")

- ask the child to point to correct pictures that help assess comprehension of grammatic morphemes (e.g., "Show me *the dog is barking*" "Show me *the ball is in the bag*" "Show me *three shoes*")

- assess comprehension of abstract statements by asking the child to explain the meaning of common proverbs (e.g., "Tell me what 'A penny saved is a penny earned' means"). It is important to remember that proverbs and other figurative language expressions are extremely culture bound.

Standardized Tests

State and federal laws frequently require the use of formal scores, gathered from formal tests, for the diagnosis of a language disorder in a preschool or elementary-aged child. Clinicians can choose from the standardized tests listed in Table 4.3.

TABLE 4.3

Commonly Used Standardized Tests of Children's Language Skills

Standardized Test	Description
Assessment of Children's Language Comprehension (R. Foster, J.J. Giddan, & J. Stark)	Used from age 3 to 6-11 to assess receptive syntax and vocabulary
Test of Auditory Comprehension of Language–3 (E. Carrow-Woolfolk)	Used from age 3 to 9 to assess comprehension of grammatic features, word classes and relations, elaborated sentence constructions
Peabody Picture Vocabulary Test–III (L.M. Dunn & L.M. Dunn)	Used from age 2-6 to adult to assess receptive knowledge of single words
Receptive One-Word Picture Vocabulary Test–Revised (M.F. Gardner)	Used from age 2-11 to 12 to assess comprehension of single words
Expressive One-Word Picture Vocabulary Test–Revised (M.F. Gardner)	Used from age 2 to 11-11 to assess production of single words
Boehm Test of Basic Concepts (A.E. Boehm)	Used from kindergarten to second grade to assess comprehension of basic semantic concepts
Clinical Evaluation of Language Fundamentals–3 (E. Semel, E. Wiig, & W. Secord)	Used from age 6 to 21-11 to assess receptive and expressive syntax, morphology, and semantics
Detroit Test of Learning Aptitude–Primary–2. (D.D. Hammill & B.R. Bryant)	Used from age 3-6 to 9-11 to assess motoric, cognitive, linguistic, attentional domains
Multilevel Informal Language Inventory (C. Goldsworthy & W. Secord)	Used from age 4 to 12 to assess expressive semantics, morphology, and syntax
Test for Examining Expressive Morphology (K.G. Shipley, T. Stone, & M. Sue)	Used from age 3 to 8-11 to assess production of various morphemes
Test of Early Language Development–3 (W.P. Hresko, D.K. Reid, & D.D. Hammill)	Used from age 2-7 to 7-11 to assess production and comprehension of syntactic and semantic structures
Test of Language Development–Primary–3 (P.L. Newcomer & D.D. Hammill)	Used from age 4 to 8-11 to assess expressive and receptive semantics, syntax, and morphology
Language Processing Test–Revised (G.J. Richard & M.A. Hanner)	Used from age 5 to 11 to assess verbal reasoning and expressive vocabulary
Test of Language Development–Intermediate:3 (D.D. Hammill & P.L. Newcomer)	Used from age 8-0 to 12-11 to assess receptive and expressive syntax and semantics and articulation
Test of Word Finding–2 (D.J. German)	Used from age 6-6 to 12-11 to assess single-word retrieval skills
The WORD Test–Elementary–Revised (R. Huisingh, M. Barrett, L. Zachman, C. Bladgen, & J. Orman)	Used from age 7 to 11 to assess expressive vocabulary and semantic skills
Bankson Language Test–2 (N.W. Bankson)	Used from age 3-0 to 6-11 to assess pragmatics, semantic knowledge, and morphology and syntax
Test of Pragmatic Skills–Revised (B.B. Shulman)	Used from age 3 to 8-11 to assess nonverbal and verbal pragmatic skills
Utah Test of Language Development–4 (M.J. Mecham)	Used from age 3 to 9-11 to assess language expression and comprehension
Token Test for Children (F. DiSimoni)	Used from age 3 to 11-11 to assess auditory comprehension of spatial and temporal concepts
Comprehensive Receptive and Expressive Vocabulary Test (G. Wallace & D.D. Hammill)	Used from age 4 to 17-11 to assess receptive and expressive oral vocabulary

✎ Concepts To Consider

Briefly describe two guidelines for assessing infants and two guidelines for assessing preschool and elementary-aged children.

_____

_____

_____

_____

_____

_____

_____

Assessment of Adolescents

■ Language disorders often persist from the early childhood years into adolescence. Research increasingly shows that such language problems, unless treated, will usually carry over into adulthood and have an impact upon the person's life in multiple areas: academic, vocational, and social/personal.

■ The area of adolescent language is receiving increased attention in speech–language pathology because of its far-reaching effects (Nippold, 1998). (*Note*: In referring to adolescents, the terms *student* and *client* are used interchangeably.)

Description of Language Disorders in Adolescents

■ Certain characteristics are commonly found in adolescents with language problems. These characteristics include difficulty in the areas of syntax, semantics, pragmatics, and reading and writing.

■ *Syntactic problems:*

– limited length of sentences; sentences shorter than would be expected

– difficulty in using complex sentences containing subordinate clauses

– difficulty using cohesion devices or connectives (e.g., the use of such expressions as *moreover, furthermore, therefore, for example*)

- lack of agreement (e.g., noun-verb agreement)

- persistent use of syntactic errors

- limited use of low-frequency structures (e.g., passive sentences like "The book was written by the author," or such noun phrase postmodifications as "a flower called the tulip" or "Mrs. McKibbin the math teacher")

■ *Semantic problems:*

- word-retrieval problems in conversational speech resulting in dysfluencies such as repetitions, revisions, and false starts

- problems with word-definition skills; possibly especially evident in defining scientific and technical words

- word-relation problems; difficulty understanding and correctly using words that are related by similar or contrastive meanings (synonyms and antonyms)

- difficulty in understanding and correctly using figurative language (e.g., idioms, metaphors, and proverbs)

- difficulty in learning and using peer-group slang

- difficulty in understanding and correctly using words with abstract and multiple meanings (e.g., *rock, pound*)

- difficulty in using precise terms with clear referents (as demonstrated by excessive use of such terms as *this, that, thing, stuff*, etc.)

■ *Pragmatic problems:*

- difficulty modifying statements or adding new information (restatement of the same information without modification for listener)

- maze behavior (false starts and repeated attempts to express the same idea; e.g., "You know, the um, the, you know, it was the um . . . the thing")

- inappropriate use of gestures and other nonverbal cues

- difficulty maintaining a topic of conversation

- difficulty distinguishing facts from opinions

- tactless expressions; difficulty being indirect when necessary (e.g., "You look really bad" rather than "It must have been a difficult night last night")

- difficulty asking relevant questions and making relevant comments during conversation; may make inappropriate interruptions, and may use non sequiturs

- difficulty using the correct register (e.g., the use of a more formal register with teachers and other authority figures than with peers)

■ *Reading and writing problems:*

- grammatical errors (e.g., "The whale were in the sea")

- difficulty comprehending material that is read

- spelling difficulties

- use of nontechnical language instead of technical language

- poor formation of letters (may be related to fine-motor problems)

- lack of punctuation skills (e.g., misuse and/or omission of such things as periods and commas)

- poor organization of narratives and essays, leaving the reader confused

- sparse information, lack of appropriate detail

General Assessment Guidelines and Procedures

■ Begin by screening language to determine if a more detailed assessment is needed; do this through brief language sampling or through formal screening measures such those listed in Table 4.4.

■ Obtain a case history.

■ Use social assessment methodologies. For example, conduct interviews with parents, teachers, and peers about the adolescent's everyday communication patterns.

■ Evaluate syntactic, semantic, morphologic, and pragmatic aspects of receptive and expressive oral language.

■ Evaluate reading and writing skills and assess how those skills relate to the demands of the classroom.

TABLE 4.4

Commonly Used Standardized Screening Tests for Adolescents

Screening Test	Description
Screening Test of Adolescent Language (E. M. Prather, S. Beecher, M. L. Stafford, & E. Wallace)	Used from age 6 to 12 to assess vocabulary, language processing, auditory memory, verbal expression
Clinical Evaluation of Language Fundamentals–Revised Screening (E. Semel, E. Wiig, & W. Secord)	Used from age 5 to 16 to assess auditory comprehension, pragmatics, and expressive and receptive morphology, syntax, and semantics
Classroom Communication Screening Procedure for Early Adolescents (C. S. Simon)	Used from age 9 to 14 to assess following directions, verbal expression skills, and metalinguistic skills
Adolescent Language Screening Test (D. L. Morgan & A. M. Guilford)	Used from age 11 to 17 to assess phonology, morphology, pragmatics, semantics, and syntax

■ Relate written and oral communication skills to potential vocational needs and demands.

■ Consider factors related to second-language acquisition, bilingualism, and use of a social dialect.

■ Create treatment targets based upon test results; ensure that those targets will result in improved functional written and oral communication.

■ Remember that adolescent language assessment may take more time than assessment of language in a younger child because of the need to obtain extended narratives, writing samples, and interviews with people in the adolescent's environment.

Specific Assessment Guidelines and Procedures

■ When assessing adolescents, clinicians can use a combination of formal and informal measures to assess syntactic, pragmatic, semantic, and reading and writing problems, which are common in adolescents with language disorders.

■ Clinicians should obtain an extended speech and language sample in order to analyze language as it occurs naturally in the environment.

■ It is necessary to obtain a sample of a conversation between the client and the following interlocutors: a teacher, one or more peers, and a family member or members.

■ To assess *syntactic skills:*

— assess the use of vague, wordy, and roundabout expressions instead of more precise (thus shorter) expressions

— assess the use of connectives or cohesion devices; note the contexts in which the student should have used such devices but did not

— assess agreement (e.g., noun-verb agreement) in oral and written language

— conduct an analysis of syntactic skills through the use of speech and language samples, narratives, and writing samples

— assess sentence length in *C-units* (communication units) or *T-units* (terminable units) (Both C-units and T-units contain an independent clause and subordinate clauses, but the C-units also may be incomplete sentences produced in response to questions. Count the number of words per unit and calculate both the mode—the most frequently observed length—and the mean.)

■ To assess *semantic skills*, such as:

— *word definition skills*—obtain a list of words from the student's teachers and textbooks; ask the student to define them

- *word-retrieval problems* in conversational speech—take note of such dysfluencies as pauses, revisions, false starts, repetitions, and others; notice which words are retrieved with difficulty

- *word-relation problems*—have the student define and contrast synonyms (e.g., *pretty–beautiful*) and antonyms (*pretty–ugly*)

- *difficulty in using precise terms* during conversation, narrative tasks, and writing—take note of the frequency with which the student uses such vague expressions as *stuff, thing, this, that, you know*

- *difficulty in understanding and correctly using figurative language*—make a list of common idioms, proverbs, and metaphors and then ask the student what they mean (e.g., *don't count your chickens before they hatch; fit as a fiddle; kicked the bucket*)

■ To assess *pragmatic skills:*

- assess the frequency with which the client asks you to repeat information, suggesting poor listening skills

- assess the use of correct register depending on the situation (e.g., use of slang register with peers and more formal register with authority figures)

- note any inappropriate body language during conversation (e.g., standing too close, using inappropriate gestures)

- introduce various topics and evaluate the student's ability to maintain those topics over successive utterances

- ask the student to read a story and then retell it; ask the student to orally narrate a story; evaluate the student's ability to correctly sequence events in a manner understandable to the listener

- count the frequency of maze behaviors such as false starts and repeated attempts to express the same ideas

- note interruptions, irrelevant comments, and non sequiturs

- make vague and nonspecific statements; evaluate whether the student requests clarification

■ To analyze *reading and writing skills:*

- ask the student to read grade-level material; analyze the type and frequency of reading errors made

- ask questions about the material read to evaluate reading comprehension

- analyze multiple writing samples for:

- difficulty forming letters and other handwriting problems

- spelling errors

- punctuation errors

- errors in syntax

- cohesion and overall organization

- appropriateness of content, including the adequacy of information offered and details given

Standardized Tests

■ A problem with many formal, published adolescent language tests is that they contain sections that evaluate aspects of language that develop at much younger ages in normal children. For example, some adolescent language tests evaluate students' production of Brown's grammatical morphemes (Nippold, 1998).

■ Thus, many clinicians prefer to use nonstandardized, informal testing for adolescents with language problems. However, state and federal laws frequently require the use of formal scores, gathered from formal tests, for the diagnosis of a language disorder in an adolescent. Some formal tests available on the market are listed in Table 4.5.

Summary

☑ Language assessment is used to observe and measure children's language behaviors. The purpose of assessment is to ascertain whether a clinically significant problem exists and what direction to take in treatment if a problem does exist.

☑ Assessment can involve the use of standardized instruments as well as informal, nonstandardized measures of language.

☑ Children of different age levels require: (a) common foundational assessment procedures such as hearing screening and a case history, and (b) specialized procedures reflecting special needs of children in certain age groups.

TABLE 4.5

Commonly Used Standardized Language Tests for Adolescents

Standardized Test	Description
Clinical Evaluation of Language Fundamentals–3 (E. Semel, E. Wiig, & W. Secord)	Used from age 6 to 21-11 to assess receptive and expressive syntax, morphology, and semantics
Woodcock Language Proficiency Battery–Revised (R.W. Woodcock)	Used from age 2 to 95 to assess oral and written language
Bilingual Syntax Measure (M.K. Burt & H.C. Dulay)	Used with 3rd through 12th graders to assess expressive syntax in English and Spanish
Comprehensive Receptive and Expressive Vocabulary Test (G. Wallace & D.D. Hammill)	Used from ages 4 to 17-11 to assess receptive and expressive oral vocabulary
Expressive One-Word Picture Vocabulary Test–Upper Extension (M. Gardner)	Used from age 12 to 15-11 to assess single-word naming skills
Receptive One-Word Picture Vocabulary Test–Upper Extension (M. Gardner & B. Brownell)	Used from age 12-0 to 15-11 to assess single-word receptive vocabulary skills
The Word Test–Adolescent (L. Zachman, M. Barrett, R. Huisingh, J. Orman, & C. Blagden)	Used from age 12-10 to 17-11 to assess expressive semantic skills
Test of Adolescent and Adult Language–3 (D.D. Hammill, V.L. Brown, S.C. Larsen, & J.L. Wiederholt)	Used from age 12-0 to 24-11 to assess auditory comprehnsion and oral and written language skills
Test of Problem Solving–Adolescent (L. Zachman, M. Barrett, R. Huisingh, J. Orman, & C. Blagden)	Used from age 12-0 to 17-11 to assess verbal problem-solving ability and sentence production
Fullerton Language Test for Adolescents (2nd ed.) (A.R. Thorum)	Used from age 11-0 to adult to assess semantic, morphologic, and syntactic skills
Test of Language Development–Intermediate:3 (D.D. Hammill & P.L. Newcomer)	Used from age 8-0 to 12-11 to assess receptive and expressive syntax and semantics
Test of Adolescent/Adult Word Finding (D.J. German)	Used from age 12 to 80 to assess naming of verbs and nouns, categories, description, and sentence completion

TREATMENT PRINCIPLES AND PROCEDURES

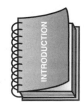

A wide variety of programs and procedures is available for serving children with language problems. Currently, clinicians are using different service delivery models in order to provide the most cost-effective, comprehensive services possible for children with language problems. These service delivery models include individual therapy, therapy in small groups, therapy carried out in the classroom setting with a small group or with the whole class, and therapy carried out by people (e.g., parents, interpreters) who have been trained by the clinician. In this section, we describe: (a) general language treatment principles, (b) specific language intervention techniques and programs that may be modified according to the age and individual needs of the child being served, and (c) augmentative and alternative communication principles for children with severe disorders of language.

General Principles

- It is important to involve the family in therapy as much as possible. Family involvement is especially important for carryover and for generalization of target behaviors into natural settings such as the home and classroom.

- Clinicians must especially target language behaviors that create social penalties for children (Johnson, 1996). For example, an adolescent who constantly interrupts others will probably be excluded from important peer groups.

- Clinicians should use a multimodal approach to treatment. Most children benefit from hearing, seeing, and touching. Instead of focusing exclusively on the auditory modality, clinicians need to use visual and tactile stimulation to reinforce language targets being taught.

- In order to truly learn and retain language treatment targets, most children need *multiple exposures to multiple exemplars* of those targets. For instance, instead of the clinician showing a picture of a Labrador and teaching the child the word *dog,* the clinician needs to have many pictures of different dogs and perhaps even some toy dogs for the child to play with.

- Clinicians should incorporate literacy—reading and writing—activities into therapy when appropriate. Although the profession of speech–language pathology is not formally designated for the teaching of reading and writing, a relationship does exist between language development and success in reading (Johnson, 1996). Children who are regularly introduced to books and reading not only will develop better language skills, but will also perform better in the classroom (Goldsworthy, 1996).

- Clinicians who provide language treatment must always consider the child's cultural and linguistic background. The child's background affects many variables, including the language used in therapy, the appropriateness of certain materials and procedures, and so forth (Roseberry-McKibbin, 1995).

- Clinicians should focus on *academic* and *social* languages—the language needed for success in school and the language needed to be socially competent.

- Clinicians must remember that a child's chronological age is not always an indicator of what kind of treatment is appropriate. The child's *developmental level* is a much more reliable indicator of what treatment procedures and goals will be appropriate for him or her.

- Computer-assisted therapy is increasingly being used with children who have language problems. Many companies are publishing software that addresses a variety of language needs.

- Collaboration with the classroom teacher is extremely important in bridging classroom language requirements with treatment targets. Children will experience much better carryover of language targets if those targets are reinforced in the classroom. Clinicians can use classroom materials in therapy, go into the classroom to conduct therapy, and collaborate in many other ways (Klein & Moses, 1999).

■ As mentioned, it is increasingly important to be flexible regarding the type of service delivery model used. Depending on the child's needs, clinicians can use one or a combination of the following delivery models:

- one-one intervention

- small group intervention

- whole classroom intervention, in which the child is worked with as part of his or her class in the classroom setting

- indirect intervention, in which the clinician sets the goals and a peer, parent, teacher's aide, interpreter, or other person carries out the treatment

✎ Concepts To Consider

You are working as a clinician in the public schools. You have been asked to give an inservice to speech–language pathology interns in your district about language therapy for children. Describe three general principles of language therapy that you will share with those interns.

_____

_____

_____

_____

_____

_____

Specific Techniques and Programs

■ The following specific techniques and programs can be modified for both group and individual therapy. They can also be modified based upon the child's developmental level and individual needs (Hegde, 1996b).

Expansion

■ The clinician expands a child's telegraphic or incomplete utterance into a more grammatically complete utterance. For example, the child says, "Doggy bark," and the clinician says, "Yes, look at the doggy barking."

Extension

- The clinician comments on the child's utterances and adds new and relevant information (this may also be called *expatiation*). For example, a child says, "Play ball." The clinician says, "Yes, you are playing with a big, red plastic ball that bounces."

Focused Stimulation

- The clinician repeatedly models a target structure to stimulate the child to use that structure. This is usually done during a play activity that the clinician designs to focus on a particular language structure (e.g., the plural morpheme -*s*).

- The clinician uses various stimulus materials, talks about them, and repeatedly models the plural constructions (e.g., "Look, here are two *pigs*. I see two *pigs* here. Over here are some *boys* playing. The *boys* are drinking from *cups*. The *cups* have *flowers* on them.").

- The clinician does not correct the child's incorrect responses but instead models the correct target (e.g., the child says, "I see two duck swimming." The clinician says, "Yes, *two ducks* are swimming in the pond.").

Incidental Teaching

- This method teaches functional communication skills through the use of typical, everyday verbal interactions that arise naturally out of situations. The child selects the activity, situation, or topic, and the clinician works language teaching into it (Reed, 1994).

- This method can also be used by parents or others who work with the child. For example, a child may elect to play with a toy farm and create situations in which animals are carrying out actions such as eating, walking, and others.

- If the clinician is teaching progressive -*ing*, he or she can use the farm animals and their actions (as the child plays) as stimuli for eliciting the -*ing* form. Thus, the clinician might say, "See, the cow is *eating* grass. Now you have the piggy *oinking* and the kitty *meowing*. Look—you have the farmer *driving* the tractor!"

Joint Routines or Interactions

- These routinized, repetitive activities are frequently used in early language stimulation with young children. Clinicians can use routines such as peek-a-boo to establish interaction with a child.

■ The clinician can also design his or her own routines of action (e.g., always starting therapy sessions by telling the same short story, which contains certain target language structures) and encourage the child to use the repetitive words, phrases, and sentences.

Joint Book Reading

■ The clinician stimulates language in children through the use of systematic storybook reading. Joint book reading allows for repetitive use and practice of the same concepts and phrases. It is also helpful for establishing joint attention (in which the clinician and the child are focused on the same thing).

■ The clinician selects appropriate storybooks with attractive, colorful, culturally appropriate pictures. He or she reads the same story several times during several sessions so that the children memorize it.

■ The clinician uses prosodic features frequently to draw attention to specific language structures. For example, the clinician might emphasize the past-tense -*ed* morpheme through increased emphasis on words containing that morpheme (e.g., "The man *looked* out the window and *opened* his eyes wide when he *viewed* the snowman.")

■ When the children are quite familiar with the story, the clinician stops at points containing target language structures and prompts the children to supply the appropriate words, phrases, or sentences (e.g., "The woman was driving her ____"). Clinicians can manipulate the activity by pausing at different junctures so children supply different language structures or produce progressively longer utterances.

■ Children can be asked eventually to "read" (recite from memory, but looking at the text and pictures) and pause while other children supply words, phrases, or sentences. Joint book reading helps develop vocabulary acquisition as well as a sense of story grammar in children.

Mand-Model

■ This variation of the incidental teaching method teaches language through the use of typical adult-child interactions in a play-oriented setting. The clinician, using attractive stimulus materials, designs a naturalistic interactive situation. He or she then establishes joint clinician-child attention to a particular material such as a set of paints.

■ Next, the clinician *mands* a response from the child (e.g., "Tell me what you want" or "Tell me what this is"). If the child gives no response or a very limited response, the clinician models the complete, correct response.

■ If the child does not imitate the entire modeled sentence, the clinician prompts (e.g., "Tell me the whole sentence"). The child is praised for imitating or for responding correctly without modeling and is given the item he or she wanted.

Milieu Teaching

■ Milieu teaching is a collection of child language intervention procedures that are used to teach language in functional, natural, and conversational communicative contexts. It can be described as a naturalistic child language teaching method, which uses such techniques as incidental teaching, mand-model, and others.

■ Milieu teaching can occur in a variety of settings, such as the therapy room, the child's classroom, and the child's home.

Narrative Skills Training

■ This techniques targets the more advanced language skill of producing narratives. *Narratives* are speakers' descriptions of events (episodes, stories) and experiences. Narratives should be produced in a cohesive, logically consistent, temporally sequenced manner. In order to train narrative skills, clinicians can:

- let the children act out the stories (e.g., stage a drama)
- use scripts based on such events as grocery shopping, birthday parties, eating in a restaurant
- get children involved in routinized, daily activities (e.g., discussing the calendar and the weather)
- repeatedly tell or read the same stories so that children memorize the characters, events, words, and temporal sequences
- pause before important phrases or descriptions when retelling stories, so that children can supply them
- ask children to tell stories or narrate events with and then without the help of pictures, scripts, or both
- ask children to narrate new events or experiences (not rehearsed or scripted)

Story Grammar

■ Children with language disorders frequently have difficulty with the structure of narratives. Clinicians can teach and model the following elements of story grammars (Larson & McKinley, 1995):

- setting statements (the introduction to the story, the physical setting, the characters, the temporal context)

- initiating events (episodes that begin the story)

- internal response (the characters' thoughts, emotions, reactions)

- theme of the story (the main idea)

- goals of the characters (what the characters are trying to accomplish)

- attempts (actions the characters take to achieve their objectives)

- direct consequences (results of actions)

- conclusion (how everything turns out, lessons or morals learned from the story)

Parallel Talk

■ The clinician plays with the child and describes and comments upon what the child is doing and the objects the child is interested in. For example, the clinician says, "You are putting the lady in the truck" or "That cow you have is brown and white."

Recasting

■ This expansion of a child's utterance into a different type of sentence is excellent for children who are working on more complex grammatical forms. The child's own sentence is repeated in modified form, but the clinician changes the modality or voice of the sentence rather than simply adding grammatical or semantic markers (Johnson, 1996).

■ For example: Child: "The baby is hungry." Clinician: "Is she hungry?" (Changed to question form.) Child: "The dog chases the cat." Clinician: "The cat is chased by the dog." (Changed to passive voice.)

Reauditorization

■ The clinician repeats what the child says during language stimulation activities. Reauditorization may be combined with other techniques such as modeling (often without requiring imitation).

■ For example, the child says, "Am swinging"; the clinician repeats, "Am swinging." More evidence is needed to demonstrate the efficacy of reauditorization.

Self Talk

■ The clinician describes his or her own activity as he or she plays with the child. Using language structures that are appropriate for that child, the clinician might say something like, "Look, I'm putting the dress on the doll. See, I'm putting the dress on her.")

Whole-Language Approach

■ This philosophical approach to language holds that learning written language should be like learning oral language. Proponents of the whole-language approach believe that children learn literacy in the same way they learn spoken language: through being immersed in a literate environment, communicating through print, and getting supportive feedback.

■ The whole-language approach focuses on acquiring *meaning*, not on teaching specific subskills or language components. Whole-language theorists and practitioners believe that *interconnections* between language components are more important than the components individually (Gillam, 1995).

■ The clinician introduces new ideas and concepts but maintains the same theme for continuity. The clinician is a facilitator, not an instructor. The whole-language approach needs efficacy research and experimental evaluation of the teaching strategies promoted.

Augmentative and Alternative Communication

Basic Principles

■ Some children have language disorders related to conditions such as autism, mental retardation, traumatic brain injury, cerebral palsy, and others. *Augmentative and alternative communication* (AAC) methods supplement oral communication and provide alternative means of communication for those children with extremely limited oral communication skills.

■ AAC methods and materials that benefit children with the above-mentioned problems may also benefit adults and children with apraxia, aphasia, cerebral palsy, laryngectomy, glossectomy, tracheostomy, spinal cord injury, and others.

■ AAC devices can be *low-technology devices*, such as notepads or message boards, which do not use electronic instruments. *High-technology devices,* or methods that use electronic instruments such as computers, may also be used.

■ When AAC users want to communicate messages, they use *displays*, which are systems or devices that show the message to their communication partner.

Displays range from communication boards to computer screens and generally involve symbols.

■ Symbols used by AAC users may be iconic or noniconic. *Iconic symbols* look like the object or picture they represent. For example, a hieroglyphic picture of a house is an iconic symbol indicating the word *house*.

■ *Noniconic symbols* are arbitrary, abstract, and geometric. They do not resemble the objects they represent and must be specifically taught. Flexible plastic shapes and chips are examples of noniconic symbols.

■ Regardless of the type of AAC device used, users of the device send messages through two means: direct selection and scanning. In *direct selection* the user selects a message by touching a key pad, touching an item or object, depressing an electronic key, pointing, or other direct means.

■ In *scanning* the user is offered available messages by a mechanical device or communication partner. The messages are offered sequentially until the AAC user indicates the messages he or she wants to communicate.

■ Speech–language pathologists may, as part of treatment, help children learn to use AAC devices in a variety of settings outside the treatment room. These settings include the home, classroom, and various places in the community (Glennen & DeCoste, 1997).

■ In both assessment and treatment of children who use AAC devices, a team approach is extremely important. The team members may include a speech–language pathologist, physical therapist, occupational therapist, psychologist, social worker, engineer, vocational counselor, teacher, and nurse (Silverman, 1995; Glennen & DeCoste, 1997). The team may work with the child to use one of several forms of AAC: gestural (unaided), gestural-assisted (aided), or neuro-assisted (aided) methods (Hegde, 1996b).

Gestural (Unaided) AAC

■ In gestural (unaided) AAC, no instruments or external aids are used. Rather, the child uses gestures and other patterned movements, which may be accompanied by some speech. Gestures play a major role in communication of messages. Widely used current gestural (unaided) forms of AAC are described as follows:

■ *Pantomime* involves mostly the use of gestures and dynamic movements that involve the entire body or parts of the body. The child uses transparent messages, facial expressions, and dramatizations of meanings. *Transparent messages* are those that are likely to be understood with no additional cues by an observer without special training (Glennen & DeCoste, 1997; Silverman, 1995).

■ *Eye-blink encoding* is a simple system in which the child learns to communicate a message by a specific number of blinks. For example, one blink means no; two blinks means yes.

- *American Indian Hand Talk* (AMER-IND) is a sign language system developed by North American Indians. AMER-IND is not phonetic; rather, gestures and movements are used as pictorial representations of concepts and ideas.

- *American Sign Language* (ASL) consists of manual signs for the 26 letters of the alphabet as well as signs for words and phrases. Recognized as a separate language, ASL may be used alone or with oral speech.

- *Limited manual sign systems* are composed of several different systems with a limited number of gestures and signs. These are often used by patients in medical settings to communicate self-care and other basic needs, and to say yes and no.

- *Left-Hand Manual Alphabet* is composed of concrete gestures that approximate printed letters of the alphabet. It is most appropriate for people with right-sided paralysis.

Gestural-Assisted (Aided) AAC

- In gestural-assisted (aided) AAC, gestures or movements are combined with an instrument or message-display device. Gestures are used: (a) display messages on a mechanical device such as a computer monitor, or (b) to scan or select messages displayed on a nonmechanical device such as a communication board.

- Mechanical devices tend to involve high technology and sophisticated electronics. These devices are often run by software, and they generate printed messages or speech. Nonmechanical devices use no electronic technology; there is no message storage, speech output, or printed output.

- Messages on both mechanical and nonmechanical devices take various forms. Six common types of symbols are used:

  - *picsyms*, a set of graphic symbols that represent nouns, verbs, and prepositions

  - *pic symbols* (pictogram ideogram communication), white drawings on a black background

  - *blissymbols,* a set of semi-iconic and abstract symbols that can be taught to speakers of any linguistic and cultural background

  - *sig symbols,* a set of ideographic or pictographic symbols based on ASL and often used in conjunction with ASL

  - *rebuses,* pictures that represent events or objects along with words, grammatic morphemes, or both

  - *Premack-type symbols, or carrier symbols*, which are abstract plastic shapes; each shape is associated with a word or phrase, and children may arrange the plastic shapes as one would printed words

Neuro-Assisted (Aided) AAC

■ Neuro-assisted (aided) AAC is useful for children who have such profound motoric impairments and limited hand mobility that they cannot use a manual switching device. This type of AAC uses bioelectrical signals such as muscle-action potentials to activate and display messages on a computer monitor.

■ Electrical activity of the muscles associated with their contraction is used to activate switching mechanisms. Electrodes attached to the child's skin pick up electrical discharges that are then amplified so they can activate special kinds of switches (called *myoswitches*) or specific displays.

■ The user receives feedback (e.g., onset of sound or light) when a switch or display is activated. The user then learns, through biofeedback, to use muscle-action potentials for activating messages.

■ Equipment for users of neuro-assisted (aided) AAC is expensive and can be challenging to maintain.

Facilitated Communication

■ Facilitated communication is a technique of language treatment for children with severe impairments such as autism or cerebral palsy. The facilitator uses physical contact with the child's hand, wrist, or elbow to facilitate pointing on a message board, writing, or typing.

■ The use of facilitated communication is highly controversial. Some researchers and clinicians in the American Speech-Language-Hearing Association (ASHA) and the American Psychological Association hypothesize that the messages the child sends may actually be messages the facilitator wants to send. Other experts believe that facilitated communication is an exciting, valid approach with great potential to help children with severe language problems. Research on validity and reliability of facilitated communication is greatly needed.

Summary

☑ Clinicians can use many different service delivery models and treatment programs and procedures to serve children with language problems.

☑ Treatment must always be individualized to meet the needs of each child, with family and classroom involvement being an intrinsic part of therapy.

☑ Some children have extremely limited oral communication skills because of conditions such as autism and cerebral palsy. For these children, augmentative and alternative communication methods can supplement oral communication or provide alternative means of communication.

CHAPTER HIGHLIGHTS

▶ Language problems in children are caused by or associated with a number of factors. Children who demonstrate language-learning disabilities may appear normal except for their language problems, which cannot be associated with any known etiology or condition.

▶ Children can also have language problems associated with specific, known, physical and sensory disabilities such as mental retardation, autism, and brain injury. It is important to provide individualized assessment and treatment based on those children's particular needs. A comprehensive team approach is especially critical, because those children often have multiple needs aside from speech and language problems.

▶ Some children have language problems related to physical and social-environmental factors. These factors include poverty, neglect and abuse, maternal and/or paternal drug or alcohol use, and attention-deficit disorder. Speech–language pathologists are seeing increasing numbers of children with language problems related to these factors. Early intervention and prevention are critical components of treatment.

▶ Assessment of language skills involves observation and measurement of a child's language behaviors to determine whether a clinically significant problem exists. Assessment can involve screening; the use of formal, standardized measures; the use of informal, nonstandardized measures; or a combination of these.

▶ Formal, standardized measures provide clinicians with a means of quantifiably comparing a child's performance to the performances of large groups of children in a similar age category. Many clinicians rely on these measures because they yield quantitative data (e.g., percentile ranks), which many state laws require before a child can receive treatment in the public school system.

▶ Because of the problems inherent in using formal, standardized measures, however, clinicians have increasingly turned to informal, nonstandardized measures. These include client-specific measures, baselines as extended measurements, forms of authentic assessment such as dynamic and portfolio assessment, social assessment methodologies, and language sampling.

▶ Clinicians are increasingly serving infants and toddlers who have an established risk of language disorders or who experience conditions that put them at risk for developing language disorders. Working with families and with interdisciplinary teams is critical in providing comprehensive, appropriate services.

(continues)

▶ Many children with language problems are identified in preschool or in elementary school. These children usually have difficulties with most or all parameters of language: morphology, syntax, phonology, semantics, and pragmatics. In elementary school, problems in written language and thus in academics are usually seen.

▶ Language problems from childhood frequently carry over into adolescence. Assessment of adolescent language can be challenging because language problems affect all aspects of the adolescent's life: social-personal, academic, and, potentially, vocational.

▶ Treatment of language disorders must be individualized to meet children's needs. Many different service delivery models, programs, and procedures exist for meeting those needs. Clinicians are increasingly collaborating with classroom teachers to provide carryover of language treatment targets into classroom settings. Children with severe language disorders may use augmentative and alternative communication devices to assist them.

▶ Add your own chapter highlights here:

_____

_____

_____

_____

KEY TERMS

American Indian Hand Talk (AMER-IND)
American Sign Language (ASL)
ataxic
athetoid
attention-deficit disorder
augmentative and alternative communication (AAC)
autism
autism spectrum disorder
baselines
blissymbols
brain injury
C-units

carrier symbols
cerebral palsy
client-specific measures
diffuse
diplegia
direct selection
displays
dynamic assessment
echolalia
expansion
extension
eye-blink encoding
fetal alcohol effects
fetal alcohol syndrome
focal
focused stimulation
function words

gestural (unaided) AAC
gestural-assisted (aided) AAC
hemiplegia
iconic symbols
incidental teaching
joint book reading
joint routines or interactions
language-learning disability
Left-hand manual alphabet
limited manual sign systems
literate lexicon
mand-model

mean length of
  utterance (MLU)
milieu teaching
monoplegia
narrative skills training
narratives
neuro-assisted (aided)
  AAC
noniconic symbols
palsy
pantomime
parallel talk
paraplegia
peer assessment

pervasive developmental
  delay
pic symbols
picsyms
portfolio assessment
Premack-type symbols
quadraplegia
reauditorization
rebus
recasting
scanning
self assessment
self talk
sig symbols

spastic
specific language
  impairment
story grammar
T-units
teacher and parent
  assessment
transparent messages
traumatic brain injury
type-token ratio
whole-language
  approach

STUDY AND REVIEW QUESTIONS

Fill in the Blank

1. Children who have language problems associated with mental retardation and autism frequently manifest _echolalia_, or parrot-like repetition of what others say to them.

2. Children with traumatic brain injury can have either _focal_ injury, which is restricted to one area of the brain, or _diffuse_ injury, which involves multiple areas due to widespread damage.

3. The term _fetal alcohol effects_ refers to signs in babies (e.g., mild physical and cognitive deficits) that have been linked to the mother's drinking alcohol during pregancy; the term _fetal alcohol syndrome_ _____ refers to a pattern of defects that develop in infants born to some women who drink heavily during pregnancy.

4. Clinicians who use the technique of _extension_ comment on the child's utterances to add additional meaning or new and relevant information; clinicians who use the technique of _reauditorization_ _____ repeat what the child says during language stimulation activities.

5. _Autism_ is a condition in which children lack responsiveness to and awareness of other people, and prefer solitude and objects to human communication; _mental retardation_ is a condition in which children have depressed language and cognitive skills and are usually delayed in language acquisition.

6. Some LLD young children use _telegraphic_ speech, in which instead of saying, "I am having a great time," the child might say, "I have great time." The child preserves the meaning of the utterance while omitting the smaller grammatical elements.

7. Two increasingly used types of informal language assessment are _dynamic_ assessment, which looks at learner modifiability, or a child's ability to learn when provided with instruction, and _portfolio_ assessment, which involves collecting samples of a child's work or performance over a period of time and observing the growth that occurs when instruction is provided.

8. Clinicians can analyze language samples by using a(n) _Type-token ratio_, in which the number of different words in the sample is divided by the total number of words in the sample.

9. Adolescents with _semantic_ problems would have difficulty understanding and correctly using words with abstract and multiple meanings (e.g., *pound*) and word-retrieval problems in conversational speech.

10. Augmentative communication devices frequently use _iconic_ symbols, which look like the object or picture they represent, or _blissymbol_ _____, a set of abstract and semi-iconic symbols that can be taught to speakers of any language background.

Multiple Choice

11. A clinician is working with parents on home language stimulation activities for their language-delayed 3-year-old daughter. The parents are using a technique in which they play with their child and describe and comment upon what she is doing and the objects she is interested in. For example, the parents might say, "You are making the car go fast" or "That pig is pink." The parents are using the technique of:

    A. self talk.

    B. expansion.

    C. expatiation.

    D. parallel talk.

    E. joint reference.

12. You are seeing a 6-year-old child with a language-learning disability. This child has adequate language comprehension but does not initiate interactions with others. Treatment should focus on:

A. increasing mean length of utterance.

B. working on bound morphemes.

C. increasing assertiveness in conversation.

D. increasing sentence complexity.

E. increasing narrative skills.

13. You are seeing a 9-year-old boy whose *Peabody Picture Vocabulary Test–3* score was 1 year above age level. However, this boy often interrupts others and irritates his listeners; as a result, he is avoided by many peers. Treatment should focus on:

A. discourse.

B. syntax.

C. morphology.

D. semantics.

E. phonology.

14. You are working with an adolescent who has receptive and expressive language problems. He is getting Ds in most of his classes at the junior high school and has few friends. In therapy, it would be best to focus on:

A. increasing auditory memory skills.

B. increasing his use of complex sentences containing subordinate clauses.

C. increasing his social use of language and collaborating with his classroom teachers.

D. increasing his ability to understand and use figurative language.

E. increasing his word-retrieval and word-definition skills.

15. A child who shows slow, writhing, involuntary movements has which type of cerebral palsy?

A. spastic

B. mixed

C. ataxic

D. hemiplegic

E. athetoid

16. Which one of the following is NOT TRUE?

    A. Standardized language tests have the advantage of providing clinicians with a means of quantifiably comparing a child's performance to the performance of large groups of children in a similar age category.

    B. Another advantage of standardized language tests is that they sample behaviors adequately, providing multiple contexts for sampling target language behaviors.

    C. Authentic assessment can involve both dynamic and portfolio assessments.

    D. In language sampling, some clinicians calculate a type-token ratio, which represents the variety of different words a child uses expressively.

    E. Clinicians are increasingly turning to informal, nonstandardized measures because many standardized tests are biased against linguistically and culturally diverse children.

17. In assessing infants and toddlers, it is important to:

    A. assess risk factors for language disorders.

    B. assess a child's play activities.

    C. assess infant-caregiver interaction.

    D. A, C

    E. A, B, C

18. You move to a new elementary school and begin seeing the children on the caseload at this school. One child, who is being treated to "increase semantic skills," has five goals listed on her IEP. Which one of these goals is inappropriate?

    A. increase types and numbers of words the child uses in the classroom

    B. increase specific word usage and decrease usage of nonspecific words such as *this, that, thing*

    C. decrease overextensions of words

    D. increase use of appropriate discourse skills, turn taking, conversational repair strategies

    E. increase comprehension of vocabulary words used in the classroom

19. A child with traumatic brain injury would most likely manifest which of the following symptoms?

A. comprehension problems, word-retrieval problems, syntactic problems

B. reading and writing difficulties, difficulties with reasoning and organization

C. hypersensitivity to touch, insistence on routines, lack of interest in human voices, comprehension and word-retrieval problems

D. A, B

E. A, B, C

20. Which of the following is NOT TRUE with regard to treatment of children with language disorders?

A. Because many children with language disorders have difficulties with auditory processing, clinicians should conduct therapy primarily through the auditory modality.

B. Collaboration with classroom teachers is becoming increasingly important in helping children generalize treatment target behaviors.

C. It is helpful, when appropriate, to incorporate reading and writing (literacy) activities into therapy.

D. A child's chronological age is not always the best predictor of what kind of treatment will be appropriate; developmental level is a more reliable indicator.

E. Service delivery models can be flexible, ranging from one-one intervention with the clinician to indirect intervention in which the clinician trains significant others to carry out language activities with the child.

REFERENCES AND RECOMMENDED READINGS

Battle, D. E., & Anderson, N. (1998). Culturally diverse families and the development of language. In D. E. Battle (Ed.), *Communication disorders in multicultural populations* (2nd ed.), pp. 213–246. Newton, MA: Butterworth-Heinemann.

Bloom, L., & Lahey, M. (1978). *Language development and language disorders*. New York: Macmillan.

Casby, M. W. (1997). Symbolic play of children with language impairment: A critical review. *Journal of Speech and Hearing Research, 40*(3), 468–479.

Chapman, R. S. (1992). *Processes in language acquisition and disorders*. St. Louis, MO: Mosby-Year Book.

Crystal, D., Fletcher, P., & Garman, M. (1976). *The grammatical analysis of language disability: A procedure for assessment and remediation*. London: Edward Arnold.

England, C. A. (1994). Assessing students with attention deficit hyperactivity disorder: Student interactions within social context. *California Speech and Hearing Association, 20*(5), 4–6.

Fey, M. E. (1986). *Language intervention with young children*. Boston: College-Hill Press.

Fey, M. E., Catts, H. W., & Larrivee, L. S. (1995). Preparing preschoolers for the academic and social challenges of school. In M. E. Fey, J. Windsor, & S. F. Warren (Eds.), *Language intervention: Preschool through the elementary years* (vol. 5, pp. 3–38). Baltimore, MD: Paul H. Brookes.

Fey, M. E., Windsor, J., & Warren, S. F. (1995). *Language intervention: Preschool through the elementary years*. Baltimore, MD: Paul H. Brookes.

Friedlander, D., & Martinson, K. (1996). Effects of mandatory basic education for adult AFDC recipients. *Educational Evaluation and Policy Analysis, 18*(4), 327–337.

Gallagher, T. (Ed.). (1991). *Pragmatics of language: Clinical practice issues*. San Diego, CA: Singular Publishing Group.

Gillam, R. (1995). Whole language principles at work in language intervention. In D. F. Tibbits (Ed.), *Language intervention beyond the primary grades: For clinicians by clinicians* (pp. 219–255). Austin, TX: PRO-ED.

Glennen, S. L., & DeCoste, D. C. (1997). *Handbook of augmentative and alternative communication*. San Diego, CA: Singular Publishing Group.

Goldsworthy, C. L. (1996). *Developmental reading disabilities: A language based treatment approach*. San Diego, CA: Singular Publishing Group.

Hegde, M. N. (1995). *A coursebook on language disorders in children*. San Diego, CA: Singular Publishing Group.

Hegde, M. N. (1996a). *Pocket guide to assessment in speech–language pathology*. San Diego, CA: Singular Publishing Group.

Hegde, M. N. (1996b). *Pocket guide to treatment in speech–language pathology*. San Diego, CA: Singular Publishing Group.

Johnson, B. A. (1996). *Language disorders in children: An introductory clinical perspective*. Albany, NY: Delmar Publishers.

Kanner, L. (1943). Autistic disturbances of affective contact. *Nervous Child, 2*, 217–250.

Klein, D., & Briggs, M. (1986). *Observation of communicative interaction*. DHS Publication No. MCJ 06351-01-0. Washington, DC: U.S. Government Printing Office.

Klein, H. B., & Moses, N. (1999). *Intervention planning for children with communication disorders: A guide for clinical practicum and professional practice* (2nd ed.). Needham Heights, MA: Allyn & Bacon.

Larson, V., & McKinley, N. (1995). *Language disorders in older students: Pre-adolescents and adolescents*. Eau Claire, WI: Thinking Publications.

Lee, L. (1974). *Developmental sentence analysis*. Evanston, IL: Northwestern University Press.

Leonard, L. (1991). Specific language impairment as a clinical category. *Language, Speech, and Hearing Services, in Schools, 22*, 66–68.

Long, S., & Fey, M. (1993). Computerized profiling (Macintosh Version 1.0, MS-DOS Version 7.1). San Antonio, TX: Psychological Corporation.

Miller, J., & Chapman, R. (1983). *SALT: Systematic analysis of language transcripts*. Madison: Language Analysis Laboratory, Waisman Center, University of Wisconsin.

Mordecai, D., & Palin, M. (1982). Lingquest 1 & 2 [computer software]. Napa, CA: Lingquest Software.

Nelson, N. W. (1998). *Childhood language disorders in context: Infancy through adolescence* (2nd ed.). Needham Heights, MA: Allyn & Bacon.

Nicolosi, L., Harryman, E., & Kresheck, J. (1996). *Terminology of communication disorders: Speech-language-hearing* (4th ed.). Baltimore, MD: Williams & Wilkins.

Nippold, M. (1998). *Later language development: The school-age and adolescent years* (2nd ed.). Austin, TX: PRO-ED.

Paul, R. (1995). *Language disorders from infancy through adolescence: Assessment and intervention*. St. Louis, MO: Mosby-Year Book.

Reed, V. A. (1994). *An introduction to children with language disorders* (2nd ed.). New York: Macmillan College Publishing Company.

Roseberry-McKibbin, C. (1995). *Multicultural students with special language needs: Practical strategies for assessment and intervention*. Oceanside, CA: Academic Communication Associates.

Roseberry-McKibbin, C., & Brice, A. (1998). *Service delivery issues in serving clients from low-income backgrounds*. Paper presented at the national meeting of the American Speech-Language-Hearing Association, San Antonio, Texas.

Rossetti, L. M. (1996). *Communication intervention birth to three*. San Diego, CA: Singular Publishing Group.

Silverman, F. H. (1995). *Communication for the speechless* (3rd ed.). Needham Heights, MA: Allyn & Bacon.

Tibbits, D. F. (Ed.) (1995). *Language intervention beyond the primary grades: For clinicians by clinicians*. Austin, TX: PRO-ED.

Tyack, D., & Gottsleben, R. (1974). *Language sampling, analysis, and training*. Palo Alto, CA: Consulting Psychologists Press.

Walker, L., & Thompson, E. (1982). Mother-infant play interaction scale. In S. Humenick-Smith (Ed.), *Analysis of current assessment strategies in the health care of young children and child rearing families* (p. 56). Norwich, CT: Williams & Wilkins.

Westby, C., & Cutler, S. K. (1994). Language and ADHD: Understanding the bases and treatment of self-regulatory deficits. *Topics in Language Disorders, 14*(4), 58-76.

Ylvisaker, M. (1995). Intervention for students with traumatic brain injury. In D. F. Tibbits (Ed.), *Language intervention beyond the primary grades: For clinicians by clinicians* (pp. 313-372). Austin, TX: PRO-ED.

ANSWERS TO STUDY AND REVIEW QUESTIONS

1. Echolalia

2. Focal, diffuse

3. Fetal alcohol effects, fetal alcohol syndrome

4. Extension, reauditorization

5. Autism, mental retardation

6. Telegraphic

7. Dynamic, portfolio

8. Type-token ratio

9. Semantic

10. Iconic, Blissymbols

11. D. If parents are using a technique in which they play with their child and describe and comment upon what she is doing and the objects she is interested in (e.g., the parents might say, "You are putting the dolly to sleep" or "You have the red dog book"), the parents are using the technique of parallel talk.

12. C. A 6-year-old child with a language-learning disability and adequate language comprehension but difficulty initiating interactions with others would best be served by treatment focusing on increasing assertiveness in conversation.

13. A. Discourse, or the connected flow of language in interaction, is the area in which this student needs the most help.

14. C. Adolescence is a time when the use and comprehension of appropriate social language is critical. In addition, collaboration with classroom teachers would yield directions for use of specific classroom materials and ideas that could be used in therapy to target deficient language skills while increasing academic performance.

15. E. A child who shows slow, writhing, involuntary movements has athetoid cerebral palsy.

16. B. Standardized tests tend to sample language behaviors inadequately, providing only one or two contexts that sample each behavior.

17. E. All of the above are important in assessing infants and toddlers.

18. D. Increasing use of appropriate discourse skills, turn taking, and conversational repair strategies would be appropriate targets for a child working on pragmatic skills, not semantic skills.

19. D. Hypersensitivity to touch, insistence on routines, and lack of interest in human voices are generally characteristic of children with autism, not children with traumatic brain injury

20. A. It is critical to use a multimodal approach to treatment because most children with language disorders will learn more quickly and retain more information this way.

CHAPTER 5

Articulatory-Phonological Development and Disorders in Children

PREVIEW OUTLINE

The ability to communicate clearly is a gift that most people take for granted. But sometimes clear communication with others is disrupted by one or more variables that cause a child to be misunderstood by members of his or her speech community. Sometimes this leads to only minor problems; other times, children experience emotional, social, and even academic difficulties related to disturbed speech patterns.

To describe these children, many authors use the term *articulation and phonological disorders*; some prefer either *articulation disorder* or *phonological disorder*. *Articulation disorder* refers to speech-motor-control problems; *phonological disorder* refers to the fact that phonology is a part of the language system, and speech requires language knowledge (Bleile, 1995). For purposes of this chapter, we have used the term *articulation and phonological disorders* (abbreviated Ar-Ph disorders) to acknowledge that many children present with reduced intelligibility due to a combination of speech-motor and phonological (language knowledge) factors. In this chapter, we describe foundational principles of articulation and phonology, acquisition and normal development of Ar-Ph skills, disorders of Ar-Ph, assessment of Ar-Ph disorders, and finally treatment of children who have Ar-Ph disorders.

FOUNDATIONS OF ARTICULATION AND PHONOLOGY

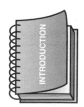

In order to understand normal development and disorders of Ar-Ph, it is necessary to understand basic definitions used to describe development and disorders. It is also helpful to understand the place-voice-manner and distinctive feature paradigms, which provide a way to classify the speech sounds of the English language. In this section, definitions and concepts from Chapter 2 are reviewed and summarized as part of the foundation for discussion of Ar-Ph development and disorders.

Basic Definitions

■ *Language* is an abstract system of symbols used to communicate meaning; it is larger than speech. *Speech* is the actual motor production of oral language.

■ Experts put forth many explanations of the differences between articulation and phonology. Fundamentally, the *articulation* approach looks at children's acquisition of individual phonemes and emphasizes speech-motor control. The *phonological* approach studies children's acquisition of sound patterns and the processes underlying such patterns. Phonology focuses on the underlying knowledge of the sound system of a language.

■ A *phoneme* is a class of speech sounds; it is an abstract name given to variations of a speech sound. Because they make a difference in meaning, phonemes are often described as the smallest unit of sound that can affect meaning. For example, *rat* and *fat* have different meanings because of the different initial phonemes /r/ and /f/.

■ A phoneme is a group, class, or family of sounds whose variations are called *allophones*. For example, although the phoneme /k/ sounds the same perceptually to the listener, it is produced in slightly different manners in the words *kitten*, *bucket*, and *cook*. These slightly different manners or variations are called allophones.

■ The term *phonemic* refers to the abstract system of sounds, whereas the term *phonetic* refers to concrete productions of specific sounds. Thus, the idealized and abstract description of /t/ is phonemic and is put in slashes. The specific sound production by a speaker would be indicated in brackets [t].

■ The English language has 46 speech sounds, which may be classified as vowels or consonants (see Chapter 2 for a more in-depth description). *Vowels* are always voiced, and the mouth is more open in vowel production than it is in consonant production.

■ Vowels are classified according to the tongue positions needed to produce them (front, central, back, high, mid, low). Vowels are also classified according to lip position; for instance, the vowels /o/ and /u/ are produced with lip rounding, while the vowel /i/ is produced with slight lip retraction.

■ When two vowels are combined, they form *diphthongs*, which are produced by a continuous change in the vocal tract shape (Peña-Brooks & Hegde, 1999). The /eɪ/ sound in *shake* and *lace* is a dipthong, as is the /aɪ/ sound in words such as *high* and *why*.

■ Vowels may be described according to the *distinctive feature paradigm*. Consonants may be described according to the distinctive feature paradigm and the *place-voice-manner paradigm*.

TABLE 5.1

The Chomsky-Halle Distinctive Features of English Consonants

	w	f	v	θ	ð	t	d	s	z	n	l	ʃ	ʒ	j	r	tʃ	dʒ	k	g	ŋ	h	p	b
Voiced	+	−	+	−	+	−	+	−	+	+	+	−	+	+	+	−	+	−	+	+	−	−	+
Consonantal	−	+	+	+	+	+	+	+	+	+	+	+	+	+	−	+	+	+	+	+	+	+	+
Anterior	+	+	+	+	+	+	+	+	+	+	+	−	−	−	−	−	−	−	−	−	−	+	+
Coronal	−	−	−	+	+	+	+	+	+	+	+	+	+	−	+	+	+	−	−	−	−	−	−
Continuant	+	+	+	+	+	−	−	+	+	−	+	+	+	+	+	−	−	−	−	−	+	−	−
High	−	−	−	−	−	−	−	−	−	−	−	+	+	+	−	+	+	+	+	+	−	−	−
Low	−	−	−	−	−	−	−	−	−	−	−	−	−	−	−	−	−	−	−	−	+	−	−
Back	−	−	−	−	−	−	−	−	−	−	−	−	−	−	−	−	−	+	+	+	−	−	−
Nasal	−	−	−	−	−	−	−	−	−	+	−	−	−	−	−	−	−	−	−	+	−	−	−
Strident	−	+	+	−	−	−	−	+	+	−	−	+	+	−	−	+	+	−	−	−	−	−	−
Vocalic	−	−	−	−	−	−	−	−	−	−	+	−	−	−	+	−	−	−	−	−	−	−	−

Note. From *Introduction to Communicative Disorders*, 2nd ed. (p. 120), by M. N. Hegde, 1995, Austin, TX: PRO-ED. Copyright 1995 by PRO-ED, Inc.. Reprinted with permission.

Distinctive Features Paradigm

■ One method of classifying vowels and consonants is based on distinctive features. Linguists who developed the distinctive features theory wanted to describe all the phonemes used in the languages of the world.

■ These linguists believe that the phoneme is not the basic unit of speech. They propose that a phoneme is a *collection of independent features*. A distinctive feature is a unique characteristic of a phoneme that distinguishes one phoneme from another (Chomsky & Halle, 1968).

■ Distinctive feature theory uses a binary system; the features are either present or absent (+ or −). For example, *voicing* is a distinctive feature. The phoneme /g/ is assigned a plus value for voicing; the phoneme /t/ is assigned a minus value for voicing. Table 5.1 lists English consonants and their distinctive features.

Place-Voice-Manner Paradigm

■ Consonants are produced by constricting the oral cavity. Consonants are traditionally classified according to three parameters: place, voice, and manner (see Table 5.2; Chapter 2 also describes these parameters):

TABLE 5.2

Place-Voice-Manner Classification of English Consonants

Place of Articulation	Manner of Production						
	Nasals	Stops	Fricatives	Affricates	Liquids	Glides	Laterals
Bilabial	ⓜ	p ⓑ					ⓦ
Labiodental			f ⓥ				
Linguadental			θ ⓓ̵				
Lingua-alveolar	ⓝ	t ⓓ	s ⓩ		ⓛ		ⓛ
Linguapalatal			ʃ ③	tʃ ⓓ̌	ⓡ	ⓙ	
Linguavelar	ⓝ̇	k ⓖ					
Glottal			h				

Note. Voiced sounds are circled. From *Introduction to Communicative Disorders*, 2nd ed. (p. 117), by M. N. Hegde, 1995, Austin, TX: PRO-ED. Copyright 1995 by PRO-ED, Inc. Reprinted with permission.

– *place* of articulation describes the location of the constriction (e.g., bilabial, linguadental)

– *voicing* describes the presence or absence of vocal fold vibrations in the production of consonants

– *manner* of articulation describes the degree or type of constriction in the vocal tract

Manner of Articulation Categories

▪ *Stops* are produced by completely stopping the airflow. The air pressure is built up in the oral cavity and then released in a manner resembling a small explosion (plosive manner). Thus, stops are also known as *stop-plosives* and consist of the phonemes /p/, /b/, /t/, /d/, /k/, /g/.

▪ *Fricatives* are produced by severely constricting the oral cavity and then forcing the air through it, creating a *hissing* or *friction* type of noise. The /f/, /v/, /ð/, /θ/, /s/, /z/, /ʃ/, /ʒ/, /h/ sounds are fricatives.

▪ Affricates are a combination of stops and fricatives. The two English affricates are /ʧ/, /dʒ/.

▪ *Glides* are produced by gradually changing the shape of the articulators. The two English glides are /w/, /j/.

■ *Liquids* are produced with the least restriction of the oral cavity. The two English liquids, /r/ and /l/, are also called *semivowels*. The /l/ sound is also called a *lateral* because in producing this sound, air escapes through the sides of the tongue.

■ *Nasals* are produced while keeping the velopharyngeal port open so the sound produced by the larynx passes through the nose. Nasal resonance is thus added to the three nasal sounds of English, /m/, /n/, and /ŋ/.

Place of Articulation Categories

- *bilabials*, produced primarily by the two lips, are /p/, /b/, /m/, /w/

- *labiodentals*, produced by the lips and teeth, are /f/, /v/

- *linguadentals*, produced by the tongue making contact with the upper teeth, are /ð/ and /θ/

- *lingua-alveolars*, produced by raising the tip of the tongue to make contact with the alveolar ridge, are /t/, /d/, /s/, /z/, /n/, /l/

- *linguapalatals*, produced by the tongue coming in contact with the hard palate, are /ʃ/, /ʒ/, /tʃ/, /dʒ/, /r/, /j/

- *linguavelars*, produced by the back of the tongue raising to contact the velum, are /k/, /g/, /ŋ/

- the *glottal* sound, produced by keeping the vocal folds open and letting the air pass through them, is /h/

Summary

☑ Speech is the motor production of oral language. The articulation approach to speech looks at children's acquisition of individual phonemes and emphasizes motor control.

☑ The phonological approach studies children's acquisition of sound patterns within the language system. Consonants and vowels make up the two major categories of speech sounds.

☑ Consonants and vowels can be described according to the distinctive features paradigm, and consonants can also be described according to the place-voice-manner paradigm.

ACQUISITION OF ARTICULATORY AND PHONOLOGICAL SKILLS: NORMAL DEVELOPMENT

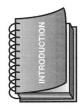

Normal Ar-Ph development is a phenomenon that most people take for granted. But sometimes children do not develop Ar-Ph skills at the expected pace for their age. In order to understand what Ar-Ph errors are age-approriate and what Ar-Ph errors indicate problematic development, it is necessary to understand theories of development and normal milestones of development in infants and children.

Theories of Development

Early studies of children's articulatory and phonological development consisted mainly of *diary studies*, which described individual children (frequently the children of the researchers). Those early studies focused primarily on environmental influences and on universals of acquisition.

■ Today's theories and models of development account much more for the child as a learner with unique learning strategies and individual patterns of production. The following is a brief summary of major theories or models of children's articulatory and phonological development (Parker, 1994; Stoel-Gammon & Dunn, 1985; Vihman, 1998):

Structural Theory

■ Proponents of the structural theory, such as Jakobson (1968) and Chomsky and Halle (1968), based their assumptions on linguists' structural theory of language.

■ According to the structural theory, phonological development follows an innate, universal, and hierarchical order of acquisition of distinctive features. The child begins with the maximal contrasts of /p/ and /a/, and differentiates and fine tunes them into more subtle contrasts.

■ Jakobson stated that babbling was not continuous with early speech, thus proposing the hypothesis of *discontinuity* between early babbling and subsequent speech development.

■ Currently, there appears to be little support for the idea of discontinuity or for the idea of development of feature contrasts. Further, because of the variability among individual children, the idea of invariable universals of development is not supported.

Behavioral Theory

■ The behavioral explanation of speech sound acquisition is based on conditioning and learning (Mowrer, 1960; Olmsted, 1971). This explanation treats the acquisition of speech like acquisition of any other skill. Thus, it is presumed that the acquisition of speech does not require such special phenomena as innate universals. The behavioral theory prevailed from the 1950s to the early 1970s (Bernthal & Bankson, 1998).

■ The behavioral theory emphasizes that the child develops the adultlike speech of his or her community through interactions with the caretaker. The theory holds that the child's babbling is gradually shaped into adult forms through principles of classical conditioning that occur primarily during caretaker-child interactions.

■ Some experts argue that this theory does not account for an infant's creativity or capacity to produce new patterns. In addition, the evidence is not compelling that caretakers selectively reinforce the child's sounds in the prelinguistic period.

Biological Theory

■ Locke (1983, 1990) stated, in the biological theory, that the foundation of phonological acquisition consists of innate dispositions to certain motor actions. For instance, a babbling child has a universal phonetic repertoire because of motoric constraints and the shape and size of the vocal tract.

■ According to the biological theory, the child's environment has an influence only around the time that the first word emerges. But production constraints remain until the child is approximately 18 months old, when he or she begins to produce characteristics of the adult language of the environment.

■ A problem with the biological theory is that, according to recent research, infants from a single linguistic background manifest individual differences even in the babbling stage. If universal constraints were so firmly set, this would not occur.

Cognitive Theory

■ Proposed by Ferguson (1978, 1986), Menn (1983), and Macken and Ferguson (1983), this theory holds that children face various challenges in their attempts to acquire the adult phonological system.

- Each child uses unique strategies in this process. The strategies depend in large part on the child's natural predispositions. Rather than targeting segments, the child appears to be targeting whole words. The child's individual creativity contributes greatly to this process.

- The cognitive theory has been criticized for overemphasizing the creative, individual aspects of phonological acquisition. Other factors such as maturational learning constraints and the language of the child's environment are not given enough consideration (Vihman, 1998).

Prosodic Theory

- Waterson's (1971, 1981) prosodic theory is based on Firth's linguistic theory. In these theories, researchers focus on words instead of segments. Children are believed to have incomplete perception of the phonetic features of adult words in early life.

- Waterson describes early word groups as schemata that share certain overall features. These features are derived from the adult form and include syllable structure, intonation pattern, nasality, continuance (presence of fricatives), and voicing (Vihman, 1998).

- According to Waterson, children's perception and production are imperfect at first and must undergo development and changes to arrive at an adultlike system.

- Waterson's approach is a useful complement to phonological process-based analysis. It especially captures the "gestalt" underlying certain productions of children that are very irregular when compared in a segment-by-segment fashion with the adult model (Vihman, 1998).

Natural Phonology Theory

- Developed by Stampe (1969), this theory proposes that instead of acquiring the phonological rules of the language they are exposed to, children are born with a universal and innate set of rules, or *phonological processes*. These processes delete or change phonological units.

- Children's task, according to Stampe, is to suppress those processes that do not occur in their languages. For example, in German, word-final obstruents (stops, affricates, and fricatives) are devoiced. In German, *Hund* (*dog*) is pronounced [hunt]. German-speaking children do not need to suppress the process of word-final obstruent devoicing, because that process is compatible with their community language. English-speaking children do need to suppress that process, however, to match the adult pronunciation of their community. Thus, in English, children need to learn to voice word-final /d/ as in the word *glad*.

■ Stampe believed that children represent or store speech forms correctly. What leads to the use of phonological processes is *output constraints*, or constraints on production that lead to simplification of the adult model.

■ The concept of the universal or innate status of child phonological processes or rules is very controversial (Vihman, 1998). Also, there is no empirical evidence that children have full and accurate perception from the earliest stages of speech production.

Generative Phonology Theory

■ Smith (1973) developed this model based upon a description of the phonology of his son at 2–4 years. According to Smith, the child does not have a psychologically real, productive system that underlies his or her forms.

■ The child's system is viewed in its own right. The child "rewrites" or maps the adult forms onto his or her system. Generative phonology states that people operate on a highly organized system of phonological rules in putting together the morphemes of language (Yavas, 1998).

■ According to Smith, children have a set of ordered universal tendencies that are either innate or learned very early in their life. Like the natural phonology theory, the generative phonology theory holds that a child stores speech forms correctly but has production constraints that lead to the use of phonological processes.

■ As stated with the natural phonology theory, there is no empirical evidence that children have full and accurate perception from the earliest stages of speech production. In addition, many researchers do not believe in the innate status of child phonological processes and rules.

✏ Concepts To Consider

Which theory of phonological development makes the most sense to you? Why?

_____

_____

_____

_____

_____

_____

_____

Infant Development: Perception and Production

Perception

- Various types of research methodology have been used to study infant perception. The two major ones are the *high-amplitude sucking paradigm* and the *visually reinforced head turn*. These methodologies observe infants' reactions to changes in their environment (for a further description, see Vihman, 1998).

- Research on infant perception has shown that:

  - 4- to 17-week-old infants can discriminate between the vowels [u] and [i], [a], and [I]

  - 2-month-old infants can discriminate between [ba] and [ga]

  - 2- to 3-month-old infants can discriminate between [ra] and [la]

  - 1- to 4-month-old infants can discriminate between [va] and [sa], [sa] and [sha], and [pa] and [ba]

  - 6- to 8-month-old infants can discriminate between [sa] and [za]

- It has generally been found that infants under 1 year of age are able to distinguish sounds that are not used in their language. However, this ability begins to decline around 12 months of age. With increasing experience of the sounds of their own language, babies eventually lose their ability to distinguish between sounds that are not used in their language.

Production

- The infant's vocal tract is significantly different from the adult's. Structural differences (e.g., a high larynx, a tongue placed far forward in the oral cavity) constrain an infant's productions especially during the first 4 months of life. Between 4 and 6 months of age, when the epiglottis and velum grow further apart, the infant becomes capable of producing a much greater variety of sounds.

- Oller (1980) proposed approximate, overlapping stages of development of prelinguistic, nonreflexive vocalizations:

  1. *Phonation stage* (birth–1 month). Speechlike sounds are rare, and most vocalizations are reflexive (e.g., burping, coughing, crying). Some nonreflexive vowels or syllabic consonants may occur.

  2. *Cooing or gooing stage* (2–3 months). Most of the infant's productions are acoustically similar to /u/. Some velar consonantlike sounds may occur.

  3. *Expansion stage* (4–6 months). The infant is "playing" with the speech mechanism, exploring his or her capabilities through such productions as growls, squeals, yells, and raspberries (bilabial trills). Some CV-like combinations and vowel-like sounds may be produced.

4. *Canonical or reduplicated babbling stage* (6–8 months). The infant produces strings of CV syllables, such as [mamamama], [dadadada], or [dedede]. Although the infant does not have sound-meaning correspondence, the timing of the CV syllables approximates that of adult speech. By about 8 months, children with hearing losses fall behind hearing peers in language development.

5. *Variegated or nonreduplicated babbling stage* (8 months–1 year). The infant continues to use adultlike syllables in CV sequences, but a variety of consonants and vowels appear in a single vocalization (e.g., [duwabe]).

Infants make a gradual progression through these stages and into the production of first words. This process is continuous and represents an important transition from the prelinguistic to the linguistic stage of phonological development, which begins around the 1st year, when the first meaningful word is produced (Lowe, 1994).

Normal Articulation Development in Children

■ The articulation development approach looks at children's development of single phonemes (Peña-Brooks & Hegde, 1999). For example, one might ask when most children master the /r/ sound. The articulation, or *segmental acquisition*, approach focuses on the age of mastery for single phonemes of English (Stoel-Gammon & Dunn, 1985) based on speech-motor control.

■ To assess when mastery of sounds occurs, researchers have generally used cross-sectional and longitudinal methods.

Research Methods

Cross-Sectional Studies

■ *Cross-sectional* research studies are used to establish norms of articulation development.

■ *Norms* are the typical behaviors of a representative group of children. The main research question is this: At what age do children master different speech sounds?

■ In cross-sectional research, a certain number of children are selected from each age level targeted for the study. The children's speech production is sampled by various test stimuli and by spontaneous conversation.

■ At each age level, the specific sounds mastered by a majority of children are determined. The different sets of sounds that are mastered by children of different ages then make up the norms.

■ Studies disagree somewhat about the age at which children master speech sounds because of the studies' differences in research methods. For example, some studies consider a sound mastered when 75% of the children produce it correctly, whereas others consider a sound mastered when 90% of the children produce it correctly.

- Norms are based on statistical averages that apply to large groups of children. Thus, norms are useful only as broad guidelines; they are of little help in predicting the performance of an individual child. Individual children vary greatly in their articulatory skills.

- Also, norms are generally based on studies of White, monolingual, English-speaking children. Therefore, they may be invalid for use with linguistically and culturally diverse children.

Longitudinal Studies

- The second type of study, using a *longitudinal method*, observes the process of learning. One or several children are observed for an extended period of time. Speech samples are recorded frequently to trace the development of speech sound learning.

- While longitudinal studies do not yield norms, they help us understand various stages and processes of sound acquisition in greater depth than cross-sectional studies do.

Research Findings: Speech Sound Acquisition

- As stated, norms for speech sound acquisition differ depending on the research methods used as well as the definition of *mastery*, which differs across investigators.

- Table 5.3 summarizes the most commonly reported normative data for mastery of phonemes (these data are based on White, monolingual, English-speaking children).

- The combination of the results of cross-sectional and longitudinal studies in speech sound acquisition have shown us the following:

  - Vowels are acquired before consonants.

  - The nasal consonants /m/, /n/, and /ŋ/ are among the earliest to be acquired. They are usually mastered between 3 and 4 years of age.

  - Stop sounds are mastered earlier than fricatives. Most stops are mastered between 3 and 4.5 years of age. The stop /p/ may be mastered the earliest.

  - Glides /w/ and /j/ are mastered earlier than fricatives. Glides are mastered between 2 and 4 years.

  - The liquids /r/ and /l/ are mastered relatively late (between 3 and 5 years).

TABLE 5.3

Age in Years-Months at Which Children Mastered Phonemes: Six Studies

Phonemes	Poole (1934)	Wellman et al. (1931)	Templin (1957)	Sander (1972)	Prather, et al. (1975)	Arlt (1976)
m	3-6	3	3	before 2	2	3
n	4-6	3	3	before 2	2	3
p	3-6	4	3	before 2	2	3
h	3-6	3	3	before 2	2	3
w	3-6	3	3	before 2	2-8	3
b	3-6	3	4	before 2	2-8	3
k	4-6	4	4	2	2-4	3
g	4-6	4	4	2	2-4	3
j	4-6	4	3-6	3	2-4	—
ng	4-6	—	3	2	2	3
t	4-6	5	6	2	2-8	3
d	4-6	5	4	2	2-4	3
f	5-6	3	3	3	2-4	3
l	6-6	4	6	3	2-4	4
v	6-6	5	6	4	4+	3-6
sh	6-6	—	4-6	4	3-8	4-6
zh	6-6	6	7	6	4	4
th (voiced)	6-6	—	7	5	4	5
th (voiceless)	7-6	—	6	5	4+	5
r	7-6	5	4	3	3-4	5
s	7-6	5	4-6	3	3	4
z	7-6	5	7	4	4+	4
ch	—	5	4-6	4	3-8	4
dj	—	—	7	4	4+	4

- Fricatives and affricates are mastered later than stops and nasals. The fricative /f/ is mastered earlier than other fricatives (around age 3). Fricatives /ð/, /θ/, /dʒ/, /s/, and /z/ are mastered the last (between 3 and 6 years).

- Consonant clusters (e.g., *br* in the word *brown*) are acquired later than most other sounds.

Normal Phonological Development in Children

Foundational Concepts

■ As stated, the articulation approach to normal development looks at children's acquisition of individual phonemes and emphasizes speech-motor control. The phonological process approach studies children's acquisition of sound *patterns* and *processes* underlying such patterns. The phonological process approach focuses on language knowledge (Bleile, 1995).

■ Researchers who utilize the phonological process approach believe that children's errors are a way of simplifying the adult model of correct articulation. Such simplifications are called *phonological processes*.

■ Phonological processes are described based on findings of longitudinal as well as large- and small-group studies. The phonological process framework helps us describe the error patterns in the speech of young children (Stoel-Gammon & Dunn, 1985).

Major Categories of Phonological Processes

■ Children may use one or more phonological process when producing a given word. For example, in the production of "hou" for "house," a child uses the single process of final-consonant deletion. But in saying "Les" instead of "Celeste," a child uses the processes of weak-syllable deletion, consonant-cluster reduction, and stridency deletion.

■ Children's phonological processes can be divided into three major categories and described as follows (Bleile, 1995; Lowe, 1994; Stoel-Gammon & Dunn, 1985; Vihman, 1998):

Substitution Processes

■ This is a group of phonological processes in which one class of sounds is substituted for another:

— In *vocalization* a vowel (usually /o/ or /u/) is substituted for a syllabic consonant (usually a liquid). For example, a child might say "bado" instead of "bottle," or "noodoo" instead of "noodle."

— In *gliding* a liquid consonant is produced as a glide. Children frequently make the following substitutions: w/l (waemp/laemp), j/l (jaɪt/laɪt), w/r (wiŋ/riŋ). Gliding can also occur in consonant clusters (e.g., pwɪti/prɪti).

— In *velar fronting* an alveolar or a dental replaces a velar; this usually occurs in word-initial position (e.g., ti/ki, doʊt/goʊt).

— In *stopping* a fricative or affricate is replaced by a stop. For example, a child might make the following substitutions: tu/ʃu, dɪs/ðɪs, bip/bitʃ, noʊd/noʊz.

- In *depalatization* a child substitutes an alveolar affricate for a palatal affricate (e.g., wats/waʧ, dzoʊk/djoʊk), or substitutes an alveolar fricative for a palatal fricative (e.g., wɪs/wɪʃ, sip/ʃip).

- In *affrication* an affricate is produced in place of a fricative or stop (e.g., ʧʌn/sʌn, ʧu/ʃu, boʧ/boʃ).

- In *deaffrication* a fricative replaces an affricate (e.g., pez/pedʒ, sɪp/ʧɪp, siz/ʧiz).

- In *backing* a posteriorly placed consonant is produced instead of an anteriorly placed consonant (velars are substituted for alveolars). For example, a child might make the following substitutions: boʊk/boʊt or gaen/daen.

- In *glottal replacement* a glottal stop (ʔ) is produced in place of other consonants (e.g. tuʔ/tuθ, baʔə/batəl).

Assimilation Processes

▨ In the following assimilation processes, the productions of dissimilar phonemes sound alike:

- *reduplication,* in which a child repeats a pattern (e.g., wɑwɑ/wɑtɚ, bɑbɑ/batəl);

- *regressive assimilation* (also called *consonant harmony*), which occurs due to the effect of a later occurring sound on an earlier sound (e.g., gʌk/dʌk, bɪp/zɪp);

- *progressive assimilation* (also called consonant harmony), in which an earlier occurring sound influences a later occurring sound (e.g., kɪk/kɪs, bup/but); and

- *voicing assimilation*, which can be either *devoicing* (e.g., pɪk, pɪg) or *voicing* (e.g., bɑd/pɑd).

Syllable Structure Processes

▨ The following syllable structure processes affect the structure of entire syllables, not just certain sounds:

- *unstressed- or weak-syllable deletion*, which involves omission of an unstressed syllable (e.g., -meɪdo/tomeɪto, -hɑɪnd/bihɑɪnd, ɛfʌnt/ɛləfʌnt);

- *final-consonant deletion*, in which the final consonant is omitted (e.g., bɛ-/bɛd, kae-/kaet);

- *epenthesis*, in which a schwa vowel is inserted between the consonants in an initial cluster (e.g., təri/tri, bəlɑek/blɑek) or after a final voiced stop (e.g., stɑpə/stɑp, godə/god);

- *consonant-cluster simplification* or *reduction*, in which a consonant or consonants in a cluster are deleted (e.g., -pid/spid, sid/spid, bɛs-/bɛst, -pun/spun);

- *diminutization*, or addition of /i/ to the target form (e.g., dɑgi/dɑg, ɛgi/ɛg);

- *metathesis*, or production of sounds in a word in reversed order; also known as a *spoonerism* (e.g., pik/kip, lɪkstɪp/lɪpstɪk, pɪsgɛti/spʌgɛti).

Summary

☑ Understanding normal Ar-Ph development necessitates an understanding of the structural, behavioral, biological, cognitive, prosodic, natural phonology, and generative phonology theories.

☑ It is also important to understand the basics of infant perception and production. In the 1st year of life, infants go through the stages of cooing/gooing, expansion, canonical or reduplicated babbling, and variegated or nonreduplicated babbling. These stages precede the development of the first word.

☑ Normal Ar-Ph development in children can be studied through the articulation or segmental acquisition approach, or through the phonological process approach. Familiarity with normal development and acquisition of Ar-Ph skills is essential to assessing and diagnosing Ar-Ph disorders.

ARTICULATORY AND PHONOLOGICAL DISORDERS

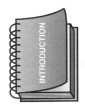

INTRODUCTION

Healthy and normal children's difficulty in producing certain speech sounds is called a functional articulation disorder. A *functional disorder* (sometimes also described as an *idiopathic disorder*), cannot be explained on the basis of neurological damage, muscle weakness or paralysis, or structural problems such as cleft palate. The term *functional* does not explain the disorder; it implies only that an *organic cause* was not found. Thus, many clinicians believe that the origin of functional articulation disorders is unknown.

Organic disorders are those that arise from various physical anomalies that affect the function or structure of the speech mechanism. There can be physical damage to the central and/or peripheral nervous system, the oral mechanism, or all of these. Treatment for organically based disorders usually should be multidisciplinary and involve members of the medical community (Air, Wood, & Neils, 1989). In this section, we describe general factors related to Ar-Ph disorders, provide a description of articulatory errors, and discuss organically based disorders that occur secondary to oral structural variables, hearing loss, and neuropathologies.

General Factors Related to Articulatory and Phonological Disorders

■ Researchers have discovered a number of factors that coexist with Ar-Ph disorders. While these factors cannot be said to be causally related to Ar-Ph disorders, they are correlated with Ar-Ph disorders.

Gender

■ There is some evidence that female children generally have slightly superior articulatory skills to those of male children. However, the evidence is weak and the reported sex differences are small or negligible (Bernthal & Bankson, 1998).

■ Nonetheless, more boys than girls tend to have articulation and phonological disorders.

Intelligence

■ Intelligence has not been shown to be causally related to Ar-Ph disorders. Children of normal intelligence may have difficulty with Ar-Ph skills.

■ Intelligence is associated with defective articulation only when intelligence is significantly below normal. Many institutionalized children with mental retardation show disordered articulation.

Birth Order and Sibling Status

■ There is some evidence that first-born and only children have better articulation skills than those who have older siblings (Bernthal & Bankson, 1998).

■ It has also been suggested that the greater the age difference between the siblings, the better the articulation of the younger child. This is because if siblings are too close to each other in age, the older one may provide a model of inadequate articulation for the younger child.

Socioeconomic Status

■ Research has shown that socioeconomic status (SES) is not a strong factor in the etiology of articulation disorders. There is no evidence that coming from a low-income background causes a child to have articulation disorders.

■ However, some studies have shown that children from lower SES backgrounds make more errors of articulation than children from middle- and upper-class backgrounds.

■ One might hypothesize that because families of low-income children tend not to have health insurance, these children cannot be readily treated for factors such as middle-ear infections and dental problems that are associated with Ar-Ph errors.

Language Development and Academic Performance

■ Research has shown that younger children with severe phonological disorders are more likely to demonstrate language problems than children with mild-moderate language delays (Bernthal & Bankson, 1998).

■ Recent evidence (e.g., Clarke-Klein & Hodson, 1995; Swank & Catts, 1994) has indicated that young children with phonological disorders may be at risk for problems with reading and spelling in the elementary school years.

Auditory Discrimination Skills

■ Researchers used to think that children with Ar-Ph disorders had poor auditory discrimination skills, which caused the disorders. Studies have produced inconsistent results; some children have scored poorly on auditory discrimination tests, whereas others have scored within normal limits.

■ Because of these equivocal research findings, it is believed that there is not a strong relationship between articulation and auditory discrimination skills. However, many clinicians still conduct intensive work on auditory discrimination skills, believing that improved auditory discrimination skills will lead to improved articulation skills.

Description of Articulatory Errors

■ Earlier in this chapter, *phonological error patterns* were described in detail. It was stated that children may manifest error patterns such as final-consonant deletion, consonant-cluster reduction, assimilation, and others. These error patterns underlie a child's lack of intelligibility.

■ The child is often able to physically produce a sound (e.g., /k/ and /g/), but if he or she displays the phonological pattern of *fronting* (e.g., *tæt/kæt, do/go*), then this child makes errors of the /k/ and /g/ sounds despite the motoric ability to produce the sounds correctly (Bernthal & Bankson, 1998).

■ Children may also make errors that can be categorized as *articulatory errors*. These errors typically involve misproductions of specific phonemes. The child is motorically unable to produce the erred phoneme (e.g., /r/, /s/), and treatment must involve teaching correct production and emphasizing speech-motor control.

■ Children may make the following articulation errors:

- *Substitutions*: Replacements of sounds; an incorrect sound is produced in place of a correct sound (e.g., tink/θink).

- *Omissions* or *deletions*: Required sounds are omitted in words (e.g., bo-/bot).

- *Labialization*: Sounds are produced with excessive lip rounding.

- *Nasalization*: Oral sounds (especially oral stops like /k/) are produced with inappropriate, usually excessive, nasal resonance.

- *Pharyngeal fricative*: Fricatives such as /h/ are produced in the pharyngeal area.

- *Devoicing*: Voiced sounds are produced with limited vocal fold vibrations or without vocal fold vibrations (e.g., dak/dag).

- *Frontal lisp*: Sibilant consonants are produced with the tongue tip placed too far forward (between or against the teeth); /s/ and /z/ are the sounds most commonly involved.

- *Lateral lisp*: Sibilant sounds such as /s/ and /z/ are produced with air flowing inappropriately over the sides of the tongue.

- *Stridency deletion*: Strident sounds are omitted (e.g., mæ-/mæʃ -tap/stap); sometimes stridency deletion is described as a phonological process.

- *Unaspirated*: Aspirated sounds (e.g., /k/, /t/) are produced without aspiration.

- *Initial, medial, final position error*: Error in the production of a beginning, medial, or final sound of a word.

- *Prevocalic, intervocalic, postvocalic error*: Errors that occur with reference to consonant position in syllables (e.g., marʧmɛlo/marʃmɛlo would involve a postvocalic error; the substitution of gag/dag would involve a prevocalic error).

✏ Concepts To Consider

Describe three factors that are related to articulatory-phonological disorders.

_____

_____

_____

_____

_____

_____

_____

_____

Organically Based Disorders

Oral Structural Variables

- Some children with deviations of the oral structure have normal Ar-Ph skills. On the other hand, Ar-Ph disorders may be found in the absence of structural anomalies. Thus, there is no demonstrable causal relationship between structural anomalies and Ar-Ph disorders. However, the following oral structural abnormalities have been associated with Ar-Ph disorders in some children.

Ankyloglossia (Tongue-Tie)

- Normally, the free tip of the tongue is mobile and permits the production of tip-alveolar sounds such as /t/, /d/. However, if the *lingual frenum*, which attaches the tongue to the base of the mouth, is too short, tongue tip mobility is reduced.

- When the frenum is thus attached too close to the tip of the tongue, this is diagnosed as a "tongue-tie" or *ankyloglossia*.

- Clipping or cutting the frenum used to be a common surgical procedure; it is more rare nowadays. Research has shown that ankyloglossia is not a frequent cause of misarticulations, and children with short lingual frenums can have normal articulation.

Dental Deviations

- *Malocclusion* refers to deviations in the shape and dimensions of the mandible and maxilla (*skeletal malocclusion*) and the positioning of individual teeth (*dental malocclusion*).

- Most children with malocclusions have a misalignment of the mandible and maxilla and the upper and lower rows of teeth. There are three basic categories of malocclusions, with many more subtypes within those categories (see Moller, 1994, for a comprehensive description).

- In *Class I malocclusion*, the arches themselves are generally aligned properly, but some individual teeth are misaligned.

- In *Class II malocclusion*, the upper jaw or maxilla is protruded and the lower jaw or mandible is receded. This is also referred to as an *overbite*. *Overjet* occurs when the child has a Class II malocclusion and the upper teeth from the molars forward are positioned excessively anterior to the lower teeth (Moller, 1994).

■ In *Class III malocclusion*, the maxilla is receded and the mandible is protruded.

Oral-Motor Coordination Skills

■ Oral-motor coordination skills are frequently evaluated through tests of *diadochokinetic rate* (maximum repetition rate of syllables in rapid succession). For example, a child might be asked to say "pʌtʌkʌ" as fast as possible in succession. The goal is to assess the functional and structural integrity of the lips, jaw, and tongue.

■ Some clinicians have observed that children who do poorly on diadochokinetic tests also have difficulty with Ar-Ph skills. However, not all children with articulation difficulties do poorly on diadochokinetic tests.

■ The relationship between diadochokinesis and speech sound production in conversational speech is unclear (Stoel-Gammon & Dunn, 1985). Research has not substantiated the hypothesis that poor oral motor coordination skills cause articulation problems.

Orofacial Myofunctional Disorders (Tongue Thrust)

■ The term *tongue thrust* has recently been expanded to be more inclusive. The current definition of *orofacial myofunctional disorders* (OMD) encompasses any anatomical or physiological characteristic of the orofacial structures (palate, cheeks, tongue, lips, jaw, teeth) that interferes with normal speech, physical, dentofacial, or psychosocial development. This includes swallow, labial and lingual rest, and speech posture differences (Kellum, 1994).

■ Usually, a child with OMD exhibits deviant swallows. In a normal swallow, the tongue tip is placed behind the alveolar ridge and the body of the tongue pushes the fluid or solid posteriorly for swallowing.

■ In the deviant swallow, the tongue tip pushes against the front teeth (usually the upper central incisors). The tongue tip may protrude between the upper and lower teeth and thus come in contact with the lower lip.

■ During speech production, the tongue also may exert some force against the front teeth, and even at rest, the tongue may be carried more forward in the oral cavity. This can contribute to an anterior open bite.

■ According to the American Speech-Language-Hearing Association (1996), OMD causes errors in the production of /s/, /z/, /ʃ/, /ʒ/, /ʧ/, and /j/; in addition, tip-dental sounds /t/, /d/, /l/, and /n/ may be misarticulated due to weak tongue tip musculature. (*Note*: Some researchers believe that OMD does not *cause* errors of articulation but rather exists in a correlational relationship with those errors.) Thus, some clinicians perform *oral myofunctional therapy* to correct the deviant swallow.

■ ASHA (1996) has stated that myofunctional therapy is appropriate and within the purview of speech–language pathologists who assess and treat the effects of OMD on swallowing, rest postures, and speech. Such speech–language pathologists traditionally work on a team composed of a dentist, an orthodontist, and a physician.

Hearing Loss

■ Various kinds of articulation problems are frequently seen in individuals with hearing loss. The degree of hearing loss is frequently related to the severity of the Ar-Ph problem.

■ Individuals who are born with a profound hearing loss generally have the most challenges with articulation, as they cannot monitor their own speech production. These individuals may have difficulties with both consonant and vowel productions, making many substitutions, distortions, and omissions of phonemes.

■ Children with mild hearing losses (10–30 dB), especially if those losses are secondary to middle ear fluid and infections, may have Ar-Ph problems. Omissions of high-frequency voiceless sounds (e.g., /s/, /t/) are common. These children may also use the phonological processes of final-consonant deletion, stridency deletion, and fronting.

Neuropathologies

Dysarthria

■ Dysarthria is a speech-motor disorder caused by peripheral or central nervous system damage. This damage causes paralysis, weakness, or incoordination of the muscles of speech. In children, dysarthria can be caused by cerebral palsy, head injury, degenerative diseases, tumors, and strokes.

■ All the speech production systems are affected: phonation, resonation, respiration, resonance, and articulation. Thus, assessment and treatment must incorporate all of those systems.

■ Dysarthric speech usually is associated with monotonous pitch, deviant voice quality, variable speech rate, and hypernasality. Reduced intelligibility is a key feature of dysarthria, with the child's speech sounding "slurred."

■ Children with dysarthria have the following common articulatory error patterns (Thompson, 1989):

　– voicing errors occur, especially those that involve devoicing of voiced sounds;

　– bilabial and velar sounds are easier than alveolar fricatives and affricates, labiodental fricatives, and palatal liquids; and

　– stops, glides, and nasals are easier than fricatives, affricates, and liquids.

▪ Treatment for childhood dysarthria is very repetitive and structured. It involves increasing muscle tone and strength, increasing range and rate of motion, and treating other parameters (e.g., respiration) that affect intelligibility.

▪ Treatment involves intensive and systematic drill, modeling, phonetic placement, and emphasis on accuracy of sound production.

▪ For children who cannot be 100% intelligible, compensatory strategies (e.g., prosthetic devices) are often used to assist in communication. For very severely involved children, alternative or augmentative communication devices may be used.

Apraxia

▪ Apraxia of speech is caused by central nervous system damage. There is no weakness or paralysis of the muscles; however, the central nervous system damage makes it difficult to program the precise movements necessary for smoothly articulated speech. Thus, apraxia of speech is described as a *motor programming disorder*.

▪ Researchers and clinicians have long debated the existence of *developmental apraxia of speech* (DAS) as a clinical entity. Children with DAS are believed to have central neural problems (Hall, Jordan, & Robin, 1993) or a disordered physiological mechanism (Klein, 1996).

▪ These problems are congenital and lead to difficulties in motor programming, although the child has not experienced frank, overt damage such as a stroke.

▪ Children who are thought to have DAS have sensorimotor problems in positioning and sequentially moving muscles for the volitional production of speech (Yavas, 1998). They frequently show groping behaviors and poor intelligibility due to inconsistent and multiple articulation errors.

▪ Children with DAS usually have the following common characteristics:

– prolongation of speech sounds

– repetition of sounds and syllables

– most difficulty with consonant clusters followed by fricatives, affricates, stops, and nasals

– more frequent occurrence of omissions and substitutions

– voicing and devoicing errors

– vowel and diphthong errors

– unusual errors of articulation including metathesis (e.g., dɛks/dɛsk) and addition of phonemes

– difficulty with volitional, oral, nonspeech movements

– deviations in prosody (e.g., rate, stress)

– resonance problems (possibly due to poor velopharyngeal control)

■ Treatment for DAS is similar to treatment for adults with apraxia. It should progress hierarchically from easy to difficult tasks.

■ DAS treatment is multimodal, involving extensive drills stressing sequences of movement involved in speech production, imitation, decreased rate of speech, normal prosody, and increased accuracy in the production of individual consonants, vowels, and consonant clusters.

■ DAS therapy often produces very slow gains, and, therefore, treatment should be intensive. Home practice and self-monitoring are essential components of DAS treatment.

Summary

✔ Articulatory errors involve misproductions of specific phonemes and are usually functionally or organically based although the specific etiology is often unclear.

✔ General factors related to articulation disorders include gender, intelligence, birth order, sibling status, socioeconomic status, language development and academic performance, and auditory discrimination skills.

✔ Organically based disorders have a variety of etiologies that are either correlated with the disorders or cause them. These include tongue-tie, dental deviations, oral motor coordination problems, orofacial myofunctional disorders (tongue thrust), and hearing loss.

✔ Children with articulation disorders based on the neuropathologies of apraxia of speech and dysarthria have unique characteristics that must be addressed in a comprehensive treatment program.

ASSESSMENT OF ARTICULATORY AND PHONOLOGICAL DISORDERS

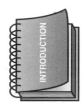

INTRODUCTION

When a child is referred for an Ar-Ph disorder, the clinician's first job is to determine whether there is a clinical problem. If there is, the characteristics of the problem need to be described. This process of identifying and describing a clinical problem is *assessment*. In this section, we discuss the components of assessment, which include carrying out general and related assessment objectives, conducting screenings, and conducting in-depth testing. In-depth testing usually involves conversational and evoked speech samples, stimulability assessment, and the administration of standardized tests. Assessment data collected through in-depth testing are scored and analyzed as a foundation for treatment.

General Assessment Objectives

■ In most cases, the clinician's general assessment objectives include:

- case history

- screening

- oral peripheral examination

- hearing screening

- language assessment if language problems are suspected

■ Further general assessment objectives include (Peña-Brooks & Hegde, 1999):

- assessing the Ar-Ph performance of the child in single word positions and in conversational speech

- assessing the presence of phonological processes that may help establish patterns in misarticulations

- evaluating a child's performance in light of developmental norms

- evaluating stimulability of speech sounds that are misarticulated

- identifying potential treatment targets

Related Assessment Objectives

■ In certain cases, clinicians may need to obtain data (if relevant) regarding:

- audiological assessment

- physical or neurological disabilities

- dental abnormalities that are negatively impacting intelligibility

- possible influences of another language or dialect

- intellectual and behavioral assessment in cases of children with such problems as behavior disorders and mental retardation

Screening

■ A screening is a brief, initial procedure that helps determine whether a child should be assessed further and in more depth. Those who pass a screening procedure are judged to have age-appropriate Ar-Ph skills. Those who fail a screening are scheduled for a comprehensive assessment.

■ There are different procedures available to screen Ar-Ph skills. If the child is willing to talk, a brief conversational sample may suffice. Sometimes clinicians may use pictures to test the production of certain speech sounds. Clinicians may also use standardized screening tests or the screening portions of full-length assessment tests of articulation. Several are listed in Table 5.4.

Assessment Procedures

Case History

■ The first step in a comprehensive evaluation is to take a case history (see Chapter 11 for a detailed description).

■ When a child has an Ar-Ph problem, the clinician may probe more deeply into such areas as:

— what the child and family think the problem is

— when the problem was first noted

— whether the problem is stable or changing

TABLE 5.4

Screening Tests of Articulation and Phonology

Test	Description
Templin-Darley Screening Test (M. C. Templin & F. L. Darley)	Uses pictures to screen production of sounds
Denver Articulation Screening Exam (A. F. Drumright)	Screens production of 30 sounds in initial and final positions of words
Predictive Screening Test (C. Van Riper & R. L. Erickson)	Attempts to predict articulatory skills at the end of second grade through screening sound production
McDonald Deep Screening Test (E. T. McDonald)	Uses 10 coarticulatory contexts to screen production of commonly misarticulated sounds such as /s/ and /r/
Quick Screen of Phonology (N. W. Bankson & J. E. Bernthal)	Screens 10 phonological processes
Assessment of Phonological Processes– Revised–Preschool Phonological Screening (B. W. Hodson)	Screens phonological processes in preschool children and yields a pass-fail score
Fluharty Speech and Language Screening Test for Preschool Children–2 (N. B. Fluharty)	The speech screening portion uses object stimuli to screen production of speech sounds

- the results of any previous treatment

- the child's general health, including especially the occurrence of ear infections

- any accidents, injuries, and diseases that could have caused brain damage

- the effects of the disorder on the child's academic and social life

■ The clinician also must assess the child's possible multilingual/multicultural status. If children speak or are exposed to other languages, the influence of such other languages should be evaluated (Klein & Moses, 1999; Roseberry-McKibbin, 1995).

Orofacial Examination

■ The clinician examines the client's facial and oral structures to rule out gross organic problems such as cleft palate.

■ In addition, the clinician notes the general symmetry of facial structures, the shape and mobility of the client's lips and tongue, and any missing teeth or dental malocclusions.

■ The clinician examines the client's hard and soft palates, looking for clefts, fistulas, or structural problems such as a high and vaulted hard palate. The client's soft-palate mobility is evaluated to make sure that the soft palate can move back and up to close the velopharyngeal port during the production of non-nasal sounds (for further details, see Chapter 11).

■ Many clinicians also perform tests of diadochokinetic skill, which evaluate the child's oral motor coordination as well as the integrity of oral structures and functions.

■ The goal of the orofacial examination is to assess the presence of any structural or functional factors that might be contributing to the Ar-Ph disorder. If one or more of these factors are present, the clinician must assess the client's potential for improvement in treatment if the factors are not addressed.

■ It may be that despite the presence of abnormal structural or functional factors (e.g., a high and vaulted palate), the child is stimulable for errored sounds and is capable of improving speech.

■ However, for some children, abnormal structure, function, or both must be addressed before treatment progress is possible. For example, the first author worked with a second-grade boy who had been in speech therapy for 4 years (with previous clinicians) with minimal progress on the treatment targets of /s, z, ʃ, ʒ/. It was found that due to the boy's thumb-sucking patterns, he had a marked Class II malocclusion with substantial overjet. He was physically unable to produce the target phonemes due to the condition of his dentition. It was determined that probably orthodontia would be required before articulation treatment could be successful.

Hearing Screening

- Generally, the child's hearing is screened by a brief audiological procedure. A hearing screening does not determine actual hearing thresholds but only suggests that hearing is or is not within normal limits.

- A child who fails a hearing screening is referred to an audiologist for a complete hearing evaluation. This evaluation may include pure-tone testing, tympanometry, or both.

Specific Components of an Assessment

Conversational Speech Samples

- It is optimal to collect 50–100 utterances as a representative sample of connected speech. Clinicians can phonetically transcribe all words or just words that contain errors. It is best to transcribe on the spot if possible.

- It is a good idea to repeat the child's unintelligible words after him or her so that if the sample is tape recorded, the clinician can understand the speech sample at a later time.

- Samples should be tape recorded in a quiet environment with a high-quality recorder and cassette tapes. Noisy toys are not recommended; if they are used, the clinician can use them on the carpet or on a table with a tablecloth to reduce noise.

- Young children might give more representative speech samples if they interact with their family members; in such cases, the clinician can observe the interaction and record notes.

- Clinicians can use broken toys, games, large pictures, storybooks, and open-ended questions to evoke speech. Especially successful topics include pets, TV shows, siblings, movies, favorite stories, and weekend or vacation activities.

Evoked Speech Samples

- Clinicians can collect speech samples not only through spontaneous conversation, but also through evoked samples. Below are three types of evoked samples that may be used to assess a child's production of sounds in single words (Bleile, 1995):

  - *Imitation*. Typically, the child imitates the clinician's model of single words. Imitation can be *immediate* (e.g., clinician: "Say truck." child: "Truck.") or *delayed* (e.g., clinician: "Truck. This truck is big and yellow. What is this?" child: "Truck."). In delayed imitation, a short phrase is placed between the clinician's model and the child's response.

     — *Naming*. The child names objects or pictures, usually after the clinician asks "What's this?"

     — *Sentence completion*. The child finishes the clinician's sentence. For example, the clinician might say "Look—here's a big, brown, barking _____." The child would fill in the word "dog" to complete the sentence.

■ It is best to evoke single-word productions in conjunction with connected speech samples. Some children may make more errors in connected speech samples when sounds are produced in a coarticulated context.

Stimulability Assessment

■ Stimulability refers to the child's ability to imitate the clinician's model. Clinicians should select the sounds the child misarticulates and assess the child's stimulability for those sounds. A stimulable child is generally able to imitate the clinician's modeled productions.

■ The clinician should ask the child to watch, listen carefully, and "say what I say." It is best initially to model sounds in isolation. Sounds can then be modeled in words and, if desired, nonsense syllables.

■ Researchers disagree about the prognostic value of stimulability. Some believe that a stimulable child will outgrow errors of articulation without therapy; others believe that a child will make faster improvement in therapy. Still other researchers believe that stimulability has questionable value in predicting improvement with or without therapy.

■ Many clinicians believe that stimulable sounds are easier to teach than nonstimulable sounds. Therefore, many clinicians use stimulable sounds as a starting point for treatment.

Standardized Tests

■ There are many standardized tests of articulatory and phonological skills. Standardized tests are, for many clinicians, convenient to give because clinicians know what the target words are. When used to test highly unintelligible children, standardized tests may be more reliable than spontaneous, connected samples.

■ Standardized tests also satisfy the requirements of many school districts, which require formal test scores. In such cases, clinicians can supplement standardized test results with conversational speech samples.

■ Most standardized tests of articulation skills assess the child's production of all phonemes in the initial, medial, and final positions of words at the single-word level. Usually, each phoneme is sampled only once in each position. Such tests yield information such as, "Johnny made th/s substitutions in the initial, medial, and final positions of words." The most commonly used standardized tests of articulation are summarized in Table 5.5.

■ Instruments that measure phonological processes assess a child's production of words in isolation and in connected speech. However, instead of focusing on individual sounds that are misarticulated, phonological process measures assess the child's use of phonological processes and the percentage of the time that those phonological processes are used. For example, a test might yield the information that "Johnny used the phonological process of final consonant deletion in 80% of all tested contexts." Commonly used tests of phonological processes are summarized in Table 5.6.

■ Most tests of Ar-Ph skills use picture stimuli. However, computerized measures are increasingly being used. Many clinicians in public school settings do not have access to computers; thus, computerized measures are more typically used in university and research settings.

TABLE 5.5

Standardized Tests of Articulation

Test	Description
Photo Articulation Test–3 (B .A. Lippke, S. E. Dickey, J.W. Selmar, & A.L. Soder)	Color pictures of objects are used to assess single phoneme productions in words
Weiss Comprehensive Articulation Test (C. A. Weiss)	Pictures are used to assess phoneme productions in words and sentences
Templin-Darley Test of Articulation (M. C. Templin & F .L. Darley)	Sound production is assessed in words, sentences, and sentence completion formats
Fisher-Logemann Test of Articulation Competence (H. Fisher & J. Logemann)	Color pictures and sentence productions are used to assess single phonemes; a place-voice-manner analysis of errors can be made from test results
Goldman-Fristoe Test of Articulation (R. Goldman & M. Fristoe)	Color pictures are used to assess productions of single phonemes in words; phonemes are also assessed at the sentence level through a story format
Arizona Articulation Proficiency Scale (J. B. Fudala & W. B. Reynolds)	Black and white pictures are used primarily to assess single phoneme productions in words
McDonald Deep Test of Articulation (E. T. McDonald)	Contextual productions of phonemes are assessed in two-word combinations and in sentences
Test of Minimal Articulation Competence (W. Secord)	Black and white line drawings are used primarily to assess single phoneme productions in words
Iowa Pressure Test (H. L. Morris, D. D. Spriestersbach, & F. L. Darley)	Items from the *Templin-Darley Test of Articulation* are used primarily to assess fricatives and plosives, thus indirectly assessing the adequacy of velopharyngeal closure

TABLE 5.6

Tests of Phonological Processes

Test	Description
Phonological Process Analysis (F. Weiner)	This uses 136 picture stimuli to assess 16 phonological processes
Assessment of Phonological Processes–Revised (B. W. Hodson)	Small objects are used to assess 40 phonological processes in 7 categories (paper-pencil and computerized formats are available)
Khan-Lewis Phonological Analysis (K. Khan & N. Lewis)	Forty-four words from the *Goldman-Fristoe Test of Articulation* are used to assess 15 phonological process
Bankson-Bernthal Test of Phonology (N. W. Bankson & J. E. Bernthal)	This assesses intelligibility, phonological error patterns, and consonant production
Assessment of Link Between Phonology and Articulation–Revised (R. J. Lowe)	Fifteen phonological processes are assessed through short sentences accompanied by picture stimuli
Compton-Hutton Phonological Assessment (A. J. Compton & J. S. Hutton)	Phonological error patterns are identified by assessing sound productions in word-initial and word-final positions
Natural Process Analysis (L. Shriberg & J. Kwiatkowski)	A 90-word spontaneous speech sample is used to assess 8 natural phonological processes
Computerized Profiling (S. Long & M. Fey)	A Macintosh or IBM-compatible computer is used to assess phonological processes
Macintosh Interactive System for Phonological Analysis (J. Masterson & F. Pagan)	A Macintosh computer is used to assess 27 phonological processes and analyze underlying individual patterns

✎ Concepts To Consider

Briefly describe three important components of an assessment for articulatory-phonological disorders.

_____

_____

_____

_____

_____

_____

Scoring and Analysis of Assessment Data

Independent vs. Relational Analysis

■ Clinicians can score and analyze assessment data in two ways: independent analysis or relational analysis. A more complete picture of a child's Ar-Ph skills emerges when both types of analyses are performed.

■ In *independent analysis*, a child's speech patterns are described without reference to the adult model of the language of the child's community. For example, an independent analysis might state that a child's speech contains [f, b, s, k], but would not state if these sounds were produced correctly in comparison to the adult community's standard form (Bleile, 1995; Stoel-Gammon & Dunn, 1985).

■ In a *relational analysis*, which is more commonly used in clinical settings, a child's speech is compared to the adult model of his or her speech community. For example, a statement in relational analysis might say, "The child produced a w/r substitution." This statement involves an evaluation in relation to acceptable speech in the larger community.

Standard Procedures

■ The following procedures should be followed when scoring and analyzing assessment data:

– Use the International Phonetic Alphabet to transcribe the child's speech. Use diacritics, if possible, to make a more detailed analysis of errors. This is especially critical for children from bilingual backgrounds and children with organically based problems such as cleft palate.

– Note how consistently the errors are produced and calculate the percentage of misarticulation for each phoneme in error (e.g., /k/ is misarticulated in 80% of contexts).

– List the phonetic contexts in which any of the misarticulated sounds were produced correctly (e.g., /r/ is produced correctly in word-initial gr-blends).

– Calculate the percent correct imitated productions on stimulability trials.

– Analyze the results of any standardized Ar-Ph test according to the manual's prescribed procedures.

■ List the sounds in error and classify them according to an acceptable format (e.g., omissions-substitutions-distortions; errors in the pre-, inter-, and postvocalic positions of words).

■ If the child has multiple misarticulations and it appears that a pattern analysis will be worthwhile, carry out a phonological analysis. List the phonological processes the child uses and the percentage of time those processes are used (e.g., "Susie used the phonological process of consonant cluster reduction in 60% of the possible contexts.").

■ Use published guidelines to decide if the child is using phonological processes that should have disappeared by his or her age. For example, a 4-year-old should not be using the process of reduplication. Table 5.7 summarizes guidelines given by Stoel-Gammon & Dunn (1985).

■ Calculate the child's intelligibility (in terms of percent) in light of the number of utterances or words that are understood with or without knowledge of the context. For example, the clinician could say, "In the known context of discussing a current movie, Mario's connected speech was 60% intelligible to the examiner."

■ Decide whether the child should receive treatment based on the following factors:

  – the child is making Ar-Ph errors at an age when he or she should be producing those patterns and sounds correctly;

  – the child's production differs markedly from that of peers of a similar cultural and linguistic background;

  – the child's speech is so unintelligible that it represents a clinically significant problem (e.g., there are social penalties for the child); and

  – the number of phonemes in error indicates that the child qualifies for treatment in a given clinical setting such as the public school.

■ Distinguish Ar-Ph disorders from hearing impairment, DAS, and dysarthria associated with a known neurological condition such as cerebral palsy.

■ Distinguish Ar-Ph disorders from normal, predictable errors manifested by a child who speaks a language other than English or who is exposed to models who speak a language other than English.

■ Describe associated conditions such as autism, fetal alcohol syndrome, or cleft palate and suggest additional or more intensive evaluation if necessary.

■ Make a statement of prognosis, considering whether variables such as hearing impairment, environmental factors, physical disabilities, and mental retardation may affect treatment outcome.

TABLE 5.7

Phonological Processes Disappearing Before and Persisting After Age 3.

Disappearing by 3 Years of Age	Persisting After 3 Years of Age
Reduplication	Final consonant devoicing
Weak/unstressed syllable deletion	Consonant-cluster reduction
Consonant assimilation	Stopping
Prevocalic voicing	Epenthesis
Fronting of velars	Gliding
Final consonant deletion	Depalatization
Diminutization	Vocalization

Summary

☑ There are several purposes of assessment. The first one is to determine whether the child manifests a clinically significant Ar-Ph problem. The second is to identify and describe the problem if it exists.

☑ Clinicians usually begin by screening to rule out children who do not need in-depth assessments. An in-depth assessment usually begins with a case history, orofacial examination, and hearing screening.

☑ Specific assessment components include conversational and evoked speech samples, stimulability assessment, and the administration of standardized tests. Assessment data are then scored and analyzed to provide directions for treatment.

TREATMENT OF ARTICULATORY AND PHONOLOGICAL DISORDERS

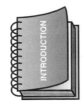

INTRODUCTION

Treatment for articulatory and phonological disorders can be organized under two major categories: *motor approaches* and *cognitive-linguistic approaches*. Bernthal and Bankson (1998) state that this dichotomy is somewhat artificial because motor and cognitive-linguistic skills are intertwined, and thus these categories are not mutually exclusive. Yet these two broad categories help clinicians conceptualize the foundation for treatment of children who are unintelligible. This treatment depends very much upon whether the child's errors reflect a lack of linguistic knowledge (phonological errors), a lack of motor skills (articulation errors), or both (Bernthal & Bankson, 1998).

(continues)

It is generally believed that motor-based approaches are best for children with several sounds in error (e.g., /r/, /s/, /l/), and that cognitive-linguistic approaches are most appropriate for highly unintelligible children with multiple sound errors. But because many children have difficulties in both areas, clinicians frequently use a combination of motor and cognitive-linguistic approaches to remediation (Klein, 1996). In this section, we describe general considerations in treatment of children with Ar-Ph disorders. We then elaborate upon motor and cognitive-linguistic approaches to treatment and briefly discuss the phenomenon of phonological awareness.

General Considerations in Treatment

- No matter what specific treatment program or combination of programs is used, most clinicians use certain basic procedures in providing treatment for children with Ar-Ph disorders. These steps usually consist of:

  - thorough assessment and analysis of the child's Ar-Ph system

  - determination of any existing patterns

  - selection and prioritization of intervention targets

  - establishment of baselines of target sounds in all contexts: words, phrases, sentences, and conversational speech

  - specific training for target patterns, sounds, or both

  - preparation of generalization and maintenance activities

- Most clinicians use a multimodal approach to treatment. This involves use of auditory, visual, and kinesthetic cues.

- Based on the individual needs of the child, clinicians must decide between training broad and training deep. *Training broad* involves treating several sounds simultaneously. Practice is limited on any specific sound, and the child receives practice on a wide, or broad, range of sounds. *Training deep* involves one or several sounds being treated intensively. Other sounds are selected only when the child has achieved mastery of the initial targets.

- Because the primary goal of treatment is effective communication, clinicians are increasingly using language- and meaning-based activities in therapy for Ar-Ph disorders. While some approaches to treatment necessarily involve drills, and sometimes drills on nonsense syllables, it is important to make activities meaningful to the child's communication in his or her daily environment.

- The concept of *communicative potency* looks at how functional words are within an individual child's communication environment. Words and phrases such as *stop, yes, give me*, and *some more* allow children greater control over their environments (Lowe & Weitz, 1994).

■ Therefore, treatment should use communicatively potent words as much as possible. Children should be taught that correct production of sounds and patterns results in improved communication with others and increased control over their environments.

■ It is very important to involve caregivers in therapy, especially in the generalization and maintenance stages. In addition, children must be taught self-monitoring skills (Peña-Brooks & Hegde, 1999).

■ Clinicians commonly use standardized tests to assess treatment progress, but this is usually ineffective because tests have only a small number of items to sample each sound or pattern. For example, most standardized tests of articulation test each phoneme only once in each word position. Using a standardized test as a measure of pretreatment skills and posttreatment gains will usually fail to show treatment gains.

■ Clinicians must always take the child's cultural and linguistic background into account. It is important to distinguish between Ar-Ph *differences* and *disorders*. Differences usually arise from the influence of the child's first language. Disorders exist when the child makes errors that are not typical for his or her cultural and linguistic speech community.

■ For example, a Spanish-speaking child typically makes ʧ/ʃ and d/ð substitutions. These differences do not constitute disorders and should not be treated as such. A child has a disorder only when his or her Ar-Ph patterns in the primary language and/or in English differ from those of peers from a similar cultural and linguistic background (Roseberry-McKibbin, 1995).

Motor-Based Approaches

General Principles

■ Articulation errors are viewed as resulting from *motor difficulties*, in which the child is physically unable to produce the sound, and from *faulty perceptual skills*. Thus, motor-based approaches to articulation therapy focus on: (a) establishing correct perception of erred phonemes, and (b) motor production of individual phonemes (e.g., separate work on /r/, /s/, /l/).

■ Those who use motor-based approaches usually describe articulation errors according to the categories of *substitutions, distortions, omissions*, and *additions*. The question asked is: Is the child producing the sound correctly or not? There is no attempt to describe underlying patterns that might be affecting classes of sounds (Klein, 1996).

■ *Van Riper's traditional approach*, first published in the mid-1930s, is the foundation for motor approaches to articulation therapy. Van Riper (1978) focused on *phonetic placement, auditory discrimination/perceptual training*, and *drill-like repetition* and practice at increasingly complex motor levels until target phonemes were automatized.

■ The underlying assumption is that motor practice leads to automatization and thus to generalization of correct productions to untrained contexts (Bernthal & Bankson, 1998). Practice and drill are critical components of treatment.

■ Practice occurs at increasingly complex motor levels until a sound is generalized into conversational speech. Thus, many clinicians who use the Van Riper approach to therapy will teach /s/, for example, in the following order: isolation, syllables, words, phrases, sentences, reading (if the child reads), and then conversation.

■ *Auditory discrimination/perceptual training* is designed to teach clients to distinguish between correct and incorrect productions of speech sounds. For example, the clinician may say, "Listen. Which is the right way to say this word? *Wabbit* or *rabbit*?" Or the clinician might have the client begin by correctly distinguishing the /w/ from the /r/ sound.

■ This is based on the assumption that auditory discrimination training is a precursor to speech sound production training. That assumption is questioned by many researchers and clinicians who believe that production training will induce correct discrimination.

■ *Phonetic placement* is used when the client cannot imitate the modeled production of a phoneme such as /r/. The clinician uses verbal instructions, modeling, physical guidance (e.g., manipulating the client's tongue with a tongue depressor), and visual feedback (e.g., mirrors, drawings) to show the client how target sounds are produced.

■ Motor-based approaches are most successful with children who have only several phonemes in error (e.g., /r/, /s/, /l/) and who are not highly unintelligible. Motor approaches work well for children who have physical difficulty producing target phonemes.

■ Motor-based approaches can be incorporated into programs that are based on cognitive-linguistic principles (e.g., the phonological process approach) for clients who have a combination of motor-based and cognitive-linguistic-based errors.

■ Commonly used motor-based approaches include McCabe and Bradley's multiple phoneme approach (MPA), Baker and Ryan's Monterey Articulation Program, McDonald's sensory-motor approach, and Irwin and Weston's paired stimuli approach (PSA).

McCabe and Bradley's Multiple Phoneme Approach

■ This behaviorally oriented treatment method (McCabe & Bradley, 1975) emphasizes that all articulation errors should be treated in all sessions. The

MPA is appropriate for children with six or more errors, and focuses on sound production in conversational speech. The MPA, unlike most other motor-based approaches, does not emphasize auditory discrimination training. The MPA has three phases.

■ *Phase I* consists of two steps: *establishment* (whose goal is the production of consonants in response to a printed letter or phonetic symbol representing it), and a *holding procedure* (designed to maintain correct production of sounds produced in isolation).

■ *Phase II* involves five transfer steps of target sounds, to: (1) syllables, (2) words, (3) phrases and sentences, (4) reading and storytelling, and (5) conversation.

■ *Phase III* has as its goal the maintenance of 90% whole-word accuracy in conversational speech produced in different speaking situations without treatment or external monitoring.

■ This approach provides an organized way of administering treatment and collecting data. Some children improve quickly and become much more intelligible with daily therapy utilizing this approach. However, it might prove difficult for preschoolers who do not recognize printed letters and who might be confused by the presentation of several sounds in each session.

Baker and Ryan's Monterey Articulation Program

■ Developed by Baker and Ryan (1971), this motor-based hierarchical and detailed program uses behavioral principles and programmed learning concepts. Imitation is heavily emphasized. There are three phases: an establishment phase, a transfer phase, and a maintenance phase.

■ The *establishment phase* has a basic program of 18 steps, 91 branching steps, and several sound evocation programs. Target sounds are produced in the following order: isolation, nonsense syllables, words, phrases, sentences, contextual reading, story narration, picture description, and finally conversational speech.

■ The *transfer phase* has 15 steps. These steps encompass home training, clinician training in different settings (e.g., conversations outside the clinic room and on the playground), and training in the classroom.

■ The *maintenance phase* is completed subsequent to the transfer phase and consists of 5 steps that involve periodic rechecks to help the child maintain accuracy in the production of newly acquired sounds.

■ Detailed and wide in scope, the Monterey approach is excellent for use with children who need a highly structured motor-articulation treatment approach. Repetition and motor practice are strongly emphasized (Bernthal & Bankson, 1998). However, the detail and technicality of the program might seem overwhelming to some clinicians.

McDonald's Sensory-Motor Approach

■ Developed around 1964, McDonald's sensory-motor approach is based on the assumption that the *syllable*, not the isolated phoneme, is the basic unit of speech production. Principles of *coarticulation* are important in this approach.

■ This system was unique in the mid-1960s because it disagreed with the established assumptions that (a) perceptual training should precede production training, and (b) treatment should begin with sounds in isolation.

■ According to McDonald, *phonetic environment* is very important in treatment; thus, training should begin at the syllable level. The clinician should administer a deep test (e.g., *McDonald's Deep Test of Articulation*) to find phonetic contexts where an otherwise misarticulated sound was produced correctly. For example, a child with an /s/ distortion might produce /s/ correctly in the context of *watch–sun*.

■ McDonald's approach has several basic steps (each step has smaller, more detailed increments; only the basics are presented here):

  – heighten the client's responsiveness to connected motor productions; begin with nonerror sounds in a variety of bi- and trisyllabic contexts (in nonsense syllables) with differing stress patterns

  – train correct production of misarticulated sounds; find a context, for example, in which /s/ is produced correctly (*watch–sun*) and have the child produce *watch–sun* in various syllable stress and phrase and sentence patterns

  – vary the phonetic contexts (e.g., *watch–sit*, *watch–saw*) and have the child practice correct production of the targets in different contexts

  – generalize by facilitating transfer to other phonetic contexts and then to natural communication activities

■ McDonald's sensory-motor approach may be helpful for children with oral-motor coordination difficulties. However, research does not support the assumption that syllabic production of nonerror productions will facilitate the correction of errored productions (Bernthal & Bankson, 1998).

Irwin and Weston's Paired Stimuli Approach

■ Developed by Irwin and Weston (1975), the PSA is based on principles of behavioral psychology and uses *operant reinforcement contingencies*. It depends on identifying a key word in which a target sound appears only once, in either initial or final position, and is produced correctly 9 out of 10 times.

■ Key words are used to teach the production of sounds in other contexts. Pictures are used to evoke the target words. A single speech sound is targeted at any one time, as opposed to approaches that target multiple speech sounds simultaneously.

- In the PSA, the clinician would take the following steps at the word level:

    – select a target sound for instruction (e.g., /r/)

    – find or create four key words, two containing the target sound in the initial position and two containing it in the final position

    – select at least 10 training words in which the target sound is misarticulated and in which the sound appears only once in the same position as the key word (e.g., *rock, run, red*)

    – select pictures as stimuli to evoke the word productions

    – put the first key word (e.g., a picture of a ring) in initial position in the center and arrange the 10 training words (pictures) around it; this is known as a *training string*

    – instruct the child to say the key word, name one of the target words, and say the key word again (e.g., *ring–rock–ring*)

    – next, ask the child to name another target word; alternate the key word and all training words in this manner

    – include three training strings in each session

    – reinforce correct productions and adhere to a training criterion of 8–10 correct productions of the training words in two successive training strings without reinforcement

- Word-level training as described above would be followed by training at the sentence and conversational levels.

- The PSA is efficient because it usually builds on behaviors already in the client's repertoire and takes little time to teach the child. The child can practice the sound in a variety of phonetic contexts (Bernthal & Bankson, 1998).

Cognitive-Linguistic Approaches

General Principles

- As previously mentioned, cognitive-linguistic approaches are sometimes used in combination with motor approaches when a child has difficulties with both the motoric and cognitive-linguistic aspects of speech sound production.

- Cognitive-linguistic approaches assume that the child has a rule-governed system with specific patterns, but that this system differs from that of the adult system in the child's community. Thus, therapy is geared toward modifying the child's underlying rule system so that it matches the adult standard (Creaghead, 1989).

- The primary goal of cognitive-linguistic approaches is to establish phonological rules in a client's repertoire. Instead of focusing on individual sounds in treatment, therapy focuses on relationships among sounds (Bernthal & Bankson, 1998).

■ Thus, the clinician is attempting to remediate *underlying patterns or rules* instead of discrete phonemes. For example, the clinician might treat the underlying pattern of *stridency deletion* instead of focusing on treating "omission of /s/, /f/, and /ʃ/," as one would in a motor approach.

■ The clinician selects sounds or target behaviors called *exemplars*. The assumption is that treatment of these exemplars will facilitate generalization to a whole class of sounds or other sounds in the same word position. In other words, the goal is to speed remediation through generalization of treatment results from a treated sound to untreated sounds (Bleile, 1995).

■ Most cognitive-linguistic treatment programs utilize *minimal pairs*, or pairs of words that differ by one feature (e.g., *shine–pine*; *bee–beach*). The goal is to show the child that sound production affects meaning.

■ The most commonly used cognitive-linguistic approaches are the distinctive features approach (DFA), the minimal pairs contrast approach, the phonological knowledge approach (PKA), and the phonological process approach (PPA).

Distinctive Features Approach

■ This goal of this approach is to establish missing distinctive features or feature contrasts by teaching relevant sounds. The DFA assumes that teaching a feature in the context of a few sounds will result in generalized production of other sounds with the same feature or features.

■ For example, a child might make the following errors: paɪn/faɪn, beɪs/veɪs, top/sop, and tʌn/sʌn. The target sounds for which the child substituted other sounds all share a common feature: stridency. Thus, the clinician might begin by teaching /f/ in hopes that the feature of stridency would generalize to /v/ and /s/ without direct training of /v/ and /s/.

■ Clinicians using the DFA try to find a child's underlying patterns (e.g., problems with the feature of stridency) and train one or several sounds in that pattern in hopes that generalization to other sounds in that pattern will occur.

■ Early distinctive feature approaches were hybrids of phonological and articulation approaches; the distinctive features used to promote generalization were phonological, and the treatment activities were motor-based (Bleile, 1995). More research is needed to fully support the DFA; currently, it is not widely used by clinicians.

Minimal Pair Contrast Approach

■ In the minimal pair contrast approach, the clinician uses pairs of words that differ by only one feature—the feature the clinician is trying to help the child to conceptualize (Klein, 1996). For example, the clinician might contrast the words *see* and *tea*.

■ The clinician focuses on these word pairs so that the child learns the *semantic* as well as the *motoric* differences between the phonemes. In other words, the child is taught that different sounds signal different meanings.

■ As an example, the clinician might remediate the phonological process of final consonant deletion by using pictures contrasting *boat* and *bow*, *bee* and *bead*, and *tea* and *teeth*. Through use of these minimal pair contrasts, the child learns that the final consonant makes a difference in word meaning.

Concepts To Consider

Although the dichotomy is artificial, many clinicians and researchers have found it useful to categorize treatment approaches into motor and cognitive-linguistic approaches. For which children might each approach be appropriate?

_____

_____

_____

_____

_____

_____

_____

Phonological Knowledge Approach

■ The PKA, proposed by Elbert and Geirut (1986), is an approach to treating phonological disorders in children. It looks at a child's *phonological knowledge*, or knowledge of the phonological organization and rules of his or her language.

■ The PKA is based on the assumption that sound productions reflect children's knowledge of phonological rules of the adult system, and it recommends that assessment include procedures (e.g., a continuous, representative, conversational speech sample) to estimate the child's phonological knowledge.

■ Those who use the PKA recommend starting treatment with the sounds that reflect the least knowledge and progressing to those reflecting greater degrees of knowledge. Thus, treatment is begun on the sounds that are most consistently misarticulated.

■ Specifically, in this *least knowledge method*, treatment targets differ from the client's existing repertoire by multiple features. Thus, treatment targets should allow the child the opportunity to acquire skills needed to produce more than single sounds.

■ For example, for a child who produces only /p/and no fricatives, /z/ might be a treatment target because it teaches many new features: place of production (alveolar vs. bilabial), voicing contrast (voiced vs. voiceless), and manner of production (stop vs. fricative).

■ This relatively new approach to treatment of phonological disorders is undergoing more efficacy research. The approach directly contradicts the traditional approach, and there is currently controversy in the literature about which approach is most effective (Klein & Moses, 1999).

Phonological Process Approach

General Tenets

■ The PPA is based on the assumption that a child's multiple errors reflect the operation of certain phonological rules and that the problem is essentially phonemic not phonetic.

■ A child's errors are grouped and described as *phonological processes* (e.g., "Johnny manifests the use of consonant-cluster reduction and weak-syllable deletion"), not as *discrete sounds* (e.g., "Johnny makes w/r, θ/s, and w/l substitutions").

■ Currently, the phonological process approach to assessment and remediation is receiving most attention in textbooks (Klein & Moses, 1999). Hodson and Paden's cycles approach is a widely used phonological process approach.

Hodson and Paden's Cycles Approach

■ In this phonological pattern approach designed to treat children with multiple misarticulations and highly unintelligible speech, error patterns are targeted for remediation based on stimulability, intelligibility, and percentage of occurrence (40% or greater).

■ Because they believe that phonological acquisition is a gradual process, Hodson and Paden recommend that error patterns not be drilled to a criterion of mastery (e.g., 90% accuracy). Rather, the clinician introduces correct patterns, gives the child limited practice with them, and returns to them at a later date (Hodson & Paden, 1991).

■ A cycle runs 5–16 weeks, and each child usually requires three–six cycles (30–40 hours at 40–60 minutes per week). Each sound in an error pattern receives 1 hour of treatment per cycle before the clinician proceeds to the next sound in the error pattern. Only one error pattern is treated in each therapy session, but all error patterns are treated in each cycle.

■ Thus, for example, cycle 1 might target the phonological processes of final-consonant deletion and fronting. During treatment session one, the clinician would spend the whole hour targeting /p/ in word-final position; during session two, the whole hour would be spent targeting /t/ in word-final position; in session three, the clinician would spent the whole hour targeting /k/ (to address the process of fronting) and so forth. During cycles 2 and 3 (if the child needs three cycles), the clinician would repeat the treatment in the above-described manner.

■ Each treatment session consists of the following activities (Hodson & Paden, 1991): (a) review of the previous session's target words, (b) auditory bombardment (listening to target words that are amplified), (c) activities involving new target words, (d) play break, (e) more activities involving new target words, and (f) repeating auditory bombardment and dismissal. Families are also given activities for home practice.

Phonological Awareness Treatment

■ Within the last several years, the profession of speech–language pathology has begun to focus on the concept of *phonological awareness*. This term refers to the explicit awareness of the sound structure of a language.

■ Phonological awareness is viewed as a subcategory of *metalinguistic awareness*, which refers to the child's ability to manipulate and think about the structure of language.

■ Some researchers have begun to link limited phonological awareness skills with later problems in reading and spelling (e.g., Ball, 1993; Catts, 1991; Clarke-Klein & Hodson, 1995; Goldsworthy, 1996; Swank & Catts, 1994). It is suggested that young children with severe phonological disorders lack, among other things, phonological awareness—and that these children are at risk for reading and spelling problems later in childhood.

■ It is recommended that in early childhood, these children receive explicit training to increase their phonological awareness. It is believed that this training may prevent later problems with reading and writing (Fey, Catts, & Larrivee, 1995).

■ Treatment activities are generally designed to increase children's awareness of the sound structure of language. Thus, treatment can include a variety of activities such as sound-blending activities, rhyming activities, and others that focus specifically on sound-structure awareness.

■ More research is needed to conclusively demonstrate (a) a causal relationship between decreased phonological awareness and later reading and spelling problems, and (b) the efficacy of phonological awareness treatment activities in preventing reading and spelling problems in later childhood.

Summary

☑ Clinicians take certain foundational steps in treating any child with an Ar-Ph disorder. Then, based upon the needs of the individual child, they may use a motor-based approach, a cognitive-linguistic approach, or a combination of those in treatment.

☑ Motor-based approaches, which focus on improving the child's perceptual and motor skills, treat sounds as isolated segments (e.g., treating /l/, /r/, /s/, etc.). Commonly used motor-based approaches include Van Riper's traditional approach, McCabe and Bradley's multiple phoneme approach, Baker and Ryan's Monterey Articulation Program, McDonald's sensory-motor approach, and Irwin and Weston's paired stimuli approach.

☑ Cognitive-linguistic approaches are geared toward finding a highly unintelligible child's underlying patterns and rule system and modifying that rule system to match the adult standard. Common cognitive-linguistic approaches include the distinctive features approach, the minimal pair contrast approach, the phonological knowledge approach, and the phonological process approach.

☑ Last, some researchers and clinicians are beginning to conduct phonological awareness treatment for young children who, it is suspected, have phonological awareness deficiencies that will cause reading and spelling problems in later childhood.

CHAPTER HIGHLIGHTS

▶ The term *articulation disorder* generally refers to speech-motor-control problems, physical difficulty producing sounds. The term *phonological disorder* is usually used to describe a highly unintelligible child who has an underlying difficulty with the phonological aspect of language knowledge. Acknowledging that many children have a combination of motor and language knowledge difficulties, many professionals use the term *articulatory-phonological disorder*.

▶ Various theories of phonological development have been proposed: structural, behavioral, biological, cognitive, prosodic, natural phonology, and generative phonology. These theories attempt to explain how children acquire phonological rules and the sounds of their speech communities.

▶ In order to diagnose articulatory-phonological delays in infants and children, many clinicians turn to developmental norms. Oller proposed five

(continues)

stages of normal infant articulatory-phonological development. Cross-sectional and longitudinal studies have yielded data about the speech sound acquisition of normally developing children. Some researchers have proposed time frames in which normally developing children use certain phonological processes for a time and then stop using those processes as they mature.

▶ Sometimes children do not develop articulatory-phonological skills normally. Those children are said to have an articulatory-phonological disorder. These disorders are generally viewed in one of two categories: *functional*, or *idiopathic* (no observable organic cause; the etiology is unknown), and *organic* (physical damage to the peripheral and/or central nervous system, the oral mechanism, or all of these).

▶ Some general factors have been associated with articulatory-phonological disorders but have not been proven to be causal in nature. These factors include gender, intelligence, birth order and sibling status, socioeconomic status, language development and academic performance, and auditory discrimination skills.

▶ Organically based articulatory-phonological disorders have been associated with oral structural variables such as ankyloglossia (tongue-tie), dental deviations such as malocclusions, poor oral-motor coordination skills, orofacial myofunctional disorders (tongue thrust), and hearing loss. Neuropathologies such as apraxia of speech and dysarthria directly cause articulatory-phonological disorders in children.

▶ Clinicians assess children for articulatory-phonological disorders using a general set of procedures. This includes, at minimum, gathering a case history, conducting an orofacial examination, and conducting a hearing screening. If relevant, clinicians may also obtain information about other variables (e.g., hearing problems, dental abnormalities, mental retardation) that occur with the articulatory-phonological disorder.

▶ When conducting a formal, in-depth assessment, clinicians may use conversational speech samples, evoked speech samples, stimulability assessments, and standardized tests. The results are scored and analyzed, and then a statement of prognosis is made. Treatment goals are created.

▶ Treatment of articulatory-phonological disorders can be artificially dichotomized into *motor approaches* and *cognitive-linguistic approaches*. Often a combination the two approaches is used. Motor approaches are usually appropriate for a child with several discrete sounds in error (e.g., /s/, /r/, /θ/) who has physical difficulty producing those sounds correctly. Motor approaches, which focus generally on remediating motor difficulties and faulty perceptual abilities, include Van Riper's traditional approach, McCabe and Bradley's multiple phoneme approach, Baker and Ryan's Monterey Articulation Program, McDonald's sensory-motor approach, and Irwin and Weston's paired stimuli approach.

(continues)

▶ Cognitive-linguistic approaches are generally appropriate for highly unintelligible children who are assumed to have underlying phonological systems that differ from those of the adult speech community. Cognitive-linguistic approaches attempt to establish phonological rules in children's repertoires and treat underlying patterns or rules instead of discrete phonemes. Commonly known cognitive-linguistic approaches include the distinctive features approach, the minimal pair contrast approach, the phonological knowledge approach, and the phonological process approach (especially that of Hodson and Paden).

▶ Add your own chapter highlights here:

_____

_____

_____

_____

KEY TERMS

affricate
affrication
allophone
ankyloglossia (tongue-tie)
apraxia
articulation
articulation disorder
auditory discrimination/perceptual training
backing
Baker and Ryan's Monterey Articulation Program
behavioral theory
bilabial
binary
biological theory
Class I, Class II, Class III malocclusion
cognitive-linguistic

approach
cognitive theory
communicative potency
consonant cluster simplification/reduction
cross-sectional
deaffrication
deletion
depalatization
developmental apraxia of speech
devoicing
diadochokinetic rate
diminutization
distinctive features approach
dysarthria
epenthesis
evoked imitation
evoked speech samples
exemplars
final consonant deletion

final position error
fricative
frontal lisp
functional disorder
generative phonology theory
glide
gliding
glottal
glottal replacement
high-amplitude sucking paradigm
Hodson and Paden's cycles approach
idiopathic disorder
immediate imitation
independent analysis
initial position error
intervocalic
Irwin and Weston's paired stimuli approach

labialization
labiodental
lateral lisp
least knowledge method
lingua-alveolar
linguadental
linguapalatal
linguavelar
liquid
longitudinal
malocclusion
manner of articulation
McCabe and Bradley's
  multiple phoneme
  approach
McDonald's sensory-
  motor approach
medial position error
metathesis
minimal pair contrast
  approach
motor approach
nasal
nasalization
natural phonology

theory
Oller's stages of infant
  production
omission
oral myofunctional
  therapy
organic disorder
orofacial myofunctional
  disorders
pharyngeal fricative
phoneme
phonemic
phonetic
phonetic placement
phonological awareness
phonological disorder
phonological knowledge
phonological knowledge
  approach
phonological process
phonological process
  approach
phonology
place of articulation
postvocalic

prevocalic
progressive assimilation
prosodic theory
reduplication
regressive assimilation
relational analysis
stimulability
stop
stopping
stridency deletion
structural theory
substitution
training broad
training deep
training string
unaspirated
unstressed- or weak-
  syllable deletion
Van Riper's traditional
  approach
velar fronting
visually reinforced head
  turn
vocalization
voicing assimilation

STUDY AND REVIEW QUESTIONS

Fill in the Blank

1. A(n) _phonemes_ is a class of speech sounds and is described as the smallest unit of sound that can affect meaning; variations are called _allophones_.

2. A clinician who described /b/ as a *voiced bilabial stop* would be describing the /b/ sound according to which paradigm? _place-voice manner paradigm_

3. The _behaviorist_ theory of articulatory-phonological development emphasizes the role of contingent reinforcement in the acquisition of speech, while the _structuralist_ theory states that phonological development follows an innate, universal, and hierarchical order of acquisition of distinctive features.

4. In Oller's stages of infant development, the cooing or gooing stage is followed by the _expansion_ stage.

5. Research in normal articulation development has basically used two types of research designs: the _longitudinal_ design, which observes the process of learning in one or several children for an extended period of time, and the _cross-sectional_ design, which selects a certain number of children from each age level targeted for the study and yields norms.

6. In the phonological process of _fronting_, an alveolar or a dental replaces a velar (e.g., *top/kop*, *det/get*); in the phonological process of _gliding of liquids_, a child might make productions such as jaɪt/laɪt, bwaun/braun.

7. In the condition of _ankyloglossia_ *or tongue-tie*, the lingual frenum, which attaches the tongue to the base of the mouth, is too short and thus tongue-tip mobility is restricted.

8. During assessment of a child with an articulatory-phonological disorder, a clinician might use _direct_ imitation (e.g., Clinician: "Say *squirrel*." Child: "Squirrel.") or _evoked_ imitation (e.g., Clinician: "*Rain*. It is falling from the sky. What is this?" Child: "Rain.").

9. _Stimulability_ refers to the child's ability to imitate the clinician's model (e.g., the clinician models /s/ production, and the child is able to accurately imitate it).

10. This cognitive-linguistic approach to treatment of articulatory-phonological disorders is well known for using pairs of words that differ by only one feature (e.g., *bow* and *boat*) to help the child learn the semantic differences between the phonemes: _minimal pairs contrast theory_

Multiple Choice

11. A child of 4½ years has θ/s, t/f, and w/r, d/ð , and j/l substitutions. You would begin therapy by addressing:

    A. θ/s substitution.

    B. t/f substitution.

    C. w/r substitution.

    D. d/ð substitution.

    E. j/l substitution.

12. Parents bring to you, for assessment, a child of 4 years and 3 months who uses the phonological processes of gliding, consonant cluster reduction, stopping, reduplication, and final consonant deletion. You would begin treatment by addressing:

A. final-consonant deletion.

B. gliding.

C. consonant-cluster reduction.

D. reduplication.

E. stopping.

13. In Oller's stages of infant phonological development, reduplicated babbling precedes:

A. nonreduplicated or variegated babbling.

B. expansion.

C. cooing.

D. phonation.

E. reduplicated expansion.

14. A child uses the phonological process of consonant-cluster reduction. Which of the following is the word you would most likely put on a word list used for treatment?

A. bus

B. stopped

C. horse

D. Lassie

E. shoes

15. The therapy technique of *phonetic placement* is used to teach or establish:

A. auditory discrimination.

B. stimulability.

C. production of a phoneme in isolation.

D. minimal pair contrasts.

E. phonological processes.

16. A speech–language pathologist's role in tongue thrust or oral myofunctional therapy currently may include:

A. none; SLPs do not work with those students.

B. working as a team member with a dentist, orthodontist, and physician.

C. evaluating and treating the effects of OMD on swallowing, rest postures, and speech.

D. A only

E. B and C

17. A child comes to you for an evaluation. She says things like gʌk/dʌk and koʊ/toʊ. This child is manifesting the phonological process of:

A. fronting.

B. stridency deletion.

C. backing.

D. glottal replacement.

E. progressive assimilation.

18. The articulation therapy approach that emphasizes the syllable as the basic unit of speech production and heavily utilizes the concept of phonetic environment is:

A. McDonald's sensory-motor approach.

B. Irwin and Weston's paired stimuli approach.

C. Baker and Ryan's Monterey Articulation Program.

D. Van Riper's traditional approach.

E. McCabe and Bradley's multiple phoneme approach.

19. Which one of the following is FALSE regarding dental deviations?

A. *Skeletal malocclusion* refers to deviations in the shape and dimensions of the mandible and maxilla.

B. *Dental malocculsion* refers to deviations in the positioning of individual teeth.

C. In *Class I malocclusion*, the arches themselves are generally aligned properly; however, some individual teeth are misaligned.

D. In *Class II malocclusion*, the maxilla is receded and the mandible is protruded.

E. *Overjet* occurs when a child has a Class II malocclusion and the upper teeth from the molars forward are positioned excessively anterior to the lower teeth.

20. Which of the following is/are TRUE with regard to treatment of articulatory-phonological disorders?

A. The *distinctive features approach* is used to find a child's underlying patterns (e.g., problems with the feature of nasality) and train one or several sounds in that pattern in hopes that generalization to other sounds in that pattern will occur.

B. *Hodson and Paden's cycles approach* involves treating children with phonological disorders in cycles in which the child is trained to a criterion of mastery for error patterns such as final-consonant deletion and fronting.

C. In *Elbert and Geirut's phonological knowledge approach*, the *least knowledge method* trains treatment targets that contain many new features that the child is missing.

D. A, B, C

E. A, C

REFERENCES AND RECOMMENDED READINGS

Air, D. H., Wood, A. S., & Neils, J. R. (1989). Considerations for organic disorders. In N. Creaghead, P. W. Newman, & W. A. Secord (Eds.), *Assessment and remediation of articulatory and phonological disorders* (2nd ed.), pp. 265–302. Columbus, OH: Merrill Publishing Company.

American Speech-Language-Hearing Association (1996). Orofacial myofunctional disorders. *Asha, 38* (2), 46–47.

Arlt, P. B., & Goodban, M. J. (1976). A comparative study of articulation acquisition as based on a study of 240 normals, age three to six. *Language, Speech, and Hearing Services in Schools, 7,* 173–180.

Baker, R. D., & Ryan, B. P. (1971). *Programmed conditioning for articulation.* Monterey, CA: Monterey Learning Systems.

Ball, E. W. (1993). Assessing phoneme awareness. *Language, Speech, and Hearing Services in Schools, 24,* 130–139.

Bernthal, J., & Bankson, N. (1998). *Articulation and phonological disorders* (4th ed.). Needham Heights, MA: Allyn & Bacon.

Bernthal, J. E., & Bankson, N. W. (Eds.). (1994). *Child phonology: Characteristics, assessment, and intervention with special populations.* New York: Thieme Medical Publishers.

Bleile, K. M. (1995). *Manual of articulation and phonological disorders.* San Diego, CA: Singular Publishing Group.

Catts, H. W. (1991). Facilitating phonological awareness: Role of speech–language pathologists. *Language, Speech, and Hearing Services in Schools, 22,* 196–203.

Chomsky, N., & Halle, M. (1968). *The sound pattern of English.* New York: Harper & Row.

Clarke-Klein, S., & Hodson, B. W. (1995). A phonologically based analysis of misspellings by third graders with disordered-phonology histories. *Journal of Speech and Hearing Research, 38,* 839–849.

Creaghead, N. A. (1989). Development of phonology, articulation, and speech perception. In N. A. Creaghead, P. W. Newman, & W. A. Secord, (Eds.) *Assessment and remediation of articulatory and phonological disorders* (pp. 35–68). Columbus, OH: Merrill Publishing Company.

Elbert, M., & Geirut, J. (1986). *Handbook of clinical phonology: Approaches to assessment and treatment.* San Diego, CA: College-Hill Press.

Ferguson, C. A. (1978). Learning to pronounce: The earliest stages of phonological development in the child. In F. D. Minifie and L. L. Lloyd (Eds.), *Communicative and cognitive abilities—Early behavioral assessment.* Baltimore, MD: University Park Press.

Ferguson, C. A. (1986). Discovering sound units and constructing sound systems: It's child's play. In J. S. Perkell and D. H. Klatt (Eds.), *Invariance and variability of speech processes.* Hillsdale, NJ: Lawrence Erlbaum.

Fey, M. E., Catts, H. W., & Larrivee, L. S. (1995). Preparing preschoolers for the academic and social challenges of school. In M. E. Fey, J. Windsor, & S. F. Warren (Eds.), *Language intervention: Preschool through the elementary years* (vol. 5), pp. 3–38. Baltimore, MD: Paul H. Brookes.

Flynn, M. C., Dowell, R. C., & Clark, G. M. (1998). Aided speech recognition abilities of adults with a severe or severe-to-profound hearing loss. *Journal of Speech, Language, and Hearing Research, 41*(2), 285–299.

Goldsworthy, C. L. (1996). *Developmental reading disabilities: A language-based treatment approach*. San Diego, CA: Singular Publishing Group.

Hall, P. K., Jordan, L. S., & Robin, D. A. (1993). *Developmental apraxia of speech*. Austin, TX: PRO-ED.

Helfer, K. S. (1998). In C. M. Seymour & E. H. Nober (Eds.), *Introduction to communication disorders: A multicultural approach* (pp. 277–305). Newton, MA: Butterworth-Heinemann.

Hodson, B. W., & Paden, E. P. (1991). *Targeting intelligible speech: A phonological approach to remediation* (2nd ed.). Austin, TX: PRO-ED.

Irwin, J. V., & Weston, A. J. (1975). The paired-stimuli monograph. *Acta Symbolica, 6*, 1–76.

Jakobson, R. (A. R. Keiler, Trans.). (1968). *Child language, aphasia, and phonological universals*. The Hague: Mouton.

Kellum, G. (1994). Overview of orofacial myology. In M. M. Ferketic & K. Gardner (Eds.), *Orofacial myology: Beyond tongue thrust*. Rockville Pike, MD: American Speech–Language-Hearing Association.

Klein, D., & Briggs, M. (1986). *Observation of communicative interaction*. DHS Publication No. MCJ06351-01-0. Washington, DC: U.S. Government Printing Office.

Klein, E. S. (1996). *Clinical phonology: Assessment and treatment of articulation disorders in children and adults*. San Diego, CA: Singular Publishing Group.

Klein, H. B., & Moses, N. (1999). *Intervention planning for children with communication disorders: A guide for clinical practicum and professional practice* (2nd ed.). Needham Heights, MA: Allyn & Bacon.

Locke, J. L. (1983). *Phonological acquisition and change*. New York: Academic Press.

Locke, J. L. (1990). Structure and stimulation in the ontogeny of spoken language. *Developmental Psychobiology, 23*, 621–643.

Lowe, R. J. (1994). *Phonology: Assessment and intervention applications in speech pathology*. Baltimore, MD: Williams & Wilkins.

Lowe, R. J., & Weitz, J. M. (1994). Intervention. In R. J. Lowe (Ed.), *Phonology: Assessment and intervention applications in speech pathology* (pp. 175–206). Baltimore, MD: Williams & Wilkins.

Macken, M. A., & Ferguson, C. A. (1983). Cognitive aspects of phonological development: Model, evidence and issues. In K. E. Nelson (Ed.), *Children's language* (Vol. 4). Hillsdale, NJ: Lawrence Erlbaum.

McCabe, R., & Bradley, D. (1975). Systematic multiple phonemic approach to articulation therapy. *Acta Symbolica, 6*, 1–18.

McDonald, E. T. (1964). Articulation testing and treatment: A sensory motor approach. Pittsburgh, PA: Stanwix House.

Menn, L. (1983). Development of articulatory, phonetic, and phonological capabilities. In B. Butterworth (Ed.), *Language production* (Vol. 2). London: Academic Press.

Moller, K. T. (1994). Dental-occlusal and other oral conditions and speech. In J. E. Bernthal & N. W. Bankson (Eds.), *Child phonology: Characteristics, assessment, and intervention with special populations* (pp. 3–23). New York: Thieme Medical Publishers.

Mowrer, O. (1960). *Learning theory and symbolic processes*. New York: John Wiley.

Oller, D. K. (1980). The emergence of the sounds of speech in infancy. In G. Yeni-Komshian, J. Kavanagh, & C. A. Ferguson (Eds.), *Child phonology: Vol. 1, Production*. New York: Academic Press.

Olmsted, D. (1971). *Out of the mouth of babes*. The Hague: Mouton.

Parker, F. (1994). Phonological theory. In R. J. Lowe (Ed.), *Phonology: Assessment and intervention applications in speech pathology* (pp. 17–34). Baltimore, MD: Williams & Wilkins.

Peña-Brooks, A., & Hegde, M. N. (1999). *Articulatory and phonological disorders in children: A dual level text*. Austin, TX: PRO-ED.

Poole, E. (1934). Genetic development of articulation of consonant sounds in speech. *Elementary English Review, 11*, 159–161.

Prather, E. M., Hedrick, D. L., & Kern, C. (1975). Articulation development in children aged two to four years. *Journal of Speech and Hearing Disorders, 40*, 179–191.

Roseberry-McKibbin, C. (1995). *Multicultural students with special language needs: Practical strategies for assessment and intervention*. Oceanside, CA: Academic Communication Associates.

Sander, E. (1972). When are speech sounds learned? *Journal of Speech and Hearing Disorders, 37*, 55–63.

Smith, N. V. (1973). *The acquisition of phonology: A case study*. Cambridge, England: Cambridge University Press.

Stampe, D. (1969). *The acquisition of phoneme representation*. Paper presented at the Fifth Regional Meeting of the Chicago Linguistic Society, Chicago, IL.

Stoel-Gammon, C., & Dunn, C. (1985). *Normal and disordered phonology in children*. Austin, TX: PRO-ED.

Swank, L. K., & Catts, H. W. (1994). Phonological awareness and written word decoding. *Language, Speech, and Hearing Services in Schools, 25*, 9–14.

Templin, M. (1957). *Certain language skills in children: Their development and interrelationships*. (Institute of Child Welfare, Monograph 26). Minneapolis: University of Minnesota Press.

Thompson, C. K. (1989). Articulation disorders in the child with neurogenic pathology. In J. Northern (Ed.), *Study guide for the handbook of speech–language pathology and audiology* (pp. 132–143). Philadelphia, PA: B.C. Decker.

Van Riper, C. (1978). *Speech correction: Principles and methods* (6th ed.). Englewood Cliffs, NJ: Prentice-Hall.

Vihman, M. M. (1998). Early phonological development. In J. E. Bernthal & N. W. Bankson (Eds.), *Articulation and phonological disorders* (4th ed.). Needham Heights, MA: Allyn & Bacon.

Waterson, N. (1971). Child phonology: A prosodic view. *Journal of Linguistics, 7*, 179–211.

Waterson, N. (1981). A tentative developmental model of phonological representation. In T. Myers, J. Laver, and J. Anderson (Eds.), *The cognitive representation of speech*. Amsterdam: North-Holland.

Wellman, B. L., Case, I. M., Mengert, E. G., & Bradbury, D. E. (1931). Speech sounds of young children. (University of Iowa Studies in Child Welfare). Iowa City: University of Iowa.

Yavas, M. (1998). *Phonology development and disorders*. San Diego, CA: Singular Publishing Group.

ANSWERS TO STUDY AND REVIEW QUESTIONS

1. Phoneme; allophones

2. Place-voice-manner paradigm

3. Behaviorist, structuralist

4. Expansion

5. Longitudinal, cross-sectional

6. Fronting, gliding

7. Ankyloglossia or tongue-tie

8. Direct, evoked

9. Stimulability

10. Minimal pairs contrast approach

11. B. The /f/ sound is developed earlier than the /s/, /r/, /θ/, and /l/ sounds, thus beginning therapy by addressing /f/ would be the best approach.

12. D. Reduplication is the earliest of the listed phonological processes to be phased out. In normally developing children, reduplication is usually phased out by approximately 2 years and 4 months of age.

13. A. In Oller's stages of infant phonological development, reduplicated babbling precedes nonreduplicated or variegated babbling.

14. B. *Stopped* is the only word that contains a consonant cluster.

15. C. Phonetic placement is used when a client cannot imitate the modeled production of a phoneme such as /s/ or /r/. The clinician uses a combination of verbal instructions and physical guidance to show the client how target sounds are produced.

16. E. ASHA (1996) has stated that this therapy is appropriate for and within the purview of speech–language pathologists, who assess and treat the effects of OMD on swallowing, rest postures, and speech. Speech–language pathologists traditionally work on a team composed of a dentist, orthodontist, and physician.

17. C. A child who says things like gʌk/dʌk and koʊ/toʊ is manifesting the phonological process of backing.

18. A. The articulation therapy approach that emphasizes the syllable as the basic unit of speech production and heavily utilizes the concept of phonetic environment is McDonald's sensory-motor approach.

19. D. The maxilla is receded and the mandible protruded in Class III malocclusion. In Class II malocclusion, the maxilla is protruded and the mandible receded.

20. E. In Hodson and Paden's cycles approach, children are *not* trained to a criterion of mastery for error patterns. Rather, the clinician introduces correct patterns, gives the child limited practice with production of those patterns, and moves on to other error patterns.

CHAPTER 6

Fluency and Its Disorders

PREVIEW OUTLINE

CHAPTER INTRODUCTION

Disorders of fluency are speech disorders. There are two main varieties of fluency disorders: stuttering and cluttering. Fluency may be impaired in such clinical conditions as aphasia, although a diagnosis of stuttering or cluttering may not be made in such cases. Disorders of fluency associated with aphasia are described in Chapter 8. In this chapter, information on stuttering and cluttering is summarized from various sources (Bloodstein, 1995; Culatta & Goldberg 1995; Guitar, 1998; Onslow, 1996; Van Riper, 1973, 1982).

STUTTERING: FOUNDATIONAL CONCEPTS

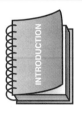

Fluent speech is usually defined as smooth, rhythmic, and flowing. Nonfluent or stuttered speech is dysrhythmic and can be defined according to various criteria. Incidence and prevalence studies of people who stutter yield information about familial and gender prevalence as well as about ethnocultural variables. Stuttering onset can be sudden or gradual but eventually is associated with various types of abnormal motor behaviors, breathing abnormalities, negative emotions, and avoidance behaviors. The loci of stuttering, or locations in the speech sequence where stutterings are typically observed, can often be predicted. Stuttering frequently varies when certain variables are manipulated, creating phenomena such as adaptation and adjacency. Theories of stuttering include environmental, genetic, and neurophysiological theories; none of these is universally accepted.

Definition and Description of Fluency

■ Fluency has not been studied as extensively as stuttering. For the most part, some rudimentary characteristics of fluency have been described. For example, fluent speech is:

- produced with relative ease (less effort and tension)

- flowing

- smooth

- continuous

– relatively rapid

– normally rhythmic

– free from an excessive amount or duration of dysfluencies

■ Characteristics of fluency contrast with those of stuttering. For example, stuttered speech contains excessive amounts of dysfluencies, durations of dysfluencies, or both.

■ Stuttered speech is produced with greater than the normal amount of effort; it is halting, and thus does not flow. Perhaps for the same reason, it is discontinuous; it is not smooth, and it may be slow because of all the dysfluencies. The rhythm of stuttered speech may be abnormal because of the various kinds of dysfluencies (Bloodstein, 1995; Starkweather & Givens-Ackerman, 1997).

Definition and Description of Stuttering

General Principles

■ It is generally agreed that stuttering is a *disorder of fluency*—it is the most researched of the fluency disorders—and historically, it has also been defined as a *disorder of rhythm*.

■ Although it is agreed that stuttering is a disorder of fluency and rhythm, clinicians have further defined it in a variety of different ways. Much of this disagreement is due to theoretical orientation, not clinical approach. A few sample definitions illustrate the variety.

Definition in Terms of Non-Speech Behaviors

■ Historically, some experts have defined stuttering in terms of variables that are not specific to speech characteristics. The following three definitions seem to emphasize various personal and social consequences of dysfluent speech.

■ First, stuttering is defined as an anticipatory, apprehensive, hypertonic, avoidance reaction. According to Johnson and associates (1959), who offered this definition, stuttering is not the same as dysfluency. Stuttering begins when a child learns to avoid speech, speaking situations, and certain kinds of audiences. It consists of anticipating trouble in speaking situations, becoming apprehensive about the prospect of speaking, experiencing tension, and, finally, avoiding the speaking situation.

■ According to this definition, a diagnosis of stuttering is not made on the basis of dysfluencies. The definition is based on the theory that avoidance is a result of parental disapproval or punishment of normal dysfluencies. The child seeks to avoid the parental disapproval of normal nonfluencies.

■ Second, stuttering is defined as what a person does to avoid stuttering. This is an alternative definition offered by Johnson (1959), but it is consistent with the view that stuttering is essentially an attempt to avoid the negative consequences of normal nonfluencies.

■ Third, stuttering is defined as a social role conflict. Sheehan (1970), who offered this definition, believed that the primary problem of stuttering is a social role conflict. The person who stutters cannot play certain social roles normally.

■ For example, stuttering people typically speak with improved fluency when they talk to young children and pets and when they play theatrical roles. However, the same people may have difficulty talking to their bosses, ordering in restaurants, and speaking to strangers. To Sheehan, this indicated a problem in playing different social roles efficiently.

Definition in Terms of Unspecified Behaviors

■ Some definitions do not specify any behaviors at all. They simply refer to stuttering in some molar or global terms. The central notion in these definitions is an expert judgment. In essence, an expert's judgment that stuttering has occurred is the definition of stuttering.

■ For example, in one view, the moment of stuttering is defined as what an expert observes in a time duration. This definition emphasizes a time duration during which something believed to be stuttering has occurred; it does not specify the behavior that is observed. Although it is widely used, this definition does not specify what stuttering is and thus does not help measure the behavior objectively.

■ Another view focuses on the stuttering event: stuttering is an event so recognized by an expert. This definition, also widely used, does not specify the behavior or action that constitutes stuttering. It is similar to the notion of a stuttering moment in that it is both nonspecific and not helpful in objective measurement.

Definition Limited to Certain Types of Dysfluencies

■ Dysfluencies play a major role in the description and diagnosis of stuttering in many definitions. However, in some definitions, only certain types of dysfluencies are included.

■ In other words, some forms of dysfluencies are of clinical significance, while other forms are considered a part of normal speech. Some classic definitions of stuttering have limited the term to part-word repetitions and speech-sound prolongations.

■ Stuttering occurs when the forward flow of speech is interrupted by a motorically disrupted sound, syllable, or word or by the speaker's reactions thereto (Van Riper, 1982, p. 15).

- This definition restricts stuttering to sound, syllable, or word repetitions and sound prolongations. An important aspect of the definition is its emphasis on speaker reactions.

- Some clinicians consider only part-word repetitions and speech-sound prolongations as stuttering; Van Riper, though, included word repetitions in his definition. However, all other forms of dysfluencies are considered non-stuttering types.

Definition Based on Psychopathology (Neurosis)

- Psychoanalysts and psychologists believe that stuttering may be due to some kind of psychopathology or that it may be a neurotic reaction. Such psychological reactions as anxiety, frustration in self-expression, and apprehension about speaking situations or speaking certain kinds of words are all self-reported by many adults who stutter. These and other psychological reactions are the basis for definitions based on psychopathology or neurosis.

- Stuttering is a form of neurosis because it is based on some form of psychopathology. Freudian psychoanalysts believe that such psychological processes as fixation at an earlier stage of psychosexual development, frustration later in life, regression to the fixated stage of development, and subsequent symptom formation (conversion) explain stuttering.

- Psychologists who hold the view that stuttering is a form of neurosis need not believe in the Freudian fixation-regression-symptom formation model, however. Some may believe that stuttering is a form of learned neurotic reaction.

Concepts To Consider

How is stuttering defined? Describe at least three definitions.

_____

_____

_____

_____

_____

_____

_____

_____

Definition Based on All Types of Dysfluencies

- Many experts tend to describe stuttering in terms of the frequency and duration of dysfluencies. Several experts tend to include all types of dysfluencies in their definitions or descriptions of stuttering: Stuttering is the production of dysfluencies of excessive frequency, excessive durations, or both.

- In that definition, stuttering includes all varieties of dysfluencies. In a later section of this chapter, different varieties of dysfluencies are described with examples. It is important to note that both excessive frequency and excessive duration of dysfluencies may be grounds for a diagnosis of stuttering.

Definition Based on Etiology

- Most definitions are descriptions of what constitutes stuttering. Very few include a hypothesized cause of stuttering. One such definition says that stuttering is that class of fluency failure that is a result of classically conditioned negative emotion; only part-word repetitions and sound prolongations fall into this category; all other forms of dysfluencies are not stutterings but are operantly conditioned (Brutten & Shoemaker, 1967).

- In this definition, two types of etiology are hypothesized for two classes of dysfluencies. Part-word repetitions and speech-sound prolongations are said to fall into one category and all other forms into another. Repetitions and prolongations are hypothesized to be a result of negative emotion; their basis is Pavlovian, or classical conditioning.

- All other forms of dysfluencies (including whole-word repetitions, interjections, pauses, etc.), according to this definition, are due to Skinnerian, or operant conditioning. Stuttering is diagnosed only on the basis of part-word repetitions and speech-sound prolongations.

Forms of Dysfluencies

- Regardless of definitional orientations, it is important to understand the different forms of dysfluencies, as they all interrupt fluency. The following are the major types of dysfluencies and their examples:

- *Repetitions*. Saying the same element of speech more than once.

  - *Part-word repetitions* (sound or syllable repetitions): Repetition of a part of a word or a sound or syllable (e.g., "S-S-S-Saturday" or "Sa-Sa-Sa-Saturday").

  - *Whole-word repetitions*: Repetition of an entire word more than once; word repeated may be of single or multiple syllables (e.g., "I-I-I am fine" or "could-could-could not do it").

– *Phrase repetitions*: Repetition of more than one word (e.g., "I am–I am–I am fine" or "could not–could not–could not do it").

■ *Sound prolongations*. Sounds produced for a duration longer than typical (e.g., "lllllike it" or "Mmmmommy").

■ *Silent prolongations*. An articulatory posture held for a duration longer than average but with no vocalization (e.g., the articulatory position held for longer than usual while producing a word such as *Wanda,* in which the *W* can be prolonged).

■ *Interjections*. Extraneous elements introduced into the speech sequence. These may be one of the following:

– sound or syllable interjections

– word interjections

– phrase interjections

■ *Pauses*. Silent intervals in the speech sequence at inappropriate junctures or of unusually long duration.

■ *Broken words*. Silent intervals within words, also known as *intralexical pauses* (e.g., "Be [pause] fore you say it").

■ *Incomplete sentences*. Often described as incomplete phrases, these are grammatically incomplete productions (e.g., "Last summer I was . . . last summer . . . we went to Paris this time").

■ *Revisions*. Changes in wording that do not change the overall meaning of an utterance (e.g., "Let us have a drink—coffee").

Theoretical and Clinical Significance of Dysfluencies

■ As the different definitions of stuttering make evident, not all experts agree on how to evaluate different forms of dysfluencies. Some think that only certain forms of dysfluencies are stutterings; others think that all forms of dysfluencies, if they exceed certain quantitative limits of duration and frequency, are stutterings (or at least disorders of fluency even if not diagnosed as stuttering).

■ There is evidence that forms of dysfluency that are traditionally not considered indicative of stuttering (e.g., whole-word repetitions or schwa interjections) may still evoke judgments of stuttering from listeners if the frequency exceeds certain limits (Hegde & Hartman, 1979a, 1979b).

■ Generally, speech that contains 5% or more dysfluencies may be judged dysfluent or stuttered by most listeners. Bloodstein, among others, has advocated that dysfluencies found in normally fluent speech, if they exceed certain limits, are grounds for diagnosing stuttering.

■ Research also has shown that listeners may have different tolerance thresholds for different forms of dysfluencies. Part-word repetitions (e.g., "buh-buh-baby") and sound prolongations are judged abnormal at lower frequencies (as low as 2% of words spoken), whereas whole-word repetitions and schwa interjections must reach at least 5% to evoke judgments of dysfluent or stuttered speech.

■ Thus, all forms of dysfluencies that exceed certain limits of frequency or duration may be judged abnormal, but some forms are judged abnormal at lower levels of frequency or duration.

Incidence and Prevalence of Stuttering

General Principles

■ The *incidence* of a given disorder or disease is its rate of occurrence in a specified group of people. Incidence is studied by the longitudinal method.

■ An incidence study starts with a healthy or normal group of subjects and repeatedly observes those individuals over a period of time, counting the number who begin to show a particular disease or disorder. Incidence is a predictive statement. Incidence studies are more expensive and time consuming than prevalence studies.

■ *Prevalence* of a particular disorder or disease is determined by counting the number of individuals who currently have it. Prevalence involves a head count. To establish the prevalence of a disorder, investigators use a cross-sectional method of study.

■ A prevalence study starts with clinical records of individuals who already exhibit a disorder. The study's investigators collect information from various sources (e.g., clinics and hospitals) and add up the number of individuals who are receiving clinical services or have received such services.

■ Prevalence does not make a predictive statement; it simply gives the current number of people who exhibit a disorder. Prevalence studies are less expensive and less time consuming than incidence studies. However, head counting often underestimates the prevalence of a disorder by missing those who have not received clinical services.

■ Most available studies of stuttering are prevalence studies; most are rough estimates. There are only a few studies of the incidence of stuttering. However, incidence and prevalence can be derived from each other.

Incidence and Prevalence in the General Population

■ A classic study of incidence was conducted in England and reported by Andrews and Harris in 1964. They studied more than 1,000 newborn babies and followed them for 15 years. This is the only longitudinal study of stuttering of such a long duration involving such a large number of subjects. This and other, less extensive, studies on the incidence and prevalence of stuttering have shown the following facts:

■ The life time expectancy of stuttering is about 5%. This means that 5% of the population has a probability of ever stuttering, even if stuttering lasts only a few days, weeks, or months.

■ The prevalence is about 1% in the general U.S. population. Somewhat higher prevalence rates have been reported for European countries. Investigations have shown that the prevalence of stuttering is higher in African Americans than in other ethnic groups in the United States (Cooper & Cooper, 1998). Experts believe that in spite of variations, no society is completely free from stuttering.

■ The risk of developing a stutter varies by age, but stuttering typically begins during early childhood. In the majority, stuttering begins between the ages of 3 and 6 years. The onset of stuttering is relatively rare after 12 years of age.

■ Adult onset of stuttering is rare. In some cases, a reemergence may occur of early childhood stuttering, from which the individual had recovered. In most cases, adult onset of stuttering is associated with neurological damage or disease. For example, some adults begin to stutter after a stroke or as a result of Alzheimer's dementia.

Spontaneous Recovery

■ Spontaneous recovery of stuttering is its disappearance without professional help. The term may be a misnomer because such recovery may be associated with the use of certain techniques. For instance, a stutterer may accidentally discover that a slower rate of speech reduces stuttering and adopt such a rate. That is not truly spontaneous recovery.

■ That some children and adolescents recover from stuttering without professional help has been documented, but the percentage of such recovery has remained controversial. Some early studies have suggested a 60% or higher spontaneous recovery rate.

■ Others believe that a realistic spontaneous recovery rate is about 30 to 35%. Even then, the rate applies to groups of stuttering children, not to individual children. It is not possible to predict whether a given child will recover spontaneously.

Prevalence and Gender Ratio

■ It is well documented that stuttering is far more common in males than in females. The most frequently cited ratio is 3:1 (male:female) for children in earlier elementary grades.

■ The ratio is larger in higher grades (perhaps 4:1). This may be because of a slightly higher spontaneous recovery of stuttering in girls or because of a greater number of new cases in boys.

■ The documented gender ratio has given rise to hypotheses about possible genetic factors in the etiology of stuttering.

Familial Prevalence

■ Familial prevalence is the frequency with which a given condition appears in successive generations of blood relatives.

■ The familial prevalence of stuttering is higher than that in the general population. If there is one stuttering person in a family, there are likely to be others among his or her blood relatives. It is estimated that the familial prevalence of stuttering is more than three times higher than that in the general population.

■ Some evidence suggests that familial prevalence is higher in families that have a female stutterer than in families that have a male stutterer. Familial prevalence and gender ratio interact; sons of mothers who stutter run a greater risk of stuttering than sons of fathers who stutter.

■ Daughters generally have a lower risk, but daughters of stuttering mothers have a higher risk than daughters of nonstuttering mothers or of stuttering fathers. Familial incidence may be explained on the basis of genetic or environmental factors; most experts tend to emphasize genetic factors.

Prevalence and Concordance Rates in Twins

■ *Concordance* is the occurrence of the same clinical condition (or normal trait) in both members of a twin pair. If both members of a twin pair have the same condition, then they are *concordant* for that condition; if only one member of a twin pair has a particular condition, then the pair is *discordant* for that condition.

■ A *concordance rate* for stuttering is based on the number of twin pairs studied and the number in whom stuttering is evident in both members. For instance, if in a hundred pairs of twins studied, stuttering is found in both members of 50 pairs, then the concordance rate would be 50%; the remaining 50% would be discordant (one twin member stutters; the other does not).

■ Differential concordance rates in ordinary siblings, identical (monozygotic) twins, and fraternal (dizygotic) twins would suggest the importance of genetic variables in stuttering.

■ The concordance rate of stuttering for identical twins is higher than that for fraternal twins; the rates reported vary across studies with a range of 30% to 80% of identical twin pairs.

■ The concordance rate for fraternal twins is higher than that for ordinary siblings; this suggests that at least a *portion* of the concordance rate for identical twins may be due to their common environment.

■ Studies of identical twins who have been separated and brought up in different environments and of children who have been adopted by families with and without stuttering members might be more definitive, but such studies either are nonexistent or have reported ambiguous results.

■ Differential prevalence data suggest that both genetic factors (which predispose the individual to stutter) and environmental events (which may trigger the disorder) play a part in the etiology of stuttering.

Concepts To Consider

List three facts about the incidence and prevalence of stuttering. What does current research state about the familial and gender prevalence of stuttering?

_____

_____

_____

_____

_____

_____

_____

_____

_____

Prevalence in Other Selected Populations

■ The prevalence of stuttering in several other specific populations has been studied. A somewhat *higher* prevalence of stuttering than that for the general population has been reported for:

  – developmentally disabled people (especially children and adults with Down syndrome); some data suggest that many in this group may clutter (see "Cluttering" section later in chapter) or clutter and stutter;

  – neurologically impaired people (especially the brain-injured and epileptic)

■ A *lower* prevalence of stuttering has been reported for deaf and hard of hearing people; at one time, it was claimed that deaf people do not stutter. However, stuttering in deaf people with oral skills has been documented; the reported lower prevalence may be due to the limited oral language skills in many individuals who are deaf.

Prevalence and Ethnocultural Variables

■ Some experts, Wendell Johnson among them, have claimed that stuttering is a culturally determined disorder. According to Johnson (1959), parents who are critical of their children's normal nonfluencies tend to encourage apprehension and avoidance reactions, which he called stuttering.

■ Johnson has further stated that societies and cultures that place a heavy emphasis on verbal skills have a higher prevalence of stuttering; Native Americans, for example, do not stutter, according to him.

■ Johnson's theory has been contradicted by data. Native Americans do stutter; as previously noted, stuttering is found in almost all societies and ethnocultural groups. The prevalence rates appear to be somewhat different in different ethnocultural groups, but those differences are hard to explain and may even be due to methodological variations across studies.

Onset and Development of Stuttering

■ Stuttering begins as the frequency of dysfluencies increases. The increase may be sudden or gradual, but the dysfluency rate remains highly variable for some time, resulting in periods of normal or near-normal fluency alternating with periods of excessive dysfluency.

■ In many cases, parents report nothing unusual about the time of onset. Excessive tension, facial grimaces, and breathing abnormalities may or may not be present at or soon after the onset.

■ The frequency of dysfluencies may stabilize and become more consistent across situations and time, although some degree of variability is a basic characteristic of stuttering, even in adults with many years of stuttering history.

■ Development of avoidance and negative emotions (described later) may occur as stuttering becomes more consistent across situations and on certain words.

Associated Motor Behaviors

■ Stuttering may be associated with various abnormal motor behaviors, including:

- excessive muscular effort

- various facial grimaces

- various hand and foot movements (e.g., wringing the hands, tapping the foot)

   – rapid eye blinking

   – knitting of the eyebrows

   – lip pursing

   – rapid opening and closing of the mouth

   – tongue clicking

- The number and severity of associated motor behaviors vary across individuals. While some children who stutter show notable associated motor behaviors, others may show none or show several that are almost undetectable. Adults who stutter generally show at least a few associated motor behaviors; some show many and severe forms of such behaviors.

- Associated motor behaviors may have been accidentally reinforced. For instance, just when a person who stutters experienced a release from stuttering, he or she may have jerked an arm. From then on, an arm jerk may be associated with stuttering. Such accidentally reinforced associated motor behaviors rarely help the stuttering persons speak fluently.

- Associated motor behaviors are not crucial for a diagnosis of stuttering. Excessive frequency or duration of dysfluencies is sufficient to diagnose stuttering. However, the presence of severe forms of frequently exhibited motor behaviors associated with increased frequency or duration of dysfluencies virtually assures a diagnosis of stuttering.

Associated Breathing Abnormalities

- In many people, stuttered speech may be associated with certain breathing abnormalities. Although not crucial for a diagnosis of stuttering, it is important to consider the following kinds of associated breathing abnormalities:

   – attempts to speak on inhalation

   – holding breath before talking

   – continued attempts to speak even when the air supply is exhausted

   – interruption of inhalations by exhalations and vice versa

   – speaking without first inhaling a sufficient amount of air

   – rapid and jerky breathing during speech

   – exhaling puffs of air during stuttered speech

   – generally tensed breathing

- The noted breathing abnormalities do not suggest an inherent respiratory disorder; they are a part of the stuttering symptom complex. Fluent speech in people who stutter is not characterized by severe forms of breathing abnormalities.

Negative Emotions and Avoidance Behaviors

■ When stuttering persists, negative emotions and avoidance of words and speaking situations tend to develop. Avoidance and negative emotions are not crucial to a diagnosis of stuttering, although they are important to consider in a comprehensive program of assessment and treatment.

■ Negative emotions associated with stuttering include anxiety and apprehension about stuttering, fear of certain speaking situations, possibly some hostility toward certain speakers, frustration in efforts to communicate, and, possibly, a sense of humiliation in certain difficult speaking situations.

■ Difficult speaking situations include speaking with strangers and formal audiences, speaking with people at counters where services or products are bought, speaking on the telephone, ordering in restaurants, speaking to authority figures, and self-introductions or introductions of other people; however, avoidance of listeners and speaking situations is typically client-specific.

■ Avoidance may occur of specific sounds and words on which stuttering is frequently experienced, resulting in circumlocution and use of nonspecific words. However, sounds and words avoided are typically client-specific. For example, one client might avoid words beginning with *b* because he stutters more when saying such words. Another client may avoid saying her boss's name because she stutters whenever she tries to say it.

■ People who stutter may anticipate or expect to have more or fewer problems in certain speaking situations. A majority of people who stutter can predict a certain amount of their stuttering; however, there is no one-to-one correspondence between the anticipation of and actual stuttering. Words not expected to be stuttered may be, and those that are expected to be stuttered may be spoken fluently.

The Loci of Stuttering

■ Certain classes of sounds, words in certain positions in a sentence, and certain kinds of words have a high probability of being stuttered. Based on such observations, it is possible to predict the loci of stuttering. The *loci of stuttering* refers to the locations in a speech sequence where stutterings are typically observed.

■ In the speech of *adults and school-age children* who stutter, stuttering is more likely to occur:

   – *with consonants than with vowels*, though some speakers stutter predominantly on vowels; this is explained partly on the basis of the greater complexity of consonantal productions than vowel productions;

   – *on the first sound or syllable of a word*; more than 90% of stutterings occur on the initial sound or syllable of a word; this suggests that stuttering is a phenomenon of either disturbed speech initiation or disturbed movement to the next element in the speech chain;

- *on the first word in a phrase or sentence*; generally, the first few words are more likely to be stuttered than the last few words in a sentence; this again suggests that the initial components in a speech sequence are more difficult than subsequent components;

- *on the first word in a grammatical clause*; this suggests that grammatical class initiation is somewhat similar to sentence initiation;

- *on longer words*; this is explained on the basis that longer words may be generally more difficult to produce than shorter words;

- *with less frequently used words*; this may be because less frequently used words tend to be longer as well;

- *on content words* (nouns, verbs, adjectives, and adverbs) more often than on function words (articles, conjunctions, prepositions, and pronouns); this tendency may partly be due to the word position; content words tend to initiate more sentences and phrases than do function words.

■ The loci of stuttering in *preschool children* are the same as those for adults and school-age children except for one factor; preschool children's stuttering tends to occur on function words (especially pronouns, conjunctions, and prepositions).

■ This contrasts with the adult and school-age stutterers' tendency to stutter more often on content words than on function words. This is partly explained on the basis that preschool children tend to initiate their phrases and sentences with certain function words, especially pronouns and conjunctions.

■ In addition, preschool children tend to exhibit many whole word repetitions. Thus, an early characteristic of stuttering is an increase in whole word repetitions.

■ Generally, dysfluencies tend to occur at the same loci in the speech of stuttering and nonstuttering people. Dysfluencies in the speech of people who do not stutter also tend to occur on initial consonants, initial words, longer words, less frequently used words, and content words.

✎ Concepts To Consider

Summarize the results of the research on the loci of stuttering.

_____

_____

_____

_____

_____

_____

_____

_____

_____

Stimulus Control in Stuttering

■ Stuttering shows certain patterns of variation that suggest a strong environmental control. Research has shown that stuttering varies systematically when certain variables are manipulated. A few important phenomena that suggest a strong stimulus control of stuttering include adaptation, consistency, adjacency, and audience size.

Adaptation

■ The *adaptation effect* is systematic reduction in the frequency of stuttering when a short printed passage is repeatedly read aloud. Research has identified several important characteristics of adaptation, which include those explained below:

  – The amount of reduction in stuttering is greatest during the first few oral readings of a passage; by about the fifth reading, most reduction will have been evident.

  – The magnitude of reduction is progressively less on subsequent readings of the same passage until the amount of reduction is negligible.

  – The greater the time interval between readings, the less the degree of adaptation.

  – There is no transfer of adaptation from one passage to another.

  – Adaptation is a temporary phenomenon; if the same passage is read after a few hours of rest, the amount of stuttering will have increased to the baseline level.

  – Silent reading of a passage does not decrease the magnitude of stuttering when that passage is subsequently read orally.

  – Lipped or whispered reading may reduce stuttering to some extent, but repeated oral reading produces the most dramatic adaptation.

  – Less severe stuttering tends to adapt more than more severe stuttering.

- Both children and adults, and those who stutter and those who do not, show adaptation.

- There is a great deal of individual difference in the amount of adaptation exhibited; most adapt to varying extents; some do not adapt at all; and some show an increase in stuttering upon repeated readings.

■ Adaptation has been explained in various ways, including the following:

- Adaptation is an experimental extinction of the stuttering response (Wischner, 1950).

- Adaptation is due to a deconfirmation of the expectancy of stuttering, which results in reduced anxiety and reduced stuttering (Johnson, 1959).

- Adaptation is due to a reactive inhibition; stuttering is reduced because it produces a reactive inhibition (fatigue), which suppresses further stuttering (Brutten & Shoemaker, 1967).

- Adaptation is due to fear reduction; each instance of stuttering reduces fear of stuttering and hence further reduces stuttering (Sheehan, 1970).

- Adaptation is due to the rehearsal effect; repeated reading of the same passage provides rehearsal of the material and hence a reduction in stuttering (Bloodstein, 1995).

■ There is no agreement on the explanation of adaptation. No theory is fully supported by data. The degree of adaptation is inconclusive evidence of the degree of improvement that will occur in therapy.

Consistency

■ The *consistency effect* is the occurrence of stuttering on the same word or loci when a passage is read aloud repeatedly. In a sense, it is the opposite of the adaptation effect: While adaptation refers to a disappearance of stuttering on certain previously stuttered words, consistency refers to stuttering on the same words upon repeated reading.

■ Aspects of the consistency effect include the following:

- About 65% of stuttering in given individuals may be consistent; that is, stuttering tends to occur on the same words or loci in repeated readings.

- Consistency remains when the subjects reread a passage after weeks of interval.

■ The consistency effect is presumed to be an indicator of the strength of the stimuli that evoke stuttering. The consistency effect is a stimulus-response phenomenon.

Adjacency

■ The *adjacency effect* is the occurrence of new stuttering on words that surround previously stuttered words. It is a striking phenomenon of stimulus control.

■ This effect is studied by having a subject read a passage multiple times, blotting out or otherwise concealing the words on which stuttering occurs, and then having the subject read the passage again to note the occurrence of new stuttering.

■ The results of such experiments have shown that:

– In several subjects, words that were fluently read during earlier readings were eventually stuttered.

– The newly stuttered words were often adjacent to those blotted-out (previously stuttered words).

– The adjacency effect is evident in adults and children who stutter.

– The adjacency effect may be horizontal (new stuttering occurs on words to the right or left of the blotted out word on which stuttering had occurred previously) or vertical (new stuttering occurs on words printed below or above the word previously stuttered).

■ The adjacency effect is yet another powerful demonstration of stimulus control of stuttering. A stimulus associated with past stuttering may serve as a stimulus for new stuttering.

Audience Size

■ The *audience size effect* refers to the observation that the frequency of stuttering increases with an increase in audience size.

■ Yet another striking phenomenon of stimulus control, the audience size effect is characterized by:

– a marked decrease in stuttering when there is no audience and the person is speaking to himself or herself;

– a corresponding increase in the amount of stuttering with a systematic increase in the number of listeners;

– a reduced amount of stuttering when a listener's hearing is visibly masked; and

– a greater amount of stuttering when listeners can hear the stutterer than when listeners can only see the stutterer.

■ The audience size effect is another demonstration of conditioning and stimulus control over stuttering. This phenomenon is sometimes explained on the basis of communicative pressure. The greater the number of listeners, the higher the communicative pressure.

People Who Stutter and Their Families

■ Various theories and viewpoints in the past held that certain "personality" variables might be the underlying cause of stuttering. This idea is especially inherent to psychoneurotic conceptions of stuttering, in which persons who stutter are thought to exhibit psychoneurotic tendencies.

■ Other conceptions, such as those of Johnson (1959), implied that parents of stutterers may hold unusually and unrealistically high standards of fluency.

■ Such parents are then likely to place undue pressure on their children or to misdiagnose stuttering based on normal nonfluency, as Johnson has hypothesized. Such views have led to an investigation of the personality of individuals who stutter and their families, especially their parents.

■ Such personality variables as anxiety, level of aspiration, obsessive-compulsive behaviors, oral and anal eroticism, passive-dependency, hostility and aggression, self-concept, social adjustment, body image, and so forth have been investigated over several decades. Various kinds of questionnaires and such projective tests as the Rorschach have been used.

■ This kind of research has shown that people who stutter:

- do not have a distinct personality that may be causally related to their stuttering;

- are not clinically maladjusted;

- are not clinically and chronically anxious (although many may have slightly elevated levels of anxiety in speaking situations, this may be an effect, not a cause, of stuttering); and

- may have low self-esteem, possibly due to their stuttering.

■ Research on parents of people who stutter has shown that they:

- do not exhibit unique personality patterns that may be causally related to stuttering in their children;

- are not clinically maladjusted or neurotic;

- may exhibit a somewhat higher standard of behavior and be somewhat more critical of their children than are parents of children who do not stutter; however, the clinical significance of this finding is unclear and a general conclusion about its importance is unwarranted.

■ In essence, neither the personality of people who stutter nor that of their parents seems to provide strong clues to the etiology of stuttering. People who stutter and their parents are not a distinct and unique group of individuals who are neurotic or maladjusted. In most respects, they are like people who do not stutter and their parents.

✎ Concepts To Consider

Define the adaptation, consistency, and adjacency effects discussed in the literature on stuttering.

_____

_____

_____

_____

_____

_____

_____

Theories of Stuttering

Foundational Concepts

- There are environmental, genetic, and neurophysiological theories of stuttering. However, no theory explains all aspects of stuttering.

- Theories are likely to remain incomplete until the nature of causation is determined. Existing theories are at best hypotheses that require the support of additional research. Hence, none is universally accepted as an explanation of stuttering. Several theories are described below.

- The basic premise of genetic and neurophysiological theories of stuttering is that the person who stutters has a genetic basis for stuttering and that his or her neurophysiological speech system is deviant compared to that in nonstuttering individuals.

- Theories within this group differ in their emphasis on genetic and neurophysiological variables. Some place a greater emphasis on genetic variables, while others emphasize neurophysiological organization involved in speech production.

- Other theories about stuttering include those that focus on the role of learning and conditioning as well as those that view stuttering as a form of psychoneurosis.

Genetic Hypothesis

■ There is much speculation about the role genes play in the genesis of stuttering. A potential genetic basis of stuttering is suggested by the following observations:

  − Stuttering has a higher familial incidence.

  − There is a well-established gender ratio in the prevalence of stuttering.

  − Stuttering shows a higher concordance rate among identical twins.

■ Although various kinds of data suggest a possible genetic basis in a certain number of individuals, no gene or chromosomal abnormality responsible for stuttering has been identified. Also, no particular mechanism of inheritance of stuttering has been clearly established. Furthermore, in about half the number of cases, familial incidence may be negative.

■ Evidence does not suggest a simple, Mendelian type of inheritance. Data do not support sex-linked, autosomal, or recessive inheritance patterns. Some investigators believe that patterns of familial prevalence suggest inheritance due to a single gene.

■ Others believe that inheritance may be based on multiple genes (polygenic inheritance) that predispose an individual to stutter. Currently, no genetic transmission theory is universally accepted (Bloodstein, 1995).

Neurophysiological Hypotheses

■ Several variations exist of the basic neurophysiological position that people who stutter have an abnormal neurophysiological or neuromotor organization.

■ The *laryngeal dysfunction hypothesis* states that stuttering is due to aberrant laryngeal functions. The etiology of aberrant laryngeal function may be defective neuromotor control of the laryngeal mechanism, as no local laryngeal pathology has been documented in people who stutter.

■ Evidence supporting the laryngeal dysfunction hypothesis includes the following:

  − *slightly delayed voice onset time* (VOT) in some people who stutter; VOT is measured by giving a visual or auditory signal to produce a simple vocal response (e.g., saying /a/) and measuring the time between the offset of the stimulus and the onset of the vocal response; delay is in milliseconds and fades with repeated trials;

  − *increased tension in the laryngeal muscles* associated with stuttered speech, measured by such techniques as electromyography;

- – *aberrant muscle behavior* during stuttered speech (e.g., simultaneous activation of laryngeal abductors and adductors, which are normally active reciprocally); and

- – *excessive laryngeal muscle activity* during stuttered speech, also measured by such techniques as electromyography.

■ Whether laryngeal abnormality, especially the delayed vocal reaction time, is due to potential respiratory problems is an unresolved issue. Vocal responses involve respiratory responses as well. Problems in respiratory control of the speech mechanism could result in delayed vocal response.

■ *Hypotheses on the brain and speech and language mechanisms and stuttering* suggest that the brain, which controls the speech mechanism, may not be working properly in speakers who stutter. Related hypotheses suggest that the auditory portion of the brain may not be functioning properly or that there may be an auditory feedback problem.

■ Evidence suggesting potential brain dysfunction in people who stutter includes the following:

  - – Some studies suggest that people who stutter may not have a *dominant hemisphere* to process language. This lack of dominance for language may cause inefficient or even confused neuromotor control of the speech mechanism, resulting in stuttering.

  - – Some *electroencephalographic* studies suggest that the brain waves, especially the alpha waves, may be abnormal in some people who stutter. However, the evidence on abnormal brain waves is contradictory. While some studies report abnormal patterns of brain waves, others report essentially normal patterns.

  - – Limited evidence suggests that in some people who stutter, *cerebral blood flow* may be reduced. Such a reduction has been noted in the frontal lobe involved in speech-motor control and the left temporal lobe.

  - – Some *cineradiographic* studies of face and oral structures suggest that even when speech is fluent, movements involved in speech are slower than normal in people who stutter; the brain may not be initiating and regulating speech activity in a smooth, efficient, and coordinated manner.

  - – Some studies on the *central auditory function* in people who stutter suggest potential involvement of the auditory portion of the brain although the specific pathology is unclear. Studies on central auditory processing suggest that some people who stutter may have subtle central auditory problems. Such evidence has been reported with the ipsilateral competing message test, the acoustic reflex amplitude function, and the staggered spondaic word test. However, contradictory evidence suggests essentially normal central auditory function in most people who stutter.

- Unspecified *auditory feedback problems* are suggested by studies investigating delayed auditory feedback and auditory masking noise, both of which reduce most types of dysfluencies. Based on such outcomes, some experts have suggested a potential involvement of the auditory mechanism in the etiology of stuttering. Investigators have speculated that people who stutter may have a basic delay in processing auditory information, and thus delayed auditory feedback helps them achieve greater fluency. Masking noise was once hypothesized to prevent stuttering people from hearing their own voice or masking a defective auditory feedback mechanism. That hypothesis has been discredited by studies that show that stuttering is reduced under even mild masking that does not prevent auditory feedback. Some experts attribute increased fluency under altered auditory conditions to a decreased speech rate, which is dramatically evident in delayed auditory feedback.

Learning, Conditioning, and Related Hypotheses

- In contrast to neurophysiological theories, learning, conditioning, and a few other somewhat related theories emphasize the importance of environmental variables in the etiology of stuttering. These theories also have several variations, including those described below.

Stuttering as an Operant Behavior

- Some studies suggest that stuttering may be an operant behavior. An operant is a behavior that can be changed by changing its consequences.

- Some studies have shown that stuttering frequency may be decreased by corrective feedback (e.g., saying, "No," or, "Wrong," for every dysfluency), response-contingent electric shock or noise, time-out, or response cost. The evidence on the effect of shock on stuttering is somewhat controversial, while the evidence on the effects of time-out and response cost is more uniform and positive.

- Studies generally have shown that any stimulus can decrease stuttering. For example, the word "tree" presented response-contingently can reduce the frequency of stuttering. Such studies do suggest that stuttering may be an operant because to show that a behavior is an operant, one only needs to show that its frequency may be altered by certain consequences.

Stuttering as Speech Disruption Due to Classically Conditioned Negative Emotion

- Brutten and Shoemaker (1967) have proposed that stuttering consists of fluency disruption due to classically conditioned negative emotion.

- They limit the term *stuttering* to part-word repetitions and sound prolongations that are based on negative emotion. The negative emotion may be classically conditioned to speaking situations, sounds, words, or audience factors. In this theory, all other forms of dysfluencies (e.g., whole word repetitions, interjections, pauses) are operant behaviors that can be changed by changing their consequences.

■ Stutterings as defined in the theory are not operant behaviors and can be reduced only by counter-conditioning more positive emotional reactions that replace those negative emotions.

Stuttering as Avoidance Behavior

■ This view, too, has several variations. An early and systematic theory of stuttering based on avoidance is that of Johnson (1959).

■ His *diagnosogenic theory* states that when parents punish a child's normal nonfluencies, the child develops anticipatory, apprehensive, and hypertonic avoidance reactions that are indeed stutterings. Johnson (1959) asserted that dysfluencies are normal as they are found in almost all speakers, and, hence, stuttering could not be diagnosed based on a feature of normal dysfluency.

■ It is only when a child begins to *avoid* the consequences of normal nonfluencies that the stuttering problem emerges. Johnson further asserts that stuttering is a cultural phenomenon created by parents who overly emphasize fluency.

■ Consistent with that position, Johnson believed that such cultures as those of Native Americans, who did not emphasize fluency, did not have people who stutter. It is now well known that Native Americans do stutter and that there is no conclusive evidence of parental punishment of normal nonfluency being the origin of avoidance behaviors (Bloodstein, 1995).

Stuttering as Approach-Avoidance

■ Sheehan's (1970) early version of stuttering theory emphasizes an approach-avoidance conflict. He believed that a stuttering person's hesitations and repetitions indicate a conflict between a desire to approach speaking situations and an equally strong desire to avoid them.

■ Fluent speech is possible when the drive or desire to speak is stronger than the drive to avoid speech. When the drive to avoid speech is the stronger of the two, the person does not talk at all. However, when the two drive states are equal in strength, stuttering results.

Stuttering as a Reaction of Tension and Fragmentation

■ Bloodstein (1995) has proposed that stuttering is essentially a response of tension and fragmentation in speech. Stuttering is not unlike normal nonfluency (dysfluency), though it is typically greater in quantity and more disruptive in quality. Such a response of tension and fragmentation may come about because of a child's belief that speech is a difficult task.

- Unlike Johnson, who proposed that the origin of stuttering (avoidance behavior) is parental disapproval of normal nonfluency, Bloodstein thinks that stuttering may have many origins, most of them related to various kinds of severe communicative pressure that leads to repeated communicative failures. This view is generally known as the *anticipatory struggle hypothesis* (Bloodstein, 1995).

Stuttering Due to Demands Exceeding Capacities

- This view of stuttering implies an interaction between a child's inherent linguistic, cognitive, motoric, or emotional capacity for effective and fluent communication and environmental demands made on the child for realizing such communication.

- The theory essentially states that stuttering can result when a child faces demands for communication that he or she cannot meet because of limited capacities. This view, known as the *demands and capacities model*, is not unlike other approaches such as that of Bloodstein (1995), which states that continued and severe communicative pressure can result in chronic communicative failure.

Concepts To Consider

Summarize the key points of the neurophysiological and the learning and conditioning hypotheses of stuttering.

_____

_____

_____

_____

_____

_____

_____

Stuttering as a Form of Psychoneurosis

- The hypothesis that states that stuttering may be a psychological disorder has a long history. A particular form of this hypothesis was proposed by Freudians, who considered stuttering a form of psychoneurosis.

- This hypothesis states that stuttering is due to an underlying psychopathology and that stutterings themselves are merely symptoms of deep-seated psychological conflicts.

These conflicts are generated and maintained by such psychological processes as infantile fixation, later frustration, regression to the fixated stage, and symptom formation. In this sense, stuttering is similar to other forms of neurosis including anxiety, phobia, and hysterical (conversion) reaction. Such unconscious but socially unacceptable urges as oral or anal gratification may find socially acceptable forms of expression such as repetitions or prolongations. The main problems with the psychoanalytic explanation of stuttering are that it is unverifiable and that treatment based on it is generally ineffective.

Summary

- ☑ Fluent speech is generally rhythmic, smooth, and produced with ease. Stuttered speech contains excessive amounts of dysfluencies, durations of dysfluencies, or both. Various definitions of stuttering exist.

- ☑ The incidence and prevalence of stuttering have been studied in relation to the general population, spontaneous recovery, prevalence and gender ratio, familial prevalence, and prevalence and concordance rates in twins and other selected populations.

- ☑ Stuttering onset may be gradual or sudden. It is usually characterized by abnormal associated motor behaviors, breathing abnormalities, negative emotions, and avoidance behaviors.

- ☑ Several phenomena such as adaptation, consistency, adjacency, and audience size suggest that there is a strong stimulus control of stuttering.

- ☑ There are environmental, genetic, and neurophysiological theories of stuttering. No theory explains all aspects of stuttering, and hence none is universally accepted.

ASSESSMENT AND TREATMENT OF STUTTERING

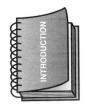

INTRODUCTION

Assessment of stuttering includes standard procedures such as a hearing screening, a detailed case history obtained from the client and/or family members, and assessment of the stuttering itself. A detailed assessment of the stuttering includes evaluation of the frequency and types of dysfluencies, variability in stuttering, associated motor behaviors, avoidance behaviors, rate of speech, and negative emotional reactions. Methods of treatment of stuttering include psychological methods, the fluent stuttering method, the fluency shaping method, the fluency reinforcement method, masking and delayed auditory feedback techniques, and the direct stuttering reduction method.

Assessment of Stuttering

■ Assessment includes procedures designed to evaluate stuttering and related behaviors. In addition to standard procedures such as hearing screening and orofacial examination, the following are important considerations (Hegde, 1996a).

■ It is important to take a detailed case history by interviewing the client, the family members, or both to obtain information on:

- the onset of stuttering and any special circumstances associated with the onset;

- familial prevalence of stuttering;

- the earliest behaviors considered stuttering by the family members, other caretakers, or teachers who initially diagnosed the stuttering;

- the initial and subsequent course of the stuttering, including its variability and stability;

- prior clinical services and the names of the specialists who provided them;

- prior treatment procedures and their initial and subsequent effects;

- education and occupation or educational and occupational plans of the client;

- general health history; and

- language and speech development, in the case of children who stutter.

■ Assessment of the frequency and types of dysfluencies or stutterings may be conducted by:

- recording an extended conversational speech sample with the clinician and with a member of the family (e.g., the child's mother as she engages the child in conversation); and

- recording an oral reading sample with reading material appropriate for the client's age, interest, reading skill level, and ethnocultural background.

■ The clinician may make an assessment of variability in stuttering by:

- having the client or a caretaker rate different speaking situations in which stuttering frequency varies;

- obtaining verbal reports from family members regarding variability in stuttering across time and situations;

- obtaining a tape-recorded sample of speech produced at home, school, or an occupational setting;

- comparing the frequency of dysfluencies produced in the clinic with that produced in naturalistic settings; and

- repeating the clinic and the home measures if results of the two are discrepant.

■ Assessment of associated motor behaviors may be carried out by:

- taking note of the associated motor behaviors exhibited during assessment; and

- describing those behaviors.

■ The clinician may conduct an assessment of avoidance behaviors by:

- having the client describe sounds, words, situations, and audience types typically avoided;

- taking note of words and sounds avoided during the interview;

- asking the client to make a list of sounds or words that are especially difficult and submit this list during the next clinical visit;

- asking the client to make a hierarchy of most difficult (e.g., speaking to the boss) to least difficult (speaking to a close friend) speaking situations; and

- having family members describe a child's avoidance reactions.

■ Assessment of speech rate and articulatory rate may be carried out by:

- counting the number of words or syllables spoken per minute in at least three 2-minute samples of continuous speech (speech rate); and

- counting the number of syllables produced while discounting all stutterings and pauses that exceed 2 seconds (articulatory rate).

■ Assessment of negative emotional reactions may be carried out by:

- having the client describe his or her various negative emotions about speech, particular speaking situations, specific audiences, and so forth;

- administering the modified S-Scale by Andrews and Cutler (1974); and

- asking family members or friends about negative emotions the client typically expresses.

■ Diagnosis of stuttering may be made by using one of several diagnostic criteria:

- a dysfluency rate that exceeds 5% of spoken words when all kinds of dysfluencies are counted

- a certain frequency of part-word repetitions, speech sound prolongations, and broken words

- excessive duration of dysfluencies

- other criteria the clinician adopts

Treatment of Stuttering

■ There are several approaches to stuttering treatment, described in various sources (Bloodstein, 1995; Culatta & Goldberg, 1995; Guitar, 1998; Hegde, 1996b; Onslow, 1996; Van Riper, 1982). Most of the treatment procedures can be classified and described as follows.

Psychological Methods of Treatment

■ Psychological methods include Freudian psychoanalysis, non-Freudian psychotherapy, and counseling. Psychological methods are offered by psychiatrists, psychologists, and psychoanalysts. Various forms of counseling may be offered by some speech–language pathologists.

■ These methods involve the assumption that stuttering is a psychological disorder and that underlying psychological conflicts, which may be conscious or unconscious, are the causes of stuttering. Treatment consists of attempts to resolve those conflicts.

■ The somewhat varied methods include:

- discussion of psychological problems associated with stuttering;

- discussion of feelings, emotions, and attitudes associated with stuttering;

- discussion and resolution of potential psychological conflicts, unconscious psychosexual conflicts, and various kinds of negative reactions; and

- reeducation of the client about a more realistic and rational approach to the stuttering problem.

■ There is no strong evidence that psychotherapy or counseling is effective in treating stuttering. Speech–language pathologists who offer counseling do so in conjunction with other methods designed to enhance fluency. In such cases, it is difficult to claim effectiveness for any one method used.

Fluent-Stuttering Method

■ An established method of treating stuttering is Van Riper's fluent-stuttering approach, also called the stutter-more-fluently approach. Van Riper believed that modifying the severity and the visible abnormality of stuttering is the most realistic goal for many people who stutter. The goal of this approach is not normal fluency, but more fluent (less abnormal) stuttering. This method involves the steps described below:

■ *Teaching stuttering identification.* The client is taught to identify his or her stuttering and associated problems (e.g., feelings and attitudes) in both clinical and everyday situations.

■ *Desensitizing the client to his or her stuttering.* The client is encouraged to be open and honest with his or her stuttering and voluntarily stutter in many speaking situations to get desensitized.

■ *Modifying stuttering.* The client is taught to produce more fluent, easier, and less abnormal stuttering by the clinician, encouraging the client to:

   – face difficult speaking situations and use feared words without avoidance

   – use *cancellations* (pausing after a stuttered word and saying the word again with easy and more relaxed stuttering)

   – use *pull-outs,* or changing stuttering in mid-course (e.g., by slowing down and using soft articulatory contacts instead of blocking on sounds or words)

   – use *preparatory sets* (e.g., changing the manner of stuttering so that the client produces less abnormal stuttering)

■ *Stabilizing the treatment gains.* The client is encouraged to use the techniques of stuttering modification (cancellations, pull-outs, and preparatory sets) in all speaking situations.

■ *Counseling the client.* The client is encouraged to discuss the emotions and attitudes he or she associates with stuttering to gain a more realistic and accepting view of his or her difficulties.

■ A limitation of the fluent-stuttering method is that it rarely establishes normal fluency, as only modified stuttering is its goal.

Fluency-Shaping Method

■ The goal of fluency shaping (also called the speak-more-fluently approach) is to establish normal fluency (not fluent stuttering). Teaching the various skills of fluency (e.g., appropriate management of airflow to produce and sustain fluent speech, slower rate of speech, and gentle onset of phonation) is the main treatment task.

■ In different treatment programs, one or more of such fluency skills may be emphasized or particular combinations of skills may be targeted. The treatment targets and procedures include the following:

   – Teach airflow management (i.e., inhalation of air and immediate slight exhalation before phonation; teach maintenance of an even airflow throughout an utterance).

   – Teach gentle, soft, relaxed, and easy onset of phonation, beginning after the initiation of exhalation.

   – Teach a reduced rate of speech through syllable prolongation, not by extending pause durations; typically, the vowel is prolonged; if preferred, delayed auditory feedback can be used to reduce the rate of speech.

- Help the client achieve stutter-free speech, mostly by means of airflow management, gentle phonatory onset, and rate reduction through syllable prolongation.

- Shape normal prosodic features (e.g., increased rate, normal vocal intensity, and normal intonation after stutter-free speech is stabilized).

- Implement maintenance strategies (e.g., teaching self-monitoring skills and training family and friends to monitor and reinforce fluency in natural settings and over time).

■ Use specific treatment procedures as follows:

- Initially, skills are taught individually and in the sequence of airflow management, gentle onset, and rate reduction; the achievement of stutter-free speech; and the shaping of normal prosodic features.

- Treatment starts with what the client can handle; words, phrases, or even short sentences can be used to practice fluency skills. Treatment gradually moves to controlled conversation and finally to more spontaneous conversation in natural settings.

- Specific procedures include instruction, modeling, corrective feedback for mismanaged skills and dysfluencies, and positive reinforcement for correct responses.

■ A limitation of the fluency-shaping method is that it generates slow, deliberate, and somewhat unnatural-sounding fluency. Clients tend not to maintain the slower rate needed to sustain that fluency, as such a rate is socially and personally unacceptable.

Concepts To Consider

Compare and contrast the fluent-stuttering method and the fluency-shaping method. What are three key differences between those methods?

_____

_____

_____

_____

_____

_____

_____

_____

Fluency Reinforcement Method

A simple method that works with many young children is to positively reinforce fluent speech in naturalistic conversational contexts. This method can be combined with such targets as reduced speech rate.

■ In this method, the clinician:

- arranges a pleasant and relaxed therapeutic setting;

- evokes speech with the help of picture books, toys, and other play materials;

- positively reinforces the child for fluent utterances with verbal praise, tokens, or both;

- frequently models a slow, relaxed speaking rate that assures stutter-free speech; and

- reshapes normal prosody if a slower rate is an added target.

■ Clinical experience suggests that fluency reinforcement alone may be effective with young children, whereas with older children and adult clients, adding a slower speech rate as a target may increase the efficiency of the technique.

Masking and Delayed Auditory Feedback Techniques

■ An approach popular for many years in the past involved altered auditory feedback of speech. As noted in a previous section, when a stuttering person hears his or her own speech with a fraction of a second's delay, most of that person's dysfluencies are reduced. Similarly, auditory masking noise improves fluency.

■ Most experts now believe that both techniques may achieve their desirable effects by inducing syllable prolongation, especially the prolongation of vowels. Consequently, both techniques, especially the delayed auditory feedback (DAF), induce a slow speech with reduced prosodic features.

■ In using the DAF technique, the clinician:

- uses a DAF machine that allows for variable delays;

- determines a client-specific duration of delay that assures stutter-free speech;

- has the client practice stutter-free speech for varying lengths of time to eliminate stutterings; and

- fades the delay in gradual steps to reshape normal prosody while maintaining fluency.

■ The main advantage of DAF is its capacity to induce a slower rate of speech. Many clinicians, however, have found it unnecessary to use DAF to achieve that effect. Instruction and repeated modeling are often sufficient to induce a slow rate that assures stutter-free speech.

■ In using the masking noise technique of DAF, the clinician:

- determines a minimum level of auditory masking that induces stutter-free speech;

- has the client practice stutter-free speech for variable lengths of time, depending on the client's progress; and

- fades the masking noise to reshape normal prosody while maintaining fluency.

■ The use of masking noise has decreased over the years mainly because of the problems of maintaining fluent speech in natural settings. Even in therapy sessions, masking noise may eventually lose its effects because of adaptation to noise.

Direct Stuttering Reduction Method

■ Direct stuttering reduction methods seek to reduce stuttering directly, without teaching specific fluency skills or modifying stuttering into less abnormal forms. To reduce stuttering directly, behavioral methods of time-out or response cost may be used. These methods are described below:

■ *Time-out, or pause and talk.* This method involves a behavioral contingency of pausing after each dysfluency and then talking. The specific procedures include the clinician doing the following:

- saying "stop" or giving other signals (e.g., a light that comes on) as soon as a dysfluency is observed and making sure that the client completely ceases talking;

- avoiding eye contact with the client for about 5 seconds;

- reestablishing eye contact after the time-out duration and letting the client continue his or her speech; and

- maintaining eye contact, smiling, and employing other social reinforcers for fluent speech.

■ *Response cost.* This method involves a behavioral contingency of taking a positive reinforcer away from the client for every instance of stuttering. The specific procedure includes the following:

- reinforcing the client for every fluently spoken word, phrase, or sentence with a token that is backed up with other kinds of reinforcers;

- taking a token away and in a matter-of-fact manner immediately following a stuttering or at the earliest sign of it; and

- progressing from words and phrases to conversational speech (GILCU, or gradually increased length and complexity of utterance).

■ A limitation of direct stuttering reduction methods is limited research on response costs. An advantage is that both techniques can help establish more natural-sounding fluency.

Summary

- ☑ Assessment of stuttering includes standard assessment procedures and a detailed interview of the client, family, or both.

- ☑ Detailed assessment of the stuttering behavior itself includes assessment of frequency and types of dysfluencies, variability in stuttering, associated motor behaviors, avoidance behaviors, speech rate, and negative emotional reactions.

- ☑ Approaches to the treatment of stuttering include psychological methods, the fluent-stuttering method associated with Van Riper, and the fluency-shaping method.

- ☑ Other approaches to treatment include the fluency reinforcement method, masking and delayed auditory feedback techniques, and the direct stuttering reduction method.

CLUTTERING

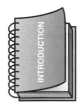

INTRODUCTION

Cluttering is a disorder of fluency that often coexists with stuttering. People described as clutterers often speak in a highly dysfluent, rapid, unclear, and disorganized manner that is jerky and monotonous. They do not manifest obvious concern about their speaking patterns. Little research exists on treatment of cluttering, although it has been found that decreasing the rate of speech and increasing the client's awareness of the problem are often effective.

Definition and Description of Cluttering

■ Compared to stuttering, less information is available on cluttering. The prevalence of cluttering in the United States is unknown, but in Germany it is reported to be 1.8% of 7- to 8-year-old children. Like stuttering, cluttering is more common in males than in females.

■ *Cluttering* is a disorder of fluency characterized by rapid but disordered articulation, possibly combined with a high rate of dysfluencies and disorganized thought and language. It tends to coexist with stuttering, but there is no strong tendency for stuttering to coexist with cluttering (Myers & St. Louis, 1992).

▨ The characteristics of cluttering are as follows:

- impaired fluency with excessive amounts of dysfluencies

- rapid repetition of syllables, along with other forms of dysfluencies

- rapid but disordered articulation resulting in indistinct (unintelligible) speech

- clearer articulation and improved intelligibility at slower rate of speech

- omission and compression of sounds and syllables

- jerky or stumbling rhythm

- monotonous tone

- spoonerisms (unintentional interchanges of sounds in a sentence, e.g., *many thinkle peep so* instead of *many people think so*)

- reportedly, a lack of personal concern about or awareness of one's speech problem

- lack of anxiety about or negative reactions to one's speech difficulty

▨ The causes of cluttering are unknown. Genetic transmission and subtle brain damage have been among suggested factors. No hypothesis or theory about its causation has received wide support. However, some experts think that it is a central language disorder (a disassociation between thought and language).

✎ Concepts To Consider

Briefly define cluttering.

_____

_____

_____

_____

_____

_____

_____

Treatment of Cluttering

■ Little or no controlled treatment research exists on cluttering. Currently, most clinicians treat cluttering as they would stuttering.

■ Reducing the rate of speech usually improves clarity as well as fluency. If thought problems or language formulation problems are dominant, teaching the client to plan sentences and other forms of expression before actually producing them might be helpful.

■ Increasing the clutterer's awareness of his speech through the use of audiotapes or videotapes can be highly effective. Many people who clutter are suprised when confronted with recordings of their speech.

■ Maintenance of fluent and well-articulated speech is the major problem in treating persons who clutter. Systematic treatment research is needed to develop unique and more effective treatment procedures for cluttering.

Summary

☑ Cluttering is a disorder of fluency characterized by rapid, imprecise, jerky, and disorganized speech.

☑ Little research exists about its treatment. Reducing the speaking rate and increasing self-awareness helps some people who clutter to sound more intelligible.

CHAPTER HIGHLIGHTS

▶ Fluent speech is flowing, smooth, and relatively rapid and effortless. Stuttering and cluttering are two main forms of fluency disorders. Stuttering may be defined as: (a) all types of dysfluencies that exceed a measure such as 5% of words spoken, (b) production of part-word repetitions and speech-sound prolongations, (c) moments or events judged to be stutterings, (d) anticipatory, apprehensive, hypertonic, avoidance reaction.

▶ Dysfluencies interrupt the flow of fluency; there are many forms including repetitions, prolongations, broken words, interjections, pauses, incomplete sentences, and revisions. When dysfluencies exceed 5% of words spoken, listeners tend to judge the speech as dysfluent or stuttered.

(continues)

▶ The incidence of stuttering in the U.S. general population is about 1%. The lifetime expectancy of stuttering is about 5%. Stuttering is more prevalent in men than in women; there is a higher concordance rate for identical twins than for ordinary siblings. Neither those who stutter nor their parents constitute a unique group whose characteristics are causally related to stuttering.

▶ In early childhood, stuttering begins as an initial increase in the amount of dysfluencies. Associated motor behaviors, breathing abnormalities, negative emotions, and avoidance behaviors tend to develop in due course and to varying extents across individuals.

▶ Stuttering occurs at such predictable loci as initial sounds and words, consonants, longer and unfamiliar words, content words in older children and adults, function words in younger children.

▶ Stuttering is under strong stimulus control, as evidenced by such phenomena as adaptation (progressive decrease in stuttering upon repeated oral reading of a passage), consistency (persistent stuttering on the same loci), adjacency (new stuttering on loci adjacent to old stuttering), and dependence on audience size (increased stuttering with increased number of listeners).

▶ Genetic explanations of stuttering include a single-gene hypothesis and a multiple-genes hypothesis, which presume that certain individuals may be predisposed to stutter. Neurophysiological hypotheses propose that stuttering people may have abnormal laryngeal control, abnormal cerebral language processing, or aberrant neuromotor control of the speech mechanism. Psychoanalytic hypotheses propose deep-seated psychopathology. Conditioning and learning hypotheses propose faulty learning and conditioning. None of the hypotheses is fully supported by experimental evidence.

▶ Assessment of stuttering includes a detailed case history; measurement of types and frequency of dysfluencies in conversational speech and oral reading; evaluation of the variability of dysfluencies; assessment of negative emotions, avoidance reactions, and associated motor behaviors; measurement of speech and articulatory rates, and application of a chosen diagnostic criterion.

▶ Treatment of stuttering includes a variety of procedures, including counseling and psychotherapy; the fluent-stuttering method (Van Riper's method aimed at reducing the abnormality of stuttering through cancellations, pull-outs, and preparatory sets); the fluency-shaping method (widely used procedures that include airflow management, gentle phonatory onset, rate reduction, and shaping normal prosody); fluency reinforcement and time-outs (teaching pausing after every instance of stuttering); response

(continues)

cost (losing a tangible reinforcer after every instance of stuttering); and delayed auditory feedback and use of masking noise.

▶ Cluttering, another disorder of fluency, includes rapid but disordered articulation, possibly combined with a high rate of dysfluencies and disorganized thought and language. Treatment of cluttering is similar to that of stuttering.

▶ Add your own chapter highlights here:

_____

_____

_____

_____

KEY TERMS

adaptation
adjacency
airflow management
anticipatory struggle
  hypothesis
anticipation or expectation
approach-avoidance
  conflict
articulatory rate
associated motor
  behaviors
audience size
avoidance and negative
  emotions
breathing abnormalities
broken words
cancellation
cerebral blood flow
cerebral dominance
cineradiography
classically conditioned
  negative emotion
cluttering
concordance rate
consistency

content words
cross-sectional method
delayed auditory feed-
  back technique
demands and capacities
  hypothesis
diagnosogenic theory
diagnostic criteria
direct stuttering reduc-
  tion
dysfluencies
electroencephalography
familial prevalence
fluency
fluency shaping
fluent stuttering
function words
gender ratio
gentle phonatory onset
incidence and preva-
  lence
incomplete phrases
interjections
laryngeal dysfunction
loci of stuttering
longitudinal method

masking noise technique
normal prosodic features
operant behavior
part-word repetitions
pauses
polygenic inheritance
preparatory sets
pull-outs
rate reduction
reinforcement of fluency
response cost
revisions
silent prolongations
situational variability
skills of fluency
speech rate
speech sound prolonga-
  tions
spoonerism
stimulus control
stuttering
stuttering moment
time-out
voice onset time

STUDY AND REVIEW QUESTIONS

Fill in the Blanks

1. Three adjectives that characterize fluency are _flowing_____, _smooth_____, and _continuous_.

2. The moment of stuttering is a time period during which some _unspecified_ behaviors, judged to be stuttering, are observed by an expert.

3. Silent prolongations are characterized by a silent _articulatory_ _posture_.

4. Incidence requires the _cross-sectional_ method to study.

5. Prevalence requires the _longitudinal_ method to study.

6. Familial prevalence of stuttering is _higher_ than that found in the general population.

7. Adaptation refers to a progressive _decrease_ in the frequency of stuttering upon _repeated_ reading of the same passage.

8. Consistency is the _opposite_ of adaptation.

9. The proponent of the anticipatory struggle hypothesis is _Bloodstein_.

10. Direct stuttering reduction strategy includes _time-out_ and _response cost_

Multiple Choice

11. The position that stuttering indicates a social role conflict was taken by:

    A. Van Riper

    B. Wischner

    C. Sheehan

    D. Bloodstein

    E. Brutten and Shoemaker

12. Research on the prevalence of stuttering has shown that:

    A. familial incidence is higher than that in the general population.

    B. sons of stuttering mothers run a greater risk than sons of stuttering fathers.

    C. blood relatives of a stuttering woman run a greater risk of stuttering themselves than those of a stuttering man.

    D. all of the above

    E. A, C

13. Stuttering in preschool children is more likely on:

    A. content words.

    B. function words.

    C. final words in a sentence.

    D. vowels.

    E. consonant clusters.

14. Facts about stuttering adaptation include:

    A. The greatest reduction in stuttering occurs only on the seventh reading.

    B. There is transfer from one passage to the other.

    C. Most of the reduction in stuttering occurs by the fifth reading.

    D. A higher magnitude of adaptation occurs with an increased time interval between readings.

    E. Most people who stutter do not show the adaptation effect.

15. Brutten and Shoemaker proposed that:

    A. stuttering is limited to part-word repetitions and sound prolongations.

    B. stuttering is due to classically conditioned negative emotion.

    C. some dysfluencies are operantly conditioned.

    D. all of the above

    E. B, C

16. Bloodstein believes that stuttering may be caused by:

    A. any belief that speech is a difficult task, resulting in tension and speech fragmentation.

    B. parental diagnosis of stuttering in normally fluent children.

C. demands exceeding a child's capacities for fluency.

D. an approach-avoidance conflict.

E. an emotionally traumatic experience in childhood.

17. The fluent-stuttering treatment:

A. aims for reduced abnormality of stuttering.

B. aims for normally fluent speech.

C. was developed by Van Riper.

D. all of the above

E. A, C

18. Cancellations, pull-outs, and preparatory sets are taught in:

A. the fluent-stuttering approach.

B. the fluency-shaping approach.

C. approach-avoidance reduction treatment.

D. none of the above

E. all of the above

19. Such skills as airflow management, gentle phonatory onset, and reduced rate of speech are targets in:

A. the fluent-stuttering technique.

B. the fluency-shaping technique.

C. counseling to reduce psychological conflicts.

D. all of the above

E. B, C

20. Cluttering involves:

A. a rapid rate of speech.

B. indistinct articulation.

C. spoonerisms.

D. all of the above

E. A, B

REFERENCES AND RECOMMENDED READINGS

Andrews, G., & Cutler, J. (1974). Stuttering therapy: The relation between changes in symptom level and attitudes. *Journal of Speech and Hearing Disorders, 39,* 312–319.

Andrews, G., & Harris, M. (1964). The syndrome of stuttering. *Clinics in developmental medicine, 17.* London: Heinemann.

Bloodstein, O. (1995). *A handbook on stuttering* (5th ed.). San Diego: Singular Publishing Group.

Brutten, G. J., & Shoemaker, D. J. (1967). *The modification of stuttering.* Englewood Cliffs, NJ: Prentice-Hall.

Conture, E. G. (1990). *Stuttering* (2nd ed.). Englewood Cliffs, NJ: Prentice-Hall.

Cooper, E. B., & Cooper, C. S. (1998). Multicultural considerations in the assessment and treatment of stuttering. In D. E. Battle (Ed.), *Communication disorders in multicultural populations* (2nd ed.), pp. 247–274. Newton, MA: Butterworth-Heinemann.

Culatta, R., & Goldberg, S. A. (1995). *Stuttering therapy: An integrated approach to theory and practice.* Needham Heights, MA: Allyn and Bacon.

Curlee, R. F., & Siegel, G. M. (Eds.). (1997). *Nature and treatment of stuttering: New directions* (2nd ed.). Needham, MA: Allyn and Bacon.

Guitar, B. (1998). *Stuttering: An integrated approach to its nature and treatment* (2nd ed.). Baltimore, MD: Williams & Wilkins.

Hegde, M. N. (1996a). *Pocketguide to assessment in speech–language pathology.* San Diego, CA: Singular Publishing Group.

Hegde, M. N. (1996b). *Pocketguide to treatment in speech–language pathology.* San Diego, CA: Singular Publishing Group.

Hegde, M. N., & Hartman, D. (1979a). Factors affecting judgments of fluency: I. Interjections. *Journal of Fluency Disorders, 4,* 1–11.

Hegde, M. N., & Hartman, D. (1979b). Factors affecting judgments of fluency: II. Word repetitions. *Journal of Fluency Disorders, 4,* 13–22.

Johnson, W., & Associates. (1959). *The onset of stuttering.* Minneapolis: University of Minnesota Press.

Myers, F. L., & St. Louis, K. O. (1992). *Cluttering: A clinical perspective.* Kibworth, England: Far Communications.

Onslow, M. (1996). *Behavioral management of stuttering.* San Diego: Singular Publishing Group.

Sheehan, J. G. (1970). *Stuttering: Research and Therapy.* New York: Harper & Row.

Silverman, F. H. (1996). *Stuttering and other fluency disorders* (2nd ed.). Englewood Cliffs, NJ: Prentice-Hall.

St. Louis, K. O. (1986). *The atypical stutterer.* New York: Academic Press.

Starkweather, W., & Givens-Ackerman, J. (1997). *Stuttering.* Austin, TX: PRO-ED.

Van Riper, C. (1973). *The treatment of stuttering.* Englewood Cliffs, NJ: Prentice-Hall.

Van Riper, C. (1982). *The nature of stuttering.* Englewood Cliffs, NJ: Prentice-Hall.

Wall, M. J., & Myers, F. L. (1995). *Clinical management of childhood stuttering* (2nd ed.). Austin, TX: PRO-ED.

Wischner, G. J. (1950). Stuttering behavior and learning: A preliminary theoretical formulation. *Journal of Speech and Hearing Disorders, 15,* 324–335.

ANSWERS TO STUDY AND REVIEW QUESTIONS

1. Any three of the following: flowing, smooth, continuous, relatively rapid, normally rhythmic, relatively effortless

2. Unspecified

3. Articulatory posture

4. Cross-sectional

5. Longitudinal

6. Higher

7. Decrease, repeated

8. Opposite

9. Bloodstein

10. Time-out, response cost

11. C. The position that stuttering indicates a social role conflict was taken by Sheehan.

12. D. Research on the prevalence of stuttering has shown all of the above—that familial incidence is higher than that in the general population, that sons of stuttering mothers run a greater risk than sons of stuttering fathers, and that blood relatives of a stuttering woman run a greater risk than those of a stuttering man.

13. B. Stuttering in preschool children is more likely on function words.

14. C. One fact about stuttering adaptation is that most of the reduction in stuttering occurs by the fifth reading.

15. D. Brutten and Shoemaker proposed all of the above—that stuttering is limited to part-word repetitions and sound prolongations, that stuttering is due to classically conditioned negative emotion, and that some dysfluencies are operantly conditioned.

16. A. Bloodstein believes that stuttering may be caused by any belief that speech is a difficult task, resulting in tension and speech fragmentation.

17. E. The fluent-stuttering treatment aims for reduced abnormality of stuttering and was developed by Van Riper.

18. A. Cancellations, pull-outs, and preparatory sets are taught in the fluent-stuttering approach.

19. B. Such skills as airflow management, gentle phonatory onset, and reduced rate of speech are targets in the fluency-shaping technique.

20. D. Cluttering involves all of the above—a rapid rate of speech, indistinct articulation, and spoonerisms.

CHAPTER 7

Voice and Its Disorders

PREVIEW OUTLINE

CHAPTER INTRODUCTION

The area of voice and its disorders is becoming a topic of increasing interest to communicative disorders professionals and members of the public alike. Society is increasingly recognizing the value of a clear, professional-sounding, and pleasing voice for optimal communication. Communicative disorders professionals, due to more sophisticated instrumentation, are learning more about how to treat voice disorders and help patients achieve maximally competent voice production. In this chapter, we discuss normal aspects of voice, evaluation of voice disorders, disorders of resonation, disorders of phonation, and aspects of treatment.

VOCAL ANATOMY AND PHYSIOLOGY

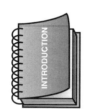

Optimal voice production is based upon intact anatomy and physiology of the larynx and surrounding structures. The human voice undergoes certain changes throughout the life span; between birth and death, everyone experiences vocal changes. In this section, the topics of laryngeal anatomy and physiology and voice changes through the life span are discussed. (*Note*: Chapter 1 contains more detailed information about laryngeal anatomy and physiology and the neurological mechanisms that control vocalization. These concepts are briefly reviewed in this chapter.)

The Larynx

Basic Principles

- The larynx is a biological valve located at the top of the trachea. It helps close the entry into the trachea so food, liquids, and other particles do not enter the lungs. The larynx connects superiorly to the oral cavity and vocal tract and inferiorly to the lungs and trachea.

- The larynx builds air pressure below it to assist in the performance of biological functions such as getting rid of body wastes, coughing, doing heavy lifting, and child bearing.

- The larynx houses the vocal folds, which vibrate to produce voice. The vocal folds *adduct* (move toward the midline) or *abduct* (move away from the midline). The opening between the vocal folds is called the *glottis*.

- The *ventricular* or *false* vocal folds lie above the "true" vocal folds described above. They do not usually vibrate during normal phonation and are used only during activities such as lifting and coughing.

- The *aryepiglottic folds* lie above the ventricular folds. They separate the pharynx and the laryngeal vestibule and help preserve the airway.

- *Cranial nerve VII* innervates the posterior belly of the digastric muscle of the vocal folds. The primary cranial nerve involved in laryngeal innervation is *Cranial nerve X* (vagus nerve). The primary branches of the vagus nerve that innervate the larynx are the superior laryngeal nerve (SLN) and the recurrent laryngeal nerve (RLN).

- The *superior laryngeal nerve* has internal and external branches. The internal branch provides all sensory information to the larynx, and the external branch supplies motor innervation solely to the cricothyroid muscle.

- The *recurrent laryngeal nerve* supplies all motor innervation to the interarytenoid, posterior cricoarytenoid, thyroarytenoid, and lateral cricoarytenoid muscles. It supplies all sensory information below the vocal folds.

Key Structures and Cartilages

Hyoid Bone

- The larynx is suspended from the hyoid bone. Many extrinsic laryngeal muscles are attached to the hyoid bone. Figure 7.1 illustrates the hyoid bone in relation to other key laryngeal structures.

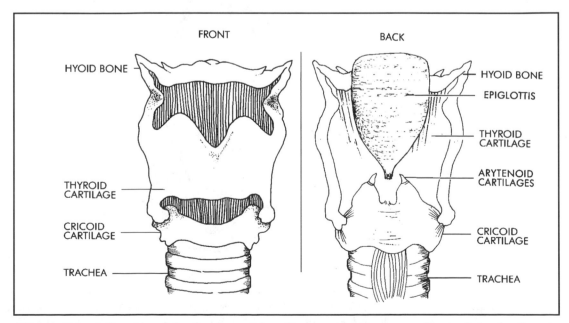

Figure 7.1. A front and back view of key laryngeal structures. From *Introduction to Communicative Disorders*, 2nd ed. (p. 264), by M. N. Hegde, 1995, Austin, TX: PRO-ED. Copyright 1995 by PRO-ED, Inc. Reprinted with permission.

Epiglottis

▪ This leaf-shaped cartilage is attached to the hyoid bone.

▪ The epiglottis protects the trachea by closing down inferiorly and posteriorly over the laryngeal area, directing liquids and food into the esophagus during swallowing.

Thyroid Cartilage

▪ The largest of all the laryngeal cartilages, the thyroid cartilage is sometimes called the *Adam's apple*. It is particularly prominent in men. The thyroid cartilage shields other laryngeal structures from damage.

  – It is composed of two lamina, or plates of cartilage, that are joined at midline and form an angle. Figure 7.2 shows the thyroid cartilage and its relation to the vocal folds.

Cricoid Cartilage

▪ This is the second-largest laryngeal cartilage and is sometimes called the uppermost tracheal ring (however, it is quite different from the other tracheal rings).

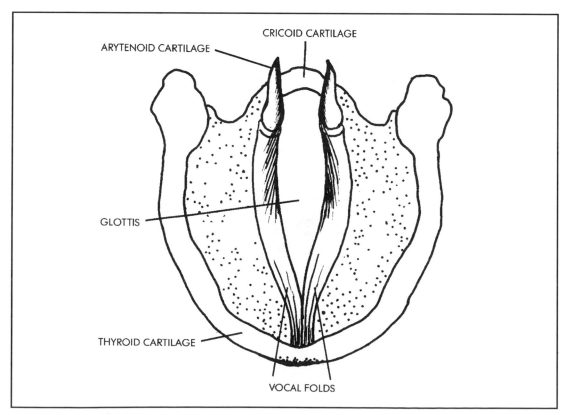

Figure 7.2. The thyroid cartilage and surrounding structures. From *Introduction to Communicative Disorders*, 2nd ed. (p. 265), by M. N. Hegde, 1995, Austin, TX: PRO-ED. Copyright 1995 by PRO-ED, Inc. Reprinted with permission.

■ The cricoid cartilage completely surrounds the trachea. It is linked with the paired arytenoid cartilages and the thyroid cartilage.

Arytenoid Cartilages

■ These are positioned on the supraposterior surface of the cricoid cartilage on either side of the midline.

■ The arytenoid cartilages are shaped like pyramids. The *vocal processes* are the most anterior angle of the base of the arytenoids; the true vocal folds attach at the vocal processes.

Corniculate Cartilages

■ These sit on the apex of the arytenoids and are small and cone-shaped.

■ They play a minor role in vocalization.

Cuneiform Cartilages

■ These are tiny, cone-shaped cartilage pieces under the mucous membrane that covers the aryepiglottic folds.

■ They play a very minor role in the phonatory functions of the larynx.

Intrinsic Laryngeal Muscles

■ These pairs of muscles have both of their attachments to structures within the larynx (see Figure 7.3). With one exception, all are adductors. The intrinsic laryngeal muscles are primarily responsible for controlling vocalization.

■ The sets of intrinsic laryngeal muscles are:

- thyroarytenoids
- cricothyroids
- posterior cricoarytenoids (the only abductors)
- lateral cricoarytenoids
- transverse arytenoids
- oblique arytenoids

Extrinsic Laryngeal Muscles

■ These muscles have one attachment to a structure outside the larynx and one attachment to a structure within the larynx. All extrinsic laryngeal muscles are attached to the hyoid bone.

■ These muscles elevate or lower the position of the larynx in the neck. They give the larynx fixed support.

■ The *infrahyoid* laryngeal muscles lie below the hyoid bone; their primary function is to depress the larynx. They are sometimes called the *depressors*. They have a strong impact upon vocal pitch. The infrahyoid muscles are listed below (one can remember them by the acronym TOSS):

– thyrohyoids
– omohyoids
– sternothyroids
– sternohyoids

■ The *suprahyoid* laryngeal muscles lie above the hyoid bone; their primary function is to elevate the larynx. They are sometimes called *elevators*. The suprahyoid muscles are:

– digastrics
– geniohyoids
– mylohyoids
– stylohyoids
– genioglossus
– hyoglossus

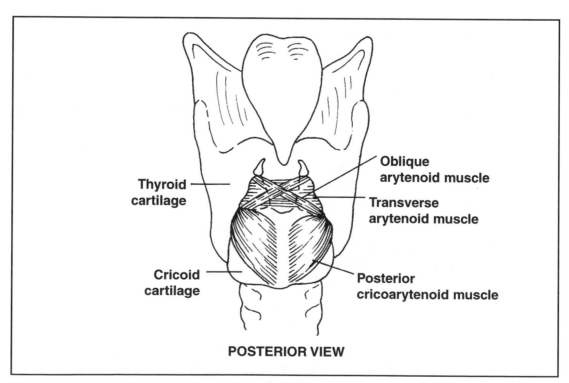

POSTERIOR VIEW

Figure 7.3. Intrinsic laryngeal muscles: oblique arytenoids, transverse arytenoids, posterior cricoarytenoids. From *Anatomy and Physiology for Speech, Language, and Hearing* (p. 186), by J. A. Seikel, D. W. King, and D. G. Drumright, 1997, San Diego, CA: Singular Publishing Group, Inc. (401 West A Street, Suite 325, San Diego, CA 92101-7904, 800-521-8545). Copyright 1997 by Singular Publishing Group, Inc. Reprinted with permission.

Concepts To Consider

List and briefly describe two key laryngeal cartilages, two sets of intrinsic laryngeal muscles, and two sets of extrinsic laryngeal muscles:

_____

_____

_____

_____

_____

_____

_____

_____

_____

_____

Voice Changes Through the Life Span

Infancy Through Adolescence

Mean Fundamental Frequency (MFF)

- There is a gradual and discernible decline in MFF from birth on. As people grow older, their voices become lower in pitch.

- Most studies suggest that boys' and girls' voices are similar before adolescence. During adolescence, changes in pitch become noticeable.

- The MFF of 7- and 8-year-old children ranges from 281 to 297 Hz.

- The MFF of 10- and 11-year-old children ranges from 238 to 270 Hz.

- Nineteen-year-old females have an MFF of 217; nineteen-year-old males have an MFF of 117.

Maximum Phonation Time (MPT)

- This refers to a client's ability to sustain "ah." Usually, the client is asked to breathe deeply and "say ah for as long as you can."

- Three- and 4-year-old children have an MPT ranging from 7.50 to 8.95 seconds. Five- to 12-year-old children have an MPT ranging from 14.97 to 17.74 seconds.

Changes Resulting from Puberty

- Girls' voices may lower by 3–4 semitones.

- Boys' voices may lower by as much as an octave. Boys may show pitch breaks, huskiness, and hoarseness as their pitch lowers due to laryngeal growth.

Adulthood

- Men have an MFF of 100–150 Hz. Women have an MFF of 180–250 Hz.

- Adults ages 18–39 have an MPT ranging from 20.90 to 24.60 seconds.

The Geriatric Voice

- Females 70–94 years old have an MFF of 201 Hz; males 70–89 years old have an MFF that ranges from 132 to 146 Hz.

- Adults ages 66–93 years have an MPT ranging from 14.20 to 18.10 seconds.

Summary

- ☑ The human larynx is used as a biological valve for helping humans perform certain functions. It also houses the vocal folds, which vibrate to produce voicing.

- ☑ Key structures in the laryngeal area include the hyoid bone, epiglottis, thyroid cartilage, cricoid cartilage, arytenoid cartilages, corniculate cartilages, and cuneiform cartilages. There are two groups of laryngeal muscles: the intrinsic and extrinsic laryngeal muscles.

- ☑ There are three sets of vocal folds: the aryepiglottic folds, the ventricular or false vocal folds, and the true vocal folds, which vibrate to produce voice.

- ☑ Cranial nerve X, with its superior and recurrent laryngeal nerve branches, which innervate the larynx, is the key cranial nerve in laryngeal function.

- ☑ The voice changes throughout the life span. Mean fundamental frequency declines from birth on, with more dramatic changes for the male in adolescence. Maximum phonation time grows greater between childhood and adulthood. It usually decreases as people age.

VOCAL PITCH, VOLUME, AND QUALITY

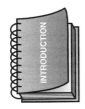

Pitch, volume, and quality are important characteristics of the voice. People's personality, intelligence, and competence are often judged by these parameters. Voice disorders tend to affect vocal pitch, volume, and quality. Experienced clinicians listen for disturbances in these aspects of voice when evaluating clients with voice disorders.

Pitch

■ The perceptual correlate of frequency, pitch is largely based on the frequency with which the vocal folds vibrate. This rate is often described as the *fundamental frequency*. Fundamental frequency is generally considered an individual's habitual or typical pitch.

■ Pitch is determined by mass, tension, and elasticity of the vocal folds. Higher pitch results when the vocal folds are thinner, more tense, or both; lower pitch results when the folds are thicker, more relaxed, or both.

■ *Frequency perturbation*, or *jitter*, refers to variations in vocal frequency that are often heard in dysphonic patients. Jitter can be measured instrumentally as a patient sustains a vowel. Patients with voice problems such as tremor or hoarseness might show a large amount of jitter (Colton & Casper, 1996).

Volume

■ The perceptual correlate of intensity, volume or loudness is determined by the intensity of the sound signal; the more intense the sound signal, the greater its perceived loudness.

■ The sound is a disturbance in air particles; it is in the form of waves that move forward and backward in a medium such as air or water. The extent of such movements is *amplitude*. The greater the amplitude, the louder the voice.

■ *Amplitude perturbation*, or *shimmer*, can be measured instrumentally as a patient sustains a vowel. Patients who have difficulties with regularity of vocal fold vibration (e.g., roughness) might show large amounts of shimmer.

Quality

Definition

Voice quality is the perceptual correlate of complexity. It refers to the physical complexity of the laryngeal tone, which is modified by the resonating cavities (Aronson, 1990). The determination of voice quality is frequently subjective.

Types of Vocal Quality

Hoarseness

■ The voice shows a combination of breathiness and harshness, which results from irregular vocal fold vibrations. In such cases, the fundamental frequency of the speaker varies randomly due to aperiodic vibration.

■ Hoarse voices often sound breathy, low-pitched, and husky. There may be pitch breaks and excessive throat clearing.

Harshness

■ The voice is described as rough, unpleasant, and "gravelly" sounding. It is associated with excessive muscular tension and effort. The vocal folds are adducted too tightly, and the air is then released too abruptly.

Strain-Strangle

■ Phonation is effortful, and the patient sounds like she or he is "squeezing" the voice at the glottal level. Initiating and sustaining phonation and both difficult.

■ Talking fatigues patients, and they experience much tension when they speak.

Breathiness

■ The breathy voice results from the vocal folds being slightly open, or not firmly approximated, during phonation. Air escapes through the glottis and adds noise to the sound produced by the vocal folds (see Figure 7.4).

■ Breathiness can be due to *organic* (physical) or nonorganic (nonphysical, or *functional*) causes. Patients often complain that they feel like they're running out of air.

■ Breathy voices are often soft, with little variation in loudness. Patients frequently show restricted range.

Glottal Fry

■ Also called *vocal fry*, glottal fry is heard when the vocal folds vibrate very slowly. The resultant sound occurs in slow but discrete bursts and is of extremely low pitch. The voice sounds "crackly."

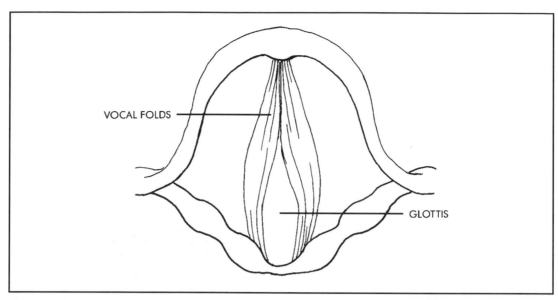

Figure 7.4. Partially open vocal folds, allowing to escape through the open glottis and create a breathy voice. From *Introduction to Communicative Disorders*, 2nd ed. (p. 268), by M. N. Hegde, 1995, Austin, TX: PRO-ED. Copyright 1995 by PRO-ED, Inc. Reprinted with permission.

Diplophonia

■ This means "double voice." It occurs when one can simultaneously perceive two distinct pitches during phonation.

■ Diplophonia usually occurs when the vocal folds vibrate at different frequencies due to differing degrees of mass or tension. A client with a unilateral polyp, for example, might sound diplophonic.

Stridency

■ A patient with a strident voice sounds shrill, unpleasant, somewhat high-pitched, and "tinny."

■ Physiologically, stridency is often caused by hypertonicity or tension of the pharyngeal constrictors and elevation of the larynx. Tense patients may sound strident.

Summary

☑ Pitch (the perceptual correlate of frequency) and volume (the perceptual correlate of intensity) are important vocal parameters that clinicians must evaluate in all voice patients.

(continues)

☑ Vocal quality, the perceptual correlate of complexity, is often affected by pathological changes of the laryngeal mechanism. Patients can manifest such vocal qualities as hoarseness, harshness, strain-strangle, breathiness, glottal fry, diplophonia, and stridency.

☑ Experienced clinicians evaluate patients' pitch, volume, and quality in making a determination of whether a voice disorder exists.

EVALUATION OF VOICE DISORDERS

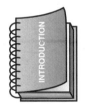

INTRODUCTION

A thorough voice evaluation is critical to creation of an individualized, successful treatment program. When conducting evaluations, clinicians must remember to carry out a thorough oral peripheral examination, hearing screening, and speech–language sample. Gathering a complete case history is important. A team-oriented approach to evaluation is always necessary; the team can consist of specialists from medicine, education, and professional voice pedagogy. Clinicians, depending upon their settings and the availability of technology, use both instrumental and perceptual tools to evaluate patients' voices.

Case History: Purposes and Goals

■ Obtain information about variables such as onset, duration, causes, and variability of the voice problem. Ask for the perceptions of the patient as well as significant others about these variables.

■ Obtain information about any associated symptoms or problems such as slurring of speech, difficulty swallowing, excessive coughing, and others.

■ Identify factors (e.g., health, environment, family history) that might be contributing to the problem.

■ Gather information regarding previous therapy, medical intervention, or other attempts to deal with the voice problem.

■ Obtain patient and significant others' descriptions of daily vocal use and possible abuse or misuse patterns.

■ For culturally and linguistically diverse clients, obtain their specific perceptions of what constitutes a "normal-sounding" voice in their particular culture (DeJarnette & Holland, 1998).

A Team-Oriented Approach

■ A multidisciplinary, team-oriented approach is critical to a thorough evaluation.

■ Before beginning therapy, it is always necessary to have a medical evaluation of the vocal mechanism; this is performed by an otolaryngologist. In some cases, it may also be necessary to refer the patient to a neurologist before treatment is initiated.

■ The team will always include the speech–language pathologist, but teams may be oriented diferently, as follows, for example (Andrews, 1995):

  – A *medical team* would consist of a general practitioner, neurologist, otolaryngologist, radiologist, orthodontist, social worker, psychiatrist or psychologist, pulmonary specialist, and gastroenterologist.

  – An *educationally oriented team* would consist of a classroom teacher, school nurse, school psychologist, and counselor.

  – A team oriented toward professional voice users could consist of voice scientists, psychologists, and vocal pedagogy teachers such as singing and vocal coaches.

Instrumental Evaluation

■ All forms of instrumental evaluation are used to view the vocal folds. A description of each type of evaluation follows.

Indirect Laryngoscopy (Mirror Laryngoscopy)

■ The specialist uses a bright light source and a small, round, 21–25 mm mirror, angled on a long, slender handle, to lift the velum and press gently against the patient's posterior pharyngeal wall area.

■ The specialist maneuvers the mirror to view the laryngeal structures during phonation (usually the patient's production of "eeeee") and during quiet respiration. Figure 7.5 shows a patient undergoing indirect laryngoscopy.

Direct Laryngoscopy

■ This procedure is performed by a surgeon when the patient is under general anesthesia in outpatient surgery. The laryngoscope is introduced through the mouth into the pharynx and positioned above the vocal folds.

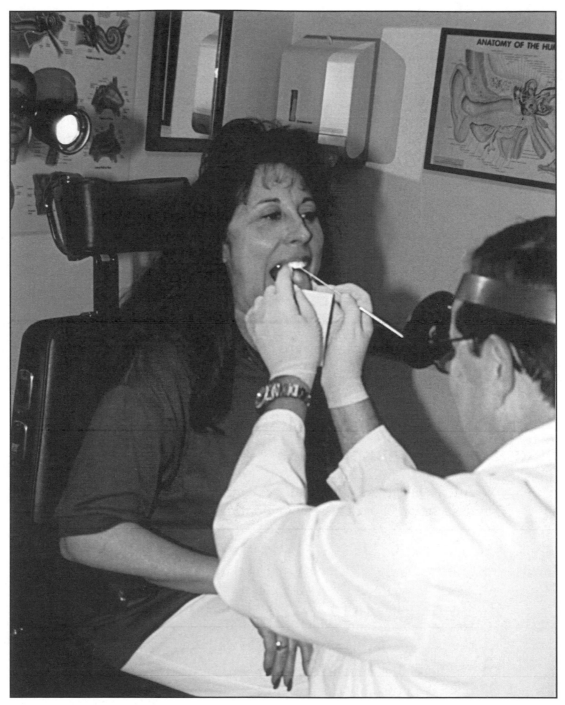

Figure 7.5. Indirect laryngoscopy. From *Clinical Management of Voice Disorders*, 3rd ed. (p. 53), by J. L. Case, 1996, Austin, TX: PRO-ED. Copyright 1996 by PRO-ED, Inc. Reprinted with permission.

■ The patient cannot phonate, thus vocal function cannot be determined. However, the surgeon can obtain a direct microscopic view of the larynx.

■ Direct laryngoscopy is valuable when a biopsy is required due to suspicions of laryngeal cancer.

Flexible Fiber-Optic Laryngoscopy

■ This procedure utilizes a thin, flexible tube containing a lens and fiberoptic light bundles.

■ The specialist inserts the tube through the nasal passage, passes it over the velum, and maneuvers it into position above the larynx. The fibers transmit the laryngeal image to the specialist's eyepiece.

■ The patient is able to speak and sing. The specialist can obtain an excellent, prolonged view of the vocal mechanism and photograph rapid vocal fold movement.

Endoscopy

■ There are two kinds of endoscopes: *flexible* and *rigid*. The rigid endoscope is introduced orally; the flexible endoscope is introduced nasally, using a 3.6-mm tube (see Figure 7.6).

■ There is a light at the tip of the scope; this light is fiber optic and comes from an external light source.

■ The structures are illuminated by the light and viewed by the specialist at the other end of the endoscope through a window lens.

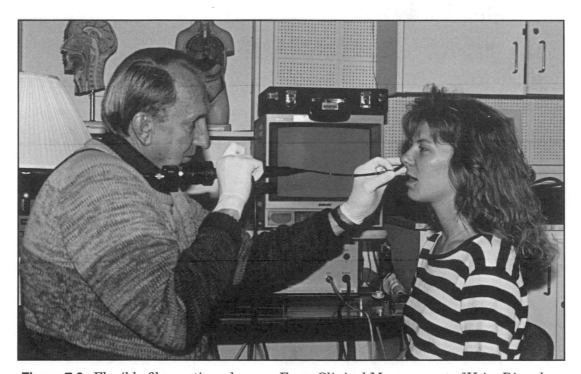

Figure 7.6. Flexible fiber-optic endoscopy. From *Clinical Management of Voice Disorders*, 3rd ed (p. 55), by J. L. Case, 1996, Austin, TX: PRO-ED. Copyright 1996 by PRO-ED, Inc. Reprinted with permission.

■ The endoscope can be attached to a videocamera (*videoendoscopy*). A stroboscopic (*flashing*) light source can also be used.

■ With the flexible endoscope, the specialist can view the velopharyngeal mechanism, including velopharyngeal valving. The endoscope (also called a nasopharyngoscope) can be lowered further to view the laryngeal mechanism (see Figure 7.7).

■ Because the patient can perform a variety of phonatory tasks, endoscopy can be used to study laryngeal anatomy and physiology in detail, including the mucosal wave (Colton & Casper, 1996).

Videostroboscopy

■ Videostroboscopy can be helpful in differentiating functional and organic voice problems. It can also be used to detect laryngeal neoplasms (tumors).

■ The specialist can perform videostroboscopy by using a flexible fiber-optic laryngoscope, rigid endoscope, or both.

■ The strobe light is a pulsing light that permits the optical illusion of slow-motion viewing of the vocal folds during a variety of tasks. The observer per-

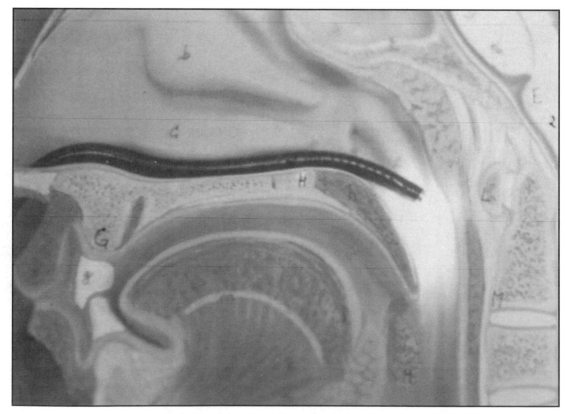

Figure 7.7. Model showing placement of nasopharyngoscope. From *Clinical Management of Voice Disorders*, 3rd ed (p. 55), by J. L. Case, 1996, Austin, TX: PRO-ED. Copyright 1996 by PRO-ED, Inc. Reprinted with permission.

ceives the rapidly presented images as a complete picture of cycle-to-cycle vibration (vibratory pattern of phonation).

■ The specialist places a microphone on the patient's neck along the thyroid cartilage to record the voice signal. Then he or she introduces the scope, switches on the stroboscopic light, and asks the patient to phonate.

■ The resulting image on the monitor screen is projected through optic devices such as a camera lens, an endoscope, and pixels on the monitor screen.

■ The stroboscopic image yields information about periodicity or regularity of vocal fold vibrations, vocal fold amplitude (horizontal excursion), glottal closure, presence and adequacy of the mucosal wave, and the possible presence of lesions or neoplasms (Colton & Casper, 1996).

Electroglottography (EGG)

■ This noninvasive procedure yields an indirect measure of vocal fold closure patterns.

■ Surface electrodes are placed on both sides of the thyroid cartilage, and a high-frequency electric current is passed between the electrodes while the patient phonates. The laryngeal and neck tissue conducts the current.

■ A glottal wave form results, and the specialist is able to observe vocal fold vibration. EGG can also detect breathy and abrupt glottal onset of phonation.

■ Researchers and practitioners disagree about the efficacy of EGG as a diagnostic technique; many variables can impact its accuracy. It is currently recommended as a cross-validation tool with other measures of vocal fold functioning.

Electromyography (EMG)

■ This invasive procedure directly measures laryngeal function to study the pattern of electrical activity of the vocal folds and view muscle activity patterns.

■ The specialist inserts needle electrodes into the patient's peripheral laryngeal muscles; the resulting electrical signals are judged as either normal or indicative of pathology.

■ When the specialist interprets the electrical signals, he or she is looking for: (a) reduced or increased speed of muscle activation, (b) extraneous bursts of muscle activity, or (c) onset or termination of muscle activity.

■ EMG is useful when attempting to determine vocal fold pathology, especially that caused by neurological and neuromuscular diseases. It is also useful in verifying excessive muscle activity prior to the injection of BOTOX (botulinus toxin; described later) for patients with spasmodic dysphonia (Colton & Casper, 1996).

Aerodynamic Measurements

■ Aerodynamic measurements refer to the airflows, air volumes, and average air pressures produced as part of the peripheral mechanics of the respiratory, laryngeal, and supralaryngeal airways (Bless & Hicks, 1996).

■ Specialists use aerodynamic measurements to evaluate dysphonia, monitor voice changes and treatment progress, and differentiate between laryngeal and respiratory problems.

■ Many specialists want to assess patients' lung volume because breath support for optimal voice may be lacking. Specific measures can be made of the following parameters:

- *tidal volume* (amount of air inhaled and exhaled during a normal breathing cycle)

- *vital capacity* (the volume of air that the patient can exhale after a maximal inhalation)

- *total lung capacity* (total volume of air in the lungs)

■ Various instruments can be used to obtain aerodynamic measurements. Some of the most common include *wet spirometers, dry spirometers, manometric devices*, and *plethysmographs*. (For further description of these forms of instrumentation, see Andrews, 1995; Boone & McFarlane, 1994; Colton & Casper, 1996).

 Concepts To Consider

Describe two types of instrumental evaluation that might be appropriate for a patient with laryngeal lesions that might be indicative of laryngeal cancer.

_____

_____

_____

_____

_____

_____

Pitch Measurements

■ Many instruments can be used to measure pitch. One of the most popular is the *Visi-Pitch* (see Figure 7.8).

■ To use it, the patient speaks into a microphone, and the Visi-Pitch displays his or her frequencies visually on a computer monitor. The Visi-Pitch can indicate the patient's frequency range, optimal pitch, and habitual pitch. It can give a printout of these factors.

■ The Visi-Pitch enjoys widespread use among clinicians because it is noninvasive and affordable, and it gives instant visual feedback to both clinician and patient. As mentioned, printouts give documented, quantitative measurements of a patient's pitch characteristics.

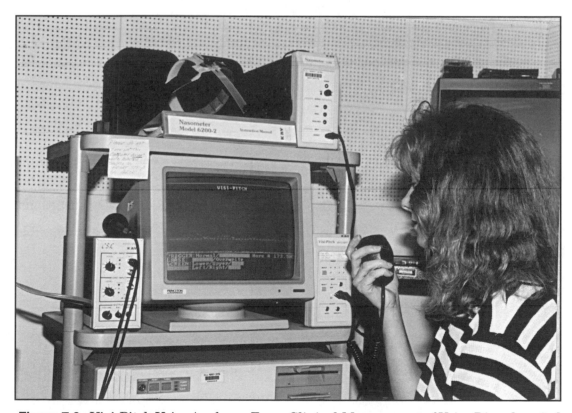

Figure 7.8. Visi-Pitch Voice Analyzer. From *Clinical Management of Voice Disorders*, 3rd ed (p. 80), by J. L. Case, 1996, Austin, TX: PRO-ED. Copyright 1996 by PRO-ED, Inc. Reprinted with permission.

Perceptual Evaluation

Basic Principles

■ In perceptual voice evaluation, the clinician makes subjective judgments of many vocal parameters, including the patient's pitch, volume, vocal quality, resonance, respiration, and ability to sustain phonation.

■ Many rating scales are available for making these judgments; Table 7.1 is an example of a scale that the clinician can use for making subjective judgments.

Pitch Assessment

■ To assess pitch, clinicians make subjective judgments about the following:

- the patient's habitual pitch, or typical conversational pitch;

- whether the client is using optimal pitch (judged to be the most appropriate, comfortable pitch for that individual);

- whether the pitch is appropriate to the client's gender and age, rather than too high or too low; and

- whether the patient is *monopitched*, with lack of appropriate inflections as judged by members of his or her mainstream culture.

Loudness Assessment

■ To assess loudness, clinicians make subjective judgments about the following:

- parameters such as harshness, hoarseness, breathiness, and vocal tension;

- whether the client's loudness is appropriate to daily situations; and

- whether the client's voice is too soft or too loud due to possible physical factors (e.g., asthma, a hearing loss).

Resonance Assessment

■ To assess resonance, clinicians subjectively judge the presence of:

- *hyponasality* (when nasal resonance is absent on nasal sounds); and

- *hypernasality* (when too much nasal resonance is present on non-nasal sounds).

TABLE 7.1

Summary of Voice Assessment Data Using a Rating Scale

University Speech and Hearing Center

Client _____ Age _____ Sex _____

Clinician_____ Date/time _____

	Normal	Mild	Moderate	Severe	Profound
1. Voice quality	1	2	3	④	5

Breathy/Harsh/Hoarse

The voice was judged hoarse on 90% of the utterances produced in conversational speech.

2. Pitch	1	2	3	④	5

Too high/Too low

The client's pitch was judged too high on 80% of the utterances produced in conversational speech.

3. Loudness	1	2	③	4	5

Too loud/Too soft

The client's voice was judged too loud during most of the assessment time.

4. Nasal resonance	1	2	③	4	5

Hypernasal/Hyponasal

The client's voice was judged hypernasal on 45% of the utterances produced in conversational speech.

5. Oral resonance	1	②	3	4	5

Reduced oral resonance

The client spoke with limited mouth opening; on most of the utterances, the oral resonance was reduced.

6. Muscle tension	1	2	③	4	5

Hypertense/Hypotense

The client's muscles of the face, neck, and chest were judged hypertense during conversational speech

7. Abusive vocal behaviors	1	2	3	④	5

Client has a history of vocally abusive behaviors including loud and excessive talking, loud cheering at games, and screaming and yelling while playing with friends.

Comments and Recommendations: The client speaks with excessive muscular tension and effort; voice is excessively hoarse most of the time; there is a history of frequent and severe abusive vocal behaviors. Voice therapy is recommended to reduce the frequency and severity of such behaviors.

Note. The comments are for illustration only; a given client may not exhibit all the problems described. From *Introduction to Communicative Disorders*, 2nd ed. (p. 264) by M. N. Hegde, 1995, Austin, TX: PRO-ED. Copyright 1995 by PRO-ED, Inc. Reprinted with permission.

Respiration Assessment

■ To assess respiration, many clinicians look for the following types of breathing:

- *Clavicular breathing.* When the patient inhales, the shoulders elevate. Often there is strain and tension. Clavicular breathing is inefficient.

- *Diaphragmatic-abdominal breathing.* This appropriate, efficient breathing utilizes the abdominal region and the lower thoracic cavity. There is little to no chest or shoulder movement. Diaphragmatic-abdominal breathing is ideal for professional voice users, including singers, teachers, and public speakers.

- *Thoracic breathing.* The patient who uses thoracic breathing exhibits characteristics of both clavicular and diaphragmatic-abdominal breathing. There is no observable abdominal or upper thoracic expansion upon inspiration.

Phonation Assessment

■ To assess a patient's ability to sustain phonation, clinicians use simple measures such as the following:

- *Maximum phonation time (MPT).* As mentioned earlier, MPT is a measurement of the patient's ability to sustain phonation (e.g., "ah") during one exhalation. The clinician generally gives the patient three trials and compares the patient's MPT (in seconds) with norms. MPT enables the clinician to observe adequacy of respiration, glottal efficiency, and the possible presence of vocal pathology such as nodules.

- *s/z ratio.* This procedure is used to help determine whether there is laryngeal pathology present. The patient is asked to produce two long /s/ phonemes, then two long /z/ phonemes. The clinician divides the longest /s/ by the longest /z/. An s/z ratio of more than 1.4 is indicative of possible laryngeal pathology.

- For example, a patient may sustain /s/ for 15 seconds and /z/ for 9 seconds. This would yield an s/z ratio of 15/9, or 1.6, indicating possible laryngeal pathology.

Summary

☑ A comprehensive, multidisciplinary team assessment of the voice patient is necessary as a foundation for appropriate treatment. A key component of assessment is a thorough case history.

☑ Instrumentation procedures that various specialists can use to assess a patient's voice include indirect or mirror laryngoscopy, direct laryngoscopy, flexible fiber-optic laryngoscopy, endoscopy (flexible or rigid), videostrobo-

(continues)

scopy, electroglottography, and electromyography. Instruments can also be used to obtain aerodynamic and pitch measurements.

☑ In a perceptual evaluation (which can occur alone or accompany instrumental evaluation), clinicians often use rating scales and informal tasks to assess pitch, loudness, vocal quality, resonance, respiration, and the ability to sustain phonation.

☑ Ideally, each patient will be evaluated through a combination of measures that will permit both qualitative and quantitative baseline measures and documentation of progress in voice therapy.

DISORDERS OF RESONANCE AND THEIR TREATMENT

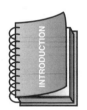

INTRODUCTION

Resonance is the modification of sound by structures through which the sound passes. The resonating structures that lie below and above the larynx (e.g., the oral and nasal cavities) modify the laryngeal tone. Voice disorders of resonance include an absence of a desired resonance, inadequate resonance, or inappropriate resonance. Appropriate resonance or lack thereof is based in part on cultural and linguistic norms. Among some cultural and linguistic groups (e.g., Americans living in the United States), there is little tolerance for hypernasality in conversational speech. Some Asians, speakers of Chinese, for example, may have slightly more hypernasality than Americans perceive as normal or desirable. Clinicians must always take patients' cultural and linguistic backgrounds into account when judging resonance.

Hypernasality

■ Hypernasality is the most common resonance disorder presented by patients who come for services. A person who exhibits hypernasality, or excessive nasality, sounds like he or she is speaking through the nose.

■ Hypernasality results when the velopharyngeal mechanism does not close the opening to the nasal passage during the production of non-nasal sounds. The air and sound escape through the nose, adding unnecessary nasal resonance to non-nasal speech sounds.

■ Hypernasality can occur due to functional or organic factors. In the case of functional hypernasality, there is no physical reason for the hypernasality; the patient has made a habit of "talking through the nose." Functional nasality is often found in the speech of deaf people; they have adequate velopharyngeal mechanisms but are unable to monitor the sound of their own voices.

■ Patients who are hypernasal due to organic factors have a physical problem that may need to be corrected surgically. *Cleft palate* is a major cause of hypernasality. Patients with inadequate cleft repairs are often severely hypernasal.

■ *Velopharyngeal inadequacy*, another cause of hypernasality, means that the velopharyngeal mechanism is inadequate to achieve closure; the nasal cavities are not sealed off appropriately from the oral cavity. Major causes of velopharyngeal inadequacy are:

- *Decreased muscle mass of the velum* (not enough velar tissue) to achieve closure.

- *Adenoidectomy or tonsillectomy*. This occurs especially when a child's velopharyngeal mechanism initially did not have sufficient muscle mass. The adenoids and tonsils are masses that can help compensate for an otherwise inadequate velopharyngeal mechanism. When these masses are surgically removed, the basic velopharyngeal inadequacy may become apparent.

- *Paresis (weakness) or paralysis of the velum*, which reduces its mobility so it is unable to assist in achieving adequate closure. Velar paresis and paralysis frequently occur secondarily to cerebral palsy, stroke, head injury, debilitative diseases such as Parkinson's disease, and other conditions of neuropathology.

- Assessment of hypernasality can include subjective, perceptual judgments as well as use of instrumentation such as the Nasometer (described later).

Hyponasality

■ Hyponasality, or *denasality*, is a lack of appropriate nasal resonance on nasal sounds /m, n, ng/. Patients often substitute oral sounds for nasal sounds (e.g., "<u>b</u>aby" instead of "<u>m</u>aybe").

■ Hyponasality can be temporary, due to conditions such as colds and allergies. It can also occur due to obstructions in the nasal cavity (e.g., nasal polyps or papilloma), enlarged adenoids, or a deviated septum. Hyponasal patients may be mouth breathers. Deaf people, due to their inability to monitor their own voices, are sometimes hyponasal (Boone & McFarlane, 1994).

■ Assessment of hyponasality also can include subjective, perceptual judgments as well as use of instrumentation such as the Nasometer (described later).

Assimilative Nasality

- Assimilative nasality occurs when the sound from a nasal consonant carries over to adjacent vowels. For example, in the word *banana*, the /æ/ sounds appear hypernasal because they are next to the nasal /n/.

- In assimilative nasality, the velar openings begin too soon and last too long, thus nasalizing vowels that occur next to nasal phonemes (Shipley, 1990).

- Assimilative nasality can be functionally or organically based; assessment and treatment depend on etiology.

Cul-de-Sac Resonance

- *Cul-de-sac* (bottom of the sack) *resonance* is produced by backward retraction of the tongue; the tongue is carried too far posteriorly in the oral cavity.

- The oral cavity is partially closed at the back and open in the front. Because the tongue blocks some of the sound waves generated by the larynx from reaching the oral cavity, the perceptual result is distorted voice and resonance.

- Deaf people and those with neurological disorders often have difficulty making proper tongue adjustments, resulting in cul-de-sac resonance. People with no organic deviations also may acquire the habit of carrying the tongue too far back in the oral cavity while speaking.

Concepts To Consider

Describe the differences between hypernasality and hyponasality. What are some causes of each?

_____

_____

_____

_____

_____

_____

_____

_____

_____

Treatment Principles

Medical Intervention

■ It is always imperative, as a first step, to determine whether the disorders of resonance are due to functional or organic factors. Clearly, organically-based resonance problems must be treated medically before therapy can be successful (Case, 1996).

■ Medical treatment can take the form of surgery, prostheses, or both. For example, a child with a cleft palate may undergo surgery to repair the cleft and then be fitted with a prosthesis. (A more detailed description of medical intervention is presented in the section on craniofacial anomalies in Chapter 13.)

Treatment of Hypernasality

■ Biofeedback can be effective in treating hypernasality. Electronic instruments instantaneously display the amount of oral and nasal resonance as the patient talks. Such visual displays give the patient immediate feedback.

■ The *Nasometer*, an instrument created by Kay Elemetrics, allows the patient to receive visual feedback through a computer display. Feedback includes the target level of *nasalance* (oral-nasal ratio) and the amount of nasalance the patient is producing. The patient's productions can be shaped so they increasingly reflect an oral-nasal resonance balance that is within normal limits.

■ Specific treatment techniques for hypernasality include:

– employing *visual aids* such as a piece of tissue or a mirror, which can be put under a patient's nose so he or she can see appropriate vs. inappropriate nasal airflow during phonation;

– *ear training*, or helping patients learn to monitor their own productions (instruments such as the Nasometer and even a tape recorder (video or audio) are helpful);

– *increasing the patient's mouth opening* so that oral resonance is enhanced;

– *increasing the patient's loudness*, which can be accompanied by *respiration training*;

– *improving the patient's articulation*, which often results in his or her voice being perceived as less hypernasal; exaggerating consonants can contribute to a perception of less hypernasality;

– *changing the patient's speaking rate*; the clinician must first assess whether increasing or decreasing the rate decreases hypernasality; and

      — *decreasing pitch*, which can contribute to greater oral resonance, especially if the patient's habitual pitch is too high.

Treatment of Hyponasality

■ As with hypernasality, hyponasality can often be effectively treated through feedback such as that provided by the Nasometer and video or audio recordings.

■ Specific techniques that can decrease hyponasality involve increasing the patient's awareness of the nasal cavity as a resonator. These techniques include:

      — *Focusing*, or directing of the tone into the facial "mask," which is the area above the maxillary sinuses and around the nasal bridge. The clinician demonstrates and then has the patient say words with nasal sounds (e.g., *moon, me*) in an exaggerated way. This produces vibrations in the mask. The patient is asked to feel the vibrations, focusing his or her attention in the mask area. Appropriate resonance is then shaped from that point of reference.

      — *Nasal-glide stimulation.* The clinician selects words with many glides and nasals (e.g., *lawnmower, many, manners, lemon*). The patient practices saying those words in various combinations. The combination of glides and nasals helps direct resonance more appropriately into the nasal cavity and gives the patient auditory and kinesthetic feedback about proper utilization of the nasal cavity.

      — *Visual aids.* A piece of tissue or a mirror can be put under the patient's nose so he or she can see appropriate vs. inappropriate nasal airflow during phonation.

Summary

☑ Resonance is an important component of voice and must be evaluated as part of a thorough voice assessment. Difficulties with resonance include hypernasality, hyponasality, assimilative nasality, and cul-de-sac resonance.

☑ Treatment may include medical intervention if necessary; the patient with medical-physical needs will not progress until those needs are dealt with.

☑ When the clinician has ascertained that physical factors have been accounted for and treated appropriately, then he or she can use appropriate treatment techniques to help patients achieve optimal resonance patterns.

DISORDERS OF PHONATION AND THEIR TREATMENT

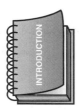

Many disorders of phonation are associated with physical factors. Some patients have cancer of the larynx; others have progressive diseases of the central nervous system. Some patients present with pathological changes in the vocal folds due to vocally abusive habits, with consequent perceptual sequelae such as hoarseness, breathiness, harshness, and low pitch. In this section, we describe some of the major physical factors associated with voice disorders of phonation. Basic treatment principles are also discussed.

Carcinoma and Laryngectomy

Basic Principles

- The larynx is one of the most common sites of cancer, accounting for approximately 3–5% of human cancer. Laryngeal cancer is found more frequently in men than in women and is considered a multifactorial disease.

- Alcohol, tobacco, exposure to environmental toxins (e.g., irradiation, asbestos), gastroesophageal reflux, and a combination of these cofactors all can contribute to laryngeal cancer.

- Early warning signs of laryngeal cancer include hoarseness, difficulty swallowing, and pain in the laryngeal area. Successful treatment of laryngeal cancer is highly dependent upon early detection and intervention.

Medical Treatment

- Medical treatment depends on the site, type, and extent of the cancer. Tumors can be *supraglottic* (above the vocal folds), *glottic* (at the level of the vocal folds), or *subglottic* (below the vocal folds). *Metastasis* (spread of the cancer to other regions) and *node involvement* are also major considerations.

- Doctors classify and treat laryngeal cancer based upon three primary categories: *T* (primary site of tumor), *N* (involvement of the lymph nodes), and *M* (metastasis). Thus, the patient's medical chart will probably feature a TNM designation to describe the site(s) and extent of the cancer.

- There are three basic types of medical treatment for laryngeal cancer: surgery, chemotherapy, and radiation.

- A *laryngectomy*, or surgery to remove the larnyx, can consist of a *total laryngectomy* (in which the entire larynx is removed) or a *hemilaryngectomy* (in which only the diseased part of the larynx is removed). Patients with advanced laryngeal cancer involving lymph nodes and metastasis may undergo total laryngectomy with *radical neck dissection*, in which the lymphatic system in the neck is removed. The person who has had his or her larynx removed is known as a *laryngectomee.*

- *Chemotherapy* may be used alone or in conjunction with other measures to increase the survival of patients with advanced cancer when the original tumor is large and metastasis is a risk. Side effects of chemotherapy include weight and hair loss, nausea, and weakness.

- *Radiation therapy*, used alone or combined with surgery, may be used for some patients. Doctors often use radiation therapy, before surgery is attempted, to try to eliminate the cancer. Some patients prefer radiation therapy to laryngectomy if given a choice. Side effects of radiation can include skin burns, risk of cavities, edema, swallowing problems, diminished taste, sore throat, and *xerostomia* (dry mouth due to trauma to the salivary glands).

General Issues in Rehabilitation of the Laryngectomee

- A team approach is critical in rehabilitation. Laryngectomees and their families need support from the surgeon, speech–language pathologist, social worker, nurse, vocational counselor, nutritionist, and maybe a counselor or psychologist to deal with accompanying emotional issues.

- Experienced, rehabilitated laryngectomees can be substantially helpful in providing information and support both pre- and postsurgically. Some cities have established support groups for laryngectomees and their families.

- Consultation and support, both written and verbal, are needed pre- as well as postsurgically. Patients and families who do not receive presurgical support tend to suffer more depression and isolation than those who receive information and support prior to surgery. Clinicians must remember that spouses and significant others need support just as the patient does.

Types of Alaryngeal Speech

- Because after a laryngectomy the vocal folds are gone, normal voicing is not possible and breathing is different. To allow the patient to breathe, the surgeon creates a *stoma* or opening in the lower part of the neck and connects it with the trachea. The patient now breathes through that opening.

- Figure 7.9 illustrates the anatomy and physiology of the head and neck before and after a total laryngectomy. Because of this altered anatomy and physiology, a new source of sound is needed for voicing.

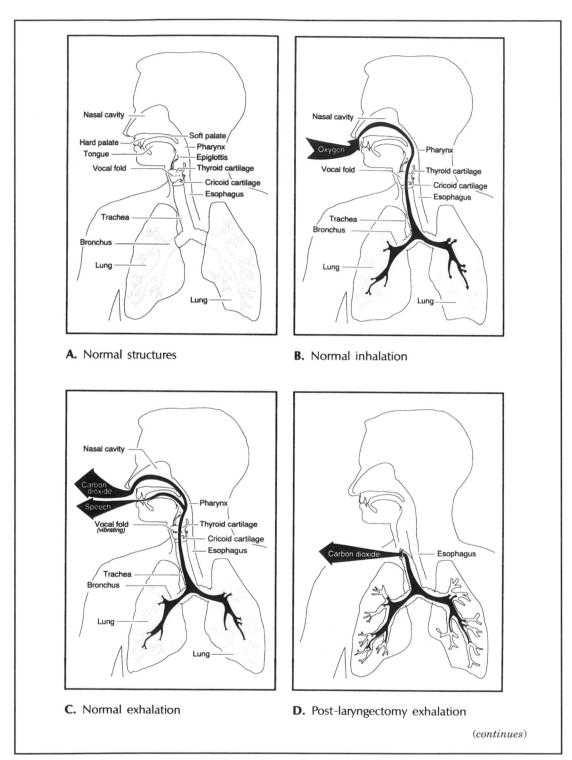

A. Normal structures

B. Normal inhalation

C. Normal exhalation

D. Post-laryngectomy exhalation

(continues)

Figure 7.9. Before and after laryngectomy: physiology of the head and neck. From *Manual of Voice Treatment: Pediatrics Through Geriatrics* (pp. 312–313), by M. L. Andrews, 1995, San Diego, CA: Singular Publishing Group, Inc. (401 West A Street, Suite 325, San Diego, CA, 92101-7904, 800-521-8545). Copyright 1995 by Singular Publishing Group, Inc. Reprinted with permission.

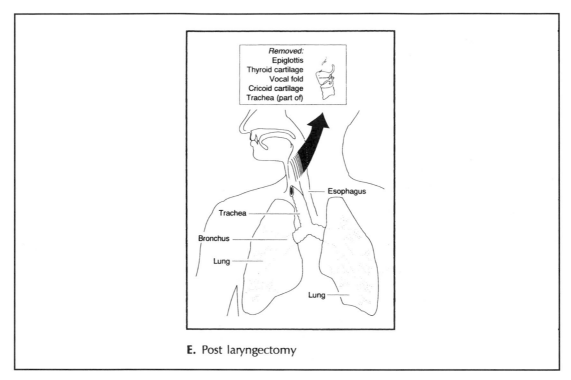

E. Post laryngectomy

Figure 7.9. *Continued.*

■ There are three ways that laryngectomees produce vocalizations: *external devices, esophageal speech*, and *surgical modifications or implanted devices* in the laryngeal area.

■ A widely used external device is the *artificial larynx*, a mechanical, hand-held device that generates sound. Many types of artificial larynxes exist on the market. The patient presses the artificial larynx against the neck, and turns on the unit with his or her thumb. The sound generated by the vibrator is transferred to the mouth, and the patient then articulates in a slightly exaggerated manner to increase intelligibility.

■ The esophagus is also a source of sound. Patients can be taught *esophageal speech*, in which they literally speak on burps or belches. There are two methods of esophageal speech:

   — In the *injection method*, the patient impounds the air in the mouth as in saying /t/ or /p/. The impounded air is pushed back into the esophagus and then expelled, producing vibrations of the soft tissues of the esophagus—particularly the *cricopharyngeus* muscle. The patient shapes the resulting belch into speech.

   — In the *inhalation method*, the patient is taught to inhale rapidly while keeping the esophagus open and relaxed. The inhaled air passes through the esophagus and sets its tissues into vibratory motion. The resulting sound is shaped into speech.

■ *Surgical modifications and implanted devices* can also serve as sound sources. In the popular *Blom-Singer tracheoesophageal puncture* (TEP), the tracheo-esophageal wall, which separates the trachea and esophagus, is punctured. A shunt or tunnel is opened to connect the two structures. To keep the tunnel open, the Blom-Singer prosthetic device (see Figure 7.10) is inserted into it. The device, which is a small 1.8–3.6-cm plastic or silicone tube, is designed to prevent the passage of fluid and food into the trachea. To speak, the patient exhales and occludes the stoma with a finger; the pulmonary air enters through the anterior opening of the tube, passing from the trachea to the esophagus. This sets the esophagus into vibration, resulting in sound production. The patient modifies the sound into speech.

✎ Concepts To Consider

You have been asked to give an inservice to physicians about medical treatment of patients who have undergone a laryngectomy. Briefly describe three things that you will tell them.

_____

_____

_____

_____

_____

_____

_____

Physically and Neurologically Based Disorders of Phonation

Granuloma

■ A *granuloma* is a localized, inflammatory, vascular lesion, which is usually comprised of granular tissue in a firm, rounded sac. Granulomas frequently develop on the vocal processes of the arytenoid cartilages in the posterior laryngeal area. They can be unilateral or bilateral. An example is shown in Figure 7.11.

■ Granulomas can be caused by vocal abuse, intubation during surgery, injury to the larynx, and gastroesophageal reflux. Granulomas are most often associated with contact ulcers.

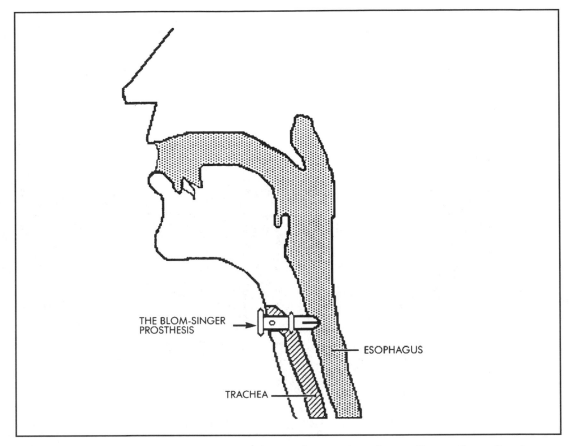

Figure 7.10. The Blom-Singer prosthetic device in place. From *Introduction to Communicative Disorders*, 2nd ed. (p. 278), by M. N. Hegde, 1995, Austin, TX: PRO-ED. Copyright 1995 by PRO-ED, Inc. Reprinted with permission.

- Patients with granulomas often sound breathy and hoarse; they feel the need to frequently clear their throat. The degree of dysphonia depends on the granuloma size and how much it interferes with glottal efficiency.

- Granulomas are treated by surgery, voice therapy, or both.

Hemangioma

- *Hemangiomas* are similar to granulomas, but hemangiomas are soft, pliable, and filled with blood. They occur in the posterior glottal area.

- Hemangiomas are usually caused by intubation or hyperacidity due to gastroesophageal reflux. They can also be congenital.

- Usually hemangiomas are surgically excised. Follow-up voice therapy is often necessary to improve vocal quality.

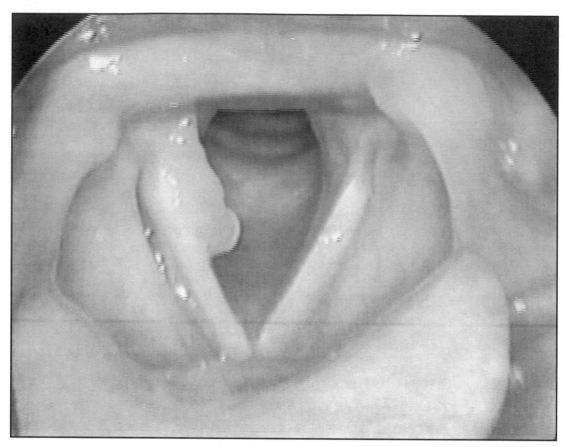

Figure 7.11. Contact ulcer with granuloma. From *Clinical Management of Voice Disorders*, 3rd ed. (p. 171), by J. L. Case, 1996, Austin, TX: PRO-ED. Copyright 1996 by PRO-ED, Inc. Reprinted with permission.

Leukoplakia

■ *Leukoplakia* are benign growths of thick, whitish patches on the surface membrane of the mucosa. These growths may extend into the subepithelial space.

■ Leukoplakia occur due to tissue irritation, especially that caused by smoking, alcohol, and vocal abuse. They may appear on the anterior third of the vocal folds and under the tongue.

■ Though benign, leukoplakia are considered precancerous and must be monitored to ensure that they do not develop into squamous cell carcinoma.

■ Patients with leukoplakia may sound hoarse, low-pitched, breathy, and soft in volume. Diplophonia may also be present. Treatment usually involves a combination of surgery, voice therapy, and eliminating exposure to tissue irritants.

Hyperkeratosis

■ *Hyperkeratosis* refers to a rough, pinkish lesion that can appear in the oral cavity, larynx, or pharynx. Hyperkeratosis of the vocal folds may involve the epithelial cover of the folds as well as the superficial layer of the lamina propria. These lesions are often benign but may be precursors to malignancy.

■ Hyperkeratotic growths occur due to tissue irritation and may arise in response to such causes as smoking, gastroesophageal reflux, and vocal abuse.

■ The voice symptoms presented by patients range from mild to severe hoarseness or harshness, reduced loudness, and low pitch. Treatment involves eliminating the tissue irritants, possible ablative surgery, and voice therapy.

Laryngomalacia

■ A congenital condition also known as *congenital laryngeal stridor, laryngomalacia* involves soft, "floppy" laryngeal cartilages, particularly the epiglottis.

■ The epiglottis is very soft and pliable due to abnormal development. When the child breathes, the epiglottis resists the airstream, causing *stridor,* or rough, breathy noise upon inhalation.

■ Because this condition usually resolves spontaneously by the time the child is 2 or 3 years old, no treatment is normally required after the initial diagnosis. However, in severe cases, the child may have substantial breathing problems, which will require treatment.

Papilloma

■ Papillomas are sometimes called *juvenile papillomas* because they tend to occur primarily in children (although they can occur in adults as well). When children reach puberty, papillomas often cease to be a problem.

■ Papillomas are wart-like growths caused by the human papilloma virus. They are pink and/or white and can be found anywhere in the airway (including but not limited to the larynx) (see Figure 7.12).

■ Hoarseness, breathiness, and low pitch are the most frequent perceptual symptoms of papilloma. Airway obstruction is a major and potentially life-threatening concern.

■ At present, most patients with papilloma are treated through multiple surgeries; some patients have had 30–100 surgeries for papilloma removal.

■ Repeated surgeries strip the mucosa and create vocal fold scar tissue, which impacts vocal quality. Children often sound even more hoarse and low-pitched

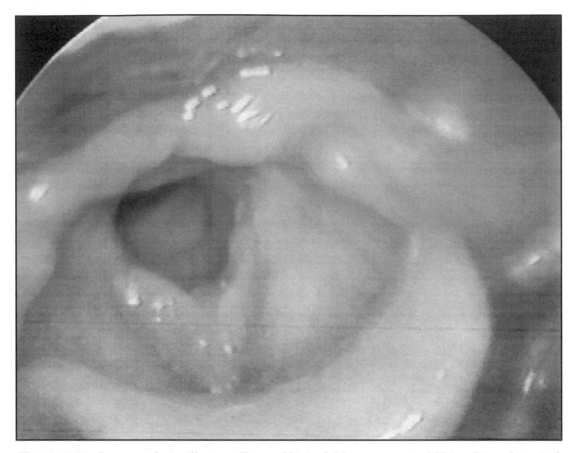

Figure 7.12. Laryngeal-papillomas. From *Clinical Management of Voice Disorders*, 3rd ed. (p. 346), by J. L. Case, 1996, Austin, TX: PRO-ED. Copyright 1996 by PRO-ED, Inc. Reprinted with permission.

than before. Laryngeal webbing (discussed later) can also occur. However, doctors are most concerned about airway preservation, and thus sequelae like hoarseness and laryngeal webbing are not considered high-priority problems.

- Treatments include *cup forceps surgery* (diminishing in popularity), *Interferon* medication, and *CO_2 laser surgery* (widely used). Carefully performed CO_2 laser surgery helps preserve mucosa and surrounding tissue while ablating the papillomas. Interferon can be effective but has potentially serious side effects including induced autoimmune diseases.

- Voice therapy can be helpful after surgical treatment. Therapy can involve relaxation exercises, teaching the patient to use amplification devices, and helping the patient decrease supraglottic hyperfunction. Therapy does not prevent recurrences of the papilloma, but it can help patients make the best use of their weakened and scarred vocal mechanism.

Laryngeal Trauma

■ Seen more frequently in children than in adults, laryngeal trauma refers to many kinds of injury to the larynx. Causes of laryngeal trauma include burns (thermal or chemical), motor vehicle accidents, sports-related accidents, and attempted strangulations and gunshot wounds. Young children may suffer trauma by swallowing sharp objects.

■ Patients who suffer laryngeal trauma generally undergo immediate surgery designed to reconstruct the vocal mechanism. The postsurgical necessity of voice therapy will vary from patient to patient, depending on the degree of dysphonia displayed. Voice therapy success depends largely on the proficiency of the remaining or surgically reconstructed laryngeal mechanism.

Laryngeal Web

■ A laryngeal web is a membrane that grows across the anterior portion of the glottis.

■ There are two basic types of laryngeal webs: *congenital*, or present at birth; and *acquired* due to trauma to the inner edges of the vocal folds. The vocal folds can be traumatized by forceful or prolonged intubation, surgery, severe laryngeal infections, or accidental injury.

■ Treatment for infants with congenital webs involves immediate surgery followed by tracheostomy.

■ Treatment for webbing in adults involves surgery to remove the web. After surgery, the surgeon will place a *laryngeal keel* (a fingernail-sized, rudder-shaped device) between the vocal folds to prevent them from growing back together. The patient generally undergoes 6–8 weeks of voice rest while the keel is in place. After the keel is removed, voice therapy may be required to assist in return of normal phonation (Boone & McFarlane, 1994).

Paradoxical Vocal Fold Motion (PVFM)

■ In PVCM, also called *laryngeal dyskinesia*, the true vocal folds adduct instead of abducting during inhalation and may remain closed throughout the respiratory cycle (see Figure 7.13). Sometimes the ventricular folds may also adduct.

■ Patients with PVFM often mistakenly appear asthmatic and sometimes undergo tracheotomy to relieve symptoms. Some patients display stridor and dysphonia; others display only stridor.

■ PVFM has been attributed to both psychological and physiological causes. Some experts view it as a conversion disorder in patients with psychological

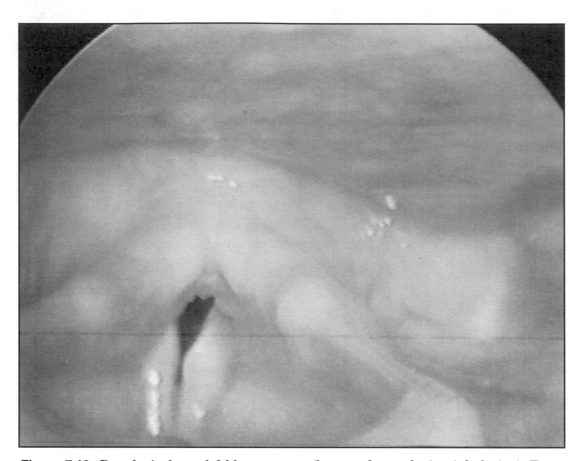

Figure 7.13. Paradoxical vocal fold movement (larynx shown during inhalation). From *Clinical Management of Voice Disorders*, 3rd ed. (p. 352), by J. L. Case, 1996, Austin, TX: PRO-ED. Copyright 1996 by PRO-ED, Inc. Reprinted with permission.

problems. Other experts believe that it may be due to psychological, pharmacological, or neurogenic variables.

■ Treatment may include a combination of psychological, medical, and behavioral approaches. Some patients respond well to voice therapy involving endoscopy and direct feedback, in which they learn the nature of the disorder as well as how to relax the entire vocal mechanism (Colton & Casper, 1996).

Gastroesophageal Reflux (GER)

■ GER occurs when gastric contents spontaneously empty into the esophagus. Patients may experience heartburn, acid indigestion, sore throat, and hoarseness. There can also be consequent pathological vocal fold changes such as *contact ulcers* (bilateral ulcerations on the medial surfaces of the vocal processes of the arytenoid cartilages).

■ Treatment options include antacids, propping up the head at night, prescription medications, and changes in dietary habits. Medical personnel should usually be involved.

Paralysis and Ankylosis

■ Because the vocal folds are composed primarily of muscle, they can be paralyzed when their nerve supply is cut off. Muscles that are not stimulated by the nerves do not move, resulting in paralysis.

■ Vocal folds can become paralyzed due to the following:

- accidental injury of the recurrent laryngeal nerve during certain *surgical procedures* (e.g., a thyroidectomy, in which a cancerous thyroid gland is surgically removed);

- progressive, debilitative *neurological diseases*, such as amyotrophic lateral sclerosis;

- *malignant diseases*, causing tumors outside the larynx to impact vocal fold mobility;

- *intubation trauma*, causing compression of the recurrent laryngeal nerve, dislocation of the arytenoids, and other difficulties;

- *laryngeal trauma* that is so severe it is irreparable (e.g., gunshot wound);

- *stroke*; and

- *vagus nerve deficits*.

■ Even in patients who can achieve a near-normal sounding voice despite vocal fold paralysis, coughing is not vigorous because of the difficulty in achieving the necessary amount of subglottal pressure for the vocal folds to close firmly. Some patients demonstrate dysphagia, breathiness, and reduced pitch and volume.

■ In *unilateral paralysis*, only one vocal fold is paralyzed and assumes a static position. In some cases, the normal fold may move toward the paralyzed fold to make contact; the voice in such cases may sound almost normal. In other cases, the paralyzed fold may be so far away from midline that the healthy fold cannot make contact to achieve closure. This causes aphonia.

■ *Bilateral paralysis*, or paralysis of both vocal folds, may lead to a wide-open glottis, causing aphonia. However, paralyzed folds can vibrate; thus, if the two paralyzed folds are positioned close to each other, they can approximate closure. The patient may then have a near-normal voice.

■ In *ankylosis*, or stiffening of the joint(s), the movement of the arytenoids is restricted because of a bone-joint disease such as arthritis. Cancer can also cause ankylosis. The vocal folds are attached to the arytenoids; when the arytenoids are stiff, the vocal folds don't close fully.

■ There are a number of treatment techniques available for patients with vocal fold paralysis. In cases of unilateral paralysis, doctors create a bulge in the paralyzed fold so that the healthy fold meets it more readily. Substances used to create the bulge include *Teflon, collagen, Gelfoam*, and *autologous fat* (the patient's own fat).

■ One popular new technique used to achieve vocal fold medialization is *thyroplasty I*. The surgeon creates a small window in the thyroid cartilage, medializes the vocal fold, and places a small Silastic implant to keep the paralyzed fold medialized (Brown, Vinson, & Crary, 1996).

■ In *nerve-muscle pedicle reinnervation*, the surgeon takes a pedicle of a neck strap muscle with innervation and sutures it either into the adductors for medialization purposes or into the posterior cricoarytenoids in order to promote abduction (Case, 1996).

■ Depending on the type of paralysis, the following treatment techniques have been used to help patients achieve firmer vocal fold closure:

   – elevation in pitch

   – increase in loudness

   – increased breath support, as well as breathing more often between phrases

   – pushing approach, in which the patient activates the glottal effort closure reflex by pushing against an object to increase vocal fold medialization

   – hard glottal attacks

   – head turning or positioning, in which the patient changes head position to see which position creates the best voice

Spasmodic Dysphonia

■ Spasmodic dysphonia (SMD) is a focal laryngeal dystonia. Although it has traditionally been considered psychologically based, most experts today believe that SMD has neurogenic causes with possible emotional side effects. The onset of SMD usually occurs in adults; the average age of onset is 38 years. There are two types.

■ *Abductor spasmodic dysphonia* is created by intermittent, involuntary, fleeting vocal fold abduction when the patient tries to phonate. Loudness is reduced and the patient is occasionally aphonic, with breathy or whispered speech. Treatment options include BOTOX (Botulinus toxin) injections, speech therapy involving relaxation techniques and continuous voicing, and pharmacological intervention.

■ *Adductor spasmodic dysphonia*, the most common type, is characterized by overpressure due to prolonged overaddiction or tight closure of the vocal folds. The voice may sound quite choked and strangled. Popular current treatment techniques include:

   – *CO_2 laser surgery*. The paralyzed fold is thinned with a CO_2 laser beam. This creates a 2-mm-wide groove whose healing and scarring action pulls the vocal fold away from the midline, widening the glottis. Repeated surgeries may be needed.

— *Recurrent laryngeal nerve (RLN) resection*. Here, the RLN is cut in order to paralyze the vocal fold on that side. This reduces vocal fold hyperadduction. RLN resection has met with mixed success.

— *BOTOX injections*. BOTOX, a neurotoxin injected directly by needle into the vocal folds, creates a flaccid paralysis, and hyperadduction ceases. Injections are usually repeated every 3–6 months. BOTOX is currently the treatment of choice among many specialists.

— *Voice therapy*. Voice therapy can include inhalation phonation, increased pitch, relaxation, head turning, counseling, the yawn-sigh approach, and soft, breathy phonation onset using /h/. (*Note*: Pushing techniques are counterproductive for patients who have RLN; recurrence of spasticity can occur.)

Neurological Diseases

Multiple Sclerosis (MS)

- Patients with MS experience progressive and diffuse demylination of white matter, with corresponding preservation of axons at the brainstem, cerebellum, and spinal cord.

- Patients may have impaired prosody, pitch, and loudness control, harshness, breathiness, hypernasality, articulation breakdown, and nasal air escape.

- Pharmacological intervention may include ACTH (adrenocorticotrophic hormone) to reduce acute symptoms. Corticosteroids such as Prednisone may also be used.

Myasthenia Gravis

- This neuromuscular autoimmune disease produces fatigue and muscle weakness. There is a decreased amount of acetylcholine at the myoneuronal junction.

- Patients often sound hypernasal, breathy, hoarse, and soft in volume. Dysphagia and distorted articulation may also be present.

- Myasthenia gravis is often treated with corticosteroids, which improve strength and endurance of the bulbar musculature.

Amyotrophic Lateral Sclerosis (ALS)

- ALS, or *Lou Gehrig's disease*, is a progressive, fatal disease involving degeneration of the upper and lower motor neuron systems.

- Patients with ALS often sound breathy, low pitched, and monotoned. There is poor respiratory control.

■ ALS does not respond well to medications, but Riluzole has been shown to slow muscle deterioration in some patients.

■ Because ALS is progressive, many clinicians focus treatment efforts on augmentative/alternative forms of communication that can be used even in the later stages of the disease.

Parkinson's Disease

■ Parkinson's is caused by a lack of dopamine (a neurotransmitter) in the substantia nigra of the basal ganglia. It can be idiopathic (occurring in isolation or primary form) or secondary to other conditions such as dementia.

■ Patients with Parkinson's disease often sound breathy, low pitched, and monotoned.

■ Treatment includes *L-dopa* (levodopa) to increase dopamine in the substantia nigra; voice treatment may also be indicated. The currently popular *Lee Silverman Voice Treatment* program emphasizes stimulating patients to increase respiratory and phonatory efforts and to sustain those efforts over time (Ramig, Bonitati, Lemke, & Horii, 1994).

Treatment Techniques for Patients with Neurological Diseases

■ Because patients with neurological diseases tend to manifest dysarthria, with some exceptions, treatment techniques often follow principles based upon therapy for dysarthria.

■ Although patients will differ and have individual needs, many of them will benefit from the following therapy strategies designed to improve the efficiency of the overall system and increase general intelligibility:

— improve articulation through exaggerating consonants and slowing rate of speech;

— improve resonance through increasing mouth opening, decreasing posterior tongue tension, and improving velopharyngeal closure;

— improve prosody to decrease monopitch;

— improve respiration through relaxation, increasing efficiency of breathing (e.g., teaching diaphragmatic-abdominal breathing), and teaching the patient to breathe as often as necessary; and

— improve vocal fold approximation through activities already mentioned (see "Paralysis and Ankylosis").

✎ Concepts To Consider

Describe two neurologically based disorders of phonation. What types of treatment might be appropriate for those disorders?

_____

_____

_____

_____

_____

_____

_____

Abuse-Based Disorders of Phonation

Vocally Abusive Practices

■ Many disorders of voice occur due to vocally abusive behaviors. The sophisticated vocal mechanism works well when used properly. But it is extremely sensitive to abuse, which often causes a variety of voice problems.

■ *Abusive behaviors* that can damage the vocal mechanism are: excessive shouting; screaming; cheering; excessive talking; coughing; hard glottal attacks; throat clearing; strained and explosive vocalizations; excessive laughing and crying; speaking with inappropriate pitch, loudness, or both; and speaking in noisy environments.

■ The majority of vocally abusive behaviors are associated with excessive muscular effort, tension, and consequent irritation of the vocal folds. Excessive effort and tension can cause physical damage to the vocal folds and create physical pathologies. The voice problems that result from vocally abusive behaviors are due to such physical damage to and pathological states of the larynx.

■ Therapy, medication, surgery, or a combination of those treatments are generally used to correct voice disorders resulting from pathological changes to the vocal folds due to abuse. However, if patients continue the abusive practices and do not change their vocal habits, pathological changes to the vocal folds with consequent voice problems are likely to recur.

Vocal Nodules

■ Vocal nodules are small nodes that develop on the vocal folds and protrude from surrounding cells (see Figure 7.14). In the beginning, the nodules are

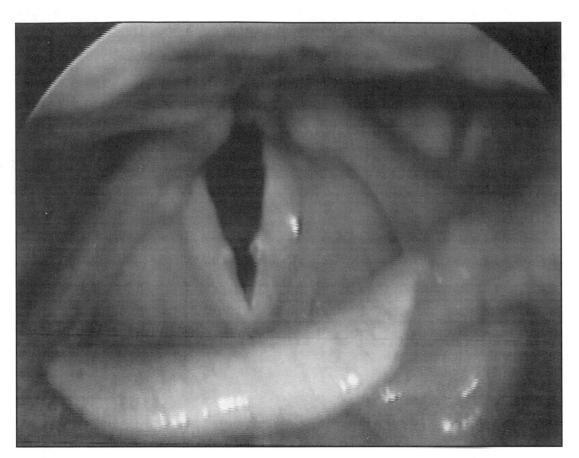

Figure 7.14. Vocal folds with nodules. From *Clinical Management of Voice Disorders*, 3rd ed. (p. 129), by J. L. Case, 1996, Austin, TX: PRO-ED. Copyright 1996 by PRO-ED, Inc. Reprinted with permission.

reddish or pinkish. As they develop over time, they appear white or grayish because they become fibrous.

■ Vocal nodules can be unilateral; however, they are typically bilateral and sit opposite each other on the two folds. Nodules typically appear at the junction of the anterior and middle-third portion of the folds.

■ Nodules are well defined in the beginning stages but become more diffuse later because of inflammation of the surrounding tissue. Nodules develop over time as the result of prolonged vocally abusive behaviors.

■ Vocal nodules increase the mass of the vocal folds. Consequently, the folds vibrate at a slower rate, resulting in lower pitch. The nodules also make smooth vocal fold approximation impossible, contributing to breathiness and hoarseness of voice.

■ Vocal nodules are seen most frequently in children who scream and yell on playgrounds and in adults whose career and/or leisure activities involve vocally abusive practices (e.g., yelling at sports events). Singers are especially susceptible to vocal nodules.

■ Vocal rest usually clears up the nodules. But prolonged abuse of the vocal folds will result in larger and more persistent nodules. Unless the patient changes his or her abusive behaviors, the nodules will rarely disappear.

■ Persistent nodules are frequently treated in two ways: voice therapy (described later) and/or surgery. Surgery involves tissue excision, or removal of the nodules through microdissection or laser.

■ Recently, some doctors have been using cold steel lasers or microspot CO_2 (heat) lasers, whose beam is so small that heat cannot penetrate the surrounding tissues. The goal of laser and microdissection is to remove the nodules while disturbing as little of the mucosa and surrounding tissue as possible.

Polyps

■ Polyps, like nodules, are masses that grow and bulge out from surrounding tissue. Polyps are softer than nodules and may be filled with fluid or have vascular tissue. Polyps tend to be unilateral as opposed to the typically bilateral nodules. Figure 7.15 shows a vocal polyp.

■ *Sessile polyps* have a broad base on the vocal fold; *pedunculated polyps* are attached to the vocal folds by a stalk.

■ It is believed that traumatic use of the vocal folds results in submucosal hemorrhage (bleeding within the folds), which leads to the formation of tumorlike polyps. Polyps can grow over time or can be created after just one instance of severe vocal abuse (e.g., screaming if attacked).

■ Polyps are more frequently seen in adults than in children, who are more susceptible to developing vocal nodules. Patients with polyps usually sound breathy and hoarse. They may also have *diplophonia* ("double voice," in which two different pitches are heard simultaneously) because the healthy fold vibrates at a different rate than the fold with the polyp.

■ Polyps may disappear with voice rest and changes in vocal habits, or they may persist and become worse with time and no treatment. Techniques for treating patients with vocal polyps are described later.

Contact Ulcers

■ Contact ulcers are sores or craterlike areas of ulcerated, granulated tissue that develop (usually bilaterally) along the posterior third of the glottal margin.

■ The causes of contact ulcers include:

   – *The slamming together of the arytenoid cartilages* that occurs during low-pitched phonation accompanied by hard glottal attack and sometimes by

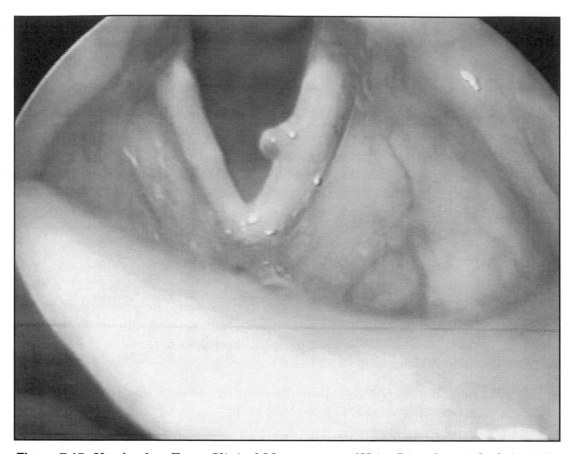

Figure 7.15. Vocal polyp. From *Clinical Management of Voice Disorders*, 3rd ed. (p. 347), by J. L. Case, 1996, Austin, TX: PRO-ED. Copyright 1996 by PRO-ED, Inc. Reprinted with permission.

increased loudness. Frequently, contact ulcers are seen in hard-driving patients who speak forcefully and talk excessively.

– *Gastroesophageal reflux* (discussed earlier), in which stomach acid is forced into the esophagus. The acid pools in and irritates the area between the arytenoid cartilages; this can occur especially at night when one is sleeping.

– *Intubation* for surgery, especially if intubation is prolonged or the tube is too large for the patient's larynx. Seventy percent of children who are intubated have a lacerated glottal area; this can cause permanent scarring and dysphonia.

■ Patients with contact ulcers may complain of vocal fatigue and pain in the laryngeal area. They frequently sound hoarse and often clear their throats.

■ Depending on the etiology, contact ulcers may require medical treatment (e.g., medication for gastroesophageal reflux). Surgery is not recommended; because the area is already ulcerated and highly irritated, healing is usually poor. Voice therapy techniques (described later) are geared toward taking the extra effort out of phonation.

Vocal Fold Thickening

■ Prolonged use of vocally abusive behaviors such as throat clearing, screaming, and others can cause the vocal folds to thicken slowly and gradually. The vocal folds usually thicken along the anterior two-thirds of the glottal margin.

■ Vocal fold thickening results in a breathy voice with lowered pitch. Vocal fold thickening is often a precursor to nodules or polyps. When these appear, the voice becomes increasingly hoarse. Vocal fold thickening can be reduced through elimination of the vocally abusive behaviors.

Traumatic Laryngitis

■ *Traumatic laryngitis* differs from *infectious,* or *organic,* laryngitis, which occurs due to infections, colds, or allergies (of bacterial or viral origin). Traumatic laryngitis is created when the patient engages in vocally abusive behaviors such as continual yelling.

■ Vocally abusive behaviors irritate the vocal folds, which get swollen. Consequently, the voice is hoarse and may be low pitched with pitch breaks.

■ Voice therapy usually consists of vocal rest and strategies for changing the vocally abusive behaviors.

Treatment for Abuse-Based Voice Disorders

Basic Principles

■ As described above, abuse-based voice disorders are the result of a chain of causes and effects:

> vocally abusive behaviors, which cause
> ↓
> laryngeal tissue changes, which in turn cause
> ↓
> voice disorders, which then may cause
> ↓
> personal, social, emotional, and occupational problems
> that cause additional stress and more vocal strain

■ The clinician's goal, in voice therapy, is to help the patient achieve the best-sounding voice possible. This can involve either *restoration* of the previous healthy voice, or *compensation*, by which the patient produces the best voice possible given damage already done to the laryngeal mechanism (Brown et al., 1996).

- As mentioned, treatment for abuse-based voice disorders usually involves *voice therapy, medication, surgery*, or a combination of these.

- Patients with voice disorders due to vocal abuse and consequent pathological changes in the vocal mechanism must reduce or eliminate vocal abuses and learn to regularly use healthy vocal habits. Laryngeal lesions and resulting voice problems will recur unless patients permanently alter their ways of speaking.

- Clinicians can facilitate medical evaluations, awareness of vocally abusive habits, and the learning of new, healthy habits that will ensure optimal vocal health and voice production.

Fundamental Steps in Therapy

- Most adults and children who undergo voice therapy benefit from the foundational treatment steps listed below.

- Make a thorough evaluation of the voice disorder.

- Always have a medical evaluation completed before starting voice therapy.

- Maintain a cooperative working relationship with a laryngologist; be knowledgeable about laryngeal surgical procedures and medications and their effects on and interactions with voice treatment methods.

- Have periodic medical examinations completed during the course of voice therapy.

- Combine, in most cases, techniques designed to reduce vocally abusive behaviors with those that facilitate efficient and normal voice production.

- Individualize the facilitating techniques to each patient.

- Help patients understand the nature of their disorder, what habits are maintaining the disorder, and the harmful results of the vocally abusive behaviors.

- Give adults readings, illustrations of vocal anatomy and physiology, and explanations.

- Design a program to help patients reduce abusive behaviors and establish vocally appropriate behaviors.

- Help all patients understand what their specific treatment goals are.

- Work closely with patient's significant others (e.g., parents, siblings, spouses) to help reduce vocally abusive behaviors and to reinforce healthy vocal behaviors.

- Establish baselines of vocally abusive behaviors and the frequency of abnormal voice productions in and outside the clinic.

- Ask patients (or parents of young children) to measure their vocally abusive behaviors for a few days and graph their frequency on a daily basis to establish the baselines of vocally abusive behaviors in natural settings.

■ Encourage patients to monitor their own voice production both inside and outside the clinic setting.

■ Consistently use audio recordings for feedback, ear training, and development of patients' ability to self-monitor; video recordings are even better.

■ Use visual monitoring and feedback such as that provided by the Visi-Pitch.

■ Support patients, especially adults, in identifying and making needed lifestyle changes such as avoiding smoke (including secondhand smoke) and alcohol, drinking enough water, and taking appropriate allergy medications.

Specific Treatment Techniques

■ Not every client will need every technique. Clinicians can select individually appropriate techniques that are designed to reduce vocally abusive habits and replace them with positive, nonabusive practices that will promote optimal vocal health. See the following list for examples:

— Use the *open mouth approach*. Teach the patient to speak with a wider mouth opening; this helps increase volume and improve the oral-nasal resonance balance. Use a mirror if necessary.

— Help the patient speak with *appropriate pitch and volume.*

— Teach the patient to *reduce the frequency of coughing* and throat clearing.

— Teach the patient to *relax the body* and the oral-laryngeal area when speaking; reduce tension.

— Use the *chant-talk method*, in which words are spoken in a connected manner, with soft glottal attack, even stress, prolongation of sounds, and the absence of stress for individual words.

— Use *digital manipulation* of the larynx, which will lower pitch and decrease laryngeal tension. Here, the clinician gently places his or her thumb and fingers on either side of the patient's thyroid cartilage and gently pushes downward while the patient phonates. The clinician can then fade the model, and the patient can perform the manipulation.

— Use *respiration training* to teach thoracic and diaphragmatic-abdominal breathing to increase breath support for vocalization.

— *Encourage voice rest*, which can range from no vocalizations at all for a time period to specific, planned periods of the day when the client does not vocalize.

— Teach *gentle voice onset*, in which the client initiates phonation using an /h/ or /h/ + vowel (e.g., "ha" or "hi"). Voice initiation is gentle, relaxed, and whispered.

— Teach the *yawn-sigh method* to relax the oral-laryngeal mechanism and increase the mouth opening. The client inhales on a wide yawn, which is followed by an expiratory sigh and phonation.

– For clients with pharyngeal focus, or voices coming from too deep in the throat, teach *appropriate focus* in the facial mask (referred to earlier).

✎ Concepts To Consider

A 43-year-old high school football coach comes to you for an evaluation. He states that he has been hoarse for approximately 10 months. A subsequent medical evaluation reveals the presence of well-developed vocal nodules. Describe some treatment techniques you will use with this patient.

_____

_____

_____

_____

_____

_____

_____

_____

Disorders of Loudness and Pitch

Basic Principles

■ Frequently, the problems of loudness and pitch are components of other voice disorders. For example, the breathy and hoarse voice is typically low pitched. Laryngeal pathologies may prevent a loud enough voice.

■ However, several disorders of loudness and pitch occur independently of other problems. When treating patients with these disorders of loudness and pitch, clinicians must rule out physical problems such as hearing loss, asthma, and others.

Disorders of Loudness

Key Facts

■ Vocal loudness varies among individuals and is determined by variables such as culture and gender of the patient as well as health issues.

- Very few people seek professional help for loud speech unless it is part of a larger problem such as vocal nodules or polyps, which in turn create a voice problem.

- The typical patient who seeks treatment speaks too softly. Patients may speak too softly, as judged by mainstream listeners, for a variety of reasons: hearing loss, cultural mores, clinical depression, psychological trauma, or sheer habit.

Treatment

- Most patients with inadequate loudness and no contraindicating health problems can be easily trained. The clinician can help them maintain enough air pressure while speaking and can systematically reinforce progressively louder speech.

- Auditory and visual feedback such as that provided by a tape recorder, the Visi-Pitch, or a computer program can be very helpful.

Disorders of Pitch

Key Facts

- The typical pitch disorder consists of either too high or too low a pitch considering the age and sex of the speaker. Due to mainstream cultural expectations, an unusually high pitch in a man or an unusually low pitch in a woman might be considered abnormal or undesirable.

- Some patients come to therapy because they have undergone a sex-change operation and wish to produce a voice that is compatible with their new identity. These patients are considered not to have pitch disorders, but rather to have unique needs that can best be met by clinicians trained to serve the members of that population.

- Most clients with pitch disorders are men who speak with too high a pitch and wish to speak with a lower, more appropriate pitch. A high pitch in a man can be due to psychological factors, physical factors, or both.

- In *mutational falsetto,* or *puberphonia*, a young man speaks with a high pitch although the larynx has grown normally and puberty is completed. This can occur due to psychosocial factors (e.g., embarrassment about the newly developing low voice), endocrine disorders, or neurologic diseases.

- For patients with puberphonia, it is optimal for treatment to be initiated in the teens or early twenties. Some atrophy of the vocal muscles may occur if the mutational falsetto persists untreated.

- Pitch disorders due to *hormonal changes* may impact some patients, especially women. Menstruation, menopause, use of oral contraceptives, and virilization (increased masculinity) of the female voice have all been associated with pitch changes.

■ Pitch changes before and during menstruation are not usually a major problem. However, such changes are troublesome to professional singers. Lowered levels of estrogen and progesterone before menses can cause vocal fold thickening, with consequent hoarseness and lowered pitch.

■ Drugs containing male hormones are sometimes used to treat cancer. For example, uterine cancer is often treated with testosterone. Such drugs can thicken the vocal folds and decrease vocal pitch; those changes may be irreversible.

Treatment

■ In patients with a pitch that is too high, especially young men with puberphonia, the larynx is often elevated, with accompanying tension of the laryngeal musculature.

■ Because of this tension, relaxation, yawn-sigh, the open-mouth approach, and digital manipulation are often successful in lowering pitch. The use of nonspeech vocalizations such as coughing and glottal fry can also be helpful.

■ Visual and auditory feedback such as that provided by tape recordings and instruments such as the Visi-Pitch are quite helpful to patients with pitch problems.

■ Some patients may need psychological counseling in conjunction with voice therapy. This is dependent upon the needs and background of the individual.

■ Clients from linguistically and culturally diverse backgrounds should be asked to describe their perception of a voice with normal pitch; the clinician should then conduct the therapy accordingly (DeJarnette & Holland, 1998).

Psychogenic Voice Disorders

Basic Principles

■ Psychogenic, or "functional," voice disorders occur when the voice is abnormal in the presence of normal laryngeal structures. A laryngoscopic examination reveals essentially normal vocal structures; however, during attempted phonation, the vocal folds may remain fully or partially abducted.

■ In *hysterical*, or *conversion aphonia*, there is usually no evidence of a structural pathology. There is no known physiological or neurological basis for the patient's voice loss. The loss can be sudden or gradual.

■ Patients with conversion aphonia often experience voice loss after an emotionally traumatic event such as a violent crime. The voice loss may represent an unconscious attempt to avoid dealing with the traumatic event. The voice problem is thus viewed as a conversion reaction, or translation of the emotional trauma into another set of symptoms.

Treatment

▪ Aphonia in the absence of any organic cause has been treated with either counseling/psychotherapy or behavior therapy.

▪ For *counseling/psychotherapy*, clinicians will often refer the patient to a professional psychologist, psychiatrist, or marriage and family counselor. During therapy sessions, clients are encouraged to speak freely about themselves and their problems. With the support of a sympathetic listener, clients are expected to resolve their psychological conflicts and return to normal phonation.

▪ Clinicians who employ *behavior therapy* treat conversion aphonia by modifying the client's behaviors. Specific therapy techniques can include:

- Masking, or the *Lombard effect*; when the patient receives masking noise and is asked to vocalize, he or she may do it reflexively; the clinician should tape-record this.

- Progressive relaxation techniques and reduction in muscle tension.

- Encouraging coughing, grunting, throat clearing, laughing, humming, and other non-speech vocalizations.

- Prolonging a cough into a normal vowel.

- Inhalation phonation.

- The yawn-sigh approach.

- Production of vowels, monosyllabic words, and polysyllabic words.

- Progression to simple phrases, oral reading.

- Engaging in simple conversation alone with the clinician.

- Engaging in conversations with an increased variety of interlocutors in an increased variety of settings.

- Generalization to daily communication activities.

▪ For many patients with conversion aphonia, the prognosis for return to normal voice is quite good. Clinicians must, after gathering an extensive case history and viewing the overall situation, make accurate decisions about the most effective course of treatment for conversion aphonia patients.

Summary

☑ Patients often seek evaluation and treatment for voice disorders that have been caused by physical changes to the larynx. One major physical change, for some patients, involves laryngeal cancer.

☑ Patients who have surgery for total removal of the larynx need specific rehabilitation to learn alaryngeal speech. Other patients present voice disorders that result from physical changes caused by abusive vocal habits, neurological problems, and irritation by environmental agents.

☑ Disorders of loudness and pitch can be caused by organic or functional factors. Treatment will depend upon the etiology of the problem, as well as the patient's cultural perception of what constitutes a normal voice.

☑ Patients who have psychogenic voice disorders have frequently undergone emotional trauma with consequent loss of voice. For many of these patients, behavioral therapy, counseling/psychotherapy, or a combination is quite successful in voice restoration.

CHAPTER HIGHLIGHTS

▶ Having a normal, optimal-sounding voice depends on the health and intactness of the larynx and its structures. Key structures include the major laryngeal cartilages: thyroid cartilage, cricoid cartilage, arytenoid cartilages, and the corniculate and cuneiform cartilages. Cranial nerve X, the vagus nerve, is the nerve primarily responsible for innervation of the larynx.

▶ Key laryngeal muscles include the intrinsic laryngeal muscles: thyroarytenoids, cricothyroids, posterior cricoarytenoids, lateral cricoarytenoids, and interarytenoids. The extrinsic laryngeal muscles include: (a) the infrahyoids or laryngeal depressors—thyrohyoids, omohyoids, sternothyroids, and sternohyoids—and (b) the suprahyoids or laryngeal elevators—digastrics, geniohyoids, mylohyoids, stylohyoids, genioglossus, and hyoglossus.

▶ Each individual's voice undergoes changes during his or her life span. These changes involve mean fundamental frequency and maximum phonation time.

▶ Vocal pitch (frequency) and volume (intensity) are important parameters of the voice. Vocal quality is greatly impacted by patients' daily vocal habits.

(continues)

▶ Evaluation of voice disorders should be comprehensive and based on a multidisciplinary, team approach. A medical evaluation should be conducted before therapy is initiated.

▶ Optimally, a voice evaluation should include: (a) gathering a thorough case history, (b) conducting additional assessments such as an oral peripheral examination and hearing screening, (c) instrumental analysis, and (d) perceptual analysis of vocal characteristics.

▶ Disorders of resonance include hypernasality, hyponasality, assimilative nasality, and cul-de-sac resonance. For the patient with resonance problems, it is critical to rule out organic causes such as velopharyngeal inadequacy. Therapy will not succeed unless the physical basis for the resonance problem is resolved.

▶ Disorders of voice are often associated with physical factors involving pathological changes of the laryngeal mechanism. These factors include carcinoma, physical changes due to vocal abuse, neurological problems, and vocal fold irritation created by environmental agents. Treatment often involves medication, surgery, therapy, or a combination of these approaches.

▶ Disorders of loudness and pitch are associated with functional causes, organic causes, or both. Common problems associated with pitch and loudness include mutational falsetto, hormonal changes, and hearing loss.

▶ Psychogenic voice disorders occur when the voice is abnormal in the presence of normal laryngeal structures. Hysterical or conversion aphonia is often attributed to an underlying emotional etiology. Patients with psychogenic voice disorders can often be successfully treated with a variety of behavioral strategies. However, some patients may require psychotherapy or counseling.

▶ Add your own chapter highlights here:

_____

_____

_____

_____

_____

KEY TERMS

abduct
adduct
aerodynamic measurements
amplitude
amyotrophic lateral sclerosis (ALS)
ankylosis
artificial larynx
aryepiglottic folds
arytenoid cartilages
assimilative nasality
autologous fat
Blom-Singer prosthetic device
Blom-Singer tracheo-esophageal puncture
BOTOX
breathiness
case history
chant talk method
contact ulcers
corniculate cartilages
CO_2 laser surgery
cranial nerve VII
cranial nerve X
cricoid cartilage
cul-de-sac resonance
cuneiform cartilages
diaphragmatic-abdominal breathing
digital manipulation
diplophonia
direct laryngoscopy
electroglottography
electromyography
endoscopy
epiglottis
esophageal speech
extrinsic laryngeal muscles
flexible fiber-optic laryngoscopy
functional
fundamental frequency

gastroesophageal reflux (GER)
gentle voice onset
glottal fry
glottis
granuloma
harshness
hemangioma
hemilaryngectomy
hoarseness
hyoid bone
hyperkeratosis
hypernasality
hyponasality
hysterical (conversion) aphonia
indirect laryngoscopy
infectious laryngitis
infrahyoids
inhalation method
injection method
Interferon
intrinsic laryngeal muscles
jitter
L-dopa
laryngeal dyskinesia
laryngeal keel
laryngeal trauma
laryngeal web
laryngectomee
laryngectomy
laryngomalacia
larynx
Lee Silverman Voice Treatment program
leukoplakia
Lombard effect
maximum phonation time (MPT)
mean fundamental frequency (MFF)
metastasis
monopitch
multiple sclerosis

mutational falsetto (puberphonia)
myasthenia gravis
nasalance
Nasometer
nerve-muscle pedicle reinnervation
nodules
organic
papilloma (juvenile)
paradoxical vocal fold motion
Parkinson's disease
pitch
polyps (sessile and pedunculated)
psychogenic voice disorders
quality
radical neck dissection
recurrent laryngeal nerve (RLN)
shimmer
spasmodic dysphonia (SMD)
stoma
stridency
strain-strangle
subglottic
superior laryngeal nerve (SLN)
supraglottic
suprahyoids
s/z ratio
team approach
thoracic breathing
thyroid cartilage
thyroplasty I
tidal volume
TNM designation
total laryngectomy
total lung capacity
traumatic laryngitis
velopharyngeal inadequacy

ventricular (false) vocal folds	Visi-Pitch	vocal processes
videoendoscopy	vital capacity	volume
videostroboscopy	vocal fold thickening	xerostomia
	vocal folds	yawn-sigh

STUDY AND REVIEW QUESTIONS

Fill in the Blank

1. The *infrahyoid* laryngeal muscles lie below the hyoid bone; they are sometimes called *depressors*. These muscles are called the _thyrohyoid_, _omohyoid_, _sternothyroid_, and _sternohyoid_.

2. The *suprahyoid* laryngeal muscles lie above the hyoid bone; they are sometimes called *elevators*. The suprahyoid muscles are: _digastric_, _geniohyoid_, _mylohyoid_, _stylohyoid_, _genioglossus_, and _hyoglossus_.

3. Cranial nerve ___X___, the ___vagus___ nerve, has two branches: the _superior laryngeal nerve_ and the _recurrent laryngeal nerve_.

4. When a young man speaks with a pitch that is perpetually too high despite complete laryngeal maturation, he has a condition called _puberphonia or mutational falsetto_.

5. The patient who has no evidence of structural pathology of the laryngeal mechanism yet loses his or her voice and cannot vocalize is said to have _hysterical or conversion aphonia_.

6. Sometimes specialists assess the lung volume of voice patients because breath support is inadequate. Specialists can measure _total lung volume_, or the total volume of air in the lungs; other measurements can include _tidal volume_, or the amount of air inhaled and exhaled during a normal breathing cycle, and _vital capacity_, or the volume of air that the patient can exhale after a maximal exhalation.

7. The most efficient type of breathing is not _clavicular breathing_, in which the shoulders elevate on inhalation, but _diaphragmatic/abdominal_, in which the patient uses the abdominal region and lower thoracic cavity.

8. The two basic types of esophageal speech include the _inhalation_ method, in which the patient is taught to keep the esophagus open and relaxed while inhaling rapidly, and the _injection_ method, in which the patient impounds the air in the oral cavity, pushes it back into the esophagus, and vibrates the cricopharyngeus muscle.

9. Pediatric patients can present with organically based disorders of phonation caused by conditions such as _laryngomalacia_, a congenital condition involving soft, "floppy" laryngeal cartilages, and _juvenile papilloma_, which are wartlike growths caused by a virus that frequently necessitate multiple surgeries.

10. In a recently studied phenomenon called _paradoxical VF motion_ the true vocal folds adduct instead of abducting during inhalation and may remain closed throughout the respiratory cycle. This is also called _laryngeal dyskinesia_.

Multiple Choice

11. The cranial nerve primarily responsible for innervating the larynx is:

    A. nerve V

    B. nerve II

    C. nerve X

    D. nerve VI

    E. nerve IV

12. The procedure that uses a pulsing light to permit the optical illusion of slow-motion viewing of the vocal folds is:

    A. electroglottography

    B. stroboscopy

    C. electromyography

    D. videofluoroscopy

    E. nasoendoscopy

13. A 67-year-old man comes to you for an evaluation. He states that his voice has been getting "weaker" for the last 5–6 months. Upon oral peripheral examination, you find that he has fasciculations (tremors) of the tongue and some general facial weakness. The first thing you would do is:

    A. refer him to a psychologist for an evaluation.

    B. take detailed notes and tell him to come back in 6 months.

C. begin voice therapy, focusing on strengthening exercises.

D. refer him to a pulmonary specialist.

E. refer him to a neurologist for an evaluation.

14. The cartilages that are pyramid shaped and have the vocal processes attached to them at the most anterior angle are the:

A. arytenoid cartilages.

B. cuneiform cartilages.

C. corniculate cartilages.

D. cricoid cartilages.

E. hyoid cartilages.

15. Which of the following are TRUE?

A. Nineteen-year-old females have a mean fundamental frequency of 217 Hz.

B. Nineteen-year-old males have an MFF of 117 Hz.

C. Most 18–39-year-old adults have a maximum phonation time of 15–18 seconds.

D. A, B

E. A, B, C

16. Variations in vocal frequency, or frequency perturbation, are known as:

A. jitter.

B. shimmer.

C. amplitude perturbation.

D. fundamental frequency variation.

E. frequency changes.

17. You have an 8-year-old boy in therapy for vocal nodules. You would begin therapy for this boy by:

A. prescribing 2 weeks of voice rest.

B. monitoring him by seeing him once every 2 months for the next year.

C. focusing on identification and reduction of vocal abuse behavior.

D. sending him to a counselor.

E. giving him and his parents reading materials that discuss vocal abuse.

18. The Blom-Singer prosthetic device is used by laryngectomees to:

    A. clean the surgically created fistula.

    B. shunt air from the esophagus to the trachea so that the salpingopharyngeus muscle will vibrate during inhalation.

    C. assist in the development of competent esophageal speech.

    D. prevent particles of food from entering the trachea.

    E. shunt the air from the trachea to the esophagus so that the patient can speak on pulmonary air entering the esophagus.

19. A patient with a "double voice," the perception of or two distinct simultaneous pitches during phonation, has:

    A. glottal fry.

    B. diplophonia.

    C. strain-strangle.

    D. cul-de-sac resonance.

    E. harshness.

20. Patients who might be treated with CO_2 laser surgery, recurrent laryngeal nerve resection, BOTOX, voice therapy, or a combination would probably have:

    A. contact ulcers.

    B. paradoxical vocal fold motion.

    C. hemangioma.

    D. spasmodic dysphonia.

    E. myasthenia gravis.

REFERENCES AND RECOMMENDED READINGS

Andrews, M. L. (1995). *Manual of voice treatment: Pediatrics through geriatrics*. San Diego, CA: Singular Publishing Group.

Aronson, A. (1990). *Clinical voice disorders: An interdisciplinary approach* (3rd ed.). New York: Thieme.

Bless, D. M., & Hicks, D. M. (1996). Diagnosis and measurement: Assessing the "WHs" of voice function. In W. S. Brown, B. P. Vinson, & M. Crary (Eds.), *Organic voice disorders: Assessment and treatment* (pp. 119–170). San Diego, CA: Singular Publishing Group.

Boone, D. R., & McFarlane, S. C. (1994). *The voice and voice therapy* (5th ed.). Englewood Cliffs, NJ: Prentice-Hall.

Brown, W. S., Vinson, B. P., & Crary, M. (Eds.). (1996). *Organic voice disorders: Assessment and treatment*. San Diego, CA: Singular Publishing Group.

Case, J. L. (1996). *Clinical management of voice disorders* (3rd ed.). Austin, TX: PRO-ED.

Colton, R., & Casper, J. K. (1996). *Understanding voice problems: A physiological perspective for diagnosis and treatment* (2nd ed.). Baltimore, MD: Williams and Wilkins.

DeJarnette, G., & Holland, R. W. (1998). Voice and voice disorders. In D. E. Battle (Ed.), *Communication disorders in multicultural populations* (2nd ed., pp. 275–308). Newton, MA: Butterworth-Heinemann.

Fawcus, M. (Ed.). *Voice disorders and their management* (2nd ed.). San Diego, CA: Singular Publishing Group.

Prater, R. J., & Swift, R. W. (1984). *Manual of voice therapy*. Boston: Little, Brown.

Ramig, L. O., Bonitati, C. M., Lemke, J. H., & Horii, Y. (1994). Voice treatment for patients with Parkinson's disease: Development of an approach and preliminary efficacy data. *Journal of Medical Speech–Language Pathology, 2*, 191–209.

Shipley, K. G. (1990). *Systematic assessment of voice: Methods and procedures for evaluating voice disorders*. Oceanside, CA: Academic Communication Associates.

Stemple, J. C., Glaze, L. E., & Gerdeman, B. K. (1995). *Clinical voice pathology: Theory and management* (2nd ed.). San Diego, CA: Singular Publishing Group.

ANSWERS TO STUDY AND REVIEW QUESTIONS

1. Thyrohyoids, omohyoids, sternothyroids, and sternohyoids (TOSS)

2. Digastrics, geniohyoids, hylohyoids, stylohyoids, genioglossus, and hyoglossus.

3. X, vagus, superior laryngeal nerve, recurrent laryngeal nerve

4. Puberphonia or mutational falsetto

5. Hysterical or conversion aphonia

6. Total lung capacity, tidal volume, vital capacity

7. Clavicular breathing, diaphragmatic-abdominal breathing

8. Inhalation, injection

9. Laryngomalacia, juvenile papillomas

10. Paradoxical vocal fold motion, laryngeal dyskinesia

11. C. Cranial nerve X, the vagus nerve, is primarily responsible for laryngeal innervation.

12. B. Stroboscopy is the only procedure that uses a pulsing "strobe" light for perceived slow-motion viewing of the vocal folds.

13. E. The first thing a clinician must do with a patient who exhibits potential signs of a neurological problem is refer the patient to a neurologist.

14. A. The pyramidal arytenoid cartilages are attached anteriorly to the vocal processes. There is only one cricoid cartilage; the hyoid is a single bone from which the larynx is suspended.

15. D. Most 18–39-year-old adults have a maximum phonation time of 20.90–24.60 seconds.

16. A. Jitter is the same thing as frequency perturbation. Shimmer refers to amplitude perturbation.

17. C. Voice rest for an 8-year-old boy is somewhat unrealistic. There is no indication that he needs a counselor. He is old enough to identify and reduce vocally abusive behaviors.

18. E. The Blom-Singer device is used to shunt air from the trachea to the esophagus so that the patient can speak on that air.

19. B. The term *diplophonia* refers to the perception of a "double voice."

20. D. The above-listed treatment techniques are commonly used with patients who have spasmodic dysphonia.

PREVIEW OUTLINE

CHAPTER INTRODUCTION

Several disorders of communication are caused by neuropathologies, or brain trauma. In this chapter, we provide an overview of the nature, assessment, and treatment of such communicative disorders, which include aphasia, apraxia of speech, dysarthrias, dementia, right hemisphere syndrome, traumatic brain injury, and swallowing disorders (dysphagia).

Aphasia, a neurologically based language disorder, is often caused by strokes. There are different types of aphasia, depending upon the area(s) of the brain in which the stroke(s) occurred. Apraxia is a neurogenic speech disorder characterized by sensorimotor problems in volitional production of speech, while the dysarthrias (all types) are a group of motor speech disorders that result from impaired muscular control of the speech mechanism due to nervous system pathology. Dementia is an acquired neurological syndrome that is usually accompanied by progressive deterioration in intellectual functioning. Right hemisphere syndrome describes a group of characteristics—mostly related to perceptual and attentional deficits—demonstrated by patients with neurological insult to the right hemisphere. Traumatic brain injury refers to injury to the brain due to external force or physical trauma, and dysphagia refers to swallowing disorders, which are not necessarily related to communication disorders.

APHASIA

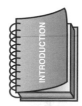

Aphasia, a neurologically based language disorder, is caused by various types of neuropathologies (most commonly stroke). Types of aphasia can be classified broadly as fluent, nonfluent, and subcortical aphasia. Assessment of patients with aphasia may involve standardized tests and functional assessment tools. Treatment of aphasia generally focuses on auditory comprehension, verbal expression, reading, and writing. Aphasia may or may not be accompanied by alexia, agraphia, or agnosia.

Foundational Concepts

■ *Aphasia* is a neurologically based language disorder, contrasted with such neurologically based speech disorders as apraxia and dysarthria.

■ Aphasia is caused by various kinds of neuropathologies. The third leading cause of death in the United States, strokes, or cerebrovascular accidents

411

(CVA), are the most common causes of aphasia. More than half a million people suffer a stroke each year.

■ Strokes may be ischemic or hemorrhagic. *Ischemic strokes* are caused by a blocked or interrupted blood supply to the brain. Blockage or interruption may be caused by two kinds of arterial diseases: thrombosis or embolism.

■ A *thrombus* is a collection of blood material that blocks the flow of blood. An *embolus* is a traveling mass of arterial debris or a clump of tissue from a tumor that gets lodged in a smaller artery and thus blocks the flow of blood.

■ *Hemorrhagic strokes* are caused by bleeding in the brain due to ruptured blood vessels. Ruptures may be *intracerebral* (within the brain) or *extracerebral* (within the meninges, resulting in subarchnoid, subdural, and epidural varieties).

■ Other causes of aphasia include brain trauma, intracranial tumors, and infections. Tumors may be *primary intracranial* (grown within the brain) or *secondary*, or *metastatic* (grown elsewhere but migrated and attached to brain tissue and still growing). Infections may be bacterial or viral.

Definition and Classification of Aphasia

■ There are numerous definitions of aphasia. Some are nontypological and others are typological. *Nontypological definitions* suggest a single disorder. Other definitions are based on cognitive functions. *Typological definitions* classify aphasia into types (Hegde, 1998).

■ Darley's (1982) definition of aphasia as "an impairment, as a result of brain damage, of the capacity for interpretation and formulation of language symbols" (p. 42) illustrates a nontypological definition. The definition suggests a unitary language disorder due to recent brain injury.

■ There are several typological definitions. For example, Goodglass and Kaplan (1983) define aphasia as the "disturbance of any or all of the skills, associations and habits of spoken or written language, produced by injury to certain brain areas that are specialized for these functions" (p. 5).

■ The terms *any disturbance* and *all disturbance* can refer to different types of aphasia. Most contemporary experts classify aphasia into fluent aphasias, nonfluent aphasias, and subcortical aphasias.

■ Cognitive definitions base their description on impaired cognition. For example, Davis (1993) defines aphasia as "an acquired impairment of the cognitive system for comprehending and formulating language, leaving other cognitive capacities intact" (p. 10).

Nonfluent Aphasias

■ Varieties of nonfluent aphasias are characterized by limited, agrammatic, effortful, halting, and slow speech with impaired prosody.

Broca's Aphasia

■ This nonfluent variety of aphasia is caused by damage to Broca's area (Brodmann's areas 44 and 45) in the posterior-inferior frontal gyrus of the left hemisphere.

■ Broca's aphasia is characterized by:

- nonfluent, effortful, slow, halting, and uneven speech
- limited word output, short phrases and sentences
- misarticulated or distorted sounds
- agrammatic or telegraphic speech (often limited to nouns and verbs, with omission of articles, conjunctions, and prepositions)
- impaired repetition of words and sentences, especially the grammatic elements of a sentence
- impaired naming, especially confrontation naming
- better auditory comprehension of spoken language than production
- difficulty in understanding syntactic structures
- poor oral reading and poor comprehension of material read
- writing problems (slow and laborious writing that is full of spelling errors and letter omissions, possibly because patients are forced to use their nonpreferred left hand due to paralysis of the right hand)
- monotonous speech
- apraxia of speech
- dysarthria

Transcortical Motor Aphasia (TMA)

■ This nonfluent variety of aphasia is caused by lesions in the anterior superior frontal lobe, often below or above Broca's area, which is not affected.

■ Transcortical motor aphasia is characterized by:

- initial speechlessness
- echolalia and perseveration

- absent or reduced spontaneous speech

- nonfluent, paraphasic, agrammatic, and telegraphic speech

- *intact repetition skill*, a distinguishing characteristic

- awareness of grammaticality (patients may correct a grammatically incorrect model)

- refusal to repeat nonsense syllables

- unfinished sentences

- limited word fluency

- simple and imprecise syntactic structures

- attempts to initiate speech with the help of such motor activities as clapping, vigorous head nodding, and hand waving

- generally good comprehension of simple conversation; possibly impaired for complex speech

- slow and difficult reading aloud

- seriously disturbed writing

Mixed Transcortical Aphasia (MTA)

■ This somewhat rare variety of nonfluent aphasia is caused by lesions in the watershed area or the arterial border zone (between the areas supplied by the middle cerebral arteries and the anterior and posterior arteries, described in Chapter 1).

■ MTA is characterized by:

- limited spontaneous speech

- automatic, unintentional, and involuntary nature of communication

- severe echolalia (parrotlike repetition of what is heard)

- repetition of an examiner's statement

- severely impaired fluency

- severely impaired auditory comprehension for even simple conversation

- marked naming difficulty and neologism; impaired confrontation naming

- mostly unimpaired automatic speech (e.g., recitation of months in a year or a number series) if somehow initiated and not interrupted

- severely impaired reading, reading comprehension, and writing

Global Aphasia

■ This is the most severe form of nonfluent aphasia. It is caused by extensive lesions affecting all language areas (the perisylvian region). Widespread destruction of the fronto-temporo-parietal regions is common.

■ Global aphasia is characterized by:

- profoundly impaired language skills and no significant profile of differential skills

- greatly reduced fluency

- expressions limited to a few words, exclamations, and serial utterances

- impaired repetition

- impaired naming

- auditory comprehension limited to single words at best

- perseveration (repetition of short utterances)

- impaired reading and writing

🖉 Concepts To Consider

Describe the major characteristics of fluent and nonfluent aphasias. Describe symptoms that may be common to the two types of aphasias as well as those that are unique.

_____

_____

_____

_____

_____

_____

_____

_____

_____

_____

Fluent Aphasias

- ▇ Varieties of fluent aphasias are characterized by relatively intact fluency but generally less meaningful, or even meaningless, speech.

- ▇ The speech is generally flowing, abundant, easily initiated, and well articulated with good prosody and phrase length.

Wernicke's Aphasia

- ▇ This common variety of fluent aphasia is caused by lesions in Wernicke's area (the posterior portion of the superior temporal gyrus in the left hemisphere).

- ▇ Wernicke's aphasia is characterized by:

    - incessant, effortlessly produced, flowing speech with normal, or even abnormal, fluency (*logorrhea,* or *press of speech*) with normal phrase length

    - rapid rate of speech with normal prosodic features and good articulation

    - intact grammatical structures

    - severe word-finding problems

    - paraphasic speech containing semantic and literal paraphasias, extra syllables in words, and creation of meaningless words (neologisms)

    - circumlocution (talking around words that cannot be recalled)

    - empty speech (substitution of such general words as *this*, *that*, *stuff*, and *thing*)

    - poor auditory comprehension, especially for sentences and names of common objects; much worse comprehension of speech when there is background noise, movements, and background conversation

    - impaired conversational turn taking

    - impaired repetition skill

    - reading comprehension problems, including difficulty recognizing sounds associated with written words, meanings of printed words

    - writing problems, including excessive but meaningless writing, frequent misspellings, and neologistic writing

    - generally poor communication in spite of fluent speech

Transcortical Sensory Aphasia (TSA)

- ▇ This variety of fluent aphasia is caused by lesions in the temporo-parietal region, especially in the posterior portion of the middle temporal gyrus.

■ TSA is characterized by:

- fluent speech with normal phrase length, good prosody, normal articulation, and apparently appropriate grammar and syntax

- paraphasic and empty speech

- severe naming problems and pauses due to those problems

- good repetition skills but poor comprehension of repeated words

- echolalia of grammatically incorrect forms, nonsense syllables, and words from foreign languages (unlike patients with TMA)

- impaired auditory comprehension of spoken language

- difficulty in pointing, obeying commands, or answering simple yes/no questions

- normal automatic speech (e.g., counting)

- tendency to complete poems and sentences started by the clinician

- good reading (aloud) but poor comprehension of material read

- generally better oral reading skills than other language skills

- writing problems that parallel those in expressive speech

Conduction Aphasia

■ This variety of fluent aphasia is caused by lesions in the region between Broca's area and Wernicke's area, especially in the supramarginal gyrus and the arcuate fasciculus. Lesion sites of conduction aphasia are controversial.

■ Conduction aphasia is characterized by:

- disproportionate impairment in repetition (a distinguishing characteristic); especially impaired repetition of longer words, function words, and longer phrases and sentences

- variable speech fluency across patients; generally less fluent than patients with Wernicke's aphasia

- paraphasic speech

- marked word-finding problems, especially for content words

- empty speech because of omitted content words

- efforts to correct errors in speech, though not always successful

- good syntax, prosody, and articulation

- severe to mild naming problems

- near normal auditory comprehension, especially for routine conversational speech

- being better at pointing to a named stimulus than at confrontation naming

- highly variable reading problems; better comprehension of silently read material

- writing problems in most cases

- buccofacial apraxia (difficulty in performing buccofacial movements when requested) in most patients

Anomic Aphasia

■ This variety of fluent aphasia is controversial and may be caused by lesions in different regions, including the angular gyrus, the second temporal gyrus, and the juncture of the temporo-parietal lobes.

■ Anomic aphasia is a syndrome, whereas *anomia* is a naming difficulty (a symptom) common to most forms of aphasia.

■ Anomic aphasia is characterized by:

- a most debilitating and pervasive word-finding difficulty, which is the distinguishing feature; however, pointing to named objects is unimpaired

- generally fluent speech

- normal syntax except for pauses (word-finding trouble)

- use of vague and nonspecific words, resulting in empty speech

- verbal paraphasia (word substitutions)

- circumlocution (beating around the bush because of lack of access to precise words)

- good auditory comprehension of spoken language

- intact repetition

- unimpaired articulation

- normal oral reading skills and good reading comprehension

- normal writing skills

Subcortical Aphasia

■ Aphasia is typically produced by cortical damage; however, aphasia due to subcortical injury has been reported in recent years.

■ Extensive subcortical damage, with possible involvement of cortical areas, may underlie this type of aphasia. Lesions in areas surrounding the basal ganglia and the thalamus have been linked to subcortical aphasia.

■ Subcortical aphasia caused by lesions in the basal ganglia and surrounding structures in the left hemisphere is characterized by:

- fluent speech, which may include pauses and hesitations

- intact repetition skills

- normal auditory comprehension for routine conversation; may be defective for complex material

- articulation problems (similar to those in Broca's aphasia)

- prosodic problems

- word-finding problems

- semantic paraphasia in some cases

- relatively preserved writing skills

- limb apraxia if the lesions extend posteriorly to deep white matter in the parietal area

■ Subcortical aphasia caused by lesions or hemorrhages in the thalamus is characterized by:

- hemiplegia, hemisensory loss, right-visual field problems, and, in some cases, coma

- initial mutism, which may improve to paraphasic speech

- severe naming problems

- good auditory comprehension of simple material and poor comprehension of complex material

- good repetition skills

- impaired reading and writing skills

Assessment of Aphasia

Foundational Concepts

■ Assessment of aphasia involves an evaluation of speech and language skills along with reading and writing skills.

■ Related cognitive functions also may be assessed, depending on the clinician's theoretical view and treatment goals. Both standardized and client-specific procedures may be used.

Standardized Aphasia Tests

▨ Aphasia screening tests include the *Aphasia Language Performance Scales* (ALPS) (Keenan & Brassell, 1975); *Sklar Aphasia Scale* (SAS) (Sklar, 1966); *Aphasia Screening Test* (Whurr, 1974); and *Bedside Evaluation and Screening Test–Second Edition* (BEST–2) (West, Sands, & Ross-Swain, 1998).

▨ Screening tests should not replace diagnostic tests and extended client-specific observations. The following are among the more frequently used diagnostic tests:

  – The *Boston Diagnostic Aphasia Examination* (BDAE) (Goodglass & Kaplan, 1983). Evaluating articulation, fluency, word-finding, repetition, serial speech, grammar, paraphasias, auditory comprehension, oral reading, reading comprehension, writing, and musical skills (e.g., singing), this test tries to classify aphasia into types.

  – The *Western Aphasia Battery* (WAB) (Kertesz, 1982). Evaluating speech content, fluency, auditory comprehension, repetition, naming, reading, writing, calculation, drawing, nonverbal thinking, and block design, this test also tries to classify aphasia into types.

  – The *Minnesota Test for Differential Diagnosis of Aphasia* (MTDDA) (Schuell, 1972). MTDDA evaluates five areas of performance: auditory disturbances, visual and reading disturbances, speech and language disturbances, visuomotor and writing disturbances, and numerical and arithmetic disturbances.

  – The *Neurosensory Center Comprehensive Examination for Aphasia* (NCCEA) (Spreen & Benton, 1977). This test evaluates such language functions as comprehension, production, reading, writing, word fluency, digit and sentence repetition, visual object naming, sentence construction, and articulation. The test also evaluates visual and tactile functions.

  – *Multilingual Aphasia Examination* (Benton & Hamsher, 1978). This test is similar to NCCEA in its contents. It evaluates such language functions as naming, repetition, fluency, auditory comprehension, spelling, and writing. It comes in English, French, German, Italian, and Spanish versions.

  – *Bilingual Aphasia Test* (BAT) (Paradis, 1987). A comprehensive test that helps evaluate skills in 40 languages with parallel forms. A patient's phonologic, morphologic, syntactic, lexical, and semantic skills in a primary and a secondary language may be assessed.

  – The *Porch Index of Communicative Ability* (PICA) (Porch, 1981). A limited measure of language, the Porch evaluates auditory comprehension, reading, oral expressive language, pantomime, visual matching, writing, and copying. However, the test requires intensive training to administer and score.

Functional Assessment Tools

■ Some assessment tools target functional communication. These are useful in evaluating daily communication in everyday settings. Functional assessment tools may be less biased than standardized tests in evaluating clients from linguistically and culturally diverse backgrounds. Changes in functional communication during treatment may be measured.

■ Most tools require the clinician to make extensive and systematic observation of their clients and rate them on variables being measured. Commonly used functional communication tools include the following:

- *Functional Communication Profile* (Sarno, 1969) evaluates 45 behaviors in five categories: movement, speaking, understanding, reading, and "other." A 9-point rating scale is used to evaluate the performance.

- *Communicative Abilities in Daily Living* (Holland, 1980) emphasizes daily communication in everyday situations. Such skills as reading, writing, estimation of time, use of verbal and nonverbal contexts in communication, role playing, social conventions, nonverbal symbolic communication, humor, absurdity, and metaphor are rated.

- The *Communicative Effectiveness Index* (Loma et al., 1989) helps assess four domains of functional communication skills, including social needs, life skills, basic needs, and health threats. Such specific skills as giving yes/no answers, expressing physical pain or discomfort, and starting a conversation are rated.

- *Communication Profile: A Functional Skills Survey* (Payne, 1994). An advantage of this test is that its sample included patients from African American, Native American/Alaska Native, Asian American/Pacific Islander, and Asian American ethnic groups. Therefore, this test is especially useful in evaluating patients from those ethnocultural backgrounds. The test uses a 5-point scale to rate the importance of selected skills in daily living.

- *Functional Assessment of Communication Skills for Adults* (ASHA FACS) (Frattali, Thompson, Holland, Wohl, & Ferketic, 1995) was developed for the American Speech–Language-Hearing Association. It helps rate social communication; communication of basic needs; reading, writing, and number concepts; and daily planning. Clinicians or others familiar with the patient may make the observations and complete the rating form.

- *Amsterdam Nijmegan Everyday Language Test* (ANELT) (Blomert, Kean, Koster, & Schokker, 1994) has two parallel forms, each containing 10 items to assess pragmatic language skills related to familiar daily living activities.

- *Revised Edinburgh Functional Communication Profile* (Wirz, Skinner, & Dean, 1990) evaluates such pragmatic communication skills as greeting, acknowledging, responding, requesting, and initiating conversation.

■ In addition to diagnostic aphasia tests, clinicians may use independent tests of specific skills such as auditory comprehension and reading.

■ Various tests of auditory comprehension include the *Token Test* (DeRenzi & Vignolo, 1962); *Auditory Comprehension Test for Sentences* (Shewan, 1979); *Functional Auditory Comprehension Task* (LaPointe & Horner, 1978); and the *Discourse Comprehension Test* (Brookshire & Nichols, 1993).

■ Tests of reading skills include the *Reading Comprehension Battery for Aphasia–Second Edition* (LaPointe & Horner, 1998); the *Nelson Reading Skills Test* (Hanna, Schell, & Schreiner, 1977); and the Gates-MacGinitie *Reading Test* (Gates, 1978).

✎ Concepts To Consider

Briefly describe two standardized tests and two functional assessment tools that can be used with patients who have aphasia.

_____

_____

_____

_____

_____

_____

_____

_____

_____

_____

An Outline of Aphasia Assessment

■ Aphasia assessment includes such standard procedures as a detailed case history, orofacial examination, and hearing screening. Beyond these basic procedures, the clinician must assess specific speech and language skills that affect a diagnosis of aphasia (Hegde, 1996a, 1998). The following outline lists the skills to be assessed.

Assessment of Repetition Skills

■ repetition of single words (single-syllable words with visible voiced consonants—e.g., *bed*—and blends and multisyllable words)

■ repetition of object names, verbs, numbers, letters, and function words

■ repetition of sentences (short and commonly used sentences—e.g., "Sit down"—first and progressively longer sentences next)

■ Repetition of a few short but infrequently used sentences

Assessment of Naming Skills

■ responsive naming (naming with contextual cues—e.g., the clinician asks, "What do you use to write?" or "What color is snow?")

■ confrontation naming (e.g., the clinician asks "What is this?" while showing a picture)

■ word fluency (recalling names that belong to a specific category—e.g., the clinician asks the client to "name all the animals you can think of")

Assessment of Auditory Comprehension of Spoken Language

■ hearing evaluation

■ visual evaluation

■ comprehension of natural commands given without gestures (e.g., "Move your chair a little closer" or "Close your eyes")

■ comprehension of multistep commands (e.g., "Pick up the pencil and the comb and place them in the box")

Assessment of Comprehension of Single Words

■ comprehension of single items ("red" or "cat") and semantic groups of items ("colors" or "animals")

■ comprehension of words that vary in number of syllables, emotionality, frequency of usage, semantic class, and phonemic similarity

Assessment of Comprehension of Sentences and Paragraphs

■ comprehension of a brief and simple story that is told

■ comprehension of more complex stories

Assessment of Reading Skills

■ comprehension of silently or orally read material (e.g., matching single printed words to pictures, matching printed words with spoken words, crossing out words that do not belong in a list)

■ completion of printed sentences (e.g., reads the printed incomplete sentence "We wear hats on our . . ." and completes it with the verbal response "head")

Assessment of Writing Skills

■ graphomotor skills (letter formation)

■ general writing skills

■ automatic writing

■ propositional writing

■ confrontation writing (e.g., the clinician says, "Write the names of these pictures")

■ writing to dictation

■ narrative writing (e.g., the clinician says, "Write a story about this picture")

■ premorbid writing samples for comparison

Assessment of Gestures and Pantomime

■ expression through gestures and pantomime

■ comprehension of gestures and pantomime

Assessment of Automated Speech and Singing

■ recitation of the alphabet, days of the week, months of the year, and numbers

■ recitation of prayers, poems, and nursery rhymes

■ singing

■ humming a tune

Treatment of Aphasia

Foundational Concepts

■ Most current research shows that aphasia treatment is effective. Many treatment approaches are available (Brookshire, 1997; Davis, 1993; Hegde, 1996b, 1998; Helm-Estabrooks & Albert, 1991; LaPointe, 1997; Rosenbek, LaPointe, & Wertz, 1989).

■ Treatment must take into account the patient's cultural and linguistic background. For example, in many minority groups, family and extended family members may be extremely helpful in assisting with home carryover of treatment targets (Wallace, 1998).

■ Prognosis for treatment is better in the case of patients:

   – who are younger and healthier

   – who are better educated and in verbally demanding occupations

   – whose lesions are smaller

   – who have no other medical or behavioral disorders

   – who have good hearing acuity

- who have normal or adequately corrected vision

- who have better motor skills

- who have better preserved language skills

- whose aphasia is less severe

- whose treatment is initiated soon after onset

- who receive effective treatment techniques in an accurate manner for a long enough duration

- whose family members are involved in treatment

- who maintain their health during the course of treatment

Treatment of Auditory Comprehension

■ Lesions within the posterior superior temporal lobe (PST) suggest a better prognosis than those outside the PST.

■ Comprehension is generally better for frequently used words, nouns, picturable words, shorter sentences, syntactically simpler sentences, active sentences, personally relevant sentences, slower speech, words that are stressed, speech in quiet surroundings, redundant messages, repeated phrases, speech preceded by alerting stimuli (e.g., "Ready?" "Listen!"). Louder speech and video presentation of stimuli are ineffective.

■ Auditory comprehension treatment is sequenced as follows:

- *Comprehension of single words*: understanding nouns and verbs (e.g., the clinician asks the patient to point to named body parts and objects, to specific named actions pictured)

- *Comprehension of spoken sentences*: question comprehension, following spoken directions, and sentence verification (e.g., the clinician asks yes/no questions and open-ended questions; following simple and more complex directions, and verifying the meaning of sentences by matching a sentence to a picture that represents it)

- *Discourse comprehension*: understanding narratives and questions (e.g., retelling a story the clinician narrates and responding to such personally relevant questions as "Do you like to watch football games?")

Treatment of Verbal Expression: Naming

■ Naming skills are the most frequently targeted expressive verbal skills. These skills are subsequently expanded into longer and grammatically more correct and communicatively more functional utterances.

- In treating naming, it is important to select words that are client specific (e.g., names of family members, activities the client engages in) and words that are functional (that enhance communication in a variety of settings).

- Naming treatment techniques include a variety of special cues that help evoke the target responses which are promptly reinforced:

  - modeling of responses

  - incomplete sentences (e.g., the clinician says, "You write with a _____")

  - phonetic cues (e.g., the clinician says, "The word starts with a *p*")

  - syllabic cues (e.g., the clinician says, "The word starts with spoo____")

  - silent phonetic cues (e.g., the clinician exhibits a silent articulatory posture for /p/ for *pen*)

  - functional descriptions of objects (e.g., the clinician says, "It is something you roll or kick")

  - descriptions and demonstrations of actions (e.g., the clinician says, "You use this to write like this" followed by writing)

  - patient's description as stimulus for naming (e.g., the clinician says, "Tell me what you do with this and then say its name")

  - patient's demonstration of function as stimulus for naming (e.g., the clinician says, "Show me how to use this and tell me its name")

  - paired objects or pictures with their printed name as stimuli for naming (e.g., the clinician shows a book and the printed word *book* and asks "What is this?")

  - patient's spelling as stimulus for naming (e.g., the clinician says, "Spell this word first and then say it")

  - patient's spelling and writing as stimuli for naming (e.g., the clinician says, "Spell this word, write the word, and then say it")

  - associated sounds as stimulus (e.g., the clinician says, "It makes an arf-arf sound")

  - rhyme as stimulus (e.g., the clinician says, "What is this? It rhymes with _____")

  - synonyms (e.g., "dwelling" to evoke "house"); antonyms (e.g., "woman" to evoke "man"); associated words (e.g., "plate" to evoke "cup"); generic words (e.g., "man" to evoke "husband"); superordinates (e.g., "flower" to evoke "rose")

Treatment of Verbal Expression: Expanded Utterances

■ *Expansion of verbal expression* involves systematically increasing the length and complexity of target responses. Names taught may be expanded into phrases and sentences that are functional and effective in naturalistic communication. The clinician initially uses modeling and subsequently fades it.

■ Action-filled pictures and stories may be used to teach narratives and discourse. Sequenced pictures also will help evoke narratives with temporal sequences.

■ Eventually, conversational speech involving topics of relevance and interest to the client is targeted for treatment. Description of daily activities (e.g., cooking) and special events (e.g., planning a vacation) may be used to promote conversational speech.

Treatment of Reading Skills

■ Target reading skills are selected based on an assessment of premorbid reading skills and the current need for reading.

■ Functional reading skills may be sequenced as follows:

- survival reading skills (e.g., reading letters, menus, bank statements, and maps)

- reading newspapers, books, and letters

- reading and comprehension of printed words read

- reading and comprehension of phrases and sentences

- reading and comprehension of paragraphs and extended material

Treatment of Writing Skills

■ Target writing skills also are selected based on an assessment of premorbid reading skills and the current need for writing.

■ Functional writing skills may be sequenced as follows:

- initially writing functional words (e.g., one's own name, names of family members)

- writing functional lists (e.g., a grocery list)

- writing short notes, reminders, addresses, and so forth

- filling out forms

- writing letters

■ Depending on current writing skills, treatment procedures include the following:

- pointing to the correct printed letter the clinician names

- pointing to printed words and phrases

- saying the sound of a printed letter shown

- saying a printed word shown

- tracing printed letters

- copying printed words and phrases

- spelling words correctly

- writing to dictation

- spontaneous writing of phrases and sentences

- spontaneous extended writing (e.g., making a grocery list, writing a note to a spouse, writing a letter to a friend)

Concepts To Consider

List one treatment technique that can be used with patients with aphasia in each of the following areas: auditory comprehension, naming, reading, and writing.

_____

_____

_____

_____

_____

_____

_____

_____

Alexia, Agraphia, and Agnosia

■ *Alexia* is loss of previously acquired reading skills due to recent brain damage. *Dyslexia*, on the other hand, is a difficulty in learning to read; this difficulty is often genetically based and is manifested beginning in childhood. Some patients with aphasia will manifest alexia.

■ *Agraphia* is the loss or impairment of normally acquired writing skills due to lesions in the foot of the second frontal gyrus, sometimes referred to as *Exner's writing area*. Various kinds of writing problems are evident in most patients with aphasia (Hegde, 1998).

■ *Agnosia* is impaired understanding of the meaning of certain stimuli even though there is no peripheral sensory impairment. Patients can see, feel, and hear stimuli but cannot understand their meaning. Impairment often is limited to one sensory modality; the meaning of stimuli may be grasped in another modality. There are several forms of agnosia (Hegde, 1998).

Auditory Agnosia

■ Auditory agnosia is caused by bilateral damage to the auditory association area and is characterized by:

  – impaired understanding of the meaning of auditory stimuli

  – normal peripheral hearing

  – difficulty in matching objects with their sound

  – normal visual recognition of objects

Auditory Verbal Agnosia

■ Auditory verbal agnosia (pure word deafness) is caused by bilateral temporal lobe lesions that isolate Wernicke's area; it is characterized by:

  – impaired understanding of spoken words

  – normal peripheral hearing

  – normal recognition of nonverbal sounds

  – normal recognition of printed words

  – normal or near normal verbal expression and reading

Visual Agnosia

■ Visual agnosia is a rare disorder caused by bilateral occipital lobe damage or posterior parietal lobe damage; it is characterized by:

  – impaired visual recognition of objects, which may be intermittent

  – normal auditory or tactile recognition of objects

Tactile Agnosia

■ Tactile agnosia is caused by lesions in the parietal lobe and is characterized by:

– impaired tactile recognition of objects when visual feedback is blocked (as with a blindfold)

– impaired naming of objects clients can feel in their hands

– impaired description of objects clients can feel in their hands

Summary

☑ Aphasia, a neurologically based language disorder, is most frequently caused by stroke. Aphasia may be categorized as fluent, nonfluent, or subcortical in nature.

☑ Assessment of patients with aphasia may include use of standardized aphasia tests. Clinicians may also use functional assessment tools, which target the patient's daily communication skills in everyday settings.

☑ Treatment of patients with aphasia generally involves the following skill areas: auditory comprehension, verbal expression (naming), verbal expression (expanded utterances), reading, and writing.

☑ Aphasia may be accompanied by alexia, agraphia, or agnosia. Types of agnosia include auditory, auditory verbal, visual, and tactile agnosia.

APRAXIA OF SPEECH

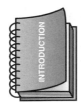

INTRODUCTION

Apraxia of speech (AOS) is a neurogenic speech disorder. Patients with AOS have sensorimotor problems in positioning and sequentially moving muscles for volitional speech production. AOS is caused by damage or injury to speech-motor programming areas (e.g., Broca's area) in the dominant hemisphere. Patients with AOS have a number of communication deficits, especially those caused by groping and struggling to speak. Assessment and treatment for patients with AOS involve detailed procedures related to evaluating and improving articulatory accuracy, speech rate, and self-monitoring.

Definition and Distinctions

■ Apraxia of speech is a neurogenic speech disorder characterized by sensori-motor problems in positioning and sequentially moving muscles for the volitional production of speech.

■ AOS is primarily an articulatory-phonologic disorder, although its etiology and characteristics are different from those of similar disorders in children. Adult patients with AOS will have acquired articulation normally. Their current articulatory problems are due to recent neuropathology.

■ However, adults with AOS have unimpaired reflex and automatic acts. The difficulty they have is mostly in executing the voluntary movements involved in speech. AOS may be associated with prosodic problems (Duffy, 1995).

■ AOS is not caused by muscle weakness or neuromuscular slowness. It is thought that a disorder of motor programming for speech causes it. More frequently, AOS and aphasia may coexist, and less frequently, dysarthria of unilateral upper motor neuron type may coexist with AOS.

■ Technically and in its pure form, AOS should not affect language skills, as it is a speech-motor programming problem. However, if AOS is accompanied by aphasia, language skills are affected by the presence of aphasia.

■ *Apraxia* is a basic disorder of volitional movement in the absence of muscle weakness, paralysis, or fatigue. As such, AOS is a special case of apraxia.

■ *Nonverbal oral apraxia* is a disorder of nonverbal movement involving the oral muscles. AOS is frequently associated with nonverbal oral apraxia.

Neuropathology of AOS

■ AOS is caused by injury or damage to speech-motor programming areas in the dominant hemisphere; such areas as Broca's and supplementary motor areas often are involved.

■ Specific types of pathology include vascular lesions that cause strokes; specifically affected are the speech programming structures and pathways. In a majority of cases, the cause is a single left hemisphere stroke; in a few, the cause is multiple strokes.

■ Frontal lesions may be associated with parietal lesions as well; temporal lobe lesions are observed occasionally but only in combination with lesions elsewhere.

■ AOS may also be caused by such degenerative neural diseases as multiple sclerosis (MS) and primary progressive aphasia. It can also be caused by left hemisphere trauma, surgical trauma, tumors in the left hemisphere, and seizure disorders.

General Symptoms of AOS

- General symptoms of AOS include impaired oral sensation in some patients. When dysarthria is a coexisting condition, facial and lingual weakness may be present. Some patients may also have limb apraxia.

- An independent nonverbal oral apraxia (NVOA) is present in many patients. In some cases, there also may be right hemiparesis and sensory deficits.

Communication Deficits in AOS

- A number of communication deficits may be present in those with AOS.
- These deficits are as follows:
  - an independent problem of auditory processing deficits in some cases;
  - general awareness of speech problems;
  - problems in volitional or spontaneous sequencing of movements required for speech with relatively unaffected automatic speech;
  - high variability of speech errors; changing patterns of errors on repeated attempts; normal production of difficult words on occasion;
  - compensatory strategy of reduced rate in some but not all patients;
  - significant articulatory problems, diagnostic of AOS, which include: substitutions (more common), distortions, and omissions of speech sounds;
  - more pronounced difficulty with consonants than vowels; more severe problems with affricates and fricatives and consonant clusters; more frequent errors on infrequently occurring sounds;
  - anticipatory substitutions (a phoneme that occurs later in the word may replace the one that occurs earlier; e.g., "lelo" for "yellow");
  - postpositioning errors (a phoneme that occurs earlier replaces the one that occurs later; e.g., "dred" for "dress");
  - metathetic errors (switched position of phonemes in words; e.g., "tefalone" for "telephone");
  - increased frequency of errors on longer words;
  - slow or delayed initiation of speech;

— trial-and-error groping and struggling associated with speech attempts;

— greater difficulty on word-initial sounds in some cases;

— easier automatic productions than volitional/purposive productions; and

— attempts at self-correction, not always successful.

▨ Patients with apraxia of speech frequently have prosodic problems, which include:

— slower rate of speech, difficulty in increasing or changing the rate when requested;

— silent pauses between words;

— impaired intonation because of increased duration of consonants and vowels, even stress on syllables, even loudness or restricted range of loudness, and limited pitch range; and

— fluency problems including silent pauses, especially at the beginning of speech initiation, and repetitions because of false starts and attempts at self-correction.

Assessment of AOS

▨ A detailed case history, careful examination of the medical records, interview of the client and his or her family members, and detailed observation of speech production are necessary to make a diagnosis of AOS in adults.

▨ Procedures designed to diagnose aphasia (problems with language production and comprehension, reading and writing) should be used when the patient shows signs of a coexisting aphasia, often Broca's aphasia (Duffy, 1995; Hegde,1996a).

▨ Assessment of speech to diagnose AOS involves the following procedures:

— tape-recording the patient's speech samples and transcribing the responses phonetically; taking note of struggle and groping, self-correction, repetition and other forms of dysfluencies, errors of articulation, delayed reaction, facial grimacing, and other behaviors that suggest apraxia;

— evoking imitative production of a speech sound;

— evoking repetitive production of syllables; (e.g., asking the patient to say "pA-pA-pA," "tA-tA-tA," and "kA-kA-kA" as long and as evenly as possible);

— evoking the repetitive production of multiple syllables (e.g., asking the patient to say "pA-tA-kA" as long and as evenly as possible);

— evoking imitative production of progressively longer words when modeling is provided (e.g., asking the patient to imitate such words as *several, tornado, artillery, linoleum, snowman, television, catastrophe, unequivocally, parliamentarian, statistical analysis, Encyclopedia Britannica*);

— evoking repeated, imitative production of words and phrases (e.g., asking the patient to say such words as *artillery, impossibility,* and *disenfranchised* five times);

— evoking the imitative production of sentences;

— evoking counting responses (e.g., asking the patient to count from 1 to 20);

— evoking picture descriptions;

— assessment of oral reading;

— administration of a complete *diadochokinetic test* to assess oral, nonverbal movement (e.g., various tongue, lip, and jaw movements) to evaluate oral apraxia or a coexisting dysarthria in case of significant muscle weakness or paralysis;

— assessment of limb movements to evaluate limb apraxia by asking the patient to perform certain actions (e.g., demonstration of how an accordion works, how one salutes or waves good-bye); and

— administration of a standardized test of apraxia (e.g., the *Apraxia Battery for Adults* (Dabul, 1979) or the *Comprehensive Apraxia Test* (DeSimoni, 1989).

Concepts To Consider

Describe the neuropathology of apraxia of speech. What are two important components of an assessment for this disorder?

_____

_____

_____

_____

_____

_____

_____

Treatment of AOS

- Treatment should be carefully sequenced to move from more automatic speech to less automatic speech and eventually to spontaneous speech.

- Treatment on simpler productions should precede that on more complex productions (e.g., visible sounds before nonvisible sounds, singletons before clusters).

- Treatment procedures should include instructions, demonstration, modeling, shaping, phonetic placement, frequent cueing, the use of rhythm, and immediate positive or corrective feedback.

- Treatment targets include articulatory accuracy, slower rate, systematic practice, gradual increase in the rate, and normal prosody.

- Treatment should be primarily concerned with speech movements as opposed to nonspeech movements.

- Treatment should include practice with a variety of sounds and sound combinations.

- Contrastive stress tasks, various cueing techniques, phonetic contrasts, carrier phrases, and singing may all be useful.

- Pushing on the abdomen to achieve vocal fold closure and phonation or use of an artificial larynx may be helpful for a speechless client.

- Emphasis on total communication (combined use of verbal expressions, gestures, writing, augmentative devices) may be desirable.

- Teaching accurate sound productions in conversational speech should be an important goal.

- Increasing the speech rate to the near-normal also should be an important goal.

- Teaching self-monitoring skills is important for maintenance.

- Techniques of treating articulation and phonological disorders are generally useful.

- In the case of severe apraxia, family members and health care workers should be asked to speak slowly, use shorter sentences, reduce background noise, talk only when the client is focused, and use total communication. In the case of most severe apraxia, augmentative communication techniques may be necessary.

Summary

☑ AOS is a neurogenic speech disorder characterized by sensorimotor problems in positioning and sequentially moving muscles for production of speech. AOS is caused by damage to speech-motor programming areas in the dominant hemisphere.

☑ Communication deficits to be assessed and treated in patients with AOS include highly variable speech errors, significant articulatory problems, increased frequency of errors on long words, prosodic problems, and groping and struggling behaviors.

☑ Assessment of patients with AOS may include detailed, individualized procedures as well as the administration of standardized tests. Treatment should be carefully sequenced to move from automatic, simple productions to less automatic, more spontaneous productions.

THE DYSARTHRIAS

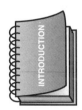

INTRODUCTION

The dysarthrias are a group of neurologically based speech-motor disorders. These disorders result from impaired muscular control of the speech mechanism, involving peripheral or central nervous system pathology. There are seven types of dysarthria: ataxic, flaccid, hyperkinetic, hypokinetic, mixed, spastic, and unilateral upper motor neuron dysarthria. Patients with dysarthria typically manifest problems in respiration, phonation, articulation, prosody, and resonance. Assessment and treatment of patients with dysarthria involve addressing those problems.

Definition of the Dysarthrias

■ Dysarthrias are neurologically based speech disorders contrasted with such similarly based language disorders as aphasia. Dysarthria also is contrasted with apraxia of speech, a neurogenic speech disorder of motor planning of speech movements with no muscular weakness or paralysis.

■ There are different types of dysarthria but all share certain characteristics. Dysarthrias are a group of speech-motor disorders resulting from impaired muscular control of the speech mechanism, involving peripheral or central nervous system pathology.

■ The oral communication problems that accompany dysarthria include respiratory, articulatory, phonatory, resonatory, and prosodic disturbances that are caused by weakness, incoordination, or paralysis of speech musculature. Dysarthrias are classified into ataxic, flaccid, hyperkinetic, hypokinetic, mixed, spastic, and unilateral upper motor neuron types (Duffy, 1995).

Neuropathology of the Dysarthrias

■ Some of the common etiological factors include degenerative neurological diseases such as Parkinson's disease, Wilson's disease, progressive supranuclear palsy, dystonia, Huntington's disease, amyotrophic lateral sclerosis (ALS), multiple sclerosis, and myasthenia gravis.

■ Dysarthria can also be caused by nonprogressive neurological conditions including stroke, infections, traumatic brain injury, and surgical trauma, as well as congenital conditions including cerebral palsy, Moebius syndrome, encephalitis, toxic effects from alcohol, drugs, and so forth.

■ Common sites of lesion include lower motor neuron, unilateral or bilateral upper motor neuron, cerebellum, and the basal ganglia (extrapyramidal system).

■ Pathophysiology and neuromuscular problems include muscle weakness, spasticity, incoordination, and rigidity. There is usually a variety of movement disorders including reduced or variable range and speed of movement, involuntary movements, reduced strength of movement, unsteady or inaccurate movement, and abnormal tone (increased, decreased, or variable).

Communicative Disorders Associated with Dysarthria

■ *Respiratory problems* include forced inspirations or expirations that interrupt speech, audible or breathy inspiration, and grunting at the end of expiration.

■ *Phonatory disorders* include:

- pitch disorders characterized by abnormal pitch, pitch breaks, abrupt variations in pitch, monopitch, diplophonia, shaky or tremulous voice;

- loudness disorders characterized by too soft or too loud speech, monoloudness, sudden and excessive variation in loudness, progressive decrease in loudness throughout an utterance, or alternating changes in loudness; and

- vocal-quality problems characterized by a harsh, rough, gravelly voice, a hoarse voice (especially the "wet" variety), a continuously or intermittently breathy voice, a strained or strangled voice, effortful phonation, or a sudden and uncontrolled cessation of voice.

■ *Articulation disorders* include imprecise production of consonants, prolongation and repetition of phonemes, irregular breakdowns in articulation, distortion of vowels, and weak production of pressure consonants.

■ *Prosodic disorders* include a variety of rate problems, including slower, excessively faster, or variable rate of speech, shorter phrase lengths, and linguistic stress problems such as reduced, even, or excessive stress. There may also be prolongation of intervals between words or syllables, inappropriate pauses in speech, and short rushes of speech.

■ *Resonance disorders* include hypernasality, hyponasality, and nasal emission.

■ *Other characteristics* include slow, fast, or irregular diadochokinetic rate and palilalia (compulsive repetition of one's own utterances with increasing rate and decreasing loudness) as well as decreased intelligibility of speech.

Classification of the Dysarthrias

Ataxic Dysarthria

■ Ataxic dysarthria results from damage to the cerebellar system. It is characterized predominantly by articulatory and prosodic problems.

■ Neuropathology that results in ataxic dysarthria includes bilateral or generalized cerebellar lesions, degenerative ataxia (e.g., Friedreich's ataxia and olivopontocerebellar atrophy), cerebellar vascular lesions, tumors, traumatic brain injury, toxic conditions (e.g., alcohol abuse and drug toxicity), and inflammatory conditions (e.g., meningitis and encephalitis).

■ The major characteristics of ataxic dysarthria include:

  – *Gait disturbances*: Instability of the trunk and head, tremors and rocking motions; rotated or tilted head posture; hypotonia

  – *Movement disorders*: Over- or undershooting of targets; discoordinated, jerky, inaccurate, slow, imprecise, and halting movements

  – *Articulation disorders*: Imprecise production of consonants; irregular articulatory breakdowns and distortion of vowels

  – *Prosodic Disorders*: Excessive and even stress; prolonged phonemes and intervals between words or syllables; slow rate of speech

  – *Phonatory disorders*: Monopitch, monoloudness, and harshness

  – *Speech quality*: Impression of drunken speech

Flaccid Dysarthria

■ Flaccid dysarthria results from damage to the motor units of cranial or spinal nerves that supply speech muscles (lower motor neuron involvement).

■ Neuropathology that results in flaccid dysarthria includes such diseases as myasthenia gravis and botulism, vascular diseases and brain stem strokes, infections (e.g., polio and infections secondary to AIDS), demyelinating diseases (e.g., Guillain-Barré syndrome), degenerative diseases (e.g., motor neuron diseases, progressive bulbar palsy, and amyotrophic lateral sclerosis), and surgical trauma during brain, laryngeal, facial, or chest surgery.

■ Specific cranial nerves that may be involved in flaccid dysarthria include the trigeminal (V), facial (VII), glossopharyngeal (IX), vagus (X), and hypoglossal (XII) nerves.

■ The major characteristics of flaccid dysarthria include:

  – various muscular disorders (e.g., weakness, hypotonia, atrophy, and diminished reflexes)

  – isolated twitches of resting muscles (fasciculations) and contractions of individual muscles (fibrillations)

  – rapid and progressive weakness with the use of a muscle and recovery with rest

  – respiratory weakness in combination with cranial nerve weakness

  – phonatory disorders including breathy voice, audible inspiration, and short phrases

  – resonance disorders including hypernasality; imprecise consonants, nasal emission, and short phrases

  – phonatory-prosodic disorders including harsh voice, monopitch, and monoloudness

  – articulation disorders which are more pronounced with lesions of cranial nerves V, VII, and XII

Hyperkinetic Dysarthria

■ Hyperkinetic dysarthria results from damage to the basal ganglia (extrapyramidal system). Dysarthria is associated with involuntary movement and variable muscle tone. Prosodic disturbances are dominant.

■ Varied causes of hyperkinetic dysarthria include degenerative, vascular, traumatic, infectious, neoplastic, and metabolic factors. Such degenerative diseases as Huntington's disease also may be associated with this type of dysarthria. Causes may be unknown in a majority of cases. The muscles of the face, jaw, tongue, palate, larynx, and respiration may be involved.

■ The major characteristics of hyperkinetic dysarthria include the following:

  – movement disorders (because of damage to the basal ganglia control circuit); abnormal and involuntary movements of the orofacial muscles;

– myoclonus (involuntary jerks of body parts), tics of the face and shoulders, tremor, chorea; abrupt and severe contractions of the extremities; writhing, involuntary movements, often in hands (athetosis); spasms (sudden and involuntary contractions of a muscle or group of muscles);

– dystonia, which results from contractions of antagonistic muscles resulting in abnormal postures; spasmodic torticollis (intermittent dystonia and spasms of the neck muscles); blepharospasm (forceful and involuntary closure of the eyes due to spasm of the orbicularis oculi muscle);

– communicative disorders, specific symptoms depending on the dominant neurological condition (e.g., chorea, dystonia, athetosis, spasmodic torticollis);

– phonatory disorders including voice tremor, intermittently strained voice, voice stoppage, vocal noise, and harsh voice;

– resonance disorders, predominantly intermittent hypernasality;

– prosodic disorders including slower rate, excess loudness variations, prolonged inter-word intervals, and equal stress;

– respiratory problems including audible inspiration and forced and sudden inspiration or expiration; and

– inconsistent articulation problems including imprecise consonant productions and distortion of vowels.

Hypokinetic Dysarthria

▪ Hypokinetic dysarthria results from damage to the basal ganglia (extrapyramidal system). It results from a variety of causes including such degenerative diseases as progressive supranuclear palsy, Parkinson's (much more commonly), Alzheimer's, and Pick's diseases.

▪ Hypokinetic dysarthria can also occur due to vascular disorders that cause multiple or bilateral strokes, repeated head trauma (such as that sustained by boxers), inflammation, tumor, antipsychotic or neuroleptic drug toxicity, and normal-pressure hydrocephalus. Parkinson's disease produces the most typical form, although dysarthria occurs only in about half the patients with that disease.

▪ Hypokinetic dysarthria is characterized by:

– tremors in the resting facial, mouth, and limb muscles that diminish when moved voluntarily;

– masklike face with infrequent blinking and no smiling;

– micrographic writing (small print);

– walking disorders (slow to begin, then short, rapid, shuffling steps);

- postural disturbances (involuntary flexion of the head, trunk, and arm; difficulty changing positions);

- decreased swallowing (accumulation of saliva in the mouth and drooling);

- phonatory disorders, including monopitch, low pitch, monoloudness, and harsh and continuously breathy voice;

- prosodic disorders, including reduced stress, inappropriate silent intervals, short rushes of speech, variable and increased rate in segments, and short phrases;

- articulation disorders, including imprecise consonants, repeated phonemes, resonance disorders, and mild hypernasality (in about 25% of cases); and

- respiratory problems, including reduced vital capacity, irregular breathing, and faster rate of respiration.

Mixed Dysarthrias

- Mixed dysarthrias are a combination of two or more pure dysarthrias. All combinations of pure dysarthrias are possible, although a combination of two types is more common than a combination of three or more. The two most common mixed forms are flaccid-spastic dysarthria and ataxic-spastic dysarthria.

- Mixed dysarthrias are characterized by:

  - symptoms characteristic of two or more individual types of dysarthria that are mixed in a given patient; and

  - the range of most to least severe symptoms of mixed flaccid-spastic dysarthria, associated with amyotrophic lateral sclerosis, include imprecise production of consonants, hypernasality, harsh voice, slow rate, monopitch, short phrases, distorted vowels, low pitch, monoloudness, excess and equal stress or reduced stress, prolonged intervals, prolonged phonemes, a strained and strangled quality, breathiness, audible inspiration, inappropriate silences, and nasal emission.

Spastic Dysarthria

- Spastic dysarthria results from bilateral damage to the upper motor neurons (direct and indirect motor pathways). Lesions in multiple areas including the cortical areas, basal ganglia, internal capsule, pons, and medulla are common.

- Spastic dysarthria is characterized by:

  - spasticity and weakness, especially bilateral facial weakness, though jaw strength may be normal and lower face weakness may be less severe;

– movement disorders, including reduced range and slowness, loss of fine and skilled movement, and increased muscle tone;

– hyperactive gag reflex;

– hyperadduction of vocal folds and inadequate closure of the velopharyngeal port;

– prosodic disorders, including excess and equal stress, slow rate, monopitch, monoloudness, reduced stress, and short phrases;

– articulation disorders, including imprecise production of consonants and distorted vowels;

– phonatory disorders, including continuous breathy voice, harshness, low pitch, pitch breaks, strained-strangled voice quality, short phrases, and slow rate; and

– resonance disorders with a predominant hypernasality.

Concepts To Consider

How is dysarthria classified? What are the major symptoms of the different types of dysarthria?

_____

_____

_____

_____

_____

_____

_____

Unilateral Upper Motor Neuron Dysarthria

■ Unilateral upper motor neuron (UUMN) dysarthria results from damage to the upper motor neurons that supply cranial and spinal nerves involved in speech production.

■ Dysarthria due to vascular disorders that produce left hemisphere lesions may coexist with aphasia or apraxia, and disarthria due to right hemisphere lesions may coexist with right hemisphere syndrome.

■ UUMN dysarthria is characterized by:

- unilateral lower face weakness, unilateral tongue weakness, unilateral palatal weakness, and hemiplegia/hemiparesis;

- articulation disorders, including imprecise production of consonants and irregular articulatory breakdowns;

- phonatory disorders, including harsh voice, reduced loudness, and strained-harshness;

- prosodic disorders, including slow rate, increased rate in segments, excess and equal stress, monopitch, monoloudness, low pitch, and short phrases;

- resonance disorders, predominantly hypernasality; and

- dysphagia, aphasia, apraxia, and right hemisphere syndrome.

Assessment of the Dysarthrias

■ Assessment of the dysarthrias involves multiple procedures because of the wide range of symptoms that must be evaluated (Duffy, 1995; Hegde, 1996a, 1998). The following procedures are appropriate in assessment.

- *Record an extended conversational speech sample* and a reading sample.

- *Use a variety of speech tasks* including imitation of syllables, words, phrases, and sentences; production of modeled syllables, words, phrases, and sentences; and sustained phonation (vowel prolongation).

- *Assess the diadochokinetic rate* or alternating motion rates (AMRs) and sequential motion rates (SMRs).

- *Assess the speech production mechanism* during nonspeech activities through the following activities:

  • observing facial symmetry, tone, tension, droopiness, expressiveness, and so forth;

  • observing the movements of the facial structures as the patient puffs the cheeks, retracts and rounds the lips, bites the lower lip, and so forth;

  • observing the patient's emotional expressions;

  • taking note of the patient's jaw movements and deviation during movement and observing the tongue movements;

  • observing the velopharyngeal mechanism and its movements;

  • assessing nasal airflow by holding a mirror at the nares as the patient prolongs the vowel /I/; and

  • assessing laryngeal functions by asking the patient to cough to take note of weak cough associated with weak adduction of the cords, inadequate breath support, or both.

– *Assess respiratory problems* by observing the patient's posture and breathing habits during quiet and speech; taking note of rapid, shallow, or effortful breathing; signs of shortness of breath and irregularity of inhalation and exhalation; and so forth.

– *Assess phonatory disorders* through the following activities:

  • having the patient say "ah" after taking a deep breath and sustain it as steadily and for as long as the air supply lasts;

  • taking note of the patient's pitch, pitch breaks, diplophonia, abrupt variations in pitch, and lack of normal pitch variations;

  • taking note of voice tremors, assessing the presence of diplophonia, and judging vocal loudness, its appropriateness, variations, decay, and alternating changes; and

  • judging the quality of voice, including hoarseness, harshness, and breathiness, taking note of strained or effortful voice production or sudden cessation of voice.

– *Assess articulation disorders* by evaluating consonant productions, duration of speech sounds, phoneme repetitions, irregular breakdowns in articulation, the precision of vowel productions, phoneme distortions, and the adequacy of pressure consonantal productions.

– *Assess prosodic disorders* by evaluating the rate of speech, phrase lengths in selected portions of speech, stress patterns in speech, pauses in speech, and the presence of short rushes of speech.

– *Assess resonance disorders* by making clinical judgments about hypo and hyper nasality and nasal emission.

– *Assess speech intelligibility* by making clinical judgments on the percentage of words or phrases understood and by using a rating scale if warranted.

– *Use such standardized tests* as the *Assessment of Intelligibility of Dysarthric Speakers* (Yorkston & Beukelman, 1981) and *Frenchay Dysarthria Assessment* (Enderby, 1983).

Treatment of the Dysarthrias

Goals and Procedures

■ Treatment of dysarthria includes a wide range of techniques partly because the communication disorders themselves have a wide range. Techniques to modify respiratory, phonatory, articulatory, and resonatory problems are all needed (Duffy, 1995; Hegde, 1996b, 1998).

■ *Treatment goals* include modification of respiratory, phonatory, articulatory, resonatory, and prosodic problems and increasing efficiency, effectiveness, and naturalness of communication.

■ Treatment goals also include increasing physiological support for speech and teaching self-correction, self-evaluation, and self-monitoring skills. Teaching compensatory behaviors for lost or reduced functions is important, and teaching the use of alternative or augmentative communication systems may be necessary.

■ *Treatment procedures* include intensive, systematic, and extensive drill, instruction, demonstration, modeling (followed by imitation), shaping, prompting, fading, differential reinforcement, and other proven behavioral management procedures. When necessary, phonetic placement and its variations can be taught. Instrumental feedback or biofeedback can be used when needed.

Specific Treatment Areas

■ The clinician needs to carry out treatment in the following areas:

■ *Modification of respiration* by:

- training, with the help of a manometer or air pressure transducer, consistent production of subglottal air pressure;

- training maximum vowel prolongation;

- shaping production of longer phrases and sentences;

- teaching controlled exhalation;

- teaching the client to push, pull, or bear down during speech or non-speech tasks;

- using a manual push on the client's abdomen;

- modifying postures that promote respiratory support, including using neck and trunk braces if helpful; and

- teaching the client to inhale more deeply and exhale slowly and with greater force during speech.

■ *Modification of phonation* by using biofeedback to shape desirable vocal intensity, and training the client in the use of portable amplification systems if the voice is too soft. Phonation modification may also include training aphonia clients in the use of an artificial larynx and teaching the client to initiate phonation at the beginning of an exhalation.

■ *Modification of resonance disorders* by providing feedback on nasal airflow and hypernasality by using a mirror, nasal flow transducer, or nasendoscope;

training the client to open the mouth wider to increase oral resonance and vocal intensity; and using a nasal obturator or nose clip.

- *Modification of articulation* by:

  - training the client to assume the best posture for good articulation;

  - using a bite block to improve jaw control and strength;

  - using such methods as simplifying the target, instruction, demonstration, modeling, shaping, and immediate feedback in teaching correct articulation;

  - using phonetic placement, slower rate, and minimal contrast pairs;

  - providing instructions and demonstrations and teaching self-monitoring skills; and

  - teaching compensatory articulatory movements (e.g., use of tongue blade to make sounds normally made with tongue tip).

- *Modification of speech rate* by using delayed auditory feedback (DAF), a pacing board, an alphabet board, a metronome, hand or finger tapping, and by reducing excessive pause durations in speech.

- *Modification of prosody* by reducing the speech rate and teaching appropriate intonation.

- *Modification of pitch* with the help of instruction, modeling, differential feedback, or with the help of such instruments as Visi-Pitch.

- *Modification of vocal intensity* through behavioral methods of modeling, shaping, and differential reinforcement of greater inhalation, increased laryngeal adduction, and wider mouth opening.

Summary

- ☑ The dysarthrias are a group of speech-motor disorders resulting from impaired muscular control of the speech mechanism, involving peripheral or central nervous system pathology.

- ☑ Dysarthrias are classified into ataxic, flaccid, hyperkinetic, hypokinetic, mixed, spastic, and unilateral upper motor neuron types.

- ☑ The oral communication problems that accompany dysarthria include respiratory, articulatory, phonatory, resonatory, and prosodic disturbances that are caused by weakness, incoordination, or paralysis of speech musculature.

- ☑ These problems are assessed and treated in most patients with dysarthria. Treatment may involve the use of augmentative devices for patients with severe dysarthria.

DEMENTIA

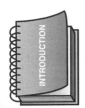

Dementia is a major health problem primarily found in people 65 years of age and older. It is an acquired neurological syndrome associated with persistent or progressive deterioration in intellectual functions (cognition, visuospatial skills), language, memory, emotion, and personality. Dementia is commonly classified as cortical, subcortical, or mixed in nature. Assessment of dementia includes informal procedures and standardized tests. Treatment usually focuses on helping clients manage their daily routines and helping families cope with the dementia.

Definition and Classification of Dementia

- Dementia, a major health care problem, may be as high as 25% in people 65 years and older. After the age of 65, the prevalence of dementia doubles every 5 years.

- In most cases, dementia is an acquired neurological syndrome associated with persistent or progressive deterioration in intellectual functions (cognition, visuospatial skills), language, memory, emotion, and personality.

- Most clinicians require that impairment should be evident in at least three of those functions. The American Psychiatric Association's definition of dementia requires that memory impairment should be evident to diagnose dementia.

- Dementia is typically progressive, but there are exceptions. It is reversible in some cases, especially when it is due to metabolic disturbances. Approximately 50% of irreversible dementia is due to Alzheimer's disease.

- Classification of dementia is controversial. A common classification includes three categories: cortical, subcortical, and mixed (Cummings & Benson, 1992).

Cortical Dementia

- In the cortical dementias, intellectual and language deterioration precede motor deficits. The opposite is true for subcortical dementia. Two major types of cortical dementia are *dementia of the Alzheimer's type* (DAT) and dementia associated with Pick's disease. In this section, DAT is described.

- In a majority of the cases of DAT, onset takes place when people are in their 70s and 80s. More women than men are affected. DAT is associated with a family history of Down syndrome and also with a history of brain injury.

■ Genetic inheritance accounts for some cases of DAT; the prevalence is 50% among the first-degree relatives. Genetic mutations in mitochondria and disturbed immune functions may also be etiological factors.

■ Neuropathology of DAT may involve the following:

– *Neurofibrillary tangles*: *Neurofibrils*, which are filamentous structures in the nerve cells, dendrites, and axons, assume unusual loops and triangles.

– *Neuritic plaques*: Also known as *senile plaques*, neuritic plaques destroy cortical and subcortical synaptic connections.

– *Granulovacuolar degeneration*: Nerve cells are destroyed by fluid-filled cavities containing granular debris.

✎ Concepts To Consider

How is dementia classified? What is the major neuropathology of dementia?

_____

_____

_____

_____

_____

_____

_____

_____

■ Symptoms of early-stage DAT (which are usually mild) include subtle memory problems (especially for remote events), somewhat pronounced difficulty in new learning, and visuospatial problems. Other early-stage DAT symptoms may include poor judgment, impaired reasoning, disorientation in new places, and depression and indifference.

■ Symptoms of later-stage DAT include:

– intensified early-stage symptoms

– severe problems in recalling remote and recent events

– intensified visuospatial problems

– widespread intellectual deterioration

– hyperactivity, restlessness, agitation, meaningless handling of objects

– problems in arithmetic calculations

- profound disorientation to place, time, and person; wandering

- problems in self-care (e.g., difficulty dressing, bathing)

- difficulty in managing daily routines

- lack of affect, tact, and judgment

- loss of initiative, indifference

- paranoid delusions and hallucinations

- aggressive or disruptive behaviors

- inappropriate humor and laughter

- seizures and myoclonic jerks (sudden muscular contractions) in the very late stage

■ Language problems associated with DAT include:

- naming problems, verbal and literal paraphasias, and circumlocution

- problems in comprehending abstract meanings

- impaired picture description

- difficulty in generating a list of words that begin with a specific letter

- repetitious speech and difficulty in topic maintenance

- empty speech, jargon, and hyperfluency

- incoherent, slurred, and rapid speech

- pragmatic language problems, including inattention to such social conventions as greetings

- reading and writing problems

- in the final stages, no meaningful speech, mutism, and complete disorientation to time, place, people, and self

Subcortical Dementia

■ Motor symptoms (e.g., tremor, rigidity, myoclonus) precede intellectual and language symptoms in subcortical dementias. Two major forms of subcortical dementia are those that are associated with Parkinson's disease and with Huntington's disease.

Subcortical Dementia and Parkinson's Disease

■ Only about 35–55% of patients with Parkinson's disease have dementia. Dementia is more common in males than in females, and onset is typically between 50 and 56 years of age. The etiology of Parkinson's disease is unknown.

■ Neuropathology of Parkinson's disease includes brain stem degeneration, frontal lobe atrophy resulting in widened sulci, and reduced dopamine due to loss of cells in the substantia nigra.

■ Symptoms of Parkinson's disease include slow voluntary movements; tremors in resting muscles, which exacerbate during stress; and muscle rigidity.

■ Other symptoms include a masklike face, reduced eye blinking, festinating gait and disturbed posture, serious memory problems, problems in abstract reasoning and problem solving, impaired word-list generation, impaired visuospatial perception, and severe naming and language comprehension problems in later stages of the disease.

■ Speech problems associated with Parkinson's disease include reduced speech volume; monotone; long and frequent pauses; slow, fast, or festinating speech rate; and dysarthric speech.

Subcortical Dementia and Huntington's Disease

■ Huntington's disease affects about 40–70 persons in a million. The typical age of onset is 35–40 years.

■ Genetic etiology is suspected. Half the offspring of a patient may have the disease.

■ Neuropathology of Huntington's disease includes a loss of neurons in the frontal and parietal regions and significant loss of neurons in the caudate nucleus, putamen, and substantia nigra.

■ Symptoms of Huntington's disease include chorea (irregular, spasmodic, involuntary movement of the neck, head, and face), increasingly uncontrollable tic-like movement disorders, gait disturbances, and progressively reduced voluntary movements.

■ Other symptoms include excessive complaining, nagging, eccentricity, irritability, emotional outbursts, a false sense of superiority, depression or euphoria, schizophrenic-like behaviors (delusion and hallucination), and suicide attempts.

■ Speech and cognitive-linguistic problems associated with Huntington's disease include deterioration in intellectual functions, impaired word-list generation, naming problems, dysarthria, and muteness in the final stages.

Other Dementias

■ A variety of dementias due to infection have been reported. Dementia due to human immunodeficiency virus (HIV) infection or Jakob-Creutzfeldt disease is commonly described in the literature. Dementia due to HIV infection is known as *AIDS dementia complex.*

■ Vascular diseases may cause bilateral cortical, subcortical, or mixed damage resulting in dementia. This type of dementia is known as *cerebrovascular dementia.*

■ Cerebrovascular dementia can be caused by multiple cerebrovascular accidents, infarctions within the deep structures of the brain, and atrophy of subcortical white matter caused by repeated infarcts (a long-standing hypertension is associated with this atrophy).

Assessment of Dementia

■ A thorough case history, clinical examination, neurological assessment including brain imaging and laboratory tests, communication assessment, and assessment of intellectual functions are a part of the diagnostic activities (Hegde, 1996a, 1998). A definitive diagnosis of dementia is possible only after an autopsy, however.

■ Neither pointing to stimuli nor automatic speech tasks are useful in diagnosing mild forms of dementia. They are best diagnosed on the basis of: verbal description, storytelling of both immediate and delayed variety, and word fluency (saying words that belong to a class, such as forms of transportation).

■ In assessing dementia, the following skills or domains are typically sampled:

  – awareness and orientation to surroundings

  – mood and affect, to assess depression or lack of emotional responses

  – speech and language

  – memory and other cognitive functions

  – abnormal thinking (e.g., hallucinations or delusions)

  – visuospatial skills

■ Various tests of aphasia may be helpful in assessing dementia. There are only a few standardized tests of dementia. The *Arizona Battery for Communication Disorders of Dementia* (Bayles & Tomoeda, 1991) has been especially designed to assess dementia associated with Alzheimer's disease. It screens speech discrimination, visual perception and literacy, visual fields, visual agnosia, mental status, linguistic expression, linguistic comprehension, and visual-spatial construction.

■ The *Blessed Dementia Scale* (Hachinsky, Illiff, Zilhka, & associates, 1975) helps evaluate changes in performance in 8 everyday activities (e.g., inability to perform household tasks or to find way indoors) and changes in 14 habits (e.g., changes in eating and dressing habits). Parents, caregivers, and medical records are the sources of information. Scores are specified for *no impairment* (below 4), *mild impairment* (4 to 9), and *moderate to severe impairment* (10 and higher).

■ The *Global Deterioration Scale* (Reisberg, Ferris, DeLeon, & Crook, 1982) also helps evaluate levels of functioning ranging from *no cognitive decline* to *very severe decline*. Information is gathered from a variety of sources.

Clinical Management of Dementia

■ The main clinical concerns are to help the client manage his or her daily routine and help the family cope with the progressively deteriorating dementia, for which there is no cure. In the early and intermediate stages, communication, memory, and behavioral management is targeted.

■ Management of daily activities may include teaching the following strategies to the client (Brookshire, 1997):

   – establishing a simple routine;

   – using various reminders: alarms, written instructions, staff reminders, self-monitoring devices, signs as reminders of activities and their times, and so forth;

   – writing down a list of things to do every morning;

   – always keeping phone numbers and possessions in a specific place;

   – writing a checklist of things to do before leaving the house;

   – always carrying a card with the names, addresses, and phone numbers of caregivers;

   – always wearing a bracelet that contains identifying information and names, addresses, and phone numbers of caregivers; and

   – writing down important information when memory begins to fail.

■ Family members and caregivers are counseled to manage the patient better by teaching them the following (Shekim, 1997):

   – before speaking, to approach the patient slowly, touch the patient gently, establish eye contact, and speak clearly and slowly;

   – to use gestures, smiling, posture, and other cues;

   – to talk about simple and concrete events and to talk in simple, short sentences;

   – point out the topic, person, or thing before speaking about it;

   – to ask yes or no questions;

- to restate important information;

- to structure the client's room and the living environment, to establish a routine;

- to always say good-bye or give other departing signals;

- to reduce emotional outbursts by analyzing the conditions under which they occur and eliminating those conditions; and

- to minimize demands made on the client.

Summary

☑ Dementia, an acquired neurological syndrome associated with progressive deterioration in many functions (especially cognition), is usually found in people over 65 years of age.

☑ Dementia is typically classified as cortical, subcortical, or mixed. A common type of cortical dementia is dementia of the Alzheimer's type. Two major forms of subcortical dementia are those associated with Parkinson's disease and with Huntington's disease.

☑ Assessment of patients with dementia includes administration of informal tasks and standardized tests. Treatment of patients with dementia focuses on helping them manage their daily routines as effectively as possible and on helping families cope with the dementia.

RIGHT HEMISPHERE SYNDROME

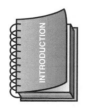

The right hemisphere specializes in processing visual and spatial information, holistic-gestalt stimuli, facial recognition, copying, and drawing. Right hemisphere damage (RHD), also referred to as right hemisphere syndrome, varies depending upon the site of lesion. Typically, however, symptoms include attentional and perceptual, affective, and communicative deficits. Assessment of patients with RHD can be both formal and informal. Treatment often addresses such problems as impaired attention, impulsive behavior, pragmatic impairments, and visual neglect.

Foundational Concepts

▦ While the left hemisphere specializes in most aspects of language, the right hemisphere specializes in processing holistic-gestalt stimuli, visual and spatial information, facial recognition, drawing, and copying. Right hemisphere functions are more diffusely organized than the left hemisphere functions.

▦ The left and the right hemispheres are susceptible to the same kinds of neuropathology, including cerebrovascular accidents, tumors, head trauma, and various neurological diseases.

▦ *Right hemisphere syndrome* varies in symptom complex. Posterior lesions do not produce motor problems, whereas frontal lobe injuries do. Those with frontal lobe injuries are hospitalized longer than those with posterior lesions.

Symptoms of Right Hemisphere Syndrome

▦ Symptoms of RHD include perceptual and attentional deficits, affective deficits, and communicative deficits. However, pure linguistic deficits are not typical of RHD. Attentional and perceptual deficits are dominant (Hegde, 1996a, 1998).

Attentional and Perceptual Deficits

▦ *Left neglect*: This is reduced awareness of the left side of the body and generally reduced awareness of stimuli in the left visual field. It consists of paying attention only to the right side of stimuli (e.g., copying only the right side of the face of a clock). Other characteristics of left neglect include failure to allow for a right margin in writing, reading only the right side of a printed page, bumping into things or people on the left side, and using only right-side pockets.

▦ *Denial of illness (anosagnosia)*: This involves denial of the existence of the paralyzed arm or leg and indifference to admitted deficits or problems.

▦ *Confabulation regarding disability*: This refers to exaggerated claims regarding a disabled body part (e.g., a man with a paralyzed hand may claim to be painting with that hand).

▦ *Facial recognition deficits*: These deficits are characterized by failure to recognize a familiar face until the person begins to speak, difficulty remembering faces shown through pictures, and difficulty distinguishing faces of older and younger or male or female people.

▦ *Constructional impairment*: This impairment includes difficulty in reproducing block designs, drawing or copying geometric shapes, and reproducing two-dimensional stick figures.

■ *Attentional deficits*: These deficits involve reduced awareness and arousal, difficulty sustaining attention, and difficulty in paying selective attention.

■ *Disorientation*: Types of disorientation include topographic disorientation (confusion about space), geographic disorientation (not knowing where one is), and reduplicative paramnesia (e.g., a patient's belief that he has two left legs or two wives).

■ *Visuoperceptual deficits*: These deficits involve difficulty recognizing line drawings; drawings that are distorted in size, dimension, or orientation; and drawings that are superimposed on another.

Concepts To Consider

You have been asked to give a workshop to physicians about recognizing right hemisphere syndrome in patients. List four things you will tell them.

_____

_____

_____

_____

_____

_____

_____

_____

_____

Affective Deficits

■ Affective deficits include difficulty in:

- understanding emotions other people express

- describing emotions expressed on printed faces in storybooks

- recognizing emotions expressed in isolated verbal productions

- understanding emotional tone of voice

- expressing emotions (not necessarily experiencing emotions)

Communicative Deficits

■ About 50% of patients with RHD have communicative deficits, which may include those described below.

- *Prosodic deficits*: These include monotone speech with flat affect as well as difficulty understanding prosodic meanings of other people's speech.

- *Impaired narrative skills*: These involve confusion between significant and irrelevant or trivial pieces of information in a picture description or conversational speech.

- *Confabulation and excessive speech*: These are characterized by excessive inference, too much attention to minor details, and saying too much, which borders on confabulation.

- *Difficulty understanding implied, alternate, or abstract meanings*: This difficulty includes failure to grasp the overall meaning of situations or stories; difficulty understanding the central message of conversation; difficulty in describing the underlying theme of a picture or a story; literal interpretation of proverbs and sayings; and problems in appreciating humor, sarcasm, and irony.

- *Pragmatic deficits*: These are characterized by problems in conversational turn-taking, topic maintenance, and maintaining eye contact as well as rambling, excessive speech with little communicative value and impulsive speech.

- *Other communicative deficits*: These include naming problems, especially of collective nouns (e.g., problem in saying "flowers," but no problem in naming a particular type of flower); difficulty comprehending complex verbal material; and impaired oral reading of sentences.

Assessment of Right Hemisphere Syndrome

■ Assessment of right hemisphere syndrome can be informal, formal, or both. For formal testing, there are published assessment tools, which include the following:

- *The Mini Inventory of Right Brain Injury* (Pimental & Kingsbury, 1989) helps evaluate such skills as visual scanning, integrity of gnosis (finger identification, tactile perception, two-point discrimination), integrity of body image, reading and writing, drawing, and affective and abstract language.

- *The Right Hemisphere Language Battery* (Bryan, 1989) helps assess comprehension of spoken and printed metaphors, inferred meanings, appreciation of humor, and discourse.

- *The Rehabilitation Institute of Chicago Evaluation of Communicative Problems in Right Hemisphere Dysfunction* (Burns, Halper, & Mogil, 1985) helps assess typical skills impaired in RHD. In addition, the protocol includes an interview schedule and observation of a patient's interaction with others.

- *The Test of Visual Neglect* (Albert, 1973) helps assess neglect by asking the patient to cross out short lines randomly printed on a page.

- *Bells Test* (Gauthier, Dehaut, & Joanette, 1989) presents tasks in which the patient is asked to circle only the bells printed on a page that also contains other objects.

- *The Behavioral Inattention Test* (Wilson, Cockburn, & Halligan, 1987) contains both paper-and-pencil tests and techniques to assess neglect in such functional tasks as reading maps, menus, and newspapers and using a telephone.

Treatment of Right Hemisphere Syndrome

- Treatment of patients with RHD is relatively new, and not much treatment research has been published. However, the treatment targets and strategies described below are generally considered appropriate (Hegde, 1996a, 1998).

  - *Denial and indifference*: The clinician provides immediate feedback on errors to increase awareness. Videotaped sessions to give visual feedback on errors are helpful.

  - *Impaired attention*: This involves drawing attention to treatment stimuli, giving specific directions to follow, repeating such directions throughout treatment, and reinforcing attention during discourse training.

  - *Impulsive behavior*: Treatment includes nonverbal signals to wait a few seconds before giving an impulsive response (e.g., a hand gesture or a tone that signals the patient to wait). *Also helpful* are such verbal stimuli as "Wait for a few seconds and then tell me."

  - *Pragmatic impairments*: Helpful techniques include videotaped conversations that show appropriate and inappropriate pragmatic behaviors to draw the patient's attention to such behaviors. The clinician may also give frequent reminders to maintain eye contact, continue talking on the same topic, and so forth.

  - *Impaired reasoning*: The clinician can use activities that require reasoning (e.g., planning a vacation) and prompt and reinforce correct and logically sequenced descriptions.

  - *Impaired inference*: Helpful treatment techniques include use of pictures that depict situations that require inference and reinforcement for correct inferences.

— *Impaired comprehension of metaphors and idioms*: Treatment involves practice in the correct interpretations of metaphors and idioms by asking the client to select printed statements or make comments that give literal, metaphoric, and implied meanings.

— *Visual neglect*: This can be addressed through use of such treatment tasks as tracking moving objects and detection of flashing lights in visual fields. The clinician can also use letter, line, or design cancellation to force the client to pay attention to the neglected side, as well as printed material that contains colored left-side margins to draw attention to the left side of each page.

Summary

- ☑ The left hemisphere specializes in most aspects of language. The right hemisphere specializes in processing holistic-gestalt stimuli, visual and spatial information, facial recognition, drawing, and copying.

- ☑ Patients with injury to the right hemisphere manifest various problems. These often include attentional and perceptual deficits, affective deficits, and communicative deficits.

- ☑ Informal and formal methods may be used to assess patients with RHD. Treatment focuses on such areas as impaired attention and behavior, pragmatic problems, impaired reasoning and inference, and visual neglect.

TRAUMATIC BRAIN INJURY

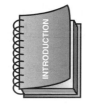 Traumatic brain injury (TBI) is injury to the brain sustained by physical trauma or external force. Injuries can be penetrating or nonpenetrating. Assessment includes formal and informal measures and is dependent upon the patient's level of post-accident consciousness. The two most common approaches to treatment of patients with TBI are the cognitive rehabilitation approach and the communication treatment approach.

Nature, Causes, and Consequences of TBI

▪ Traumatic brain injury is injury to the brain sustained by physical trauma or external force. The prevalence of TBI is about 2 million people a year in the United States.

▪ The prevalence rate is highest for the age group 15–19 years. More males than females are affected. TBI is a significant problem for people living in urban areas, many of whom are from linguistically and culturally diverse backgrounds (Wallace, 1998). About 500,000 people are hospitalized annually, and 900,000 may sustain permanent disability (Hegde, 1998).

▪ A major category of TBI is *penetrating brain injuries*. Also known as *open-head injuries*, penetrating brain injuries involve a fractured or perforated skull, torn or lacerated meninges, and an injury that extends to brain tissue. High-velocity missiles (e.g., bullets) and low-velocity impacts (e.g., blows to the head) are the most frequent causes of penetrating brain injuries.

▪ A second major category of TBI is *nonpenetrating brain injuries*. Also known as *closed-head injuries*, nonpenetrating brain injuries involve no open wound in the head, a damaged brain within the skull, and no penetration of a foreign substance into the brain. The skull may be fractured, but as long as the meninges are not torn, the injury is classified as nonpenetrating. Nonpenetrating injuries may be of acceleration-deceleration type or nonacceleration type:

   − *Acceleration-deceleration injuries* are more serious than nonacceleration injuries. A head is set into motion by physical forces; when the head begins to move, the brain inside is still static. Soon, the brain begins to move. When the head stops moving, the brain keeps moving and thus strikes the skull on the opposite side of the initial impact. The moving brain is lacerated or torn because of the bony projections on the base of the skull.

   − *Nonacceleration injuries* occur when a restrained head is hit by a moving object. These injuries may fracture the skull, but they produce much less serious consequences for the brain.

▪ Consequences of TBI include immediate or subsequent death, destruction of brain tissue, infection, and various types of hematomas (accumulation of blood in an area of the brain).

▪ Other consequences of TBI may include increased intracranial pressure; ischemic brain damage (damage due to lack of blood); seizures; and long-term physical, language, and cognitive deficits.

General Assessment of Patients with TBI

▤ In the assessment of patients with TBI, it is critical to gather a comprehensive case history, observe the client, interview family members and health care workers, and review medical records to understand the nature and extent of TBI.

▤ Initial assessment depends on the medical condition of the client and may be brief. The client regaining consciousness may be inconsistent, disorganized, disoriented, restless, distracted, and irritated. The initial assessment may be done at the bedside. Major assessment tools used in the initial and subsequent stages of recovery include those described below.

  - *The Glasgow Coma Scale* (Teasdale & Jennett, 1976) helps make an initial assessment of eye opening, motor responses (e.g., flexing the body in response to pain), and verbal responses.

  - *The Comprehensive Level of Consciousness Scale* (Stanczak & Associates, 1984) also helps assess initial status by rating posture, resting eye position, spontaneous eye opening, ocular movements, pupillary reflexes, motor functioning, responsiveness, and communicative effort.

  - *The Galveston Orientation and Amnesia Test* (Levin, O'Donnell, & Grossman, 1979) helps assess amnesia, orientation, and memory.

  - *The Rancho Los Amigos Scale of Cognitive Levels* (Hagen & Malkamus, 1979) helps assess cognition and behavior at the levels of no response, generalized response, localized response, confused-agitated, confused-appropriate, automatic-appropriate, and purposeful-appropriate.

▤ Assessment of memory impairments includes the assessment of posttraumatic amnesia (loss of memory for events following the trauma) and pretraumatic amnesia (loss of memory for events preceding the trauma). The clinician may use client-specific questions surrounding the trauma.

Assessment of Communicative Deficits Associated with TBI

▤ Pure linguistic problems may not be severe or significant in patients with TBI. Articulatory or phonological disorders may be noted only if the patient sustained injury to the cerebellum, brain stem, or peripheral nerves. A patient's verbal expressions may be grammatically correct.

▤ Assessment procedures may include selected tests of aphasia and client-specific procedures that the clinician develops (Hegde, 1996a, 1998). Initial and persistent communicative problems that need to be assessed include the following:

  - *Dysarthria*: spastic dysarthria or mixed dysarthria in some patients with TBI

- *Confused language* (may be evident initially): irrelevant, circumlocutory, incoherent, or confabulatory speech

- *Auditory comprehension problems*: possibly more pronounced for complex or abstract material

- *Confrontation naming problems*: possibly due to misperceptions or impulsive responding

- *Perseveration of verbal responses*: repetitive verbal responses

- *Pragmatic language problems:* difficulty in initiating conversation, turn-taking, selecting appropriate topics for conversation, maintaining topic and cohesion, rambling, and understanding the meaning of facial expressions and gestures

- Reading and writing difficulties

Treatment of Patients with TBI

■ Of the variety of treatment approaches advocated for patients with TBI, cognitive rehabilitation and direct communication training are the two most important (Hegde, 1996b, 1998).

■ *Cognitive rehabilitation* is preferred by some clinicians. In cognitive rehabilitation, clinicians train such components as attention, visual processing, and memory, which may not result in improved communication. Attempts to improve memory, reasoning skills, and other cognitive functions may be better integrated with communication training.

■ *Communication treatment* for patients with TBI often involves direct behavioral procedures. Systematic reinforcement of attending behaviors, appropriate discourse, topic maintenance, self-correction, and so forth, will result in their increase and a concomitant decrease in many inappropriate behaviors.

✎ Concepts To Consider

Discuss two approaches to rehabilitation of patients with TBI.

_____

_____

_____

_____

_____

_____

■ Communication treatment goals should be functional, and the initial focus should be effectiveness of communication, not grammatical correctness. Family members should be involved in treatment. Other treatment goals are described below; the clinician can be involved in:

- *increasing the patient's orientation and attention to place, person, and time* by asking questions about the patient's whereabouts; using written signs to help the patient remember the day of the week or the name of the hospital;

- *increasing the patient's memory for daily routines* through written signs that remind the patient of routines and lists of daily activities;

- *increasing the patient's memory for the names of significant people* by asking the patient to name pictures of family members;

- *decreasing the variability in activities and schedules* by initially creating a simple, structured routine with few activities for the patient;

- *increasing the patient's attention to communication partners and topics* to promote better comprehension by giving such signals as "Listen carefully, now," "I want to say something to you," "Are you listening?";

- *improving communicative attention* by introducing new topics and warning about topic changes in conversation;

- *teaching the client to ask questions* when something said is not clear to him or her by modeling such questions and statements as "What do you mean?" "I do not understand that," "Tell me more about that," and so forth;

- *withholding attention from irrelevant, inappropriate, or tangential responses* to reduce their frequency;

- *teaching narrative skills in graded steps* by initially telling a brief and simple story, asking the patient to retell it, and eventually having the client retell more complex stories;

- *integrating such pragmatic skills as topic maintenance and topic initiation into narrative skills teaching* by such prompts as "Say more" and "Give details";

- *integrating work- or school-related words, phrases, and narratives into communication training* at all levels by selecting client-specific work or school-related vocabulary and expressions for treatment;

- *using tangible reinforcers* when necessary because some patients with TBI may not respond to verbal reinforcers in the early stages of recovery;

- *teaching self-monitoring skills* by including them at all levels of training;

— *teaching compensatory strategies* to handle residual deficits (e.g., writing down instructions and important information, requesting information, requesting people to speak slowly or repeat, requesting others to write down messages, establishing simple and invariable routines, reducing environmental distractions, self-cueing, etc.);

— *training family members and others* to recognize, prompt, model, and reinforce appropriate communication and general behavior;

— *promoting community reentry* by preparing the patient for reentry to school or work; educating family members, teachers, and supervisors about the patient's strengths and weaknesses; teaching family members, teachers, colleagues, and supervisors to change their style of communication if needed; and modifying teacher or supervisor demands if necessary.

Summary

☑ TBI, or injury to the brain sustained by physical trauma or external force, can involve penetrating or nonpenetrating injuries.

☑ Patients with TBI should undergo general assessment as well as assessment of communicative deficits such as possible dysarthria, pragmatic language and auditory comprehension problems, and written-language deficits.

☑ The two primary treatment approaches for patients with TBI are the cognitive rehabilitation and communication treatment approaches. These two approaches may be integrated to help the patient reenter the community to the greatest extent possible.

SWALLOWING DISORDERS

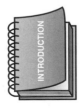

INTRODUCTION

Swallowing disorders (dysphagia) involve impaired execution of the oral, pharyngeal, and esophageal phases of a normal swallow. Dysphagia may be caused by strokes, TBI, and other factors. Assessment of dysphagia involves screening communication skills as well as evaluating the patient's ability to swallow effectively. Treatment of dysphagia may be direct, indirect, and/or medical.

Nature and Etiology of Swallowing Disorders

■ Swallowing disorders, also known as *dysphagia* or *deglutition disorders*, are technically not disorders of communication. However, except for esophageal swallowing disorders, which are handled medically, speech–language pathologists are involved in the assessment and management of swallowing disorders (Hegde, 1996a, b).

■ Dysphagia involves impaired execution of the oral, pharyngeal, and esophageal stages of swallow. The patient may have problems in chewing the food, preparing it for swallow, initiating the swallow, propelling the bolus through the pharynx, and passing the food through the esophagus.

■ There are many causes of swallowing disorders:

  – strokes, especially brain stem and anterior cortical strokes, resulting in poor motor control of structures involved in swallowing;

  – oral and pharyngeal tumors and various neurologic diseases (e.g., Parkinson's disease, amyotrophic lateral sclerosis, multiple sclerosis, myasthenia gravis, muscular dystrophy, and dystonia);

  – surgical or radiation treatment of oral, pharyngeal, and laryngeal cancer; any form of brain, head, neck, or gastrointestinal surgery;

  – traumatic brain injury; cervical spine disease;

  – poliomyelitis (polio), chronic and obstructive pulmonary disease, and cerebral palsy;

  – genetic factors (e.g., *dysautonomia*, an inherited disorder associated with autonomic imbalance, sensory deficits, and motor incoordination); and

  – side effects of certain prescription drugs (e.g., antispasticity, antipsychotic, and neuroleptic drugs).

Normal and Disordered Swallow

■ There are various phases of dysphagia involving mastication as well as the oral preparatory, oral, pharyngeal, and esophageal phases and their disorders. These phases are described below.

  – *Mastication and its disorders*: Mastication is chewing solid or semisolid food before initiating swallow. Disorders of mastication include problems in chewing food because of reduced range of lateral and vertical tongue movement, reduced range of lateral mandibular movement, reduced buccal tension, and poor alignment of the mandible and maxilla.

  – *Oral preparatory phase and its disorders*: Masticated food is prepared for swallow in the oral preparatory phase by making a *bolus* (a rounded mass of food that is ready to be swallowed). Disorders of the oral preparatory phase include difficulty in forming and holding the bolus, abnormal holding of the bolus, slippage of food into anterior and lateral sulcus, aspiration before swallow due mostly to weak lip closure, reduced tongue movement, and inadequate tongue and buccal tension.

— *Oral phase and its disorders*: This phase begins with the posterior tongue action that moves the bolus posteriorly; the phase ends as the bolus passes through the anterior faucial arches when the swallowing reflex is initiated. Disorders of the oral phase include:

- such problems in tongue movements as anterior instead of posterior movement and weak movement;

- food residue in various places (e.g., anterior and lateral sulcus and the floor of the mouth);

- premature swallow and aspiration before swallow, caused by apraxia of swallow;

- tongue thrust;

- reduced labial, buccal, and tongue tension and strength; and

- reduced range of tongue movement and elevation.

— *Pharyngeal phase and its disorders*: This phase consists of reflex actions of the swallow. Reflexes are triggered by the contact the food makes with the anterior faucial pillars. The pharyngeal phase involves velopharyngeal closure, laryngeal closure by an elevated larynx to seal the airway, reflexive relaxation of the cricopharyngeal muscle for the bolus to enter, and reflexive contractions of the pharyngeal contractors to move the bolus down and eventually into the esophagus. Disorders of the pharyngeal phase include:

- difficulties in propelling the bolus through the pharynx and into the P-E (pharyngoesophageal sphincter) segment;

- delayed or absent swallowing reflex;

- nasal and airway penetration of food;

- food coating on the pharyngeal walls;

- food residue in *valleculae* (space between the base of the tongue and the epiglottis), on top of airway, in pyriform sinuses, and throughout the pharynx;

- aspiration before and after swallow;

- delayed pharyngeal transmit time;

- reduced pharyngeal contractions;

- pharyngeal paralysis;

- reduced movement of the base of the tongue;

- reduced laryngeal movement;

- inadequate closure of the airway; and

- cricopharyngeal dysfunctions.

– *Esophageal phase and its disorders*: This swallowing phase is not under voluntary control. It begins when the food arrives at the orifice of the esophagus; food is propelled through the esophagus by peristaltic action and gravity and into the stomach. Bolus entry into the esophagus results in restored breathing and a depressed larynx and soft palate. Disorders of this phase include the following problems, which are generally caused by a weak cricopharyngeus:

- difficulties in passing the bolus through the cricopharyngeus muscle and past the 7th cervical vertebra;

- backflow of food from esophagus to pharynx;

- reduced esophageal contractions due to surgery, neurologic damage, or radiation therapy;

- formation of diverticulum (a pouch that collects food);

- development of tracheo esophageal fistula (a hole); and

- esophageal obstruction (e.g., by a tumor).

Concepts To Consider

Describe the stages of a normal swallow.

_____

_____

_____

_____

_____

_____

_____

_____

_____

_____

Assessment of Swallowing Disorders

▪ Such standard procedures as taking a detailed case history; reviewing medical records; and interviewing the patient, family, and health care workers are a part of the total assessment. In addition, the clinician may implement the following specific procedures (Hegde, 1996a):

– *Screen speech, voice, language, and writing skills* using the clinical interview. Errors of articulation, voice quality, pitch and loudness characteristics, and the presence of hyponasality and hypernasality may be noted.

– *Screen concrete and abstract language comprehension* by giving a few simple verbal commands and by asking the patient to give the meaning of common proverbs and phrases. Deviations in the use of language, if any, may be noted.

– *Conduct a laryngeal examination* with indirect laryngoscopy and/or endoscopic examination to inspect the base of the tongue, vallecula, epiglottis, piriform sinuses, vocal folds, and ventricular folds and their functioning.

– *Administer test swallows*, taking into consideration the patient's medical condition and the type of swallowing disorder. Collect the necessary materials (a laryngeal mirror, a tongue blade, a cup, a spoon, a straw, a syringe, and various foods of different consistencies).

– *Correctly position the patient for test swallows*—for example, in the case of tongue weakness and bolus manipulation problems, the patient should tilt the head downward as food is placed in the mouth and tilt the head backward when the swallow is initiated. In the case of hemilaryngectomy, delayed triggering of swallowing reflex, and inadequate laryngeal closure, the patient should tilt the head downward to hold the food in the valleculae until the reflex is triggered.

– *Appropriately place the food in the mouth*—for example, place food in the more normal side of the mouth, or use a straw or a syringe to place liquids posteriorly.

– *Use different kinds of foods in evaluating test swallows*—for example, use liquid foods or foods of thin consistency when the patient has limited oral control and foods of thicker consistency when the patient's swallowing reflex is delayed.

– *Give appropriate instructions* for head position and swallowing.

– *Manually examine the swallowing movements* by placing the index finger just below the chin, the middle finger on the hyoid, and the third and fourth fingers at the top and bottom of the thyroid to take note of the submandibular, hyoid, and laryngeal movements during swallowing or aspiration.

– *Conduct a videofluorographic assessment* (modified barium swallow) of oropharyngeal swallow involving lateral and anterior-posterior (A-P) plane examinations.

– *Conduct a manometric assessment* with the help of an esophageal manometer, which measures pressure in the upper and lower esophagus.

– *Conduct an electromyographic assessment* by attaching electrodes on structures of interest (e.g., oral, laryngeal, or pharyngeal muscles).

– *Conduct an endoscopic assessment* to examine the movement of the bolus until it triggers the pharyngeal swallow and any food residue after swallow.

– *Conduct an ultrasound examination* to measure oral tongue movement and hyoid movement.

Treatment of Swallowing Disorders

▦ Clinicians who treat patients with swallowing disorders should always take into account the patient's cultural background. Patients may have food preferences or religious beliefs that affect the type of food and the timing of feeding that occur as part of treatment (Wallace, 1998).

▦ Direct, indirect, and medical procedures are used to treat swallowing disorders. Speech–language pathologists are involved in both direct and indirect treatment (Groher, 1997; Hegde, 1996b; Logemann, 1998; Perlman & Schulze-Delrieu, 1997).

Direct Treatment of Swallowing Disorders

▦ In direct treatment, food or liquid is placed in the patient's mouth to shape appropriate swallowing. Direct treatment is designed to reduce problems that are evident in the different stages of swallow, as follows:

– *Treatment of disorders of mastication* involves teaching the patient to better handle food in the mouth. The clinician may use such procedures as:

• teaching the patient to press the tongue against the hard palate;

• teaching the patient to keep the food on the more mobile side of the tongue and/or on the stronger side of the mouth;

• applying a gentle pressure with one hand on the damaged cheek to increase cheek tension; and

• teaching the patient to keep the head tilted to the stronger side to maintain food on that side.

— *Treatment of disorders of the preparatory phase of the swallow* involves such procedures as teaching the patient to tilt the head forward to keep the food in the front of the mouth until ready to swallow, tilting the head back to promote the swallow, holding the bolus in the anterior or middle portion of the mouth, and so forth.

— *Treatment of disorders of the oral phase of the swallow* involves:

  • teaching the patient to place the tongue on the alveolar ridge and initiate a swallow with an upward and backward motion to prevent tongue thrust swallow;

  • teaching the patient to compensate by placing food at the back of the tongue and then initiating a swallow; and

  • teaching the patient to compensate for tongue elevation problems by placing food posteriorly in the patient's oral cavity, placing a straw almost at the level of the faucial arches to help the patient swallow liquid, and then tilting the patient's head back and letting gravity push the food from the oral cavity into the pharynx.

— *Treatment of disorders of the pharyngeal stage of the swallow* can be carried out by:

  • teaching the patient to tilt the head forward while swallowing, to compensate for delayed or absent swallowing reflex;

  • teaching the patient to switch between liquid and semisolid swallows so that the liquid swallows help clear the pharynx to compensate for reduced peristalsis;

  • teaching the patient to tilt the head toward the stronger side if the patient has a unilateral paralysis in lingual function and the pharynx; and

  • teaching the patient to tilt the head forward while swallowing or placing pressure on the thyroid cartilage on the damaged side to improve laryngeal closure.

Indirect Treatment of Swallowing Disorders

■ Indirect treatment of swallowing disorders does not involve food. Instead, various exercises designed to improve muscle strength are prescribed and practiced.

■ *Oral-motor control exercises* are numerous, and each is designed to reduce a particular problem. For example, various exercises are designed to:

  — increase the range of tongue movements (e.g., raising the tongue, holding the tongue as high as possible, alternating raising and lowering the tongue);

- increase buccal tension (e.g., stretching the lips as tightly as possible and saying "ee," rounding the lips tightly and saying "oh," and rapidly alternating between "ee" and "oh");

- increase the range of lateral movements of the jaw (e.g., wide opening and sideways movement of the jaw) and of tongue resistance (e.g., pushing the tongue against a tongue depressor); and

- strengthen lip closure (e.g., stretching the lips to stimulate the production of /i/; puckering the lips tightly; tightly closing the lips).

■ Some exercises are designed to *stimulate the swallow reflex* by:

- touching the base of the anterior faucial arch with a laryngeal mirror dipped in water for about 10 seconds;

- asking the patient to swallow after the stimulation without food;

- practicing liquid swallow after stimulation; and

- progressively increasing the consistency of food introduced after stimulation.

■ Some exercises are designed to *improve adduction of tissues at the top of the airway* by lifting and pushing exercises to improve laryngeal adduction to protect the airway during swallowing (e.g., holding his or her breath, the patient pushes down on the chair or pulls up on it; subsequently, the patient may lift or push with simultaneous voicing).

Medical Treatment of Swallowing Disorders

■ Surgeons are mostly involved in the medical treatment of swallowing disorders as most of the medical procedures are surgical. These procedures are described briefly below:

- *Cricopharyngeal myotomy*. In this surgical procedure, the cricopharyngeal muscle is split from top to bottom to create a permanently open sphincter for swallowing. Fibers of the inferior constrictor above and the esophageal musculature below also may be slit. Eating may be resumed within about a week. This procedure is recommended for patients with Parkinson's disease, amyotrophic lateral sclerosis, and oculopharyngeal dystrophy, whose main problem is cricopharyngeal dysfunction.

- *Esophagostomy*. This is designed for patients who cannot tolerate oral feeding. The procedure involves inserting a feeding tube into the esophagus and stomach through a hole (stoma) that has been surgically created through cervical esophagus.

- *Gastrostomy*. Also designed for patients who cannot tolerate oral feeding, this procedure involves insertion of a feeding tube into the stomach through an opening in the abdomen; blended table food is directly transported to the stomach.

- *Nasogastric feeding*. This is another surgical method for dysphagic patients who cannot tolerate oral feeding. A tube, inserted through the nose, pharynx, and esophagus into the stomach, feeds the patient.

- *Pharyngostomy*. In this variation of nonoral, surgical feeding methods, a tube is inserted into the esophagus and stomach through a hole that has been surgically created through the pharynx.

- *Teflon injection* into the vocal folds. This is a surgical implant method designed to improve airway closure during swallowing. Teflon is injected to a normal or reconstructed vocal cord or any remaining tissue on top of the airway to increase the muscle mass that will help close the airway.

Summary

☑ Dysphagia, which involves impaired execution of the oral, pharyngeal, and esophageal phases of a swallow, can be caused by many factors, including strokes and TBI.

☑ Phases of swallowing include the oral preparatory phase, oral phase, pharyngeal phase, and esophageal phase. A thorough assessment involves evaluation of all these phases.

☑ Treatment for dysphagia should take cultural factors into account. It can be direct, indirect, and/or medical. In direct treatment, food and liquid are placed in the patient's mouth to shape appropriate swallowing. In indirect treatment, food is not involved; exercises to improve muscle strength are practiced. Medical treatment may involve various surgical procedures.

CHAPTER HIGHLIGHTS

▶ Aphasia is a neurogenic language disorder caused by a stroke. Strokes have many causes, including thrombosis and embolism. Aphasia is often classified into nonfluent, fluent, and subcortical varieties.

▶ Varieties of nonfluent aphasia include Broca's aphasia, transcortical sensory aphasia, mixed transcortical aphasia, and global aphasia. Varieties of nonfluent aphasia include Wernicke's aphasia, transcortical sensory aphasia, and conduction aphasia. Fluent aphasias are generally caused by lesions in the anterior brain structures, and nonfluent aphasias are caused

(continues)

by lesions in the posterior structures; subcortical aphasia is caused by lesions in the basal ganglia and surrounding structures and the thalamus.

▶ Relatively intact auditory comprehension and agrammatic, anomic, telegraphic, dysfluent, effortful, and sparse speech characterize nonfluent aphasia. Impaired auditory comprehension and relatively fluent, jargon-filled, and grammatically correct but semantically impaired speech characterize fluent aphasia. Treatment of aphasia targets both auditory comprehension and verbal expression; functional communication is a realistic goal for many severely involved clients.

▶ Alexia is a reading disorder due to cortical damage. Agraphia is a writing disorder due to cortical damage. Agnosia is a sensory disorder in which the meaning of sensory input in one modality is not perceived (even though peripheral sensory organs are normal), while the same input in another modality may be normally perceived.

▶ Apraxia is a motor-planning disorder due to cerebral damage. Apraxia of speech is a speech-motor planning disorder due to cerebral damage; it is characterized by articulation errors and difficulty in executing volitional movements needed for speech, with relatively intact automatic movements.

▶ Dysarthria is a speech-motor disorder due to impaired muscular control of the speech mechanism, involving peripheral or central nervous system pathology and affecting respiratory, articulatory, phonatory, resonatory, and prosodic aspects of speech.

▶ Dementia is an acquired neurological syndrome associated with persistent or progressive deterioration in intellectual functions (cognition, visuospatial skills), language, memory, emotion, and personality. It is often seen in the elderly and is typically progressive but, in some cases, is reversible.

▶ Right hemisphere syndrome is a symptom complex including perceptual, attentional, affective, and communicative deficits associated with injury to the right cerebral hemisphere.

▶ Traumatic brain injury (TBI) is injury to the brain sustained by physical trauma or external force. Penetrating injury involves a fractured or perforated skull, torn or lacerated meninges, and an injury that extends to brain tissue. Nonpenetrating brain injury involves no open wound in the head, a damaged brain within the skull, and no penetration of a foreign substance into the brain; the skull may be fractured, but the injury is nonpenetrating when the meninges are intact.

▶ Dysphagia is a swallowing disorder involving impaired execution of the oral, pharyngeal, and esophageal stages of swallow. Patients with dysphagia may receive direct treatment, indirect treatment, medical treatment, or a combination.

(continues)

▶ Add your own chapter highlights here:

_____

_____

_____

_____

KEY TERMS

acceleration-deceleration
  injuries
agnosia
agraphia
AIDS dementia complex
alexia
anomic aphasia
aphasia
apraxia
apraxia of speech
ataxic dysarthria
Broca's aphasia
cerebrovascular demen-
  tia
conduction aphasia
confabulation
constructional impair-
  ment
cortical dementia
cricopharyngeal myotomy

dementia
denial of illness
dysarthria
dysphagia
esophageal phase of
  swallow
esophagostomy
flaccid dysarthria
gastrostomy
global aphasia
hyperkinetic dysarthria
hypokinetic dysarthria
infectious dementia
left neglect
mixed dysarthria
mixed transcortical
  aphasia
nonpenetrating injury
oral phase of swallow
oral preparatory phase

of swallow
penetrating injury
pharyngeal phase of
  swallow
pharyngostomy
right hemisphere syn-
  drome
spastic dysarthria
subcortical aphasia
subcortical dementia
transcortical motor
  aphasia
transcortical sensory
  aphasia
traumatic brain injury
upper motor neuron
  dysarthria
Wernicke's aphasia

STUDY AND REVIEW QUESTIONS

Fill in the Blank

1. Aphasia is a neurologically based __*lang*__ disorder, whereas
dysarthria is a neurologically based __*speech*__ disorder.

2. Broca's area is in the _____frontal_____ lobe of the left (dominant) hemisphere.

3. Wernicke's area is in the _____temporal_____ lobe of the left (dominant) hemisphere.

4. Damage to Broca's area may cause a type of _____nonfluent_____ aphasia.

5. Damage to Wernicke's area may cause a type of _____fluent_____ aphasia.

6. Interrupted or blocked blood supply to the brain can cause _____ischemic_____ strokes.

7. Transcortical motor aphasia is a variety of _____nonfluent_____ aphasia.

8. A distinguishing feature of conduction aphasia is a disproportionate impairment in _____repetition_____ .

9. Hyperkinetic dysarthria results from damage to _____basal ganglia_____ . extrapyramidal system

10. In right hemisphere syndrome, _____perceptual_____ and _____attentional_____ problems are more severe than speech and language problems.

Multiple Choice

11. Broca's aphasia is characterized by:

    A. nonfluent, effortful, agrammatic, and slow speech.

    B. fluent grammatically correct speech full of jargon.

    C. typically significant impairment in auditory comprehension.

    D. intact confrontational naming.

    E. fluent, grammatically incorrect speech.

12. Among the following standardized tests of aphasia, the one that samples speech and language skills to only a limited extent is:

    A. the *Neurosensory Center Comprehensive Examination for Aphasia*.

    B. the *Porch Index of Communicative Ability*.

    C. the *Boston Diagnostic Aphasia Examination*.

    D. the *Western Aphasia Battery*.

    E. the Functional Living Assessment.

13. Functional communication tests seek to assess:

    A. communication in natural or everyday situations.

    B. grammatically and syntactically correct communication.

    C. only the oral communication.

    D. none of the above

    E. A, B.

14. Apraxia of speech is often associated with:

    A. lesions in Broca's area.

    B. lesions in Wernicke's area.

    C. lesions in subcortical structures.

    D. lesions in the occipital area.

    E. lesions in the cerebellum.

15. Dysarthria is:

    A. a speech disorder in the absence of muscle weakness or paralysis.

    B. a speech disorder never associated with aphasia.

    C. a single disorder with a unitary etiology.

    D. a speech disorder associated with muscle weakness or paralysis.

    E. a speech disorder characterized by groping, effortful speech.

16. Of the following, the one associated with dysarthria is:

    A. even and consistent breakdowns in articulation.

    B. impaired syntactic structures.

    C. forced inspirations and expirations that interrupt speech.

    D. an invariably slower rate of speech.

    E. an increased rate of speech under pressure.

17. Speech rate modification is a significant goal in patients with:

    A. dementia.

    B. Wernicke's aphasia.

    C. dysarthria.

    D. right hemisphere syndrome.

    E. dysphagia.

18. For a diagnosis of dementia, the American Psychiatric Association's definition requires that a patient show:

    A. personality disturbances.

    B. memory impairment.

    C. impairment in language skills.

    D. all of the above

    E. A, C

19. Dominant symptoms of patients with right hemisphere syndrome include:

    A. language disorders.

    B. speech disorders.

    C. attentional and perceptual deficits.

    D. all of the above

    E. A, B

20. The oral phase of swallow:

    A. begins with the posterior tongue action to move the bolus posteriorly.

    B. ends as the bolus passes through the anterior faucial arches.

    C. neither A or B

    D. both A and B

    E. none of the above

REFERENCES AND RECOMMENDED READINGS

Albert, M. L. (1973). A simple test of visual neglect. *Neurology, 23*, 658–664.

Bayles, K. A., & Tomoeda, C. (1991). *Arizona Battery for Communication Disorders of Dementia* (research edition). Tucson, AZ: Canyonlands Publishing.

Benson, D. F., & Ardila, A. (1996). *Aphasia: A clinical perspective.* New York: Oxford University Press.

Benton, A. L., & Hamsher, K. (1978). *Multilingual Aphasia Examination* (rev. ed.). Iowa City: University of Iowa Press.

Beukelman, D. R., & Yorkston, K. M. (1991). *Communication disorders following traumatic injury: Management of cognitive, language, and motor impairments.* Austin, TX: PRO-ED.

Bhatnagar, S. C., & Andy, O. J. (1995). *Neuroscience for the study of communicative disorders.* Baltimore, MD: Williams & Wilkins.

Bigler, E. D. (Ed.). (1990). *Traumatic brain injury.* Austin, TX: PRO-ED.

Blomert, L., Kean, M. L., Koster, C., & Schokker, J. (1994). Amsterdam-Nijmegen Everyday Language Test: Construction, reliability, and validity. *Aphasiology, 8*(4), 381–407.

Brookshire, R. (1997). *An introduction to neurogenic communication disorders* (5th ed.). St. Louis, MO: Mosby-Year Book.

Brookshire, R., & Nichols, L. E. (1993). *The Discourse Comprehension Test.* Minneapolis, MN: BRK Publishers.

Brown, J. I., Bennet, J. M., & Hanna, G. (1981). *The Nelson-Denny Reading Test.* Chicago, IL: Riverside.

Bryan, K. L. (1989). *The Right Hemisphere Language Battery.* Leicester, England: Far Communications.

Burns, M. S., Halper, A. S., & Mogil, S. I. (1985). *Clinical management of right hemisphere dysfunction.* Rockville, MD: Aspen.

Cummings, J. L., & Benson, D. F. (1992). *Dementia: A clinical approach* (2nd ed.). Boston: Butterworth-Heinemann.

Dabul, B. (1979). *Apraxia Battery for Adults.* Tigard, OR: C. C. Publications.

Darley, F. L. (1982). *Aphasia.* Philadelphia: W. B. Saunders.

Davis, G. A. (1993). *A survey of adult aphasia and related language disorders* (2nd ed.). Englewood Cliffs, NJ: Prentice-Hall.

DeRenzi, E., & Vignolo, L. A. (1962). The token test: A sensitive test to detect receptive disturbances in aphasics. *Brain, 85*, 665–678.

DeSimoni, F. G. (1989). *Comprehensive Apraxia Test* (CAT). Dalton, PA: Praxis House.

Duffy, J. R. (1995). *Motor speech disorders.* St. Louis, MO: Mosby.

Enderby, P. (1983). *Frenchay Dysarthria Assessment.* San Diego, CA: College-Hill Press.

Frattali, C. M., Thompson, C. K., Holland, A. L., Wohl, C. B., & Ferketic, M. M. (1995). *Functional assessment of communication skills for adults* (ASHA FACS). Rockville, MD: American Speech-Language-Hearing Association.

Gates, W. H. (1978). *Gates-MacGinitie Reading Test*. Chicago, IL: Riverside.

Gauthier, L., Dehaut, F., & Joanette, Y. (1989). The Bells test: A quantitative and qualitative test for visual neglect. *International Journal of Clinical Neuropsychology, 11*, 49–54.

Gillis, R. J. (1996). *Traumatic brain injury: Rehabilitation for speech–language pathologists*. Boston: Butterworth-Heinemann.

Goodglass, H., & Kaplan, E. (1983). *The assessment of aphasia and related disorders* (2nd ed.). Philadelphia: Lee & Febiger.

Groher, M. E. (1997). *Dysphagia: Diagnosis and management* (3rd ed.) Boston: Butterworth-Heinemann.

Hachinsky, V. F., Illiff, L. D., Zilhka, E., & associates (1975). Cerebral blood flow in dementia. *Archives of Neurology, 32*, 632–637.

Hagen, C., & Malkamus, D. (1979). *Interaction strategies for language disorders secondary to head trauma*. Paper presented at the annual convention of the American Speech–Language-Hearing Association, Atlanta, GA.

Hanna, G., Schell, L. M., Schreiner, R. (1977). *The Nelson Reading Skills Test*. Chicago: Riverside Publishing Company.

Hartley, L. L. (1995). *Cognitive-communicative abilities following brain injury: A functional approach*. San Diego, CA: Singular Publishing Group.

Hegde, M. N. (1996a). *A pocketguide to assessment in speech–language pathology*. San Diego, CA: Singular Publishing Group.

Hegde, M. N. (1996b). *A pocketguide to treatment in speech–language pathology*. San Diego, CA: Singular Publishing Group.

Hegde, M. N. (1998). *A coursebook on aphasia and other neurogenic language disorders* (2nd ed). San Diego, CA: Singular Publishing Group.

Helm-Estabrooks, N., & Albert, M. L. (1991). *A manual of aphasia therapy*. Austin, TX: PRO-ED.

Holland, A. L. (1980). *Communicative Abilities in Daily Living*. Baltimore, MD: University Park Press.

Keenan, J. S., & Brassell, E. G. (1975). *Aphasia Language Performance Scales*. Murphreesboro, TN: Pinnacle Press.

Kertesz, A. (1982). *Western Aphasia Battery*. New York: Gruene & Stratton.

LaPointe, L. L. (Ed.) (1997). *Aphasia and related neurogenic language disorders* (2nd ed.). New York: Thieme Medical Publishers.

LaPointe, L. L., & Horner, J. (1978). The functional auditory comprehension task (FACT): Protocol and test format. *FLASHA Journal*, 27–33.

LaPointe, L. L., & Horner, J. (1998). *Reading Comprehension Battery for Aphasia*. Austin, TX: PRO-ED.

Levin, H. S., O'Donnell, V. N., & Grossman, R. G. (1979). The Galveston orientation and amnesia test: A practical scale to assess cognition after head injury. *Journal of Nervous Mental Disorders, 167*, 675–684.

Logemann, J. A. (1998). *Evaluation and treatment of swallowing disorders*. (2nd ed.). Austin, TX: PRO-ED.

Lomas, J., Pickard, L., Bester, S., Elbard, H., Finlayson, A., & Zoghaib, C. (1989). The communicative effectiveness index: Development and psychometric evaluation of a functional communication measure for adult aphasia. *Journal of Speech and Hearing Disorders, 54*, 113–124.

Love, R. J., & Webb, W. G. (1986). *Neurology for the speech–language pathologist*. Boston: Butterworths.

Lubinski, R. (1995). *Dementia and communication*. San Diego, CA: Singular Publishing Group.

Paradis, M. (1987). *The assessment of bilingual aphasia*. Hillsdale, NJ: Lawrence Erlbaum.

Payne, J. C. (1994). *Communication profile: A functional skills survey*. Tuscon, AZ: Communication Skill Builders.

Payne, J. C. (1997). *Adult neurogenic language disorders: Assessment and treatment*. San Diego, CA: Singular Publishing Group.

Perlman, A. L., & Schulze-Delrieu, K. (1997). *Deglutition and its disorders*. San Diego, CA: Singular Publishing Group.

Pimental, P. A., & Kingsbury, N. A. (1989). *Neuropsychological aspects of right brain injury*. Austin: PRO-ED.

Porch, B. E. (1981). *Porch Index of Communicative Ability* (3rd ed.). Palo Alto, CA: Consulting Psychologists Press.

Reisberg, B., Ferris, S. H., DeLeon, M. J., & Crook, T. (1982). The global deterioration scale for assessment of primary degenerative dementia. *American Journal of Psychiatry, 139*, 1136–1139.

Rosenbek, J., LaPointe, C., & Wertz, T. (1989). *Aphasia: A clinical approach*. Austin, TX: PRO-ED.

Sarno, M. T. (1969). *The functional communication profile: Manual of directions*. New York: New York University Medical Center, Institute of Rehabilitation Medicine.

Sarno, M. T. (Ed.). (1981). *Acquired aphasia*. New York: Academic Press.

Schuell, H. M. (1972). *The Minnesota Test of Differential Diagnosis of Aphasia*. Minneapolis: University of Minnesota Press.

Shadden, B. B., & Toner, M. A. (Eds.). (1997). *Aging and communication*. Austin, TX: PRO-ED.

Shekim, L. O. (1997). Dementia. In L. L. LaPointe (Ed.), *Aphasia and related neurogenic language disorders* (2nd ed.) (pp. 238–249). New York: Thieme Medical Publishers.

Shewan, C. M. (1979). *Auditory Comprehension Test for Sentences*. Chicago: Biolinguistics Clinical Institutes.

Sklar, M. (1966). *Sklar Aphasia Scale*. Los Angeles: Western Psychological Services.

Spreen, O., & Benton, A. L. (1977). *Neurosensory Center Comprehensive Examination for Aphasia*. Victoria, BC: University of Victoria.

Stanczak, D. E., & associates (1984). Assessment of level of consciousness following severe neurological insult. *Journal of Neurosurgery, 60*, 955–960.

Teasdale, G., & Jennett, B. (1976). Assessment and prognosis of coma after head injury. *Acta Neurochirargica (Wien), 34*, 45–55.

Tompkins, C. A. (1995). *Right hemisphere communication disorders: Theory and management*. San Diego, CA: Singular Publishing Group.

Wallace, G. L. (1998). Neurogenic disorders in adult and pediatric populations. In D. E. Battle (Ed.), *Communication disorders in multicultural populations* (2nd ed.), pp. 309–333. Newton, MA: Butterworth-Heinemann.

Webster, D. W. (1995). *Neuroscience of communication*. San Diego, CA: Singular Publishing Group.

West, J. F., Sands, E. S., & Ross-Swain, D. (1998). *Bedside Evaluation Screening Test–Second Edition*. Austin, TX: PRO-ED.

Whurr, R. (1974). *Aphasia Screening Test*. Obtainable from 2 Alwyne Road, London, NI2HH, England.

Wilson, B. A., Cockburn, J., & Halligan, P. (1987). *Behavioral Inattention Test*. Suffolk, England: Thames Valley Test Company.

West, J. F., Sands, E. S., & Ross-Swain, D. (1998). *Bedside Evaluation Screening Test–Second Edition*. Austin, TX: PRO-ED.

Wirz, S., Skinner, C., & Dean, E. (1990). *Revised Edinburgh functional communication profile*. Tuscon, AZ: Communication Skill Builders.

Yorkston, K. M., & Beukelman, D. R. (1981). *Assessment of intelligibility of dysarthric speakers*. Tigard, OR: C. C. Publications.

ANSWERS TO STUDY AND REVIEW QUESTIONS

1. Language, speech

2. Frontal

3. Temporal

4. Nonfluent

5. Fluent

6. Ischemic

7. Nonfluent

8. Repetition

9. The basal ganglia (or the extrapyramidal system)

10. Perceptual, attentional

11. A. Broca's aphasia is characterized by nonfluent, effortful, agrammatic, and slow speech.

12. B. Among the specified standardized tests of aphasia, the one that samples speech and language skills to only a limited extent is the *Porch Index of Communicative Ability*.

13. A. Functional communication tests seek to assess communication in natural or everyday situations.

14. A. Apraxia of speech is often associated with lesions in Broca's area.

15. D. Dysarthria is a speech disorder associated with muscle weakness or paralysis.

16. C. Of the stated disorders, the one associated with dysarthria is forced inspirations and expirations that interrupt speech.

17. C. Speech rate modification is a significant goal in patients with dysarthria.

18. B. For a diagnosis of dementia, the American Psychiatric Association's definition requires that a patient show memory impairment.

19. C. Dominant symptoms of patients with right hemisphere syndrome include attentional and perceptual deficits.

20. D. The oral phase of swallow both begins with the posterior tongue action to move the bolus posteriorly and ends as the bolus passes through the anterior faucial arches.

CHAPTER 9

Communication Disorders in Multicultural Populations

PREVIEW OUTLINE

CHAPTER INTRODUCTION

The United States has been likened to a kaleidoscope that is constantly changing colors and becoming more and more diverse. With increasing numbers of culturally and linguistically diverse (CLD) adults and children in the United States, the number of those who have disorders of communication is also increasing. Clinicians frequently find themselves attempting to effectively serve an increasingly diverse client group, but these clinicians also find that they do not have the appropriate tools. Research is scarce; an empirical foundation upon which to build assessment and treatment is lacking. But the field of communication disorders must do its best, with its current knowledge and tools, to effectively and knowledgeably serve CLD adults and children with communication disorders.

In this chapter, we begin by presenting foundational issues concerning the serving of CLD clients. We then describe speech–language characteristics of African American, Hispanic, and Asian clients and the ramifications for assessment and treatment. Next, we discuss the differentiation of language differences and language disorders in children. Included in this discussion are issues of second-language acquisition and bilingualism. Knowledge of second-language acquisition and bilingualism is critical to a fair and unbiased assessment of CLD children. We describe considerations in the use of standardized tests, alternatives to standardized tests, and important concepts in working with interpreters in the assessment process. In our section on treatment considerations, we discuss issues related to treatment of CLD children with language-learning disabilities, as well as treatment considerations for CLD adults with neurologically based disorders of communication.

FOUNDATIONAL ISSUES

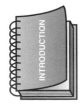

There is an increasing number of CLD people living in the United States. Speech–language pathologists need to understand basic cultural characteristics that can impact service delivery to these persons. The American Speech–Language-Hearing Association has developed policies and position statements that provide guidance for clinicians who work with CLD clients.

Demographic Data

■ The increasing diversity in the United States comes primarily from two sources: increases in birth rates among CLD groups, and immigration trends. In 1820, 92% of immigrants were of European background; in 1990, 7% of immigrants were of European descent (U.S. Bureau of the Census, 1992).

■ During the 21st century, racial and ethnic minorities will outnumber Whites; by the year 2005, Whites will have a 0.8% population decrease (Horton & Smith, 1993). Demographers project that by the year 2020, one out of every three people in the United States will be from what is currently referred to as a "minority group."

■ The number of CLD children increases constantly. It is estimated that by the year 2000, at least one third of schoolchildren in the United States will be African American, Hispanic, Asian, or Native American (Lane & Molyneaux, 1992).

■ Some states have especially great diversity; in California, for example, over 130 languages are represented in the schools. In one high school in Buffalo, New York, students from 55 countries speak 47 different languages (Goldberg, 1997).

■ The population of CLD elderly is also growing. It is estimated that between 1997 and 2000, the African American elderly population will increase by 21.5% (over 3 million). The Hispanic elderly population is projected to have an increase of 21.5% between 1987 and 2000. In 1980, approximately 325,000 Asians/Pacific Islanders were over 60 years old; that number is increasing (Payne, 1995).

■ With the growing number of CLD children and older adults, it is logical that there are more and more CLD clients who have communication disorders. Data from the 1990 U.S. Census indicate that close to 25% of the population is comprised of federally designated minorities.

■ If the prevalence of communication disorders among these groups is consistent with that for the general United States population (10%), it can be estimated that in the United States, 2.9 million African Americans, 2.2 million Hispanics, 0.72 million Asian Americans, and 0.19 million Native Americans have communication disorders (Quinn, Goldstein, & Peña, 1996). Clearly, there is a great need for information about effective service delivery to the country's culturally diverse population.

General Cultural Considerations

Basic Principles

■ When working with CLD clients of all ages, it is important to have a basic understanding of what culture is. Although there are probably hundreds of definitions, it can be agreed that culture is a dynamic, multifaceted phenomenon that is influenced by many variables.

- *Culture* can be viewed as a framework through which actions are filtered as individuals go about the business of daily living (Lynch, 1998). Culture includes the beliefs, behaviors, and values of a group of people (Battle, 1998). At the heart of culture are values; thus, when we study other cultures, it is important to examine that culture's underlying values.

- In order to understand CLD children and their families, we must first understand the cultural groups of which they are a part. A danger of attempting to understand any group, however, is that stereotyping and overgeneralizing may occur. *Stereotypes* can be viewed as a means of categorizing others based upon perceptions that are incomplete.

- Ideally, speech–language pathologists should understand *tendencies* of various cultural groups so that students and families may be viewed as individuals within the general framework of their community and culture (L. L. Cheng, personal communication, 1993).

- Professionals need to keep in mind the great heterogeneity within cultural groups. It is optimal to take a situational approach, wherein each individual is viewed as unique, with shifting needs, characteristics, and strengths.

- It is important for speech–language pathologists to develop as much cultural sensitivity as possible. This can be done through a variety of activities that focus on continually learning more about the cultures of the clients served.

- Reading literature, conducting home visits, and talking to families and community members about the cultures in question will help clinicians become increasingly sensitive to and aware of cultural variables that can impact service delivery (Roseberry-McKibbin, 1997a).

Variables Influencing Individual Behavior Within a Culture

- A number of variables influence the behavior of individuals within a culture. The combination of general cultural practices and individual characteristics of people within cultures influences service delivery to those clients and their families (Battle, 1998). Potential variables of influence upon individuals include:

  - *educational level*, which may be quite basic (e.g., several years of schooling) or sophisticated and extensive;

  - *language(s) spoken*, including the prestige of the language(s) in the area of residence and the level of skill in each language;

  - *length of residence in an area*;

  - *country of birth* (foreign born or native born), which relates to immigrant or refugee status versus being born in the United States;

    — *urban versus rural background*;

    — *gender*;

    — *religion*;

    — *age*;

    — *generational membership*;

    — *socioeconomic status or upward class mobility*;

    — *neighborhood and peer group*;

    — *degree of acculturation into mainstream American life*;

    — *outmarriage* (marriage to people from different ethnic backgrounds); and

    — *individual choice within the intrapersonal realm.*

Concepts To Consider

Discuss the issue of culture in service delivery to CLD clients and their families. What is culture? What specific variables influence an individual's behavior within a culture?

_____

_____

_____

_____

_____

_____

_____

_____

_____

_____

ASHA Guidelines Regarding Multicultural Issues

■ Due to the increasing cultural and linguistic diversity in the United States, ASHA has developed policies, position statements, and guidelines regarding service delivery to CLD clients.

■ ASHA's Office of Multicultural Affairs and its Multicultural Issues Board are active in creation and implementation of these guidelines. Copies of guidelines and policies are available; interested people can contact the national office in Rockville Pike, MD. ASHA has also created Special Interest Division (SID #14), Communication Disorders and Sciences in Culturally and Linguistically Diverse Populations.

■ It is important to have a basic knowledge of the various position statements in order to provide effective service delivery that is consistent with ASHA's policies. ASHA has published several new position statements and technical reports about service delivery to people from diverse backgrounds.

■ ASHA (1998) states that speech–language pathologists may provide ESL (English as a Second Language) instruction in the public schools if they possess the required skills and knowledge to do so.

■ ASHA (1998; Joint Subcommittee of the Executive Board on English Language Proficiency) also states that it is discriminatory not to accept individuals into the professions or into higher education programs solely on the basis of an accent or dialect. Speech pathologists with accents and/or dialects can provide effective services as long as they have the expected level of professional knowledge and can model target behaviors for clients.

Summary

☑ The increasing number of multicultural people living in the United States makes it imperative for clinicians to be sensitive to cultural issues that impact service delivery.

☑ A number of variables, such as age and generational membership, impact the behavior of individual clients from various cultures.

☑ ASHA has published guidelines regarding effective service delivery to clients from linguistically and culturally diverse backgrounds.

SPEECH–LANGUAGE CHARACTERISTICS OF CLD CLIENTS

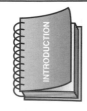

INTRODUCTION

When attempting to ascertain whether clients are manifesting language differences or language disorders, it is important to have a basic understanding of how various dialects and languages influence the production of Standard American English (SAE). It is also criti-

(continues)

cal to remember that within each language group, there is great diversity. For example, the Philippines, a country the size of Arizona, has more than 87 mutually unintelligible languages (Roseberry-McKibbin, 1997b).

Unfortunately, it is common for adults and especially children to be labeled as having a "disorder" when, in fact, they are merely manifesting language differences that are attributable to their primary language or dialect. For example, clients whose first language is Spanish, an African American Language, or an Asian language will manifest characteristics of articulation, morphology, and syntax especially that differ from patterns of SAE. Clients who speak a dialect of American English may also manifest such characteristics. In this section, we discuss dialects of American English, African American Language (AAL), Spanish-influenced English, and English influenced by Asian languages.

Dialects of American English

■ In the United States, Standard American English is used in government communications, printing, national television newscasts, and many businesses. Many consider SAE to be the official language of the United States.

■ Every language is spoken somewhat differently by different subgroups of a linguistic community. SAE has several dialects; each one has characteristic sound patterns, including typical expressions and unique accents.

■ Dialectal differences are due to several interrelated factors, including geographic region, socioeconomic level, speaking situation, and subgroup membership.

■ With regard to geographic region, people living in different parts of the United States develop variations of language use and production. Based on geographic regions, specialists have identified 10 major dialects of SAE: New York City, Eastern New England, Western Pennsylvania, Appalachian, Southern, Middle Atlantic, Central Midland, Southwest, Northwest, and North Central (see Figure 9.1).

African American Language

General Background

■ African American Language has undergone many changes in nomenclature. It has been called Black Dialect, Black English, Black English Vernacular, African American English, and Ebonics. The changes in nomenclature have been due in part to increasingly sophisticated understanding of AAL, and to changes in sociolinguistic theory.

■ Use of AAL is influenced by a number of factors, including retention of some African language patterns; geographic region; socioeconomic status, education,

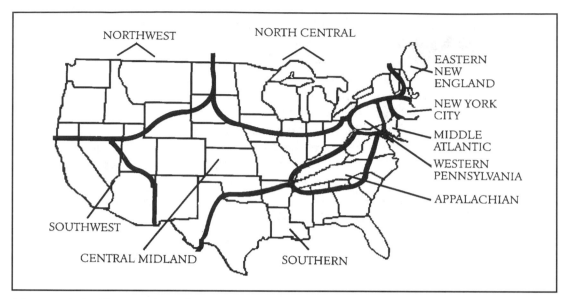

Figure 9.1. The major dialects of American English. From *Introduction to Communicative Disorders* (p. 481), by M. N. Hegde, 1995, Austin, TX: PRO-ED. Copyright 1995 by PRO-ED, Inc. Reprinted with permission.

gender, and age of the speaker; and bonding between members of the African American community (Chambers, 1983; Terrell, Battle, and Grantham, 1998; Wyatt, 1998a)

■ Dillard (1972) estimated that approximately 80% of African Americans use AAL. Middle-class African Americans may use AAL less than working-class African Americans, especially in formal settings (Iglesias & Anderson, 1998).

■ A number of West African languages have impacted modern-day African American Language: Bambara, Ewe, Fanta, Fon, Fula, Ga, Ibo, Ibibio, Kimbundu, Longo, Mandinka, Mende, Twi, Imbundu, Wolof, and Yoruba (LeMoine, 1993; Willis, 1998)

Misconceptions About AAL

■ There are some widespread assumptions and misconceptions about AAL and its speakers, listed below. It is important to be aware of these misconceptions so that AAL speakers will not be mistakenly identified as having disorders.

■ *All African Americans speak AAL.* Some African Americans speak AAL; some do not. Some code-switch back and forth between mainstream American English and AAL depending on variables such as changes in topic, listener, and communicative intent (Terrell et al., 1998; Wyatt, 1998a). African Americans who are socialized primarily with Anglos will generally speak mainstream American English (Wolfram, 1986).

■ *AAL is spoken only by African Americans.* AAL can be spoken by people of any ethnic and linguistic background. Non-African Americans may speak AAL if their primary peer group is composed of African Americans. For example, some Puerto Rican students in New York City speak AAL. Some Anglo students in Oakland, California, speak AAL.

■ *AAL is a substandard form of mainstream American English.* Some people historically took a "deficit perspective"; a major premise of this view was that African Americans were cognitively unable to learn mainstream American English (LeMoine, 1993). The *ethnolinguistic theory* of today states that AAL is a language in its own right; its roots can be traced to many languages of West Africa. AAL is systematic and rule governed.

■ *AAL does not have a regular, predictable system.* AAL is a rule-governed system in which patterns can be predicted based on rules.

■ *AAL needs to be eradicated in students who speak it.* Some experts believe that speakers of AAL should become "bilingual" or "bidialectal" so that they can fluently speak both AAL and SAE (Campbell, 1993; LeMoine, 1993). In this optimal situation, students preserve their culture, heritage, and community dialect as well as learning a style of speaking that is required in some daily situations, school learning experiences, and future places of employment.

■ *Use of standardized language tests with AAL speakers is a nonbiased indicator of actual language knowledge and skill.* Many currently used assessment instruments in schools are normed and standardized on Anglo, middle-class, monolingual English speakers. These tests have been criticized by many experts as being inappropriate for use with African American children (Washington, 1996; Wyatt, 1997).

■ Many standardized tests of morphosyntactic skill, especially in the field of speech–language pathology, are biased against AAL speakers (and students from other non-English backgrounds, also). Table 9.1 shows examples of bias against speakers of AAL on formal, standardized language tests.

■ It is recommended that alternative forms of assessment, including language sample analysis (Stockman, 1996), contrastive analysis (McGregor, Williams, Hearst, & Johnson, 1997), and description of children's functional communication skills (Campbell, 1996), be used when assessing children who speak AAL. It is also recommended that standardized tests of aphasia be appropriately modified for adults who speak AAL.

Characteristics of AAL Morphology, Syntax, and Articulation

■ When AAL speakers are tested, it is critical to know which aspects of their speech and language are reflective of AAL rules and which aspects are indicative of a disorder. Many speech–language pathologists take AAL children in

TABLE 9.1

Examples of Bias Against Speakers of African American
Language on Formal Language and Intelligence Tests

1. Grammatical judgment items.
   ▶ Examiner: Tell me whether the following sentences are correct or incorrect:
   Them girls is having a good time.
   The boys is going to the party.
   We don't have no time to talk to you.

2. Sentence repetition tasks.
   ▶ Examiner: Repeat these sentences after me. Remember to say them EXACTLY like I say them!
   Neither of the children are using the swings.
   They had been hungry.
   She looks at the big, brown dog.

3. Grammatic closure tasks.
   ▶ Examiner: I am going to say some sentences. I want you to fill in the word that is missing. For example, "A rose is a flower and a daisy is a flower. Daisies and roses are both _____." Now you do some:
   Today I play the marimba; yesterday I _____ the marimba.
   I have a cat, and you have a cat; we have two _____.
   Today Sue <u>is</u> going to the store; yesterday she _____ going to the store.

4. Receptive grammatical tasks.
   ▶ Examiner: We are going to look at some pictures. Each page has three pictures. When I say a sentence, you point to the picture that goes with the sentence I say. Here's the first picture.
   Show me "The cat<u>s</u> are playing in the garden."
   Now, show me "He play<u>ed</u> baseball."
   Point to "They <u>have been</u> painting the fence."

5. Articulation and phonological tasks. Most tests of articulation and phonology are normed on Anglo children. The speech–language pathologist must remember to take into account the unique characteristics of AAL when assessing articulation and phonology.

Note. From *Multicultural Students with Special Language Needs: Practical Strategies for Assessment and Intervention* (p. 239), by C. Roseberry-McKibbin, 1995, Oceanside, CA: Academic Communication Associates. Copyright 1995 by Academic Communication Associates. Reprinted with permission.

the public schools onto their caseloads for "remediation" of AAL. Not only is this illegal, but it is often unsuccessful, as well.

■ However, some adult speakers of AAL may elect to become bidialectal in that they become proficient in SAE as well as AAL. Being bidialectal enables these speakers to maintain their use of AAL while also being able to use SAE for purposes such as business with non-AAL speakers.

■ When speech–language pathologists are aware of what normal AAL characteristics are, they can then distinguish between a language difference and a language disorder. Table 9.2 shows characteristics of AAL morphology and syntax, while Table 9.3 shows characteristics of AAL articulation and phonology. Table 9.4 shows some examples of acceptable utterances by speakers of AAL.

Spanish-Influenced English

General Background

■ The term *Hispanic* is a label of convenience used to refer to people who were born in or trace the background of their families to one of the Spanish-speaking Latin American nations or to Spain, and reside in the United States. Hispanics may also come from Carribean countries such as Puerto Rico and Cuba.

■ *Hispanic* is used as an ethnic label by the Bureau of the Census; it does not denote a race, because most Hispanics are racially mixed, including combinations of American Indian, African Black, and European White. The majority are Mestizo, having both a European and an Indian heritage (Langdon, 1992).

Spanish-Language Characteristics and Considerations

■ The diversity among Spanish speakers is very great. Although Spanish is spoken in Spain, all of Latin America, and most of South America, there are variations, which are reflected mostly in pronunciation and some vocabulary.

■ Spanish speakers in the United States may speak different dialects or varieties of Spanish. Thus, clinicians must consider the individual client's background and origins, which are reflected in the particular variety of Spanish used, and not assume that each Spanish-speaking student can be viewed in the same way.

■ Spanish-speaking students who learn English as a second language may manifest differences with SAE in articulation of sounds and in morphosyntactic structures. There are many structural differences between English and Spanish, especially with respect to morphology (Anderson, 1996).

■ These differences are not indicative of a disorder requiring intervention, but rather are differences that are normal and to be expected. It is important for professionals who work with Spanish-speaking clients to understand some basic information regarding Spanish-influenced English (Kayser, 1998). Table 9.5 describes articulation characteristics of Spanish and the possible influences

(text continues on page 498)

TABLE 9.2

Characteristics of African American Language Morphology and Syntax

AAL Feature/Characteristic	Mainstream American English	Sample AAL Utterance
Omission of noun possessive	That's the woman's car It's John's pencil	That *the woman* car. It *John* pencil.
Omission of noun plural	He has two boxes of apples. She gives me five cents.	He got two *box* of *apple*. She give me five *cent*.
Omission of third-person singular present-tense marker	She walks to school. The man works in his yard.	She *walk* to school. The man *work* in his yard.
Omission of *to be* forms such as *is, are*	She is a nice lady. They are going to a movie.	*She a* nice lady. *They going* to a move.
Present-tense *is* used regardless of person/number	They are having fun. You are a smart man.	*They is* having fun. *You is* a smart man!
Lack of person-number agreement with past and present forms of *to be*	You are playing ball. They are having a picnic.	You *is* playing ball. They *is* having a picnic.
Present-tense forms of auxiliary *have* omitted	I have been here for two hours. He has done it again.	I been here for two hours. He done it again.
Past-tense endings omitted	He lived in California. She cracked the nut.	He *live* in California. She *crack* the nut.
Past *was* used regardless of number and person	They were shopping. You were helping me.	They *was* shopping. You *was* helping me.
Multiple negatives (each additional negative form adds emphasis to the negative meaning)	We don't have any more. I don't want any cake. I don't like broccoli.	We don't have *no more*. I don't never want *no* cake. I don't *never* like broccoli.
None substituted for any	She doesn't want any.	She don't want *none*.
Perfective construction; *been* used to indicate that an action took place in the distant past.	I had the mumps when I was 5. I have known her for years.	I *been had* the mumps when I was 5. I *been known* her.
Done combined with a past-tense form to indicate that an action was started and completed	He fixed the stove. She tried to paint it.	He *done fixed* the stove. She *done tried* to paint it.
The form *be* used as the main verb	Today she is working. We are singing.	Today *she be* working. *We be* singing.
Distributive *be* used to indicate actions and events over time	He is often cheerful. She's kind sometimes.	*He be* cheerful. *She be* kind.
Pronoun used to restate the subject	My brother surprised me. My dog has fleas.	My brother, *he* surprise me. My dog, *he* got fleas.
Them substituted for *those*	Those cars are antiques. Where'd you get those books?	*Them* cars, they be antique. Where you get *them* books?
Future-tense *is, are* replaced by *gonna*	She is going to help us. They are going to be there.	She *gonna* help us. They *gonna* be there.
At used at the end of *where* questions	Where is the house? Where is the store?	Where is the house *at*? Where is the store *at*?
Additional auxiliaries often used	I might have done it.	I *might could have* done it.
Does replaced by *do*	She does funny things It does make sense.	She *do* funny things. It *do* make sense.

Note. From *Multicultural Students with Special Language Needs: Practical Strategies for Assessment and Intervention* (pp. 52–53), by C. Roseberry-McKibbin, 1995, Oceanside, CA: Academic Communication Associates. Copyright 1995 by Academic Communication Associates. Reprinted with permission.

TABLE 9.3

Characteristics of African American Language, Articulation, and Phonology

AAL Feature/Characteristic	Mainstream American English	African American Language
/l/ phoneme lessened or omitted	tool always	too' a'ways
/r/ phoneme lessened or omitted	door mother protect	doah mudah p'otek
f/voiceless *th* substitution at end or middle of word	teeth both nothing	teef bof nufin'
t/voiceless *th* substitution in beginning of a word	think thin	tink tin
d/voiced *th* substitution at the beginning, middle of words	this brother	dis broder
v/voiced *th* substitution at the end of words	breathe smooth	breave smoov
consonant-cluster reduction	desk rest left wasp	des' res' lef' was'
differing syllable stress patterns	guitar police July	*gui*tar *po*lice *Ju*ly
Verbs ending in /k/ are changed	liked walked	li-tid wah-tid
Metathesis occurs	ask	aks ("axe")
Devoicing of final voiced consonants	bed rug cab	bet ruk cap
Final consonants may be deleted	bad good	ba' goo'
I/E substitution	pen ten	pin tin
b/v substitution	valentine vest	balentine bes'
diphthong reduction	find oil pound	fahnd ol pond
n/ng substitution	walking thing	walkin' thin

Note. Characteristics may vary depending on variables such as geographic region. From *Multicultural Students with Special Language Needs: Practical Strategies for Assessment and Intervention* (pp. 54–55), by C. Roseberry-McKibbin, 1995, Oceanside, CA: Academic Communication Associates. Copyright 1995 by Academic Communication Associates. Reprinted with permission.

TABLE 9.4

Examples of Acceptable Utterances by Speakers of African American Language

Standard American English	African American Language
That boy looks like me.	That boy, he look like me.
If he kicks it, he'll be in trouble.	If he kick it, he be in trouble.
When the lights are off, it's dark.	When the lights be off, it dark.
It could be somebody's pet.	It could be somebody pet.
Her feet are too big.	Her feet is too big.
I'll get something to eat.	I will get me something to eat.
She is dancing and the music's on.	She be dancin' an' the music on.
What kind of cheese do you want?	What kind of cheese you want?
My brother's name is Joe.	My brother name is Joe.
I raked the leaves outside.	I rakted the leaves outside.
After the recital, they shook my hand.	After the recital, they shaketed my hand.
They are standing around.	They is just standing around.
He is a basketball star.	He a basketball star.
They are in cages.	They be in cages.
It's not like a tree or anything.	It not like a tree or nothin'.
He does like to fish.	He do like to fish.
They are going to swim.	They gonna swim.
Mom already repaired the car.	Mom done repair the car.

Note. From *Multicultural Students with Special Language Needs: Practical Strategies for Assessment and Intervention* (p. 241), by C. Roseberry-McKibbin, 1995, Oceanside, CA: Academic Communication Associates. Copyright 1995 by Academic Communication Associates. Reprinted with permission.

on pronunciation of English. Table 9.6 describes morphosyntactic characteristics of Spanish and possible influences on English production.

 Concepts To Consider

List two articulation differences that Spanish and African American Language speakers might manifest that could be misinterpreted as signs of an articulation disorder (e.g., d/th). List two differences for each language background.

_____

_____

_____

TABLE 9.5

Articulation Differences Commonly Observed Among Spanish Speakers

Articulation Characteristics	Sample English Patterns
/t, d, n/ may be dentalized (tip of tongue is placed against the back of the upper central incisors).	
Final consonants are often devoiced	dose/doze
b/v substitution	berry/very
Deaspirated stops (sounds like speaker is omitting the sound because it is said with little air release).	
ch/sh substitution	Chirley/Shirley
d/voiced th, or z/voiced th (voiced *th* does not exist in Spanish).	dis/this, zat/that
t/voiceless th (voiceless *th* does not exist in Spanish).	tink/think
Schwa sound inserted before word-initial consonant clusters	eskate/skate espend/spend
Words can end in 10 different sounds: a, e, i, o, u, l, r, n, s, d	may omit sounds at the ends of words
When words start with /h/, the /h/ is silent	'old/hold, 'it/hit
/r/ is tapped or trilled (tap /r/ might sound like the tap in the English word *butter*)	
There is no /j/ (e.g., judge) sound in Spanish; speakers may substitute *y*	Yulie/Julie yoke/joke
Frontal /s/ (Spanish /s/ is produced more frontally than English /s/)	Some speakers may sound like they have frontal lisps
The ñ is pronounced like a *y* (e.g., *baño* is pronounced *bahnyo*).	
Spanish has 5 vowels: a, e, i, o, u (ah, E, ee, o, u) and few diphthongs. Thus, Spanish speakers may produce the following vowel substitutions:	
ee/I substitution	peeg/pig, leetle/little
E/ae, ah/ae substitutions	pet/pat Stahn/Stan

Note. From *Multicultural Students with Special Language Needs: Practical Strategies for Assessment and Intervention* (p. 68), by C. Roseberry-McKibbin, 1995, Oceanside, CA: Academic Communication Associates. Copyright 1995 by Academic Communication Associates. Reprinted with permission.

TABLE 9.6

Language Differences Commonly Observed Among Spanish Speakers

Language Characteristics	Sample English Utterances
Adjective comes after noun.	The *house green*.
s is often omitted in plurals and possessives.	The *girl* book is... Juan *hat* is red.
Past-tense *ed* is often omitted.	We *walk* yesterday.
Double negatives are required.	I don't have *no more*.
Superiority is demonstrated by using *mas*.	This cake is *more* big.
The adverb often follows the verb.	He drives very fast his motorcycle.

Note. From *Multicultural Students with Special Language Needs: Practical Strategies for Assessment and Intervention* (p. 67), by C. Roseberry-McKibbin, 1995, Oceanside, CA: Academic Communication Associates. Copyright 1995 by Academic Communication Associates. Reprinted with permission.

English Influenced by Asian Languages

General Background

- Asians originate from three primary geographic regions:

    - Southeast Asia: the Philippines, Laos, Cambodia, Thailand, Indonesia, Singapore, Burma, Vietnam, and Malaysia

    - South Asia: Sri Lanka, Pakistan, and India

    - East Asia: Japan, Korea, and China

- Many Asians originate from countries in the Pacific Rim. The Pacific Rim includes all nations and regions touching the Pacific Ocean.

- The "Asian/Pacific Islander" population in the United States grew by 95% between 1980 and 1990; the largest group growth was among the Hmong, who increased by 1,631% (Gall & Gall, 1993).

Speech–Language Characteristics and Considerations

- Some of the most widely spoken Asian languages in the United States include Chinese, Filipino, Vietnamese, Japanese, Khmer, and Korean.

- Many Asian languages have numerous dialects that may or may not be mutually intelligible; for example, there are over 87 mutually unintelligible dialects in China and the Philippines (Roseberry-McKibbin, 1997b; Cheng, 1998).

- Some groups have no written language and rely on oral traditions.

■ Vietnamese, Chinese, and Laotian are tonal languages; each tone change (toneme) is phonemic in nature and represents a meaning change. For example, in Mandarin, "ma" can *mean mother, horse, scold, flax,* or *curse* depending on the tone used in pronouncing it.

■ Mandarin has four tonemes; Cantonese has seven tonemes; Northern Vietnamese has six tonemes; Central and Southern Vietnamese each have five tonemes.

■ Japanese, Khmer, and Korean are not tonal languages.

■ Chinese, Vietnamese, and Laotian are basically monosyllabic.

■ Chinese and Vietnamese have no consonant blends (Cheng, 1998).

■ Many languages, such as Chinese, do not have inflectional markers.

■ Some languages (e.g., Indonesian, Japanese, and Tagalog) do not have specific gender pronouns (do not differentiate between he, she, it).

■ Asian speakers' prosody or intonation in English may sound very "choppy" and monotonous.

■ Some Asian speakers may sound hypernasal in English.

■ It is very difficult to provide generalities about Asian speakers' English patterns due to the vast variety in Asian languages and dialects. Thus, the examples in Tables 9.7 and 9.8 may or may not be representative of various students; each must be assessed on an individual basis.

Summary

☑ Knowledge of the influence of a primary language or dialect on English production is critical for differentiating language differences from language problems in CLD speakers.

☑ Speakers of African American Language, Spanish, and Asian languages have unique and predictable characteristics, based on primary-language influence, that are signs of differences and not disorders.

☑ These differences do not need to be remediated; however, some speakers may seek elective intervention so that their productions may more closely approximate Standard American English.

TABLE 9.7

Language Differences Commonly Observed Among Asian Speakers

Language Characteristics	Sample English Utterances
Omission of plurals	Here are two *piece* of toast I got five *finger* on each hand.
Omission of copula	He *going* home now. They *eating*.
Omission of possessive	I have *Phuong* pencil. *Mom* food is cold.
Omission of past-tense morpheme	We *cook* dinner yesterday. Last night she *walk* home.
Past-tense double marking	He *didn't went* by himself.
Double negative	They *don't have no* books.
Subject-verb-object relationship differences/omissions	I messed *up it*. *He like*.
Singular present-tense omission or addition	*You goes* inside. *He go* to the store.
Misordering of interrogatives	You are going now?
Misuse or omission of prepositions	She is *in* home. He goes to school 8:00.
Misuse of pronouns	*She* husband is coming. She said *her wife* is here.
Omission and/or overgeneralization of articles	*Boy* is sick. He went *the home*.
Incorrect use of comparatives	This book is *gooder* than that book.
Omission of conjunctions	You I going to the beach.
Omission, lack of inflection on auxiliary *do*	She not take it. He *do not* have enough.
Omission, lack of inflection on forms of *have*	She *have* no money. We been the store.
Omission of articles	I see little cat.

Note. From *Multicultural Students with Special Language Needs: Practical Strategies for Assessment and Intervention* (p. 81), by C. Roseberry-McKibbin, 1995, Oceanside, CA: Academic Communication Associates. Copyright 1995 by Academic Communication Associates. Reprinted with permission.

TABLE 9.8

Articulation Differences Observed Commonly Among Asian Speakers

Articulation Characteristics	Sample English Utterances	
In many Asian languages, words end in vowels only or in just a few consonants; speakers may delete many final consonants in English.	ste/step ro/robe	li/lid do/dog
Some languages are monosyllabic; speakers may truncate polysyllabic words or emphasize the wrong syllable.	efunt/elephant DIversity/diversity	
Possible devoicing of voiced cognates	beece/bees luff/love	pick/pig crip/crib
r/l confusion	lize/rise	clown/crown
/r/ may be omitted entirely	gull/girl	tone/torn
Reduction of vowel length in words	Words sound choppy to Americans	
No voiced or voiceless *th*	dose/those zose/those	tin/thin sin/thin
Epenthesis (addition of *uh* sound in blends, ends of words).	bulack/black	wooduh/wood
Confusion of *ch* and *sh*	sheep/cheap	beesh/beach
/ae/ does not exist in many Asian languages	block/black	shock/shack
b/v substitutions	base/vase	Beberly/Beverly
v/w substitutions	vork/work	vall/wall
p/f substitutions	pall/fall	plower/flower

Note. From *Multicultural Students with Special Language Needs: Practical Strategies for Assessment and Intervention* (p. 82), by C. Roseberry-McKibbin, 1995, Oceanside, CA: Academic Communication Associates. Copyright 1995 by Academic Communication Associates. Reprinted with permission.

LANGUAGE DIFFERENCES AND LANGUAGE-LEARNING DISABILITIES

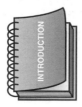

Clinicians around the United States are continually confronted with the need to distinguish language differences from language-learning disabilities (LLD). This challenging process is impacted by the unique processes of second-language acquisition and by the nature of bilingualism and language proficiency. Knowledge of basic facts about acquiring a second language can help clinicians make accurate decisions in distinguishing language differences from LLDs in CLD children (Roseberry-McKibbin, 1994).

Differentiating Language Differences from Language-Learning Disabilities

- When clinicians are confronted with CLD students who appear to be struggling in school, the first question they usually ask is: "Does this student have a language difference or an LLD?"

- In other words, can the problems be traced to cultural differences or the student's lack of facility with English, or is there an underlying language learning disability that requires special education intervention?

- Bloom and Lahey (1978) defined language as a system of symbols used to represent concepts that are formed through exposure and experience. Clinicians must ask about students' environmental and linguistic exposure and experience.

- Some CLD students do not have the environmental and linguistic exposure and experience that are assumed by schools. They may come from nonliterate backgrounds, for example, or from backgrounds where the language is oral only and has not been put in written form.

- Some clinicians do not stop to ask themselves whether students have had any of the usual mainstream experiences that are inherently assumed, like exposure to literacy.

- This is often where deficits in students are created: When students' exposure and experiences are different than those expected in the mainstream school environment, clinicians may assume that there are deficits inherent in the students themselves.

- If students' background experiences and exposure to life situations and linguistic models are different than those expected by schools, then it follows that their language, which represents their unique backgrounds, will not be consistent with that expected by the school (Cheng, 1996).

- This difference in students' backgrounds and schools' expectations can lead to misdiagnosis of students and consequent inappropriate placement into special education (Crago, Eriks-Brophy, Pesco, & McAlpine, 1997). Historically in U.S. schools, disproportionate numbers of CLD children have been placed in special education unnecessarily.

- Children who speak more than one language can be properly diagnosed as having a language-learning disability only if they manifest language-learning difficulties *in both the primary language and English*. Legally, it must be proven that the student in question has an LLD that underlies *both languages*.

- If a student has normal abilities in the primary language and is having difficulty with English, this student does not need special education remediation services such as speech–language therapy. Rather, the student needs other services, such as bilingual education, to facilitate English-language learning (Roseberry-McKibbin, 1993).

Acquiring a Second Language

- In assessing any child to differentiate a language difference from an LLD, it is necessary to know what "normal" behavior is. A major challenge confronting clinicians is that normal behavior varies widely even among monolingual children. When one is attempting to work with CLD students, the picture becomes far more complex.

- Sometimes CLD learners who are demonstrating normal second-language acquisition processes can spuriously appear to have underlying language-learning disabilities (Roseberry-McKibbin, 1994). To avoid making inaccurate diagnoses of such learners, it is important to be familiar with normal processes of second-language acquisition.

Normal Processes of Second-Language Acquisition

- *Interference.* This refers to an error in a student's second language (L2) that is directly produced by the influence of L1 (the first or primary language). Interference can occur in all areas: syntax, morphology, phonology, pragmatics, and semantics. Researchers and practitioners disagree about the extent of L1 influence on L2 production; however, it seems safe to say that a percentage of errors produced by CLD students can be directly traced to the influence of L1.

- *Silent period.* Some students, when learning an L2, go through a "silent period," in which there is much listening and comprehension and little output. It is believed that children are using this time to comprehend the new language before producing it. The silent period can last anywhere from 3 to 6 months, although estimates vary.

- *Codeswitching.* Codeswitching can be defined as the alternating or switching between two languages at the word, phrase, or sentence level; this behavior is part of natural bilingual development and is used by normal bilingual speakers worldwide (Baker, 1996).

- *Language loss.* If use of the L1 is discontinued or diminished, it is common for the second-language learner to lose skills in that first language. Because English is the dominant language of society in the United States, children often experience language loss of L1 and a gradual replacement of L1 with English or L2 (Baker, 1996).

- If a CLD student has experienced L1 loss and is still acquiring English, he or she may appear to be low functioning in both languages. Many clinicians might conclude that low functioning in L1 as well as L2 is indicative of a language-learning disability when it actually is a result of the loss of L1.

✎ Concepts To Consider

Summarize the reasons it is challenging to differentiate language differences from language-learning disabilities in CLD students.

_____

_____

_____

_____

_____

_____

Basic Interpersonal Communication Skills and Cognitive-Academic Language Proficiency

- A model of language proficiency that is useful in working with CLD children distinguishes basic interpersonal communication skills (BICS) from cognitive academic language proficiency (CALP).

- According to Cummins (1992), in CLD children BICS take approximately 2 years (in an ideal situation) to develop to a level commensurate with that of native speakers of L2. CALP takes 5–7 years to develop to a native-like level—and that frame is common for students from enriched backgrounds.

- BICS involve face-to-face communication in which conversational participants can actively negotiate meaning and have a shared reality. BICS communication is typical of that found in the everyday world outside the classroom, where language is supported by a wide range of meaningful situational and paralinguistic gestures (Cummins, 1992).

- CALP, which involves grasping the fundamentals of written language and adopting key literacy habits (Cheng, 1996), does not assume a shared reality. It may rely exclusively on linguistic cues for meaning and is more typical of the classroom.

- CALP is characteristic of situations where knowledge is not automatized and the student must actively use cognitive strategies to perform a task (e.g., writing an essay in a foreign language).

■ Many bilingual education programs help students who are "limited English proficient" (LEP) transition from English BICS to English CALP. Ideally, bilingual education would include maintenance of students' first languages and cultures and provision of second-language and culture instruction as well as subject matter (e.g., math, science).

■ This scenario appears to promote the greatest linguistic, cultural, and cognitive benefits, especially when combined with active parent and community involvement.

■ Many European countries value multilingualism so much that they are now promoting a policy of trilingualism in schools. In Switzerland, for example, students cannot graduate from high school unless they speak three languages fluently.

■ Unfortunately, some United States citizens have a negative attitude toward bilingualism and believe that it has negative cognitive and social effects on children. Thus, the availability of good bilingual programs in the United States is limited. Some states, such as California, have even passed laws that almost entirely rule out bilingual education in any form.

Simultaneous and Sequential Bilingualism

■ Researchers have broadly delineated two types of bilingualism: simultaneous and sequential. *Simultaneous bilingual acquisition* occurs when two languages are acquired simultaneously from infancy.

■ Schiff-Myers (1992) has termed this phenomenon, in which two languages are spoken to a child beginning in early infancy, *infant bilinguality*. Such children acquire two languages simultaneously in natural communication situations, and this bilingual development closely parallels monolingual development. Children who acquire two languages simultaneously in naturalistic situations seem to do so with minimal interference.

■ *Sequential bilingual acquisition* includes a greater diversity of rates and stages (Langdon with Cheng, 1992). Some students may acquire the second language with minimal interference; others may experience difficulties.

■ If a student is introduced to an L2 before the L1 competency threshold has been reached, the development of L1 may be arrested or may regress while the child is focusing on L2 development (Schiff-Myers, 1992).

■ Since, as Cummins (1992) has stated, L2 proficiency is partially a function of L1 competence, a condition of "semilingualism" may occur, in which the student does not fully develop either language. For a period of time, these students may obtain low test scores in both L1 and L2 and consequently appear LLD (Schiff-Myers, 1992).

■ Thus, when clinicians are working with CLD students in the schools, it is necessary, when a student appears to be "low functioning," to ask how the student developed both languages—simultaneously or sequentially.

■ If the languages were developed sequentially, was L1 stable and developed enough that acquisition of L2 was beneficial? If not, then the student's seemingly limited academic performance and limited skills in both languages could result from acquisition of L2 when the underlying system was not yet stable.

Summary

☑ When clinicians attempt to distinguish a language difference from an LLD in CLD students, they must take into account factors of second-language acquisition and bilingual development.

☑ Normal processes of second-language acquisition include interference, the silent period, codeswitching, and language loss. BICS and CALP are two types of language proficiency that clinicians should be aware of in assessing students.

☑ In distinguishing language differences from disorders, it is critical to ask if a child has developed two languages simultaneously or sequentially.

☑ In many cases, errors in judgment and consequent inappropriate placement of CLD students can be avoided if clinicians are aware of second-language learning factors. The greater the understanding clinicians have of these factors, the more unbiased and appropriate will be the services provided to CLD students in the schools.

ASSESSMENT OF CLD CLIENTS

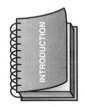

INTRODUCTION

Culturally fair and nonbiased assessment of CLD students is an issue impacting schools across the United States (Roseberry-McKibbin & Eicholtz, 1994; Seymour & Valles, 1998). A major consideration for all schools is state and federal mandates governing assessment of and intervention for CLD children. Clinicians must also look carefully at the typical practice of using standardized tests for assessment of LLD; most of these tests are biased against CLD students. Clinicians are increasingly using alternatives to standardized tests and working with interpreters from the clients' culture who can help assessment to be fair and unbiased.

Legal Considerations

■ There are a number of laws affecting service delivery to CLD students. The key law currently in practice, the Individuals with Disabilities Education Act (IDEA), specifically mandates the following:

- All children, regardless of diability, are entitled to an appropriate and free education.

- Testing and evaluation materials and procedures must be selected and administered so that they are not racially or culturally discriminatory.

- Testing and evaluation materials must be provided and administered in the language or other mode of communication in which the child is most proficient.

- Tests must be administered to a child with a motor, speech, hearing, visual or other communication disability, or to a bilingual child, so as to reflect accurately the child's ability in the area tested, rather than the child's impaired communication skill or limited English-language skill.

- Multicultural education is to be considered in guaranteeing equal educational opportunities for minorities with handicaps.

Considerations in the Use of Standardized Tests

Foundational Concepts

■ Many clinicians rely entirely on the use of standardized tests to evaluate CLD students' language abilities and to plan intervention, even though standardized tests are generally heavily biased against CLD populations (Fagundes, Haynes, Haak, & Moran, 1998; Wyatt, 1998c).

■ If clinicians continue to use these formal tests with CLD students, they should at least be aware of the tests' potential legal, psychometric, cultural, and linguistic limitations in terms of validity and reliability (Langdon & Saenz, 1996).

■ It is important to be familiar with the assumptions underlying formal, standardized tests. When clinicians are familiar with these assumptions, they can modify standardized tests so the tests are less biased.

Formal Test Assumptions

■ The development of formal tests has grown out of a framework that is Western, literate, and middle-class (Lund & Duchan, 1993; Reed, 1994). For these and many other reasons, formal tests are often very biased against CLD students.

■ Formal tests have many inherent assumptions that clinicians may be only partially aware of. These assumptions are extremely important to consider when working with CLD students (Heath, 1984; Lund & Duchan, 1993). These assumptions hold that test takers (students) will:

- follow the cooperative principle: perform to the best of their ability and try to provide relevant answers

- attempt to respond even when test tasks don't make sense

- understand test tasks (e.g., fill in the blank, point to the picture)

- have been exposed to the information and experiences inherent in a test

- feel comfortable enough with the examiner in the testing setting to perform optimally

■ These assumptions cannot be made with regard to many CLD students. For example, some students come from cultural backgrounds where it is considered respectful to be silent in the presence of an unfamiliar adult. Cultural differences may cause students not to optimally display their competence and abilities when taking standardized tests.

■ Clinicians need to remember that rules of interaction may differ from culture to culture. For example, in the African American speech community, several people may speak at once because there is greater tolerance for overlap during conversational exchanges (Wyatt, 1998b).

■ Thus, it would be important not to label an African American child as having "a deficiency in turn-taking skills" according to mainstream Euro-American standards.

■ Many formal, standardized tests that involve storytelling assume that children come from a literate narrative tradition. In such a tradition, narratives are highly structured, decontextualized, and follow specific patterns. It is assumed that the speaker must provide explicit information for and *inform* the listener.

■ However, some CLD children (e.g., African American and Native American children) come from *oral* narrative traditions where listener knowledge is assumed. The speaker's job is to *entertain* the listener; storytelling is not as structured (Klein & Moses, 1999). Clinicians must not mislabel these children as having language problems if they do not produce narratives according to a literate tradition.

Translating Standardized Tests

■ Translated versions of English tests are often used with CLD students. There are many difficulties with using translated English tests, and it is best to avoid this practice.

■ Differences in structure and content between English and the primary language raise questions of comparability of scores. Many words cannot be translated directly from one language to another. For example, some Asian languages do not have pronouns; translating "she" or "he" versus "it" into those languages is impossible.

■ Psychometric properties of tests, such as validity, reliability, sample sizes, and norming populations do not carry over to translated versions.

■ Translation assumes that CLD students have the same life experiences and background as the norming population, when they often do not.

Tests Developed in Primary Languages

■ Many clinicians believe that they can obtain valid assessments of CLD students' language skills if they use tests specifically developed in the students' primary languages. For example, Spanish-speaking students can be given Spanish tests. There are some problems with this, as well.

■ One major problem is the great heterogeneity of various minority populations. For example, many dialects of Spanish exist, and Spanish-speaking children come from such different countries as Cuba, Mexico, Puerto Rico, the Dominican Republic, and Spain. Also, Spanish-speaking students raised in different parts of the United States use different vocabulary words for some items.

■ A second difficulty is that there is little developmental data on languages other than English (Roseberry-McKibbin & Brice, 1999). Some Spanish norms for articulation have been developed (e.g., Goldstein & Iglesias, 1996; Jimenez, 1987), but few easily accessible, established language or articulation development norms exist for languages other than English.

Selecting, Administering, and Interpreting Standardized Tests

■ When professionals are considering which tests to use with CLD students, they should keep in mind the following considerations (Mattes & Omark, 1991):

– *Purpose of the test*: Is it for screening or in-depth evaluation?

– *Construct validity*: What theory was used in the test's creation? Is any theory mentioned? Is it appropriate for this particular student?

– *Appropriateness of test content*: Professionals can have native speakers review the test; they also can get help in field-testing the assessment instrument so that they can change or delete items that most of the children miss.

- *Adequacy of norms*: How was the standardization sample selected? Are the students who are being tested represented in the norming and standardization processes?

■ There are ways in which professionals can alter the administration of standardized tests so that CLD students will perform optimally in ways that reflect their true abilities (Erickson & Iglesias, 1986; Kayser, 1998; Lund & Duchan, 1993; Wyatt, 1998c):

- Omit biased items that the student will probably miss.

- Test beyond the ceiling.

- Complete the assessment over several sessions.

- Have a parent or another adult who is trusted by the child administer test items under the clinician's supervision.

- Give instructions in both English and L1.

- Rephrase confusing instructions.

- Give extra examples, demonstrations, practice items.

- Give the student extra time to respond.

- Repeat items when necessary.

- If students give "wrong" answers, ask them to explain and write down their explanations. Score items as correct if they are correct in students' cultures. Record all responses.

■ There are also ways that professionals can interpret standardized tests to effectively reduce bias (Mattes & Omark, 1991; Lund & Duchan, 1993):

- Review test results with family members and other people from the student's culture to gain additional insight into the student's performance.

- Interpret overall test results in a team setting. If professionals review and interpret results alone, errors are more likely.

- Don't identify a student as needing special education solely on the basis of test scores. Use informal measures to supplement standardized test scores.

- Ascertain if students' errors are typical of other students with similar backgrounds.

- When writing assessment reports, be sure to include cautions and disclaimers about any departures from standard testing procedures. In addition, discuss how the student's background may have influenced testing results.

Alternatives to Standardized Tests

Basic Principles

- Because the use of standardized tests poses many difficulties when professionals are evaluating CLD students, the use of nonstandardized, informal procedures and instruments for the assessment of CLD students has become increasingly frequent (Roseberry-McKibbin, 1994).

- A major advantage of informal testing is that it can be matched to students' curriculum. Another major advantage of informal testing is that it takes into account the fact that CLD students are often very capable in their own milieu and very functional in their own worlds. Formal testing seldom taps these students' individualized, functional skills in their own environments.

- The assessment wheel of a team approach to comprehensive assessment (see Figure 9.2) illustrates the necessity of combining informal assessment strategies with more formal testing for CLD students. It is important to carry out thorough assessments that include a case history, language proficiency testing, environmental observations, and dynamic assessment.

Specific Alternatives to Standardized Assessment

- Instead of relying exclusively on standardized tests for assessing CLD students, clinicians can (Kayser, 1998; Roseberry-McKibbin, 1995; Wyatt, 1998c):

  - *Use observations in a variety of naturalistic contexts*, evaluating the student's ability to interact in various everyday situations. Use of multiple observations in naturalistic settings helps clinicians obtain information about the child's communication behavior in multiple contexts (Cheng, 1991). Professionals can observe students in the classroom, at recess, at lunch, in the library, in the home, and in a variety of other settings.

  - *Use questionnaires* administered to teachers, parents, and others who interact with the student on a regular basis (Roseberry-McKibbin, 1993). Use of questionnaires gives a much broader picture of the student's communication functioning in daily contexts. It also helps the professionals doing the assessment to work as part of a team and not carry the entire responsibility for assessing the CLD student.

  - *Use authentic assessment*, which involves performances that have educational value in their own right; for example, clinicians can look at students' essays or portfolios of student work.

  - *Use a dynamic approach to assessment* in which a student is evaluated over time in a test-teach-retest format (Lidz & Peña, 1996). Because so many students come from backgrounds of reduced exposure to mainstream school concepts and vocabulary, they do poorly in formal testing situations.

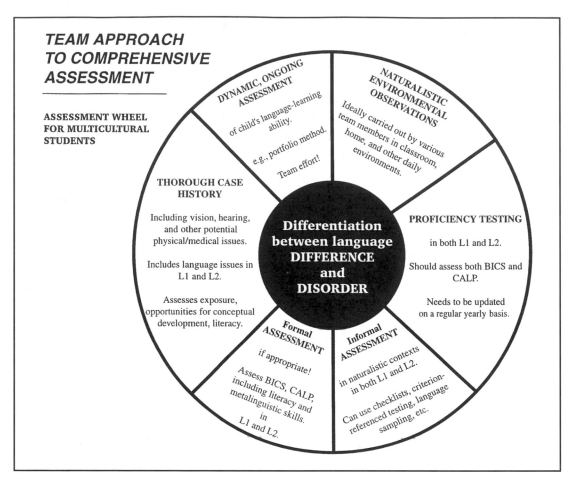

Figure 9.2. Team approach to comprehensive assessment: Assessment wheel for multicultural students. From *Multicultural Students with Special Language Needs: Practical Strategies for Assessment and Intervention* (p. 154), by C. Roseberry-McKibbin, 1995, Oceanside, CA: Academic Communication Associates. Copyright 1995 by Academic Communication Associates. Reprinted with permission.

A dynamic approach is highly preferable to a static approach in which the student is tested in one or two assessment sessions, because dynamic assessment evaluates a student's ability to learn when provided with instruction.

■ *Use narratives* appropriate to the student's background to assess the student's ability to construct narratives and remember stories she or he has heard (Gutierrez-Clellen & Quinn, 1993).

■ *Use the portfolio method of assessment,* in which samples of the student's work are gathered over time. These work samples can be analyzed to see how much learning is taking place.

■ *Use language samples* to evaluate the student's communication skills in everyday contexts with various interlocutors.

■ *Use school records* of the student's achievement and performance. Cum files (permanent records kept for each student) often contain helpful information that allows the clinician to track a student's performance over time.

Concepts To Consider

Describe the problems inherent in using standardized tests to assess the language skills of CLD children. What can clinicians do to circumvent those problems?

_____

_____

_____

_____

_____

_____

_____

_____

Working with Interpreters in the Assessment Process

■ Due to the national shortage of trained professionals who speak a language other than English, schools are increasingly turning to interpreters for assistance in assessment and treatment of CLD students. The clinician who is utilizing the services of an interpreter for assessment of CLD students has ethical responsibilities to carry out (Mattes & Omark, 1991). The clinician needs to make sure that he or she:

- makes sure that the permission for assessment form indicates that the services of an interpreter will be used during the assessment;

- makes clear in the assessment report that the services of an interpreter were used;

- recognizes the limitations of interpreted tests;

- allows interpreters to carry out only those activities for which they have been trained;

- involves others in training the interpreter when appropriate;

- gives the interpreter background information about the student who is to be tested;

- prepares the interpreter for each testing session and debriefs the interpreter afterwards;

- shows the interpreter how to use tests and makes sure the interpreter feels comfortable with the testing;

– allows the interpreter time, before the student arrives, to organize test materials, read instructions, and clarify any areas of question;

– ensures that the interpreter does not protect the student by hiding the extent of the student's limitations or disabilities;

– supervises the interpreter during the testing session and watches for possible inappropriate behaviors such as recording the assessment data incorrectly, prompting the student or giving clues, or using too many words;

– reminds the interpreter to write down all the student's behaviors seen during testing, even if the behaviors seem extraneous to the immediate task; and

– considers the interpreter's observations but doesn't place the responsibility for the placement decision on the interpreter.

Summary

☑ Federal law mandates nondiscriminatory, culture-fair testing for CLD students. However, many clinicians use standardized, formal tests that are biased against CLD students.

☑ If clinicians use those tests, they should be aware of potential forms of bias and try to control for them as much as possible.

☑ Many clinicians are increasingly turning to nonstandardized, informal assessment, which is much more valid in assessing the true language-learning abilities and skills of CLD children. Interpreters can be a valuable part of this process.

TREATMENT CONSIDERATIONS IN SERVICE DELIVERY TO CLD CLIENTS

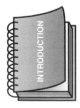

INTRODUCTION

CLD children with language-learning disabilities that underlie both the primary language and English can be served through different delivery models. Treatment should always be individualized and should be linguistically and culturally appropriate for the particular student involved. CLD adults who have neurologically based disorders of communication have unique needs that must be taken into consideration when providing services.

Children with Language-Learning Disabilities

Basic Principles

- As previously stated, students should not be diagnosed as having LLD if "problems" are observed only in English. If the student is truly LLD, problems in communication should be evident in both English and the primary language.

- An LLD affects a child's ability to learn any language. Exposure to two or more languages is not the cause of the disability. Bilingual children with underlying LLD will have difficulty learning any language (Roseberry & Connell, 1991).

- State and federal laws provide some specific guidelines for considering service options for CLD students. Many times CLD children do need assistance but do not qualify for special education.

- *It is illegal for schools to place CLD students into special education to work on improving the students' English.* Thus, only a select number of CLD students are truly eligible for special education services, including speech–language therapy.

- If CLD students do not qualify for speech–language services but need support in learning English, clinicians can help teachers find other options, such as bilingual education, English as a Second Language (ESL) programs, and others.

Service Delivery Models

- If CLD students do qualify for special education services, including speech–language therapy, the following service delivery models can be considered (Roseberry-McKibbin, 1995):

  - bilingual special education classroom;

  - monolingual, English, special education classroom with primary-language support through bilingual teacher, tutor, or others;

  - pull-out services (speech–language therapy, resource support, or both) in the primary language;

  - pull-out services in English with primary-language support;

  - consultative, collaborative service provision in which the CLD child remains in the regular classroom and the teacher receives assistance from special education personnel or ESL or bilingual staff; and

  - placement in a regular bilingual education or ESL classroom with support from special education.

Treatment Principles

- If a student is more proficient in the primary language than in English, carrying out treatment in the primary language is usually much more efficient and effective (Kiernan & Swisher, 1990; Perozzi & Sanchez, 1992).

- Ideally, intervention activities should:
  - focus on content rather than on mastery of specific grammatical forms;
  - include reading, writing, listening and talking; literacy should always be incorporated;
  - be built around whole themes, experiences, and events that have meaning to students;
  - promote effective communication and interaction among students;
  - be related to the classroom curriculum (Brice & Montgomery, 1996);
  - acknowledge students' backgrounds and experiences, and promote self-esteem; and
  - support students in learning the academic language that will help them be successful in the school setting (Brice & Montgomery, 1996; Westby, 1997).

- It is critical for intervention to involve not just therapy in a pull-out model, but also intervention in the child's classroom setting. Clinicians need to ensure, as much as possible, that they collaborate with classroom teachers to help children succeed in the academic and social setting of the classroom (Brice & Roseberry-McKibbin, 1999; Seymour & Valles, 1998).

- Clinicians should work closely with children's families and include caregivers as collaborators in the development of treatment goals (Klein & Moses, 1999). It is also very helpful to work with people from the families' cultures in order to promote treatment success (Brice, Roseberry-McKibbin, & Kayser, 1997).

Adults with Neurologically Based Disorders of Communication

Basic Issues

- The aging population is the most rapidly growing group in our country. Due to recent advances in health care, people are living longer. It is predicted that by the year 2025, approximately 60 million people will be over 65 years of age.

- As stated earlier, increasing numbers of CLD people are living longer. And research shows that CLD people as a population have a higher prevalence of neurological impairments (typically found in older people) than is found in the general population (McCrary, 1992).

■ The leading cause of neurological impairments is strokes. Strokes are associated with:

- *hypertension*, which may result in hemorrhagic strokes. Hypertension is prevalent among many CLD adults, especially African Americans.

- *arteriosclerosis*, a major etiological factor in strokes. In many CLD communities, arteriosclerosis is associated with high cholesterol levels. Also, foods that are high in salt and fat content (e.g., pork) are major causes of arteriosclerosis; these foods are popular in African American and Hispanic communities.

- *sickle cell anemia*, which primarily affects people of African and Mediterranean descent. Areas of the brain supplied by small blood vessels don't get enough oxygen, which may cause a stroke.

- *diabetes*, which affects Hispanics especially. Mexicans and Puerto Ricans have a rate of (adult onset) diabetes two to three times higher than the rate in the White population. Diabetes is associated with an increased risk of stroke (Reyes, 1995).

- *AIDS*, which is often associated with IV drug use, a pervasive problem in large urban areas.

- *alcohol abuse*, which is a serious problem in many CLD groups because so often it begins in the early to middle teen years. This places abusers at high risk for neurological impairments, such as strokes, involving linguistic and cognitive deficits (Wallace, 1998).

- *drug abuse,* which is very high in urban areas. Many inner-city residents have difficulties with drug abuse, and drugs such as crack (a vasoconstrictor) can cause strokes.

Theories Regarding Stroke Recovery in Bilinguals

■ It is important to be aware of whether a stroke patient speaks more than one language. In one actual case, a bilingual English-Russian patient had a stroke and spoke only Russian after the stroke. The hospital staff, not having checked the patient's records, thought she was using jargon.

■ Arambula (1992) has described four recovery theories, outlined below, for bilingual stroke patients.

Synergistic and Differential Recovery Theory

■ According to this theory, both languages are impaired, but not necessarily to the same degree. One language may be more affected than the other.

■ Both languages may eventually recover but not necessarily at the same rate.

■ Synergistic and differential recovery is by far the most common type; 95–98% of bilingual patients manifest this type of recovery.

Antagonistic Recovery Theory

■ According to this theory, one language returns at the expense of another previously recovered language. For example, a Spanish-speaking patient may recover Spanish and then English; however, when the English language returns, the Spanish language skills begin to disappear.

■ There have been almost no documented cases in which a patient has demonstrated antagonistic recovery.

Successive Recovery Theory

■ According to this theory, one language returns only after another has been completely restored.

■ There are few documented cases in which a patient has demonstrated successive recovery.

Selective Recovery Theory

■ According to this theory, one of the patient's languages never recovers and remains impaired. This occurs even when the other languages have recovered.

Sociocultural Considerations in Rehabilitation: Implications for Assessment and Treatment

■ It is important to consider individual patients' premorbid status as well as their functional needs within their personal life contexts. For example, many older African Americans have strong church connections (Payne-Johnson, 1992); therapy activities could address daily communication skills that are centered around church activities.

■ Clinicians must evaluate the family's culture in terms of the appropriateness of the rehabilitation goal of independence for the patient (Roseberry-McKibbin, 1997a). Encouragement of independence may be offensive in some cultures (Goldberg, 1997).

■ For example, some Hispanic families believe it is their duty to take care of the neurologically impaired patient. Requiring the patient to attend rehabilitation and become independent would be looked on as disrespectful and would cause great shame to the family (Arambula, 1992).

■ Socioeconomic status has a great impact on CLD patients' potential for utilizing rehabilitation services. Unfortunately, many elderly CLD adults tend to have little money or insurance.

■ For example, it is currently estimated that Hispanics 65 years of age and older have an average income of less than $104 a week (Arambula, 1992). Only 21%

of the Hispanic elderly have private insurance to supplement Medicare, as compared to 69% of the total population (Reyes, 1995).

■ Family relationships are an important consideration. For example, African Americans tend to be more involved than Whites in providing help across the generations, and the extended family network is much greater for African Americans than for Whites (Payne-Johnson, 1992). Clinicians can utilize family members for support.

■ It is important to assess premorbid educational levels and vocational attainments of patients, because these impact assessment and treatment. For example, according to Reyes (1995), elderly Hispanics are six or seven times more likely to be functionally illiterate (have less than 5 years of schooling) than non-Hispanics. Approximately 73% of elderly Hispanics have an educational attainment of eighth grade or less, as compared to 35% of all elderly individuals.

■ Socioeconomic status and educational attainment impact patients' acceptance of and belief in conventional rehabilitation, especially that involving technology. For example, if an elderly Asian from a low-income Hmong refugee family needs to have a CT scan to determine if he has had a stroke, the family may resist the CT scan because they have not been exposed to "high-tech" neuro-diagnostic procedures.

■ Religion also may play a role in patients' and families' acceptance of rehabilitation (Goldberg, 1997; Nellum Davis, Gentry, Hubbard-Wiley, 1998). Some families believe in folk healers, not traditional medicine. Other families believe that a disability caused by a stroke, for example, is the will of a Supreme Being and thus rehabilitation goes counter to religious beliefs.

■ It is imperative, for bilingual patients, to assess skills in both the primary language and English. Assessment should be carried out as soon as possible and should focus on the most dominant language.

■ Many standardized tests of aphasia are biased against CLD patients. Instead of using test norms, clinicians can evaluate a normal, healthy family member using a standardized test. That performance can then be used as an appropriate standard against which to compare the patient.

■ Clinicians should ascertain which is the most appropriate language to use in rehabilitation of CLD clients. Factors impacting this decision include:

   – the patient's premorbid language history

   – the availability of an interpreter

   – the patient's abilities (both oral and written) in each language

   – whether the patient will return to a home or work setting

🖉 Concepts To Consider

You are giving a workshop in a skilled nursing facility where the staff does not know anything about providing appropriate assessment and treatment for CLD adults with neurologically based disorders. Briefly describe four concepts that you would communicate in your workshop.

_____

_____

_____

_____

_____

_____

_____

_____

Summary

- ☑ A CLD child is considered to have an LLD only if he or she has language-learning difficulties that underlie both the primary language and English.

- ☑ CLD children in the schools who manifest LLD can be served through a variety of service delivery models. Treatment activities for these children should be culturally appropriate and should assist the children in becoming effective communicators in their daily environments. Family involvement is critical.

- ☑ Adults with neurologically based communication disorders, such as those resulting from strokes, may recover their languages in various ways after the stroke has occurred. Clinicians should be sensitive to these clients' bilingual status and the way it affects recovery.

- ☑ Assessment and treatment should occur in the patient's strongest language, if possible. Treatment must be functional for the individual patient's environment and appropriate for his or her cultural background.

CHAPTER HIGHLIGHTS

▶ The increasing numbers of culturally and linguistically diverse (CLD) people in the United States have created a great need for speech–language pathologists to develop cultural sensivity and knowledge about how to best provide appropriate service delivery. ASHA has developed guidelines and policies regarding optimal service delivery to people from multicultural backgrounds.

▶ Speakers of African American Language, Spanish, and the Asian languages manifest unique phonological, morphological, semantic, and syntactic characteristics and patterns that differ from those of Standard American English. These characteristics and patterns are indicative not of a disorder but of a difference.

▶ It is important to take into account the influence of the primary language or dialect so that CLD clients are not misdiagnosed as having a language disorder. Some CLD individuals may choose to participate in elective speech–language therapy so that they may improve their Standard American English skills for vocational and other purposes.

▶ A great challenge for speech–language pathologists is to differentiate between language differences and language-learning disabilities (LLDs) in children who speak more than one language. Frequently, there is a mismatch between the skills and abilities these children bring to the schools and the schools' expectations of these children. This mismatch often creates deficits in CLD students who have normal underlying language-learning ability.

▶ Part of accurately differentiating between a language difference and an LLD is knowledge of normal second-language acquisition processes. The processes of interference, the silent period, codeswitching, and language loss can appear to be symptoms of an LLD; however, these processes are normal and common. The fact of whether children are developing a second language simultaneously with or sequentially to the first language also has an impact on development.

▶ CLD children learning a second language manifest different types of language proficiency. In ideal learning situations, basic interpersonal communication skills (BICS) take approximately 2 years to develop to a native-like level; cognitive academic language proficiency (CALP) takes 5–7 years to develop to a native-like level. Awareness of the differences between these types of language proficiency can help clinicians not to misdiagnose CLD children as having underlying LLDs when, in fact, these children are following a normal time line of English-language development.

(continues)

▶ Federal law mandates that assessment of CLD children be fair, nondiscriminatory, and conducted in the children's most proficient language. Because most clinicians use standardized tests normed on English-speaking children, fair and nonbiased assessment of CLD children is a great challenge.

▶ Clinicians can make alterations in standardized testing to make that testing less biased. Optimally, however, clinicians should use nonstandardized, informal assessment measures such as dynamic assessment, questionnaires administered to adults who are familiar with the child's daily communicative functioning, and language samples. Utilizing the services of well-trained interpreters can be very helpful.

▶ Some CLD students have underlying language-learning disabilities; they are not able to learn any language adequately. There are a number of service delivery options available for these children. Treatment methods and activities should focus on improving functional communication, literacy, and knowledge of school curriculum and language, and should be culturally appropriate. It is imperative to include families in the treatment process.

▶ CLD adults tend, as a group, to be more predisposed to strokes than the general population. This is due to such related factors as diabetes, hypertension, and arteriosclerosis. CLD adults may show various patterns of stroke recovery depending on which languages they speak. Assessment and treatment of CLD adults with neurologically based communication disorders must consider many variables, such as family support, religious beliefs, educational and vocational background, socioeconomic status, and other sociocultural variables.

▶ Add your own chapter highlights here:

_____

_____

_____

_____

KEY TERMS

African American Language
antagonistic recovery theory
basic interpersonal communication
   skills (BICS)

codeswitching
cognitive academic language
   proficiency (CALP)
culture

ethnolinguistic theory
interference
language loss
selective recovery theory
sequential bilingual acquisition
silent period
simultaneous bilingual acquisition

standard American English
stereotypes
successive recovery theory
synergistic and differential recovery
  theory
toneme

STUDY AND REVIEW QUESTIONS

Fill in the Blank

1. In Vietnamese, Chinese, and Laotian, a tone change that is phonemic in nature and represents a meaning change is called a(n) _toneme_.

2. The phenomenon of _interference_ refers to an error in a speaker's second language that is directly produced by the influence of the primary language.

3. The alternating of two languages at the word, phrase, or sentence level is called _codeswitching_.

4. In _simultaneous_ bilingual acquisition, two languages are acquired at the same time beginning in infancy. In _sequential_ bilingual acquisition, one language is acquired first and the other is acquired later.

5. In the _dynamic_ approach to assessment, clinicians use a test-teach-retest paradigm to evaluate a child's ability to learn when provided with instruction.

6. The _ethnolinguistic_ theory states that African American Language is a systematic and rule-governed language in its own right, whose roots can be traced to many languages of West Africa.

7. The medical condition of _sickle cell anemia_ affects primarily people of African and Mediterranean descent, and can reduce oxygen to the areas of the brain supplied by small blood vessels, thus causing a stroke.

8. The cultural group most prone to adult-onset diabetes is _hispanic_.

9. There are several theories regarding recovery from strokes in bilingual patients. The ___Successive___ theory states that in some patients, one language returns only after another language has been completely restored.

10. Asian languages that are not tonal include ___Japanese___ and ___Khmer, Korean___.

Multiple Choice

11. Xu Fang is a 7-year-old girl in an all-English-speaking second-grade classroom at her school. She came to an all-English kindergarten speaking only Mandarin; kindergarten was her first exposure to English on a regular basis. The second-grade teacher has referred Xu for a speech–language evaluation because he says that although she interacts well with her English-speaking classmates on the playground, she is "behind" these classmates in written language skills (e.g., spelling, reading). Based on Xu's background, you can state that:

    A. because basic interpersonal communication skills take approximately 2 years to develop to a native-like level, Xu is developing on an appropriate time line.

    B. because cognitive academic language proficiency takes approximately 5–7 years to develop to a native-like level, it can be expected that Xu will lag somewhat behind English-speaking peers in written language skills.

    C. because Xu has been in an all-English speaking classroom setting for at least 2 years, her written language skills should be more developed than they are. Her difficulties are a red flag, and a speech–language assessment should be conducted.

    D. A, C

    E. A, B

12. Which of the following are normal variations of African American Language, not a sign of a disorder?

    A. f/th substitution in word-final position

    B. production of [æks] instead of [æsk]

    C. w/r substitution in all word positions

    D. A, B

    E. A, B, C

13. A 9-year-old African American male student makes the following substitutions: d/m, t/n, f/n. You would:

    A. let the classroom teacher work with the student because this is such a mild problem.

    B. do nothing, knowing that boys mature more slowly than girls

    C. do nothing, realizing that this is normal for speakers of African American Language.

    D. treat the student, because this is a sign of an articulatory-phonological disorder involving denasalization of nasals.

    E. none of the above

14. In an adolescent speaker of African American Language, which of the following utterances would be an example of the use of the perfective construction "been," indicating an action that took place in the distant past?

    A. "I been had a marble collection when I was 7."

    B. "Our family been gonna do it."

    C. "I might been coulda done it."

    D. "He been done it again."

    E. "They be cookin' a barbecue."

15. You are working with a Spanish-speaking 6-year-old girl who is in the process of learning English. Which one of the following would NOT be typical for her in terms of predictable productions based on Spanish influence?

    A. t/th substitions in word-initial positions (e.g., *tin/thin*)

    B. devoicing of final consonants (e.g., *beece/bees*)

    C. v/f substitions in word-initial and word-final positions (e.g., *vine/fine*; *roove/roof*)

    D. y/j substitutions (e.g., *yava/java*)

    E. insertion of the schwa before word-initial s-clusters (e.g., *esleep/sleep*)

16. Which of the following is/are predictable productions for speakers of Asian languages?

    A. "He be going to bed now."

    B. "I see cat the little."

    C. "Yesterday she cook a pot of soup."

    D. A, B

    E. B, C

17. A 74-year-old Asian gentleman has had a stroke, and you are seeing him for therapy. He is recovering both his primary language and his English skills, but you are working only in English. Which of the following productions would be examples, on the patient's part, of English influenced by his primary language and not the stroke?

    A. "They coming over here now."

    B. "I done got to eat breakfast now."

    C. "She have no dollar in her purse."

    D. A, B, C

    E. A, C

18. A high school teacher refers a Japanese-speaking 10th grader to you for an evaluation. The teacher says that although this boy is doing well academically, he is "hard to understand sometimes." You conduct a screening. Which of the following articulatory-phonological characteristics might be predictable based on the student's first language of Japanese?

    A. substitution of a/ae (e.g., *sock / sack, fong / fang*)

    B. final-consonant deletion (e.g., *be- / bed, po- / pot*)

    C. r/l confusion (e.g., *laise / raise, clown / crown*)

    D. B, C

    E. A, B, C

19. Which one of the following is NOT TRUE according to the Individuals with Disabilities Education Act?

    A. Testing must be administered in a way that is not racially or culturally discriminatory.

    B. Testing and evaluation materials must always be provided and administered in the child's primary language.

    C. Testing must be administered to a bilingual child so as to reflect accurately the child's ability in the area tested, rather than reflecting limited English-language skill.

    D. Mandatory consent in the primary language is required.

    E. Multicultural education is to be considered in guaranteeing equal educational opportunities for minorities with disabilities.

20. A teacher has referred a third-grade boy to you for a speech–language assessment. He and his family are Cambodian refugees, and they have

been in the United States for 8 months. Because the boy has been in refugee camps most of his life, his schooling in Cambodia was quite limited. The teacher is concerned that the boy may have an underlying language-learning disability. What would be the best combination of assessment techniques to use with him?

A. dynamic assessment, language samples in Cambodian, and observations of his interaction with family members and other Cambodian children

B. use of the *Peabody Picture Vocabulary Test–Revised* and *Test of Language Development–P:3* translated into Cambodian, dynamic assessment, and language samples in Cambodian

C. use of a district-developed test for Cambodian students in your geographic area and administration of questionnaires to the boy's teachers and family

D. use of school records of the boy's achievement and performance so far in the English-speaking classroom and use of the *Language Processing Test* translated into Cambodian by an interpreter

E. use of formal, standardized tests in English combined with observations of the boy's interactions, in Cambodian, with peers and family members

REFERENCES AND RECOMMENDED READINGS

American Speech–Language-Hearing Association. (1998). Provision of English-as-a-second-language instruction by speech–language pathologists in school settings: Position statement and technical report. *Asha, 40* (Suppl. 18), 24–27.

American Speech–Language-Hearing Association Joint Subcommittee of the Executive Board on English Language Proficiency. (1998). Students and professionals who speak English with accents and nonstandard dialects: Issues and recommendations. Position statement and technical report. *Asha, 40* (Suppl. 18), 28–31.

Anderson, R.T. (1996). Assessing the grammar of Spanish-speaking children: A comparison of two procedures. *Language, Speech, and Hearing Services in Schools,* 27(4), 333–344.

Arambula, G. (1992). Acquired neurological disabilities in Hispanic adults. In H. Langdon (Ed.) with L. L. Cheng, *Hispanic children and adults with communication disorders: Assessment and intervention* (pp. 373–407). Gaithersburg, MD: Aspen Publishers.

Baker, C. (1996). *Foundations of bilingual education and bilingualism* (2nd ed.). Bristol, PA: Multilingual Matters.

Battle, D. E. (Ed.). (1998). *Communication disorders in multicultural populations* (2nd ed.). Stoneham, MA: Butterworth-Heinemann.

Bloom, L., & Lahey, M. (1978). *Language development and language disorders.* New York: John Wiley.

Brice, A., & Montgomery, J. (1996). Adolescent pragmatic skills: A comparison of Latino students in English as a second language and speech pathology programs. *Language, Speech, and Hearing Services in Schools,* 27(1), 68–81.

Brice, A., & Roseberry-McKibbin, C. (1999). Turning frustration into success for English language learners. *Educational Leadership,* 56(7), 53–55.

Brice, A., Roseberry-McKibbin, C., & Kayser, H. (1997, November). *Special language needs of linguistically and culturally diverse students.* Paper presented at the annual meeting of the American Speech–Language-Hearing Association, Boston, MA.

Campbell, L. R. (1993). Maintaining the integrity of home linguistic varieties: Black English vernacular. *American Journal of Speech–Language Pathology, 2,* 85–86.

Campbell, L. R. (1996). Issues in service delivery to African American children. In A. G. Kamhi, K. E. Pollock, & J. L. Harris (Eds.), *Communication development and disorders in African American children: Research and intervention* (pp. 73–94). Baltimore, MD: Paul H. Brookes.

Chambers, J. W. (1983). *Black English: Educational equity and the law.* Tucson, AZ: Karoma Publishers.

Cheng, L. L. (1991). *Assessing Asian language performance: Guidelines for evaluating limited-English-proficient students* (2nd ed.). Oceanside, CA: Academic Communication Associates.

Cheng, L. L. (1996). Enhancing communication: Toward optimal language learning for limited English proficient students. *Language, Speech, and Hearing Services in Schools, 27*(4), 347–354.

Cheng, L. L. (1998). Asian- and Pacific-American cultures. In D. E. Battle (Ed.), *Communication disorders in multicultural populations* (2nd ed.), pp. 73–116. Newton, MA: Butterworth-Heinemann.

Crago, M. B., Eriks-Brophy, A., Pesco, D., & McAlpine, L. (1997). Culturally based miscommunication in classroom interactions. *Language, Speech, and Hearing Services in Schools, 28*(7), 245–259.

Cummins, J. (1992). The role of primary language development in promoting educational success for language minority students. In C. Leyba (Ed.), *Schooling and language minority students: A theoretical framework*. Los Angeles: California State University.

Dillard, J. L. (1972). *Black English: Its history and usage in the United States*. New York: Random House.

Erickson, J. G., & Iglesias, A. (1986). Speech and language disorders in Hispanics. In O. Taylor (Ed.), *Nature of communication disorders in culturally and linguistically diverse populations* (pp. 181–218). San Diego, CA: College-Hill Press.

Fagundes, D. D., Haynes, W. O., Haak, N. J., & Moran, M. J. (1998). Task variability effects on the language test performance of southern lower socioeconomic class African American and Caucasian five-year-olds. *Language, Speech, and Hearing Services in Schools, 29*(3), 148–157.

Ford, B. A., Obiakor, F. E., & Patton, J. M. (1995). *Effective education of African American exceptional learners*. Austin, TX: PRO-ED.

Gall, S. B., & Gall, T. L. (1993). *Statistical record of Asian Americans*. Detroit: Gale Research.

Goldberg, B. (1997). Tailoring to fit: Altering our approach to multicultural populations. *Asha, 39*(3), 22–29.

Goldstein, B. A., & Iglesias, A. (1996). Phonological patterns in normally developing Spanish-speaking 3- and 4-year-olds. *Language, Speech, and Hearing Services in Schools, 26*(1), 82–90.

Gutierrez-Clellen, V. F., & Quinn, R. (1993). Assessing narratives of children from diverse cultural/linguistic backgrounds. *Language, Speech, and Hearing Services in Schools, 24*(1), 2–9.

Heath, S. B. (1984). *Cross cultural acquisition of language*. Paper presented at the annual meeting of the American Speech–Language-Hearing Association, San Francisco, CA.

Horton, C. P., & Smith, J. C. (Eds.). (1993). Statistical record of Black America (2nd ed.). Detroit: Gale Research.

Iglesias, A., & Anderson, B. (1998). Dialectal variations. In J. E. Bernthal & N. W. Bankson, *Articulation and phonological disorders* (4th ed.). Needham Heights, MA: Allyn & Bacon.

Jimenez, B. (1987). The acquisition of Spanish consonants in children aged 3–5 years, 7 months. *Language, Speech, and Hearing Services in Schools, 18*, 357–363.

Kamhi, A. G., Pollock, K. E., & Harris, J. L. (1996). *Communication development and disorders in African American children: Research, assessment, and intervention*. Baltimore, MD: Paul H. Brookes.

Kayser, H. (1989). Speech and language assessment of Spanish-English speaking children. *Language, Speech, and Hearing Services in Schools, 20*, 226–244.

Kayser, H. (Ed.) (1995). *Bilingual speech–language pathology: An Hispanic focus*. San Diego, CA: Singular Publishing Group.

Kayser, H. (1998). Hispanic cultures and languages. In D. E. Battle (Ed.), *Communication disorders in multicultural populations* (2nd ed.), pp. 157–196. Newton, MA: Butterworth-Heinemann.

Kiernan, B., & Swisher, L. (1990). The initial learning of novel English words: Two single-subject experiments with minority-language children. *Journal of Speech and Hearing Research, 33*(4), 707–716.

Klein, H. B., & Moses, N. (1999). *Intervention planning for children with communication disorders: A guide for clinical practicum and professional practice* (2nd ed.). Needham Heights, MA: Allyn & Bacon.

Lane, V. W., & Molyneaux, D. (1992). *The dynamics of communicative development.* Englewood Cliffs, NJ: Prentice-Hall.

Langdon, H. W., with Cheng, L. L. (1992). *Hispanic children and adults with communication disorders: Assessment and intervention.* Gaithersburg, MD: Aspen Publishers.

Langdon, H. W., & Saenz, T. I. (1996). *Language assessment and intervention with multicultural students: A guide for speech–language-hearing professionals.* Oceanside, CA: Academic Communication Associates.

LeMoine, N. (1993). *Serving the language needs of African American students: Strategies for success.* Paper presented at the annual meeting of the California Speech–Language-Hearing Association, Palm Springs, CA.

Lidz, C. S., & Peña, E. D. (1996). Dynamic assessment: The model, its relevance as a nonbiased approach, and its application to Latino American preschool children. *Language, Speech, and Hearing Services in Schools, 4*(27), 367–372.

Lund, N. J., & Duchan, J. F. (1993). *Assessing children's language in naturalistic contexts* (3rd ed.). Englewood Cliffs, NJ: Prentice-Hall.

Lynch, E. W. (1998). Conceptual framework: From culture shock to cultural learning. In E. W. Lynch & M. J. Hanson (Eds.), *Developing cross-cultural competence: A guide for working children and their families* (2nd ed.) (pp. 23–45). Baltimore, MD: Paul H. Brookes.

Lynch, E. W., & Hanson, M. J. (Eds.). (1998). *Developing cross-cultural competence: A guide for working children and their families* (2nd ed.). Baltimore, MD: Paul H. Brookes.

Mattes, L. J., & Omark, D. R. (1991). *Speech and language assessment for the bilingual handicapped* (2nd ed.). Oceanside, CA: Academic Communication Associates.

McCrary, M. B. (1992). Urban multicultural trauma patients. *Asha, 34*(4), 37–39.

McGregor, K., Williams, D., Hearst, S., & Johnson, A. C. (1997). The use of contrastive analysis in distinguishing difference from disorder: A tutorial. *American Journal of Speech–Language Pathology, 6*(3), 45–56.

Nellum Davis, P., Gentry, B., Hubbard-Wiley, P. (1998). Clinical practice issues. In D. E. Battle (Ed.), *Communication disorders in multicultural populations* (2nd ed.), pp. 427–445. Newton, MA: Butterworth-Heinemann.

Payne, J. (1995, March). *Multicultural issues in aging.* Workshop presented at California State University, Fresno.

Payne-Johnson, J. (1992). Communications and aging: A case for understanding African-Americans who are elderly. *Asha, 34*, 41–44.

Perrozi, J., & Sanchez, M. L. C. (1992). The effect of instruction in L1 on receptive acquisition of L2 for bilingual children with language delay. *Language, Speech, and Hearing Services in Schools, 23*(4), 352–358.

Quinn, R., Goldstein, B., & Peña, E. (1996). Cultural/linguistic variation in the United States and its implications for assessment and intervention in speech–language pathology: An introduction. *Language, Speech, and Hearing Services in Schools, 27*(4), 345–346.

Reed, V. A. (1994). *An introduction to children with language disorders* (2nd ed.). New York: Macmillan.

Reyes, B. A. (1995). Considerations in the assessment and treatment of neurogenic communication disorders in bilingual adults. In H. Kayser (Ed.), *Bilingual speech–language pathology: An Hispanic focus* (pp. 153–181). San Diego, CA: Singular Publishing Group.

Roseberry, C. A., & Connell, P. J. (1991). The use of an invented language rule in the differentiation of normal and language-impaired Spanish-speaking children. *Journal of Speech and Hearing Research, 34*, 596–603.

Roseberry-McKibbin, C. (1993). *Bilingual classroom communication profile*. Oceanside, CA: Academic Communication Associates.

Roseberry-McKibbin, C. (1994). Assessment and intervention for limited English proficient children with language disorders. *American Journal of Speech–Language Pathology, 3*(3), 77–88.

Roseberry-McKibbin, C. (1995). *Multicultural students with special language needs: Practical strategies for assessment and intervention*. Oceanside, CA: Academic Communication Associates.

Roseberry-McKibbin, C. (1997a). Interviewing and counseling with linguistically and culturally diverse clients. In K. G. Shipley (Ed.), *Interviewing and counseling in communicative disorders* (2nd ed.), pp. 151–173. Needham Heights, MA: Allyn & Bacon.

Roseberry-McKibbin, C. (1997b). Understanding Filipino families: A foundation for effective service delivery. *American Journal of Speech–Language Pathology, 6*(3), 5–14.

Roseberry-McKibbin, C., & Brice, A. (1999). The perception of vocal cues of emotion by Spanish-speaking, limited English proficient children. *Journal of Children's Communication Development, 20*(2), 19–25.

Roseberry-McKibbin, C., & Eicholtz, G. (1994). Serving limited English proficient children in schools: A national survey. *Language, Speech, and Hearing Services in Schools, 25*(3), 156–164.

Schiff-Myers, N. (1992). Considering arrested language development and language loss in the assessment of second language learners. *Language, Speech, and Hearing Services in Schools, 23*, 28–33.

Seymour, C. M., & Nober, E. H. (1998). *Introduction to communication disorders: A multicultural approach*. Newton, MA: Butterworth-Heinemann.

Seymour, H. N., & Valles, L. (1998). Language intervention for linguistically different learners. In C. M. Seymour & E. H. Nober (Eds.), *Introduction to communication disorders: A multicultural approach* (pp. 89–109). Newton, MA: Butterworth-Heinemann.

Stockman, I. J. (1996). The promises and pitfalls of language sample analysis as an assessment tool for linguistic minority children. *Language, Speech, and Hearing Services in Schools, 27*(4), 355–366.

Terrell, S. L., Battle, D. E., & Grantham, R. (1998). African American cultures. In D. E. Battle (Ed.), *Communication disorders in multicultural populations* (2nd ed.), pp. 31–72. Newton, MA: Butterworth-Heinemann.

U.S. Bureau of the Census. (1992). *Statistical abstract of the United States, 1992*. Washington, DC: U.S. Government Printing Office.

Wallace, G. J. (1998). Adult neurogenic disorders. In D. E. Battle (Ed.), *Communication disorders in multicultural populations* (2nd ed.), pp. 309–334. Newton, MA: Butterworth-Heinemann.

Washington, J. A. (1996). Issues in assessing the language abilities of African American children. In A. G. Kamhi, K. E. Pollock, & J. L. Harris (Eds.), *Communication development and disorders in African American children: Research and intervention* (pp. 35–54). Baltimore, MD: Paul H. Brookes.

Westby, C. (1997). There's more to passing than knowing the answers. *Language, Speech, and Hearing Services in Schools, 28*(3), 274–287.

Willis, W. (1998). Families with African American roots. In E. W. Lynch & M. J. Hanson (Eds.), *Developing cross-cultural competence: A guide for working children and their families* (2nd ed.) (pp. 165–208). Baltimore, MD: Paul H. Brookes.

Wink, J. (1992). Immersion confusion. *TESOL Matters, 1*(6), 14–17.

Wolfram, W. (1986). Language variation in the United States. In O. Taylor (Ed.), *Nature of communication disorders in culturally and linguistically diverse populations*. San Diego, CA: College-Hill Press.

Wyatt, T. (1997). Developing a culturally sensitive preschool screening tool. *Asha, 39*(2), 50–51.

Wyatt, T. (1998a). Children's language development. In C. M. Seymour & E. H. Nober, *Introduction to communication disorders: A multicultural approach* (pp. 59–86). Newton, MA: Butterworth-Heinemann.

Wyatt, T. (1998b). Language structure and function. In C. M. Seymour & E. H. Nober, *Introduction to communication disorders: A multicultural approach* (pp. 43–58). Newton, MA: Butterworth-Heinemann.

Wyatt, T. (1998c). Assessment issues with multicultural populations. In D. E. Battle (Ed.), *Communication disorders in multicultural populations* (2nd ed.), pp. 379–426. Newton, MA: Butterworth-Heinemann.

ANSWERS TO STUDY AND REVIEW QUESTIONS

1. Toneme

2. Interference

3. Codeswitching

4. Simultaneous, sequential

5. Dynamic

6. Ethnolinguistic theory

7. Sickle cell anemia

8. Hispanics

9. Successive recovery

10. Japanese, Khmer, Korean

11. E. Xu is developing according to an appropriate time line for BICS and CALP.

12. D. Many normal speakers of African American Language produce f/th substitutions in word-final position and show metathesis in productions like aks/ask. However, a w/r substitution is not common and probably indicates an articulation problem that is not related to the use of African American Language.

13. D. The above-listed substitutions are not commonly found in speakers of African American Language, so this student has a disorder involving denasalization of nasals.

14. A. In an adolescent speaker of African American Language, the utterance "I been had a marble collection when I was 7." would be an example of the use of the perfective construction "been," indicating an action that took place in the distant past.

15. C. V/f substitions in word-initial and word-final positions (e.g., *vine/fine*; *roove/roof*) would NOT be typical for a Spanish-speaking 6-year-old girl who is in the process of learning English, in terms of predictable productions based on Spanish influence.

16. C. "Yesterday she cook a pot of soup" would be a predictable utterance for a speaker of most Asian languages. The other utterances would not be predictable based on the influence of any Asian language.

17. E. A 74-year old Asian gentleman who has had a stroke and is receiving therapy in English could say "They coming over here now" and "She have no dollar in her purse" as English utterances influenced by his primary language and not the stroke.

18. E. Predictable utterances for a Japanese-speaking 10th grader, based on his primary language of Japanese, would be substitutions of a/ae (e.g., *sock/sack, fong/fang*), final consonant deletion (e.g., *be-/bed, po-/pot*), and r/l confusion (e.g., *laise/raise, blown/crown*).

19. B. Testing and evaluation materials must be provided and administered in the child's primary language *or other mode of communication in which the child is most proficient.*

20. A. Practices that are discouraged, in evaluating CLD children, include translated English tests and formal, standardized tests administered in English. A district-developed test for Cambodian students in the geographic location might or might not include subjects who recently immigrated from Cambodia.

CHAPTER 10

Audiology and Hearing Disorders

PREVIEW OUTLINE

CHAPTER INTRODUCTION

It is estimated that in the United States, the prevalence of hearing impairment is between 14 and 40 million, depending on the definition of hearing impairment that is used. There are estimated to be approximately 3 million children in the United States who are deaf and hard of hearing (Schow & Nerbonne, 1996). *Audiology* is the study of hearing, its disorders, and the measurement and management of those disorders. The birth of the audiology profession occurred during World War II. Many servicemen had impaired hearing and needed rehabilitation; this need gave rise to the profession of audiology.

Audiologists identify, evaluate, and rehabilitate individuals with peripheral and central auditory impairments and work to prevent those impairments (American Academy of Audiology, 1997). Audiologists work in a variety of settings. Twenty percent are in hospitals or medical center facilities, and approximately 10% work in school settings. Twenty percent of audiologists work in residential health care facilities, industry, universities, and other related agencies. The remaining 50% work in nonresidential health care facilities such as physicians' practices, private clinics, and community speech and hearing centers (Stach, 1998).

Audiology as a profession has expanded into new areas of service. These areas include ear canal inspection and cerumen management, neonatal hearing screening, auditory electrophysiology (defined later), and multisensory modality monitoring in operating rooms where patients are undergoing tumor removal (especially nerve VIII tumors). In the 1990s, the profession of audiology began exploring the possibility of establishing a professional doctorate, or Au.D. In this model, students enroll in a 3–4 year program (similar to that required for dentistry and optometry). The early years are primarily devoted to academic training and the later years to clinical training. At the end of the program, students receive the Au.D. and may practice independently. At this time, some universities have started Au.D. programs; other universities with traditional master's degree programs have begun to adapt those programs to provide greater clinical training for audiology students (Stach, 1998).

ANATOMY AND PHYSIOLOGY OF HEARING

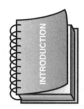

The ear is divided into three sections: the outer ear, the middle ear, and the inner ear. Efficient functioning of these sections of the ear is necessary for normal hearing. However, the auditory nervous system must also be intact in order for sound to be carried to its ultimate destination, the cortex, where it is interpreted.

The Outer Ear

- The outer ear is composed of two parts:
    - the *auricle* or *pinna*, which funnels the sound to the ear canal and helps localize sound (This is the most visible part of the ear and is composed primarily of cartilage.)
    - the *external auditory canal* (also called the *external auditory meatus*), which goes from the pinna to the *tympanic membrane* or *eardrum*.

- The external auditory canal is a muscular tube, made mostly of cartilage. The tube is not straight but curves slightly like an S. Thus, a specialist who examines the ear canal must first pull the pinna up and back to insert the *otoscope* (an instrument for examining the ear) into the canal.

- The external auditory canal is, on the average, approximately 2.5 cm (1 inch) long and resonates the sound that enters it. The canal ends at the tympanic membrane, or eardrum.

- The external auditory canal has special cells that secrete wax or *cerumen*. The cerumen filters dust and traps small insects that may try to crawl into the middle ear.

The Middle Ear

- The middle ear is an air-filled cavity. It is separated from the outer ear by the tympanic membrane.

- The three small bones in the middle ear form the ossicular chain.

- The eustachian tube connects the middle ear to the nasopharynx. See Figure 10.1.

Tympanic Membrane

- The tympanic membrane is elastic, thin, and cone-shaped. It is flexible and tough and vibrates in response to sound pressure. The entire tympanic

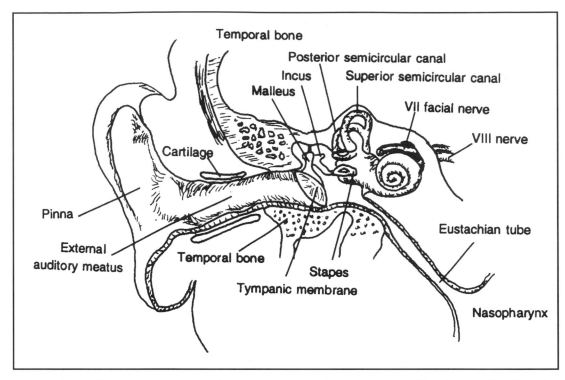

Figure 10.1. Major structures of the ear. From *Anatomy and Physiology for Speech, Language, and Hearing* (p. 534), by J. A. Seikel, D. W. King, and D. G. Drumright, 1997, San Diego, CA: Singular Publishing Group, Inc. (401 West A Street, Suite 325, San Diego, CA 92101-7904, 800-521-8545). Copyright 1997 by Singular Publishing Group, Inc. Reprinted with permission.

membrane responds to low-frequency sounds, but only certain portions respond to high-frequency sounds.

■ It is easy to damage the tympanic membrane. It can be ruptured by a Q-tip, hairpin, or other object inserted into the ear. Explosions and sudden pressure changes can also rupture the tympanic membrane.

■ A damaged or punctured tympanic membrane may heal spontaneously. However, repeated ruptures cause scar tissue, which reduces the tympanic membrane's mobility.

Ossicular Chain

■ The ossicular chain, suspended in the middle ear by ligaments, is composed of three tiny bones: the malleus, incus, and stapes.

■ The first and largest of the three bones is called the *malleus* (Latin for *hammer*) because it resembles a hammer. One end of the malleus is embedded in the tympanic membrane. Because of this attachment, the vibrations of the tympanic membrane are transmitted to the malleus.

- The malleus is attached to the second bone, which is called the *incus* (Latin for *anvil*). The malleus and incus are connected in a tight joint that permits very little movement.

- The incus is attached to the third bone, called the *stapes* (Latin for *stirrup*). The footplate, or other end of the stapes, is inserted into the oval window, a small opening that leads to the inner ear.

- The ossicular chain transmits sound efficiently and with no distortion. It also amplifies incoming sound by approximately 30 dB before transmitting it into the fluids of the inner ear.

Muscles and Reflexes

- Two small muscles in the middle ear dampen the vibrations of the tympanic membrane and the ossicular chain: the tensor tympani and the stapedius muscles.

- The *tensor tympani* is innervated by cranial nerve V (the trigeminal nerve). The *stapedius* muscle, the smallest in the body, is innervated by cranial nerve VII (the facial nerve).

- The stapedius muscle stiffens the ossicular chain so that its vibrations are reduced. The tensor tympani muscle tenses the tympanic membrane so that its vibrations are reduced.

- When a person hears very loud noises that could damage the ears, the middle ear muscles contract in a reflexive action called the *acoustic reflex*. The acoustic reflex stiffens the middle ear system, especially the tympanic membrane.

Eustachian Tube

- Also known as the auditory tube, the *eustachian tube* connects the middle ear with the nasopharynx. The eustachian tube goes from the anterior middle ear wall to the posterior wall of the nasopharynx.

- The eustachian tube helps maintain equal air pressure within and outside the middle ear. The nasopharyngeal end of the tube can be opened by yawning or swallowing. This ventilates the middle ear by letting in fresh air.

- The *tensor palatini* muscle exerts the pull that allows the eustachian tube to open during yawning, swallowing, and other actions that cause the muscle contract.

- The eustachian tube can also allow germs and infections to spread into the middle ear, causing hearing problems. This is especially common in infants, whose eustachian tubes are more horizontal than those of adults.

- Infants with a cleft of the palate frequently have eustachian tube dysfunction, making them vulnerable to conductive hearing loss (described later).

✎ Concepts To Consider

List and briefly describe the key anatomic components of the middle and inner ear.

_____

_____

_____

_____

_____

_____

_____

The Inner Ear

- The inner ear is the most complex of the three divisions of the ear. It begins with the *oval window*, which is a small opening in the *temporal bone* that houses the inner ear. Through the movement of the footplate of the stapes in the oval window, the inner ear receives the mechanical vibrations of sound.

- The inner ear is a system of interconnecting tunnels called *labyrinths* within the temporal bone. The tunnels are filled with a fluid called *perilymph*.

- There are two major structures in the inner ear, each with separate functions. The first is the *vestibular system*, which contains three *semicircular canals*. The semicircular canals are responsible for equilibrium. Thus, the vestibular system is related to movement, balance, and body posture.

- The second major structure in the inner ear is the *cochlea*. The cochlea is snail shaped and resembles a coiled tunnel. When stretched, the human cochlea measures about 3.8 cm (1.5 inches). It is filled with *endolymph*, a type of fluid.

- The floor of the cochlear duct is called the *basilar membrane*, which contains the *organ of Corti*. The organ of Corti is bathed in endolymph and contains several thousand hair cells or *cilia*, which respond to sound vibrations. Each ear contains approximately 15,500 hair cells.

- The vibrations created by the footplate of the stapes into the oval window create wavelike movements in the perilymph. Through *Reissner's membrane,* those movements are transmitted to the endolymph. The endolymph then transmits the movements to the basilar membrane.

- Different portions of the basilar membrane respond best to sounds of different frequencies. The tip of the membrane is thicker, wider, and more lax than the base.

■ At the base, the membrane is thinner, narrower, and stiffer than at the tip. Low-frequency sounds stimulate the tip, and high-frequency sounds stimulate the base. The stimulating sound signals set off waves in the fluid, which in turn create movements of the membrane.

■ The hair cells in the organ of Corti respond to the vibrations of the basilar membrane. The vibrations create a shearing force on those cells. At that point, the mechanical forces of vibrations are transformed into electrical energy, which can stimulate nerve endings.

■ This energy transformation within the organ of Corti is critical, because the nerve fibers that carry the sound to the brain do not respond to mechanical vibrations—only to electrical impluses.

The Auditory Nervous System

■ The nerve that picks up the neural impulses created by the movement of the hair cells in the cochlea is called the *acoustic nerve*. This nerve, also called *cranial nerve VIII*, is a bundle of neurons with two branches.

■ The *vestibular branch* is concerned with body equilibrium or balance. The *auditory* or *acoustic branch* supplies many hair cells of the cochlea and conducts electrical sound impulses from the cochlea to the brain.

■ The auditory division of the acoustic nerve has many endings in the cochlea. These nerve endings are in contact with the hair cells to pick up the sound vibrations that are transformed into neural impulses.

■ Approximately 30,000 nerve fibers of the auditory nerve exist in the cochlea. The auditory nerve exits the inner ear through the *internal auditory meatus*.

■ The nerve impulses carried by the right and left auditory pathways enter the brain stem. The auditory pathways up to this point (the brain stem) are considered *peripheral* (related to structures outside the brain). Beyond the brain stem, the pathways are considered *central* (within the brain).

■ At the *cerebellopontine angle*, the auditory nerve exits the temporal bone through the internal auditory meatus and enters the brain stem. At the brain stem level, most of the auditory nerve fibers from one ear *decussate* (cross over) to the opposite side, forming *contralateral* pathways.

■ Some, however, continue on the same side, forming *ipsilateral* pathways. This crossover of signals allows the brain to compare the sounds received from each of the two ears. It helps the brain localize and interpret sounds.

■ From the brain stem, the acoustic nerve fibers project sound to the temporal lobe of the brain. The temporal lobe contains the primary auditory area, which is responsible for receiving and interpreting sound stimuli. The temporal lobe, with its primary auditory area, is shown in Figure 10.2.

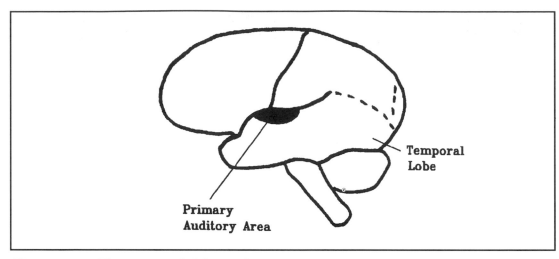

Figure 10.2. The temporal lobe and primary auditory area. From *Introduction to Communicative Disorders*, 2nd ed. (p. 425), by M. N. Hegde, 1995, Austin, TX: PRO-ED. Copyright 1995 by PRO-ED, Inc. Reprinted with permission.

Summary

☑ The outer ear, composed of the auricle and the pinna, funnels sound to the middle ear. The tympanic membrane, which separates the outer ear from the middle ear, vibrates in response to sound.

☑ Sound is then responded to by the ossicles, which conduct the sound to the inner ear. The vestibular system and cochlea are the major structures of the inner ear. Energy is transformed, in the inner ear, to electrical impulses, which stimulate the acoustic nerve.

☑ The auditory branch of the acoustic nerve carries electrical sound impulses from the cochlea to the brain, where the sound is interpreted in the primary auditory area of the temporal lobe.

ACOUSTICS: SOUND AND ITS PERCEPTION

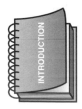

INTRODUCTION

Acoustics, a branch of physics, is the study of sound as a physical event. *Psychoacoustics* is the study of sound as the psychological experience of hearing. Speech is the most important acoustic signal for humans to perceive. (For a more in-depth discussion of acoustics, see Chapter 2.) Humans perceive sound in terms of frequency (pitch) and intensity (loudness). Hearing can be measured in terms of sound pressure or hearing level.

The Source of Sound

■ The source of sound is mechanical vibrations of an elastic object. The vibrations create waves of disturbance. The waves then travel through a gas, a liquid, or a solid—these are called *mediums*. These mediums must be elastic to carry sound. In order to be called a sound, the disturbance of the molecules must be audible.

■ There are many sources of sound: the vocal folds, the strings of an instrument, a tuning fork, and others. The vibrations of a tuning fork illustrate a source of sound. A tuning fork, when struck, vibrates at a single frequency.

■ Vibrations occur in *cycles*, or repeated patterns of movement that are measured per second. *Frequency* refers to the number of times a cycle of vibration repeats itself within a second. A tone of single frequency is called a *pure tone*. A tone of single frequency that repeats itself is called a *simple harmonic motion*. Two or more sounds of differing frequencies create a *complex tone*.

■ The vibrations that make up a complex tone may be periodic or aperiodic. As illustrated in Figure 10.3, *periodic* vibrations have a pattern that repeats itself at regular intervals. *Aperiodic* vibrations do not have such a pattern; they occur at irregular intervals (Stach, 1997).

Sound Waves

■ When an object such as a guitar string moves back and forth, it displaces nearby air molecules, causing them to move, too. This in turn causes movement in molecules lying farther and farther away from the vibrating object. These movements are called *sound waves*.

■ The molecules near the vibrating object swing back and forth while remaining where they are (they do not move from one point to another). These swings disturb adjacent molecules, which then swing back and forth, thus disturbing molecules next to them, and the process continues.

■ The to-and-fro movements of the molecules change the air pressure, because the movements consist of an instance in which the molecules are compressed together (*compression*) and an instance in which they are farther apart (*rarefaction*). As Figure 10.4 illustrates, a single cycle consists of one instance of compression and one instance of rarefaction within a second.

■ The term *Hertz* (Hz) refers to cycles per second. For example, 200 Hz means that there are 200 cycles of compression and rarefaction in 1 second. It means the same thing as 200 cps, or cycles per second.

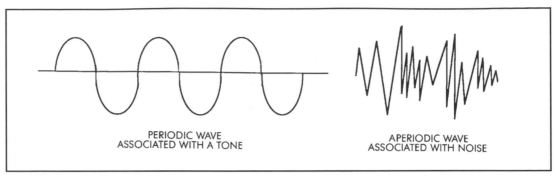

Figure 10.3. Periodic and aperiodic sound waves. From *Introduction to Communicative Disorders*, 2nd ed. (p. 416), by M. N. Hegde, 1995, Austin, TX: PRO-ED. Copyright 1995 by PRO-ED, Inc. Reprinted with permission.

Frequency and Intensity

■ The human ear is capable of responding to frequencies in the range of 20 Hz to 20,000 Hz. Some animals, such as dogs and dolphins, can hear sounds of much higher frequency.

■ Variations in the frequency of vibratory cycles cause the sensation of different pitches. *Pitch* changes are basically changes in frequency. Pitch is the perceptual correlate of changes in frequency. Pitch is perceptual; frequency is physical.

■ As well as varying in frequency, sounds vary in *intensity*. Changes in intensity are changes in the *loudness* of sounds. Loudness is a perceptual phenomenon, and intensity is a physical phenomenon.

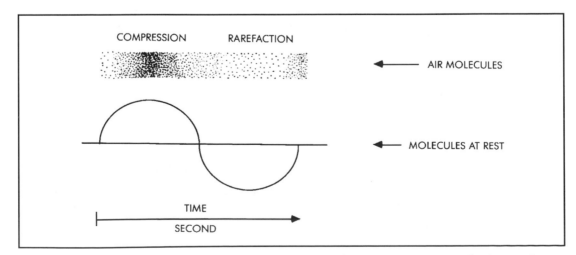

Figure 10.4. A tone of a single Hz (1 cps) containing one instance of rarefaction and one instance of compression of air molecules in 1 second. From *Introduction to Communicative Disorders*, 2nd ed. (p. 417), by M. N. Hegde, 1995, Austin, TX: PRO-ED. Copyright 1995 by PRO-ED, Inc. Reprinted with permission.

■ Intensity is related to *amplitude*, which is the extent of displacement of the molecules in their to-and-fro motion. The greater the range of displacement, the greater the amplitude of the sound. And the greater the amplitude of sound, the greater the intensity of that sound. Tones of different amplitude in the context of different frequencies are illustrated in Figure 10.5.

■ The human ear is sensitive to a wide range of intensity—perhaps 10 trillion units as measured on a linear scale that has an absolute zero point and equal numerical increments.

■ Because measuring these large numbers is cumbersome, scientists use a *logarithmic scale*. On such a scale, one number is multiplied by itself a specified number of times.

■ On a logarithmic scale, the ear is sensitive to 130 units called *decibels* (dB). A decibel is 1/10 of a Bell, the basic unit of measurement named after inventor Alexander Graham Bell.

✎ Concepts To Consider

Define the terms *frequency* and *intensity*, as they apply to acoustics.

_____

_____

_____

_____

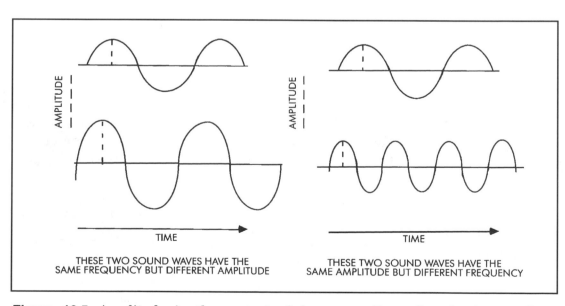

Figure 10.5. Amplitude in the context of frequency. From *Introduction to Communicative Disorders*, 2nd ed. (p. 419), by M. N. Hegde, 1995, Austin, TX: PRO-ED. Copyright 1995 by PRO-ED, Inc. Reprinted with permission.

_____

_____

_____

_____

Sound Pressure Level and Hearing Level

■ The decibel is a measure of sound pressure; it also measures the intensity of one sound against another.

■ The value of *sound pressure* is the square root of power, which is measured in *watts*. The pressure is measured in terms of *pascals*, or pa. The intensity of a sound is expressed in terms of decibels at a certain *sound pressure level*, or SPL.

■ For example, normal speech usually varies between 50 and 70 dB SPL. Very loud sounds, such as those of an airplane, may be as high as 100 dB SPL. People feel pain when sound level reaches 140 dB SPL.

■ SPL is different than *hearing level* (HL), which is the lowest intensity of a sound necessary to stimulate the auditory system. Hearing level is the decibel level used on audiometers; it is the decibel level of sound referenced to audiometric zero (Stach, 1997).

■ The auditory system is not equally sensitive to all frequencies at the same intensity. The human ear is most sensitive to sounds ranging between 1,000 and 4,000 Hz. Thus, to stimulate the auditory system, tones of 1,000–4,000 Hz can be less intense than tones of other frequencies. This differential sensitivity of the human ear to different frequencies creates complications in the measurement of hearing and hearing loss.

■ To deal with this problem, scientists first determined sound pressure levels necessary to stimulate the auditory system at different frequencies in a large number of people with normal hearing. Then those sound pressure levels were considered the 0-dB hearing level. For example, to stimulate the healthy normal ear of a young adult, a tone of 250 Hz must have a sound pressure level of 25.5 dB SPL. For the same purpose, a sound of 1,000 Hz needs only 7 dB SPL.

■ In measuring hearing with an audiometer, the actual SPL values needed to stimulate the auditory system of a normal person at those two frequencies were set at 0, although in the case of the 250 Hz tone, the SPL value is higher than in the other tone (1,000 Hz). Similarly, for all the frequencies that are tested on an audiometer, the amount of energy needed to stimulate the auditory system has been set at 0.

Summary

☑ Sound must travel through a medium and create an audible disturbance of molecules in order to be heard. Sound occurs in cycles, each of which consists of one instance of compression and one instance of rarefaction.

☑ Humans hear sounds in various frequencies at various intensity levels, and respond differentially to different frequencies. Human responses to sound can be measured by several means, including sound pressure level and hearing level.

THE NATURE AND ETIOLOGY OF HEARING LOSS

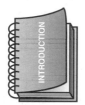

INTRODUCTION

The development of hearing begins in utero, where fetuses can respond to sound in the first trimester of development. Babies localize and discriminate sound with increasing skill as they grow older. This sound is conducted to the inner ear through either air or bone conduction. In people with hearing impairment, this process is disrupted through hearing loss of a conductive, sensorineural, or mixed nature. Some people also experience hearing loss due to auditory nervous system impairments.

Normal Hearing

Auditory Development

■ Normal hearing is made possible by the complex working of the outer, middle, and inner ear as well as the auditory nerve and auditory areas of the brain. Normal hearing also involves a set of skills that develop over time.

■ During the fetal development period, babies can hear in utero—in fact, a 20-week-old fetus responds to sound. Newborns can respond differentially to sounds of different intensity and frequency.

■ By 3–4 months of age, babies turn their head toward sources of sound. Three-month-old babies respond to the mother's voice more consistently than to anyone else's voice.

■ As babies grow older, they respond more precisely to auditory stimuli. Sounds are better discriminated and localized. By 6 months of age, an infant can localize speech that is very soft. Young babies with normal hearing can hear better than adults.

Air and Bone Conduction of Sound

- In people with normal hearing, sound is conducted to the inner ear by two means: air conduction and bone conduction.

- In the process of *air conduction*, sound waves strike the tympanic membrane. The movement of the tympanic membrane causes the ossicles to move, creating movement of the fluids of the inner ear. These movements cause vibrations in the basilar membrane of the cochlea.

- The hair cells supplied by the acoustic nerve respond to these vibrations, and the sound is carried to the brain by the acoustic nerve. In this process, sound travels through the medium of air. Thus, the process is described as air conduction.

- The process of *bone conduction* is different. The fluids of the inner ear are housed in the skull. The larger bones of the skull conduct sound, as does the ossicular chain of the middle ear. The skull bones vibrate in response to air-borne sound waves, causing movements in the inner ear fluids. Thus, bones have conducted the sound to the inner ear.

- Air and bone conduction result in the same kind of cochlear activity, in which the hair cells are displaced. Normally, air- and bone-conducted movements are integrated. It is only in certain kinds of hearing loss that the two can be distinguished.

Nature of Hearing Impairment

- Hearing impairment is an increasing health and educational problem in society. Many more people are living longer lives and thus manifesting hearing problems associated with the aging process.

- In addition, more newborn babies are at risk for hearing impairment. Advanced medical technology has enabled more fragile, high-risk, preterm infants to be saved; these infants are more vulnerable to hearing problems than healthy, full-term infants are.

- Factors that place a child at risk for hearing loss include anatomic malformations of the head and neck, maternal history of drug and/or alcohol abuse, certain maternal diseases such as rubella or syphilis during pregnancy, and family history of childhood hearing impairment.

- Hearing impairment can be very mild, creating few or no problems in communication. It can also be severe to profound, causing major difficulties in articulation, resonance, and comprehension and reception of speech. The range of hearing loss in dB HL and the corresponding categories are shown in Table 10.1.

TABLE 10.1

Range and Categories of Hearing Loss with the Corresponding dB HL

Hearing Loss	Characteristics
Up to 15 dB	Normal hearing in children. In adults the upper limit of normal hearing may extend to 25 dB.
16 to 40 dB	Mild hearing loss in children: difficulty hearing faint or distant speech; may cause language delay in children. In adults the range is between 25 and 40 dB.
41 to 55 dB	Moderate hearing loss: delayed speech and language acquisition; difficulty in producing certain speech sounds correctly; difficulty following conversation.
56 to 70 dB	Moderately severe hearing loss: can understand only amplified or shouted speech.
70 to 90 dB	Severe hearing loss: difficulty understanding even loud and amplified speech; significant difficulty in learning and producing intelligible oral language.
90+ dB	Profound hearing loss: typically described as deaf; hearing does not play a major role in learning, producing, and understanding spoken speech and language.

Note. From *Introduction to Communicative Disorders*, 2nd ed. (p. 428), by M. N. Hegde, 1995, Austin, TX: PRO-ED. Copyright 1995 by PRO-ED, Inc. Reprinted with permission.

- The term *hearing impaired* refers to the condition of being hard of hearing or deaf.

- The child who is *hard of hearing* has a loss between 16 and 75 dB; children who are hard of hearing acquire speech and oral language with variable proficiency. The adult who is hard of hearing has a loss between 25 and 75 dB.

- Children and adults who are *deaf* are those who cannot hear or understand conversational speech under normal circumstances. Their hearing loss exceeds 75 dB and in many cases is greater than 90 dB.

- The term *Deaf* with an upper-case *D* refers to deafness not as a disability but as a cultural identity (Helfer, 1998).

- People who have a hearing impairment may have one of several kinds of hearing losses: conductive, sensorineural, or mixed. Some people also manifest central auditory or retrocochlear disorders, which are special categories.

Conductive Hearing Loss

- In conductive hearing loss the efficiency with which the sound is conducted to the middle or inner ear is diminished. In pure conductive hearing loss, the inner ear, acoustic nerve, and auditory centers of the brain are all working normally. The person's bone conduction is also fairly normal (*normal bone conduction* refers to the skull bones, not the ossicular chain).

■ Even when the bones of the ossicular chain are not conducting sound, the bones of the skull will. Thus, conductive hearing loss is never profound; there is always some hearing left because of bone conduction created by the skull bones.

■ Because of this, people with conductive hearing loss can hear their own speech well. Thus, they tend to speak too softly, especially when there is background noise, which they cannot hear as well as their listeners can.

■ There are many causes of conductive hearing loss. These include abnormalities of the external auditory canal, the tympanic membrane, or the ossicular chain of the middle ear.

■ People can have birth defects, diseases, and foreign bodies that block the external ear canal. Some children born with cleft palate or other craniofacial anomalies may have *aural atresia*, in which the external ear canal is completely closed. Atresia is often associated with *microtia*, in which the pinna is very small and deformed (Bess & Humes, 1995).

■ Another birth defect, *stenosis*, results in an extremely narrow external auditory canal. In these cases, most sound waves will not strike the tympanic membrane.

■ *External otitis*, caused by bacteria or viruses, is a fairly common infection of the skin of the external auditory canal; this is a cause of conductive loss. This infection, commonly found in swimmers, results in the swelling of the tissue of the external auditory canal. Consequently, sound transmission is reduced.

■ Foreign objects in the ear canal, such as beans, paper clips, and seeds, can block the ear canal and impede hearing. *Bony growths* and tumors may appear in the external ear canal, blocking the transmission of sound to the middle and inner ears.

■ *Otitis media*, also known as *middle ear effusion*, is an infection of the middle ear that is often associated with upper respiratory infections and eustachian tube dysfunction. Figure 10.6 shows an audiogram representing a typical hearing loss seen in people with otitis media accompanied by effusion.

■ Otitis media occurs frequently in infants and children and rarely in adults. Differences in the incidence rate of otitis media have been found among racial groups. African Americans have the lowest rate; the highest rates exist among Aborigines, Alaskan Eskimos, and Native Americans. These differences in incidence rates may be related to differences in the structure and function of the eustachian tube among various racial groups (Scott, 1998).

■ Otitis media usually creates a conductive hearing loss of 20–35 dB HL, which often goes undetected by regular pure-tone screenings, which are carried out at 25 dB HL. There are three types of otitis media: serous, acute, and chronic.

■ In *serous otitis media*, the middle ear is inflamed and filled with watery or thick fluid. The eustachian tube is blocked and thus does not allow fresh air

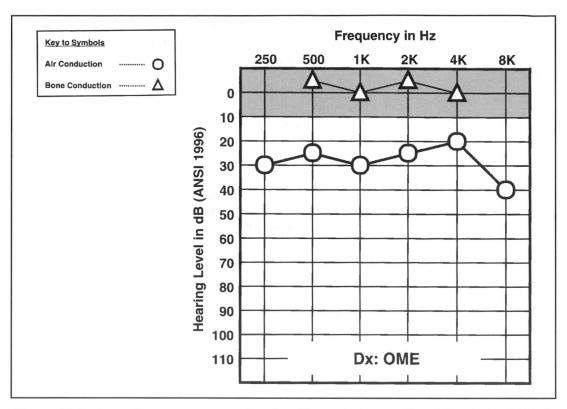

Figure 10.6. An audiogram representing the effects of otitis media with effusion (OME). From *Clinical Audiology: An Introduction* (p. 130), by B. A. Stach, 1998, San Diego, CA: Singular Publishing Group, Inc. (401 West A Street, Suite 325, San Diego, CA 92101-7904, 800-521-8545). Copyright 1998 by Singular Publishing Group, Inc. Reprinted with permission.

to ventilate the middle ear. The middle ear thus becomes airtight; soon the air inside is thinned out and the pressure is reduced.

■ The increased air pressure outside the ear begins to push the tympanic membrane inward, reducing its mobility. The retracted membrane vibrates inefficiently, resulting in conductive hearing loss. Serous otitis media is frequently treated with antibiotics and *pressure equalizing (PE) tubes*. These tiny tubes are inserted through the tympanic membrane, ventilating the middle ear and restoring hearing.

■ In *acute otitis media*, there is sudden onset due to infection. A quick buildup of fluid and pus causes moderate to severe pain. The child has a fever and may experience vertigo. The buildup of pressure in the middle ear may rupture the tympanic membrane, thus giving instant relief as pus is discharged from the ruptured membrane.

■ Acute otitis media is treated with medical and surgical procedures. In a surgical procedure known as *myringotomy*, small incisions are made in the tympanic membrane to relieve pressure.

■ In *chronic otitis media*, there is permanent damage to middle ear structures. This is frequently due to erosion of ossicles, cholosteotoma, or atrophy or perforation of the tympanic membrane (Roark & Berman, 1996).

■ When the tympanic membrane is involved, it is permanently ruptured with or without associated middle ear diseases. Many patients may have a painless, foul-smelling discharge from the ear. Antibiotics may be prescribed if an infection is present. In a surgical procedure known as *myringoplasty*, the perforated tympanic membrane is surgically repaired.

■ Mild and nonrecurrent otitis media generally does not cause permanent hearing loss. Permanent loss is more likely to result from chronic disease. However, even mild and fluctuating conductive hearing loss associated with prolonged middle ear infections in young children can adversely affect their speech and language development.

■ *Otosclerosis* is another common cause of conductive hearing loss. It may be inherited and is more common in women than in men. It is found primarily among Whites worldwide (Scott, 1998).

■ In otosclerosis, a new, spongy growth starts on the footplate of the stapes. Consequently, the stapes becomes rigid and the footplate does not move enough into the oval window to create pressure waves in the inner ear fluid. Figure 10.7 shows an audiogram representing the typical hearing loss seen in people with otosclerosis.

■ *Carhart's notch*, frequently found in patients with otosclerosis, is a pattern of bone-conduction thresholds characterized by reduced bone conduction sensitivity at 2,000 Hz (Stach, 1998).

■ A disease called *otospongiosis* causes the stapes to become too soft to vibrate. The diseased or fixated stapes is surgically removed in a procedure called a *stapedectomy*. A synthetic prosthesis of wire or Teflon replaces the removed stapes, often dramatically improving hearing post-surgically.

■ Other causes of conductive hearing loss include collapsed ear canals, impacted cerumen, ossicular fixation, and disarticulation of the articulatory chain. Figure 10.8 shows an audiogram representing the typical hearing loss seen in people with disarticulation of the articulatory chain, also called *ossicular discontinuity*.

Sensorineural Hearing Loss

■ In sensorineural hearing loss, the middle ear may conduct the sound efficiently to the inner ear, but damage to the hair cells of the cochlea or to the acoustic nerve may prevent the brain from receiving the neural impulses of sound.

■ Sensorineural loss is permanent because the damaged hair cells and the acoustic nerve are not repairable. The person with sensorineural loss experiences very mild to profound deafness.

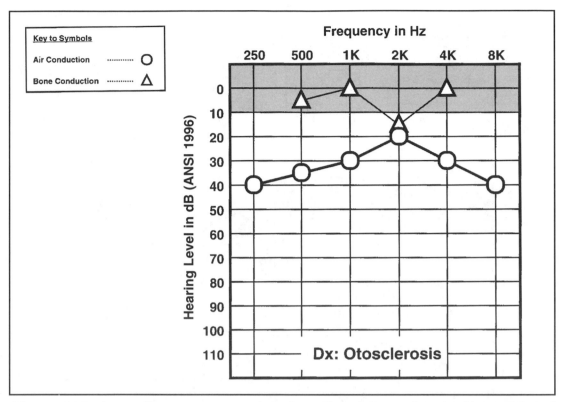

Figure 10.7. An audiogram representing the effects of otosclerosis. From *Clinical Audiology: An Introduction* (p. 132), by B. A. Stach, 1998, San Diego, CA: Singular Publishing Group, Inc. (401 West A Street, Suite 325, San Diego, CA 92101-7904, 800-521-8545). Copyright 1998 by Singular Publishing Group, Inc. Reprinted with permission.

■ Bone as well as air conduction is impaired; thus, people with sensorineural loss have difficulty hearing themselves, as well as others. This causes them to speak louder.

■ Sensorineural loss is not the same across all frequencies; some are more adversely affected than others. The higher frequencies tend to be more profoundly affected by sensorineural loss than the lower frequencies.

■ A potential symptom of sensorineural hearing loss is recruitment. *Recruitment* refers to a disproportionate increase in the growth of perception of the loudness of sound when it is presented with linear increases in intensity. Recruitment makes a person hypersensitive to intense sounds and must be considered during hearing aid fitting (Nober, 1998).

■ People with sensorineural hearing loss may experience severe effects on their speech and language. Articulation, resonance, and even voice may be affected. There are many causes of sensorineural hearing loss.

■ *Prenatal causes* of hearing loss include events that occur during pregnancy to damage fetus's hearing. Certain drugs taken by the mother, especially during the 6th and 7th week of pregnancy, can cause cochlear damage in the fetus. Children born to alcohol- and drug-addicted mothers may have sensorineural hearing loss.

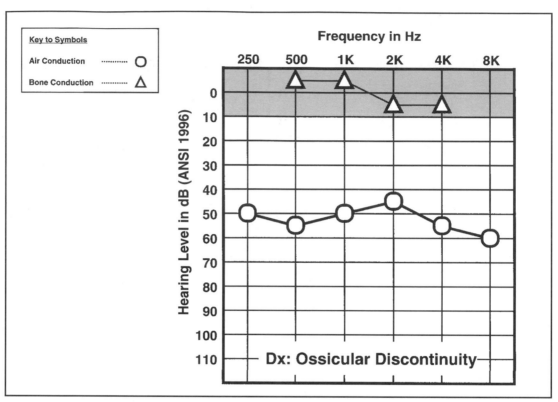

Figure 10.8. An audiogram representing the effects of ossicular discontinuity. From *Clinical Audiology: An Introduction* (p. 134), by B. A. Stach, 1998, San Diego, CA: Singular Publishing Group, Inc. (401 West A Street, Suite 325, San Diego, CA 92101-7904, 800-521-8545). Copyright 1998 by Singular Publishing Group, Inc. Reprinted with permission.

- *Ototoxic* drugs are drugs that reach the inner ear through the bloodstream and damage the cochlear hair cells or the acoustic nerve fibers in children and adults. Antibiotic drugs of the "mycin" family (kanamycin, meomycin, strepto-mycin) are especially ototoxic.

- These powerful antibiotics should be used only in cases of severe, life-threatening infections such as those related to kidney malfunctioning. In such cases, profound hearing loss may be an undesirable and unavoidable side effect.

- *Noise* is another factor that can induce sensorineural hearing loss. Prolonged exposure to intense noises (e.g., loud music, drills, airplanes, explosives) usually damages the cochlear hair cells. Noise-induced sensorineural hearing loss tends to be the worst from noise between 3,000 Hz and 6,000 Hz (see Figure 10.9).

- *Birth defects* in some children may cause sensorineural hearing loss. The auditory nerve or cochlea may not have developed normally by the time the baby is born. Portions of the inner ear may be missing.

- There are viral and bacterial diseases that can result in sensorineural hearing loss in children. Bacterial meningitis and mumps are two causes of sensorineural loss. The acronym STORCH refers to major causes of hearing loss in fetuses and newborns (Bess & Humes, 1995; Gelfand, 1997):

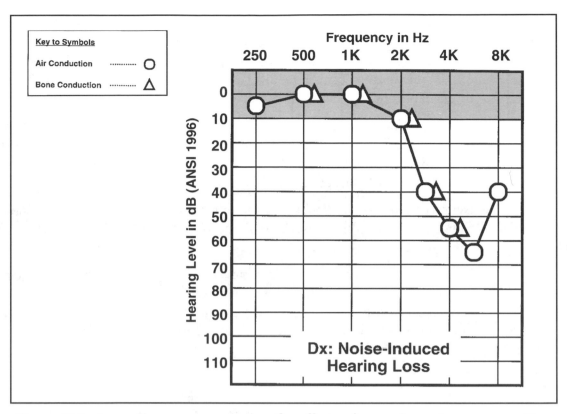

Figure 10.9. An audiogram representing the effects of excessive noise exposure. From *Clinical Audiology: An Introduction* (p. 134), by B. A. Stach, 1998, San Diego, CA: Singular Publishing Group, Inc., (401 West A Street, Suite 325, San Diego, CA 92101-7904, 800-521-8545). Copyright 1998 by Singular Publishing Group, Inc. Reprinted with permission.

- *Syphilis*, which some children contract from the mother at the time of birth, can cause inner ear damage.

- *Toxoplasmosis*, a disease transmitted through the placenta, is often contracted when the pregnant mother handles cat feces or contaminated raw eggs and meat.

- *Other*

- *Rubella*, or German measles, can be transferred to the fetus through the placenta.

- *Cytomegalovirus*, the most common cause of viral hearing loss, is a herpes-type virus transmitted by close contact with infected children and also through sexual contact.

- *Herpes simplex*, transmitted from the mother to the fetus, also can cause hearing loss.

■ A tumor called an *acoustic neuroma* can develop on the acoustic nerve and cause sensorineural loss by slowing nerve conduction of sound impulses to the brain.

■ *Presbycusis*, a hearing impairment in older people, is due to the effect of aging and is associated with sensorineural hearing loss. Presbycusis affects the high frequencies especially, resulting in a sloping, high-frequency loss (see Figure 10.10). Patients often have difficulty with recognition of speech, especially under challenging listening conditions such as noisy parties.

■ *Meniere's disease* is a condition that causes fluctuating sensorineural hearing loss, usually in adults. It is attributed to excessive endolymphatic fluid pressure in the membranous labyrinth; this causes Reissner's membrane to become distended (Gelfand, 1997).

■ Symptoms of Meniere's disease include hearing loss, spells of dizziness or vertigo, a sense of fullness in the ear, and *tinnitus*, a ringing or buzzing sound in the ears. Currently, no cure for this disease is available.

■ Some sensorineural hearing loss can be helped by medical and surgical intervention, but much cannot. Most people who have sensorineural hearing loss rely on a combination of early education (for children), amplification of sound, and speech–language therapy. These and other habilitative services are described later in the chapter.

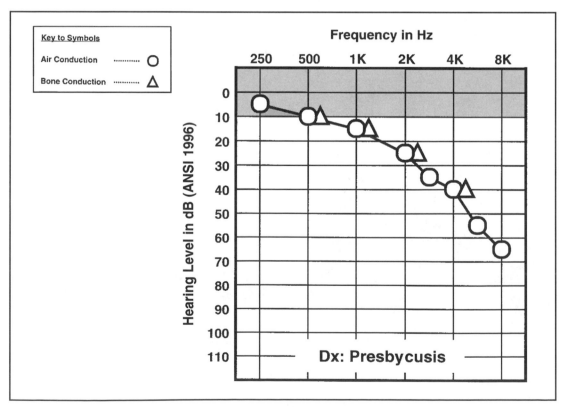

Figure 10.10. An audiogram representing the effects of presbycusis. From *Clinical Audiology: An Introduction* (p. 152), by B. A. Stach, 1998, San Diego, CA: Singular Publishing Group, Inc. (401 West A Street, Suite 325, San Diego, CA 92101-7904, 800-521-8545). Copyright 1998 by Singular Publishing Group, Inc. Reprinted with permission.

Mixed Hearing Loss

- Mixed hearing loss occurs when neither the middle nor the inner ear is functioning properly. Any of the several conditions that cause conductive and sensorineural hearing loss can, in some combination, cause a mixed loss.

- Mixed losses can be caused by the presence of two separate disorders in the same ear. For example, a child could have a sensorineural loss *and* otitis media, which created a temporary conductive loss in the same ear.

- Another cause of mixed losses could be a single pathology, such as advanced otosclerosis or a head injury, that affected both sensorineural and conductive systems (Gelfand, 1997).

- A mixed loss affects both air and bone conduction. However, air conduction is affected more than bone conduction.

- Figure 10.11 compares the typical profiles of hearing loss presented by people with conductive, sensorineural, and mixed losses.

Concepts To Consider

Define and describe the terms *conductive hearing loss* and *sensorineural hearing loss*. What are two causes of each type of loss?

_____
_____
_____
_____
_____
_____
_____
_____

Auditory Nervous System Impairments

Central Auditory Disorders

- *Peripheral hearing problems* are those problems resulting from problems in the outer, middle, or inner ear (excluding the auditory nerve). *Central auditory disorders* are those caused by a lesion or lesions in the central auditory system.

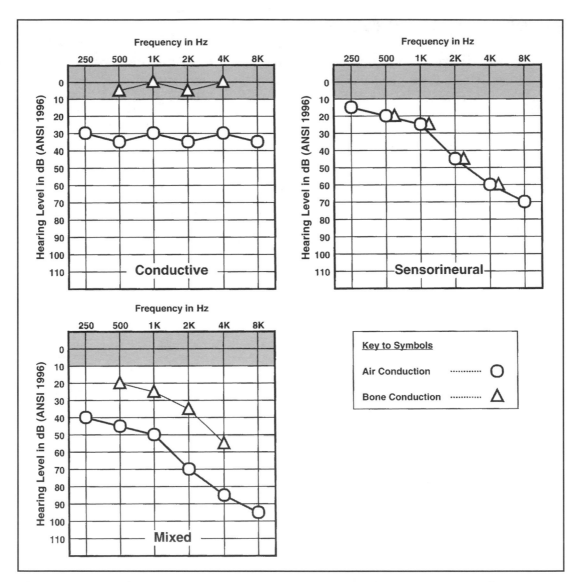

Figure 10.11. Audiograms representing the three types of hearing losses: conductive, sensorineural, and mixed. From *Clinical Audiology: An Introduction* (p. 212), by B. A. Stach, 1998, San Diego, CA: Singular Publishing Group, Inc. (401 West A Street, Suite 325, San Diego, CA 92101-7904, 800-521-8545). Copyright 1998 by Singular Publishing Group, Inc. Reprinted with permission.

■ The *central auditory system* includes the brain stem, where the auditory nerve terminates, the fibers that project sound to the auditory centers of the brain, and those brain centers themselves.

■ Central auditory disorders can be caused by tumors, traumatic brain injury, HIV, asphyxia during birth, various genetic disorders, infections such as meningitis and encephalitis, metabolic disturbances, cerebrovascular diseases, drug- or chemical-induced problems, central degenerative diseases such as Alzheimer's disease, and demyelinating diseases such as multiple sclerosis.

■ There is great controversy in the literature about the existence, nature, and treatment of central auditory disorders. Empirical evidence is limited, and many researchers do not support "central auditory disorders" as a valid diagnostic label (Cacace & McFarland, 1998), although others do.

■ In people with central auditory disorders, there may be no significant peripheral hearing loss. Routine speech recognition tests in quiet environments and typical pure-tone threshold tests are not sensitive to central auditory disorders (Hood & Berlin, 1996).

■ Difficulty understanding distorted speech is a major symptom of central auditory disorders. In some of the central auditory tests, speech may be presented at low intensity, compressed in time, masked with noise, periodically interrupted, or filtered by eliminating certain frequencies of speech. *Dichotic listening* tasks, in which the listener must process different messages presented simultaneously to both ears, are also used.

■ Although everyone has some difficulty understanding such distorted speech, those with central auditory disorders have a greater amount of difficulty.

■ For example, when there is a lesion in the temporal lobe of the brain, filtered-speech test scores may be poorer in the ear opposite the damaged side (contralateral) than in the ear on the side of the damage. People with central auditory disorders usually also have abnormal auditory discrimination because speech sounds are distorted at the cortical level (Mencher, Gerber, & McCombe, 1997).

■ Patients with central auditory disorders typically have the following characteristics (Hood & Berlin, 1996; Mencher et al., 1997):

  – poor auditory integration

  – poor auditory sequencing skills

  – poor auditory closure (e.g., recognizing that "_anta __aus" is "Santa Claus")

  – difficulty listening when background noise exists

  – poor auditory attention

  – poor auditory memory

  – poor auditory localization, or ability to locate a sound source in the environment

  – difficulty understanding rapid speech and other forms of auditory input that are characterized by reduced redundancy

  – difficulty learning to read aloud due to inability to learn correct association of visual and auditory symbols

■ Treatment for people with central auditory disorders often involves improving the patients' listening environments and implementing FM systems (described later) to enhance incoming auditory stimuli.

■ Children with central auditory disorders also profit from management techniques such as gaining the child's attention, supplementing auditory input with simultaneous visual cues, and limiting the length and complexity of incoming messages (Hood & Berlin, 1996).

Retrocochlear Disorders

■ People with *retrocochlear* pathology have damage to the nerve fibers along the ascending auditory pathways from the internal auditory meatus to the cortex (Bess & Humes, 1995). Thus, these disorders usually consist of pathology involving the cerebellopontine angle (described later) or cranial nerve VIII.

■ Retrocochlear pathology is usually caused by unilateral tumors or *acoustic neuromas*. The patient often experiences a unilateral high-frequency hearing loss that may be accompanied by tinnitus and/or dizziness (see Figure 10.12). When the affected ear is stimulated, acoustic reflexes are usually absent or present at elevated levels (Bess & Humes, 1995).

■ Patients with acoustic neuromas may also have alterations of facial sensation because the trigeminal nerve is compromised. There may be pain and headache in the ear and mastoid region. Due to compression of the brain stem

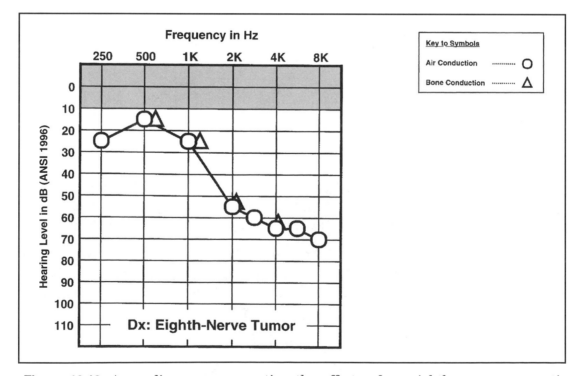

Figure 10.12. An audiogram representing the effects of an eighth-nerve or acoustic tumor. From *Clinical Audiology: An Introduction* (p. 157), by B. A. Stach, 1998, San Diego, CA: Singular Publishing Group, Inc. (401 West A Street, Suite 325, San Diego, CA 92101-7904, 800-521-8545). Copyright 1998 by Singular Publishing Group, Inc. Reprinted with permission.

and cerebellum, the patient may experience dysphagia and become hoarse (Mencher et al., 1997).

■ Symptoms of retrocochlear disorders are often subtle because patients have normal ability to detect pure tones as well as normal speech recognition in quiet. To help determine the presence of retrocochlear pathology, many audiologists use degraded speech signals, which involve speech that is interrupted, accompanied by noise, or filtered.

■ An audiological diagnosis of acoustic neuroma is challenging to make. Because hearing loss is not a complaint in patients with small tumors, audiologists often do not become involved until the tumor is so large that there is a serious hearing loss.

■ It is not difficult to confuse the symptoms of acoustic neuroma with the symptoms of Meniere's disease. Auditory brain stem responses (described later) are a frequently used electrophysiologic measure because they are the easiest to obtain and interpret, and because they assist in differential diagnosis (Mencher et al., 1997).

■ Retrocochlear disorders may be caused by *von Recklinghausen disease*, an inherited disease characterized by the presence of numerous small tumors that grow slowly and occur along various peripheral nerves. When they grow along cranial nerve VIII, they may initially be mistaken for acoustic neuroma. Patients with this disease may die if the tumors become malignant.

■ Brain stem lesions, or tumors that appear in the brain stem at levels above cranial nerve VIII, are so rare that patients often die because the tumors are undiagnosed. Even if they are detected and surgery ensues, there may be problems created by the surgery (e.g., facial paralysis). Some lesions are inoperable because they lie so deep in the brain stem.

Summary

☑ Hearing is a phenomenon that begins even before babies are born and continues to develop throughout early childhood. Through air and bone conduction, sound reaches the inner ear and is sent to the brain for interpretation.

☑ However, some people have conductive, sensorineural, or mixed hearing losses, which disrupt the transmission of sound. People with auditory nervous system impairments such as central auditory and retrocochlear disorders also experience difficulties with sound transmission.

☑ It is important to accurately assess the type of hearing impairment so that appropriate treatment may be provided.

ASSESSMENT OF HEARING IMPAIRMENT

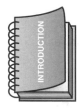

Assessment of hearing impairment has been greatly improved by new technology and sophisticated instrumentation techniques that permit increasingly accurate diagnosis of hearing problems. An initial hearing screening rules out the need for more intensive testing for most people. For those who need such testing, pure tone and speech audiometry are standard assessment procedures, as is acoustic immitance testing, which evaluates middle ear function.

Electrophysiological audiometry and medical imaging incorporate highly specialized diagnostic methods and instruments to evaluate auditory mechanism functioning. Children and infants may be tested by special methods appropriate for their age group. Once children and adults have been tested, the test results are interpreted and recommendations for treatment can be made.

Audiometry: Basic Principles

■ An *audiometer* is an electronic instrument that generates and amplifies pure tones, noise, and other stimuli for testing hearing. Advanced audiometers are totally computerized.

■ The audiometer generates tones at the frequencies (Hz) of 125, 250, 500, 750, 1,000, 1,500, 2,000, 3,000, 4,000, and 8,000 Hz. The audiologist can select the frequency and vary the intensity of the sound stimulus through use of a dial that increases or *attenuates* (decreases) the intensity of the sound.

■ The person to be tested sits in a specially constructed soundproof booth. This booth eliminates interference from ambient noise in the environment.

■ During air-conduction testing, the person wears earphones held in place by a steel headband fitting across the top of the head. The earphones deliver the sound stimulus directly to the ear. The person can respond by holding up a hand or by pressing a switch that lights up a small lamp on the audiometer.

Pure-Tone Audiometry

■ The *pure-tone* hearing test is done to determine the threshold of hearing for selected frequencies. A *threshold* is an intensity level at which a tone is faintly heard at least 50% of the time it is presented. Each tone is presented several times to reliably establish a threshold.

■ Audiologists test hearing at selected frequencies. Usually, a tone of 1,000 Hz is presented first because it is most easily detected. Next, tones of 2,000, 4,000, and 8,000 Hz are tested in that order. Finally, the tones of 500 and 250

Hz are tested. All these frequencies are tested because they are the most important ones for human speech, which falls in the range of 100 to 8,000 Hz.

■ Both ears are tested, starting with one ear. The person is asked to listen and press the response switch immediately when even a faint sound is heard.

■ Bone-conduction testing assesses the sensitivity of the sensorineural portion of the auditory mechanism. The method is as follows. A bone vibrator is placed on the forehead or behind the test ear. When the sound strikes the bones of the skull, the bones vibrate and thus stimulate the fluid in both inner ears. Thus, it is difficult to determine which ear heard the sound and which did not.

■ To overcome this problem, the audiologist uses a procedure called *masking*, in which noise is sent through a headphone at a level that is strong enough to mask the tone heard in the opposite ear.

■ Even in air-conduction testing, masking is used when hearing in one ear is markedly better than hearing in the other ear. The better ear is masked when the poorer ear is tested so that the person does not respond simply because the sound is heard in the better, nontested ear.

Speech Audiometry

■ A person's pure-tone thresholds do not indicate how well he or she understands speech. *Speech audiometry* measures how well a person understands speech and discriminates between speech sounds.

■ The audiologist first determines a *speech reception threshold*, defined as the lowest level of hearing at which the person can understand 50% of the words presented. To make this determination, a list of *spondee words* is used; these words are two-syllable words with equal stress on each syllable (e.g., *baseball*, *hotdog*).

■ The spondee words are either played through a tape recorder or spoken by the audiologist. When the person hears the words through the headphones, he or she writes them down or says them out loud. The *spondee threshold* (ST) is the lowest hearing level (in dB) at which the person correctly identifies 50% of the words.

■ Another assessment made by an audiologist is based on a *word discrimination* or *word recognition* test. This test establishes how well a person discriminates between words by having the person correctly repeat monosyllabic words such as *cap* and *day*.

■ Because the purpose of this test is to determine speech comprehension rather than speech threshold, the words are presented at a level of loudness that is comfortable for the person being tested.

■ The speech discrimination score is the percentage of presented words that the person correctly repeats. This score helps identify people who can hear but not understand speech. People with sensorineural hearing loss are most likely to show this problem.

Acoustic Immitance

▪ *Acoustic immitance* refers to a transfer of acoustic energy. An energy transformation takes place when a sound stimulus reaches the external ear canal and strikes the tympanic membrane.

▪ The tympanic membrane and middle ear structures offer *impedance*, or resistance, to the flow of sound energy. *Admittance*, a counterpart of impedance, is a measure of the amount of energy that flows through the system.

▪ Both very low and very high impedance suggest pathology within the auditory system. For example, a child with middle ear fluid may demonstrate high impedance. An adult with a broken ossicular chain may show low impedance. Tympanometry and acoustic reflex thresholds are two common acoustic immitance measures.

▪ *Tympanometry* is a procedure in which acoustic immitance is measured with an electroacoustic instrument called an *impedance bridge* or *impedance meter*.

▪ This instrument allows the audiologist to place a sound stimulus in the external ear canal with an airtight closure and measure changes in the acoustic energy as the sound stimulates the auditory system. The instrument also helps create either negative or positive changes within the ear canal. Acoustic immitance is altered by such air pressure changes.

▪ The impedance meter can also measure *acoustic reflex*, a simple reflex response of the muscles attached to the stapes bone. The acoustic reflex is elicited in both ears by a relatively loud sound presented to either ear. The reflex response involves a stiffening of the ossicular chain, presumably to protect the ear from potential damage.

▪ Acoustic reflex testing is valuable in detecting middle ear diseases, including those that are not associated with hearing loss.

✎ Concepts To Consider

Briefly compare and contrast pure-tone audiometry, speech audiometry, and acoustic immitance. What is the purpose of each of these types of hearing testing?

_____

_____

_____

_____

_____

_____

_____

_____

Other Methods

Electrophysiological Audiometry

- *Electrophysiological audiometry* is an objective measure of auditory mechanism functioning. In response to sound, the cochlea, acoustic nerve, and auditory centers of the brain generate measurable electrical impulses. These impulses are recorded as changes in the background electrical activity of the brain.

- Such electrical changes produced by sound stimuli are called *auditory-evoked potentials*. Usually, abnormal patterns of electrical activity in reaction to a sound stimulus indicate a hearing loss.

- *Electrocochleography* is the measurement of the electrical activity of the cochlea in response to sound. The electrocochleogram (ECoG) generated by this testing is a response consisting primarily of the compound action potential that occurs at the distal portion of cranial nerve VIII. Electrocochleography is most useful in monitoring cochlear function in operating rooms to simplify the placement of electrodes (Stach, 1998).

- *Auditory brain stem response* (ABR) is a technique used to record the electrical activity in the auditory nerve, the brain stem, and the cortical areas of the brain. It is useful in detecting brain stem diseases. It is also very helpful in testing the hearing of newborn infants.

- If the blood supply to the cochlea is interrupted or the nerve is severed or otherwise damaged when surgeons are operating on tumors or other masses near nerve VIII, either results in hearing loss for the patient.

- It is most helpful for an audiologist to be present during such surgeries. The audiologist uses auditory-evoked potential monitoring to measure the function of nerve VIII and provide feedback to the surgeon during the surgery (Stach, 1998).

Medical Imaging

- *Computerized axial tomography* (described further in Chapter 13) is an important tool in otological diagnosis. It can help detect small tumors as well as brain lesions (e.g., infections, strokes) that cause hearing impairment.

■ *Magnetic resonance imaging* (also described in Chapter 13) is best for imaging the internal auditory canals, base of the skull, and pituitary gland regions to evaluate the possible presence of pathology affecting the auditory system. MRI is especially helpful in detecting acoustic neuromas or tumors.

Hearing Screening

■ It is time consuming to test patients with a complete battery of hearing tests. However, it is important to identify those people who may have a hearing problem. Hearing screening is a quick, preliminary way to determine whether the person being tested has normal hearing or may have a hearing problem and need further, more in-depth testing.

■ The three major groups of individuals who undergo hearing screening are newborns, schoolchildren, and adults in professions in which they are exposed to potentially hazardous levels of noise (Stach, 1998).

■ In hearing screening, pure tones are presented at 20–25 dB. Only the frequencies of 500, 1,000, 2,000, and 4,000 Hz are tested. Testing usually takes place in a quiet room and may be done with individuals or groups.

■ Some people undergo acoustic immitance testing as a part of screening. In public schools, this is rare; usually, schoolchildren undergo pure-tone audiometric screening only.

Assessment of Infants and Children

■ It is important to detect hearing loss in infants as soon as possible, because early intervention can reduce its effects on speech and language acquisition.

■ Various committees and health boards such as the Joint Committee on Accreditation of Health Organizations and the Department of Health and Human Services are encouraging all hospitals to include universal newborn hearing screening programs (Robinette, 1997).

■ Because infants and some young children cannot give voluntary responses, hearing assessment procedures depend mostly on reflexive responses elicited by loud sounds. These sounds may include electronic instruments, toys, or bells. Testing of this type is most effective in eliciting reflexive responses from infants between birth and 6 months of age.

■ *Localization audiometry*, often used with older infants, involves presenting a sound and seeing if the infant will turn his or her head toward the sound. This response is measured by presenting sound from different directions and noting the infant's response.

■ In *operant audiometry*, a child's hearing is tested by conditioning voluntary responses to sound stimuli. Operant audiometry is best for children who are challenging to test through traditional audiometric means. Children with mental retardation, attention-deficit disorder, and behavioral disorders often benefit from operant audiometry procedures.

Interpretation of Hearing Test Results

■ Before audiologists make recommendations about the habilitation of a person with hearing impairment, they consider audiological test results and information gathered from a variety of sources. These sources include:

- a case history and interview

- a comprehensive speech and language assessment

- otological records from the patient's otologist

- any general medical reports that include information relative to the patient's hearing and overall health

- for children, reports from regular and special education teachers

■ Hearing losses can be judged as follows:

- mild (16–40 dB)

- moderate (41–55 dB)

- moderately severe (56–65 dB)

- severe (66–89 dB)

- profound (90+ dB)

■ *Unilateral losses* are those found only in one ear, whereas *bilateral losses* affect both ears. The degree of loss may be the same in both ears, or there may be a difference between the ears.

■ *Audiograms* are graphs that display the results of air- and bone-conduction tests (see Figure 10.13). A typical audiogram shows the hearing level in dB for both bone- and air-conducted tones for the tested frequencies.

■ Figure 10.13 shows an example of conductive hearing loss. The bone-conducted hearing is normal bilaterally because the sound is delivered directly to the inner ear through bone conduction. However, when sound is delivered to the outer ear, there is a hearing loss. The *air-bone gap* indicates that the loss is conductive.

■ When the hearing is not significantly better in one ear, there is no need to use masking noise. Therefore, in Figure 10.14, unmasked bone-conduction thresholds are represented by different symbols. The audiogram shows that the person's hearing is better for some frequencies than others, which is typical of sensorineural hearing loss.

■ Figure 10.15 shows an audiogram representing a mixed hearing loss. A sensorineural component is evident because the thresholds are higher than

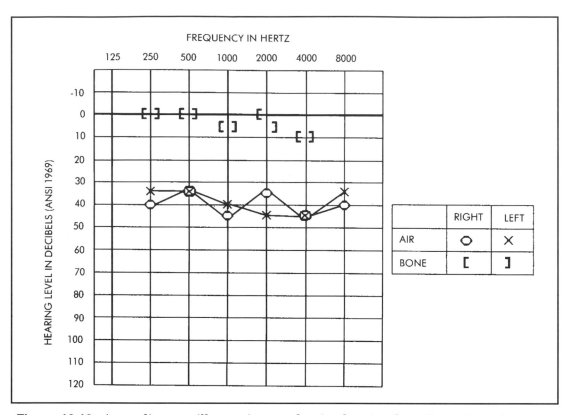

Figure 10.13. An audiogram illustrating conductive hearing loss. From *Introduction to Communicative Disorders*, 2nd ed. (p. 440), by M. N. Hegde, 1995, Austin, TX: PRO-ED. Copyright 1995 by PRO-ED, Inc. Reprinted with permission.

normal when the sound is delivered directly to the cochlea via bone conduction. However, the air-conduction thresholds are also elevated. The difference between the air- and bone-conduction thresholds indicates a probable conductive hearing loss as well.

▨ Figure 10.16 illustrates an audiogram of a noise-induced hearing loss. The difference in air- and bone-conduction thresholds indicates the sensorineural nature of the loss. There is also an important diagnostic sign of noise-induced loss: a greater loss between 3,000-6,000 Hz.

Summary

☑ Primary methods of assessing hearing impairment include pure-tone and speech audiometry, acoustic immitance, and electrophysiological audiometry.

☑ Whether children or adults are assessed, it is important to accurately interpret hearing test results so that appropriate management of the hearing impairment can be undertaken.

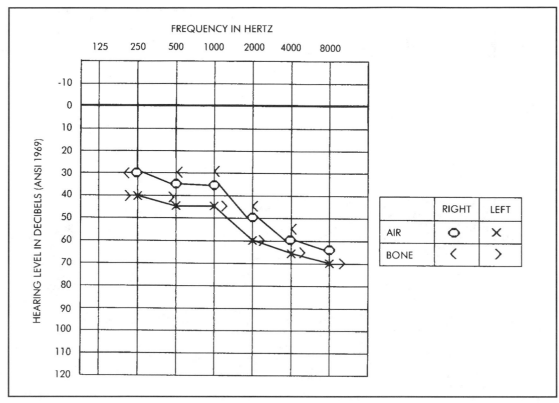

Figure 10.14. An audiogram showing a sensorineural loss. From *Introduction to Communicative Disorders*, 2nd ed. (p. 441), by M. N. Hegde, 1995, Austin, TX: PRO-ED. Copyright 1995 by PRO-ED, Inc. Reprinted with permission.

MANAGEMENT OF HEARING IMPAIRMENT

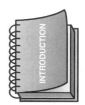

Hearing impairments can range from mild to profound, and management of hearing impairment reflects this continuum. Depending upon the type and extent of the hearing loss, people with hearing impairment will often manifest difficulties in articulation, language, voice, fluency, and resonance. Amplification devices such as hearing aids, cochlear implants, tactile aids, and assistive devices are often used in aural rehabilitation of individuals with hearing impairment. These individuals may also undergo communication training, which involves methods such as auditory training, speech reading, cued speech, oral language training, and speech, rhythm, and voice training. There are two broad approaches to communication training: verbal approaches, which involve speech, and nonverbal approaches, which involve sign language.

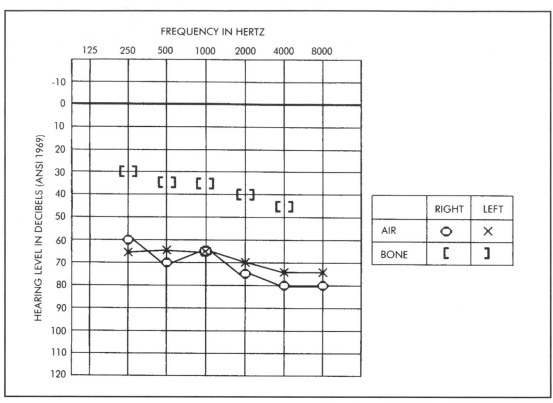

Figure 10.15. An audiogram showing a mixed hearing loss. From *Introduction to Communicative Disorders*, 2nd ed. (p. 442), by M. N. Hegde, 1995, Austin, TX: PRO-ED. Copyright 1995 by PRO-ED, Inc. Reprinted with permission.

Communication Disorders of People with Hearing Impairment

General Principles

- Without normal hearing, children may learn signs, gestures, and other modes of manual communication. However, spoken language is affected.

- Hearing supports the acquisition and production of speech and language in several ways. Hearing makes infants aware of environmental and speech sounds. Hearing also makes it possible to understand spoken language. Those who cannot hear and understand speech usually need special assistance.

- Hearing is also necessary in monitoring one's own production of speech and language. Self-monitoring enables people to monitor *how* they speak as well as what they say. People with hearing impairments have challenges in monitoring their speech, language, and voice productions.

- The extent of adverse effects of hearing impairment on speech, language, and voice depends on many variables—especially the *age of onset* of the hearing loss and the *degree of the loss*.

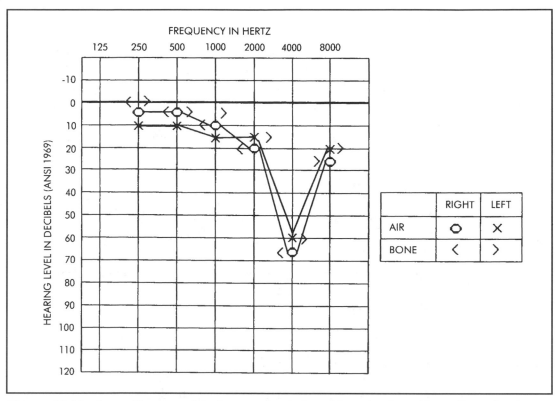

Figure 10.16. An audiogram showing a noise-induced hearing loss. From *Introduction to Communicative Disorders*, 2nd ed. (p. 443), by M. N. Hegde, 1995, Austin, TX: PRO-ED. Copyright 1995 by PRO-ED, Inc. Reprinted with permission.

■ *Congenital* hearing loss, or loss present at birth, has a greater impact than hearing loss acquired later in adult life. Children with *prelingual deafness* become deaf before they acquire speech and language, while children with *postlingual deafness* have a hearing impairment that occurs after age 5.

■ Prognosis for speech and language improvment in hard-of-hearing and deaf children depends on several factors:

 – how early in life professional help is given

 – the quality and scope of services the child receives

 – the extent to which the parents help their deaf child

 – the presence of other disabling conditions (e.g., blindness, brain damage)

■ In judging the impact of the hearing impairment on the patient's daily life, audiologists can have adults and older children carry out self-assessments. These typically involve questionnaires in which people with hearing impairment evaluate the impact of the hearing loss on many aspects of their daily life and functioning.

Speech Disorders

■ Children with hearing impairments have difficulty learning the speech sounds because they cannot hear these sounds well if at all. People who are profoundly deaf distort many vowels and almost all consonants. Omissions, substitutions, and distortions of sounds are common.

■ It is common for people with hearing impairment to manifest the following speech problems:

– distortion of sounds, especially fricatives and stops

– comission of initial and final consonants

– consonant cluster reduction

– substitution of voiced consonants for voiceless consonants (e.g., g/d)

– omission of /s/ in almost all positions of words

– substitution of nasal consonants for oral consonants (e.g., *mat/bat*)

– increased duration of vowels

– imprecise production of vowels (e.g., diphthongization of vowels)

– epenthesis, or adding a schwa sound to consonant blends (e.g., sətap/stap)

Language Disorders

■ Some individuals who are deaf use language well; for example, there are accomplished writers who are deaf. However, many prelingually deaf people are likely to exhibit problems with language.

■ Language problems of many prelingually deaf people include:

– use of a limited variety of sentence types

– use of sentences of reduced length and complexity

– difficulty comprehending and producing compound, complex, and embedded sentences

– occasional irrelevance of speech, including non sequiturs (utterances that do not relate to the topic at hand)

– providing insufficient background information to the listener

– limited oral communication, including lack of elaborated speech and reluctance to speak

– difficulty understanding proverbs, metaphors, and other abstract utterances

– slower acquisition of grammatic morphemes

- omission or inconsistent use of many morphemes including past tense and plural inflections, third-person singular -*s*, indefinite pronouns, present progressive -*ing*, articles, prepositions, and conjunctions

- poor reading comprehension

- writing that reflects oral language problems (e.g., deviant syntax, limited variety of sentence types, omission of grammatic morphemes)

Voice, Fluency, and Resonance Disorders

■ Problems in voice, fluency, and resonance depend heavily on the degree of hearing loss and the amount of intervention a person has experienced.

■ Voice, fluency, and resonance problems in many people who are deaf include:

- hypernasal resonance on non-nasal sounds

- hyponasal resonance on nasal sounds

- abnormal phrasing, flow, and rhythm of speech

- monotone speech with lack of appropriate intonation

- improper stress patterns, including excessive pitch inflections

- restricted pitch range

- inappropriately high pitch

- rate of speech that is too slow or too fast

- pauses at inappropriate junctures

- inefficient breathing, including breathiness

- deviations in voice quality, including hoarseness and harshness

✎ Concepts To Consider

Describe two characteristics each of the speech, language, voice, and resonance of people who are deaf.

_____

_____

_____

_____

_____

Aural Rehabilitation: Basic Principles

■ *Aural rehabilitation* is an educational and clinical program implemented primarily by audiologists. It is designed to help people with hearing losses achieve their full potential.

■ Aural rehabilitation includes several key components (Kelly, Davis, & Hegde, 1994; Schow & Nerbonne, 1996; Stach, 1998):

- an evaluation of the hearing loss

- an assessment of the communicative needs of the person (including the patient's self-assessment)

- determination of the availability of human and financial resources to support hearing habilitation

- prescription and fitting of a hearing aid

- auditory training

- use of amplification systems in communication and educational training sessions

- focus on communication patterns in the environment

- addressing the impact of social, vocational, psychological, and educational factors of the hearing loss

- counseling the person with the hearing impairment and his or her family

- recommending additional services if needed

- periodic reevaluation of the client's status

■ Many specialists are involved in aural rehabilitation. They include:

- the *audiologist*, who is primarily responsible for the aural rehabilitation components listed above;

- the *otologist*, who monitors the health of the ear (This medical specialist performs such ear surgeries as stapedectomy and tympanoplasty and prescribes medication for middle ear diseases.);

- the *speech–language pathologist*, who provides treatment for articulation, language, resonance, voice, and fluency;

- in schools, the *educator of the deaf*, a special educator who teaches communication methods such as American Sign Language as well as academic subjects to children with hearing impairments; and

– the *vocational counselor*.

■ Professionals carrying out aural rehabilitation have historically focused intensive efforts on speech reading and auditory training. Today, there is a greater focus on hearing aid fitting and orientation, the environment and communication patterns within the environment, and early identification and intervention (Schow & Nerbonne, 1996; Stach, 1998).

Amplification

■ An important part of aural rehabilitation of people with hearing impairment is amplification of sound and speech. Sound and speech can be amplified through several means, including hearing aids, cochlear implants, and auditory trainers.

■ When children and adults with hearing losses are considered as candidates for amplification, there are two major considerations. First, do they truly need the amplification? Second, are they motivated to use the amplification and care for any amplification devices properly? Patient motivation is a major factor in deciding upon appropriate amplification.

Hearing Aids

■ Most traditional hearing aids are small, electronic devices that are worn inside the ear unilaterally or bilaterally depending upon the needs of the person. Hearing aids amplify sound and deliver it to the ear canal. An ear mold, though not part of the hearing aid itself, is necessary for using the aid.

■ There are four basic types of hearing aids:

– *the eyeglass variety*, in which the hearing aid is built into the frame of the eyeglasses;

– *body aids*, worn under a person's shirt or blouse;

– *the behind-the-ear model*, which fits behind the ear and has an internal receiver; and

– *the in-the-ear model*, which fits in the ear canal.

■ *Analog hearing aids*, a common type of aid, create patterns of electric voltage that correspond to the sound input. All analog hearing aids have the same basic components: a microphone, an amplifier, a receiver, a power source (batteries), and volume control.

■ Hearing aid *transducers* include the *microphone*, which picks up sound, and the *receiver*, which delivers the sound to the ear. These transducers convert one form of energy into another.

▓ The microphone converts the sound energy into electrical energy; the receiver, housed in the ear mold, converts the electrical energy back into sound waves. The *amplifier*, to which the electrical signals are fed, amplifies those signals and delivers them to the receiver.

▓ The more recently developed *digital hearing aid* contains microcomputer technology. Whereas the microphone of a traditional analog hearing aid creates a continuously variable voltage pattern that is analogous (similar) to the sound input, a digital aid rapidly samples the input signal and converts each sample into a binary system of zeros and ones. Those numbers are then processed by a computer housed in a unit worn on the body.

▓ There are several advantages of digital aids:

– They are more flexible than the analog aids and can be modified to adapt to each patient's pattern of hearing loss and communicative needs.

– Digital processing helps amplify selected frequencies for which loss is greater.

– Digital aids are more effective than analog aids in reducing irritating loud noises, such as dogs barking and vacuums running.

– Digital aids provide a better *signal-to-noise ratio*; they are more effective than analog aids in clearly separating speech from background noise, which also is more effectively suppressed.

▓ Advances in technology have greatly improved the quality of hearing aids. These advances include highly sensitive microphones, ear molds that are custom made for each person, and amplifiers that amplify sound with minimal to no distortion.

▓ State-of-the-art hearing aids are *programmable*, in that they can be programmed to provide different types of amplification depending upon the setting (Helfer, 1998). For example, the wearer could choose among different hearing aid settings depending upon whether he or she was at a party (with background noise) or watching TV alone at home (Gelfand, 1997).

▓ A recent development in hearing aid technology is *computerization*. Hearing aid specifications, automated testing procedures, prescriptive fitting methods, and hearing aid selection formulas are now available from computer software (Mueller & Strouse, 1996).

▓ Most hearing aids (such as those previously described) are air-conduction aids. *Bone-conduction hearing aids* amplify sound for the patient using a bone-conduction vibrator. The vibrator can be built into the temple portion of the patient's eyeglasses or held in place with a spring headband (Gelfand, 1997).

▓ Bone-conduction hearing aids are used in place of air-conduction aids when the patient manifests certain pathologies such as atresia of the ear canal or other physical problems that make an air-conduction aid inadvisable.

■ Selection of a hearing aid is a process involving several steps:

- an ear examination by an otologist to identify any physical condition of the ear that may contraindicate the use of amplification;

- diagnostic tests administered by an audiologist to help determine the extent and type of hearing loss;

- a hearing aid evaluation, conducted by an audiologist, in which various models are tested to determine the best aid for the individual's needs; and

- evaluation of whether the patient needs *monaural* (one ear only) or *binaural* (both ears) amplification.

■ Several decades ago, it was deemed unethical for audiologists to sell hearing aids for profit. ASHA did not permit audiologists to sell hearing aids until the 1970s. Today, a hearing aid can be purchased from several sources, including audiologists and hearing aid dealers.

Cochlear Implants

■ Hearing aids are an invaluable tool for many people with hearing losses. However, some people with profound hearing losses cannot benefit from hearing aids. The recent technology of cochlear implants may profit those individuals.

■ *Cochlear implants* are electronic devices. They are surgically placed in the cochlea and other parts of the ear, and they deliver the sound directly to the acoustic nerve endings in the cochlea. Although the patient may be profoundly deaf, there is often a large residual population of primary cochlear neural elements; a cochlear implant can take advantage of those residual elements (Thedinger, 1996).

■ Cochlear implants differ from hearing aids primarily in that the hearing aid delivers amplified sound to the ear canal, but cochlear implants deliver electrical impulses, converted from sound, directly to the auditory nerve. Basically, cochlear implants replace the nonfunctioning inner hair cell transducer system (Thedinger, 1996).

■ Cochlear implants can be thought of as "prosthetic cochleas." They have four elements:

- A *microphone* is mounted on an ear mold and worn in the ear canal or on the body. It picks up the sound and converts it into electrical impulses.

- The microphone is connected to a *processor*, which is contained in a small box that can be worn on a belt or placed in a pocket. The battery-operated processor suppresses extraneous noise and selects sounds salient to comprehending speech.

- Those sounds are then sent to an *external transmitter*, a magnetic coil worn on the skull (in a manner similar to that of an external hearing aid). Behind the external transmitter, directly under the skin, an internal magnetic coil is implanted. The two magnetic coils are attracted to each other.

- A ground electrode is implanted in an area outside the cochlea; active electrodes are placed inside of it. Through the skin, the external transmitter sends a signal to the *implanted receiver* (the internal coil and the electrodes), which stimulates the auditory nerve.

■ Unlike earlier cochlear implants that had only one channel (one active electrode), more recent implants have multiple channels or electrodes. Implants with multiple channels stimulate different areas of the cochlea and attempt to produce various tonal perceptions (Thedinger, 1996).

■ As previously stated, cochlear implants today are used only with people who have minimal or no hearing and cannot profit from hearing aids. Cochlear implants enhance patients' speech-reading performance (see "Speech Reading" later in chapter), give patients general sound awareness, and help patients recognize environmental sounds (Gelfand, 1997). Perhaps someday cochlear implants will be beneficial in helping patients understand and produce speech as well.

■ Candidates for cochlear implants are selected after extensive examinations carried out by teams of specialists. These specialists include audiologists, speech pathologists, deaf educators, psychologists, and otologists.

■ Because placing a cochlear implant is a surgical procedure involving general anesthesia, there is a minimal risk of postsurgical infection and nerve damage involving facial paralysis.

■ Prelingual children who receive cochlear implants can make substantial progress. Cochlear implants help maximize these children's potential and may positively impact the auditory system's ability to mature.

■ Recent research has shown that some adults with severe to profound hearing losses may also benefit from cochlear implants (Flynn, Dowell, & Clark, 1998). It must be noted, however, that many members of the community of deaf people have shown resistance to cochlear implants (Helfer, 1998).

■ The *central electroauditory prosthesis* (CEP) is a more current development in implant technology. The CEP directly stimulates the cochlear nucleus of the auditory nerve at the brain stem level.

■ When the cochlea and its hair cells are damaged to such an extent that a cochlear implant will not work, implants of electrodes may carry the sound to the auditory nerve fibers at the brain stem. More research is needed to establish the usefulness of the CEP.

Tactile Aids

■ Tactile aids are a type of *sensory substitution method* used for individuals who are deaf (Gelfand, 1997). These aids are devices or methods that promote the comprehension of speech by means of touch. Thus, tactile (touch) sense is substituted for hearing.

■ Tactile aids are sometimes used for individuals with profound deafness; they may also be used for individuals who are both deaf and blind.

■ Because the human skin does not respond well to sounds of different frequencies, tactile aids have vibrators that generate patterns of stimuli that represent different speech sounds.

■ Simple tactile aids have a single channel that transforms acoustic signals into mechanical signals and stimulates the skin. These aids help their wearers to detect environmental sounds. More complex multichannel tactile aids have multiple stimulators that stimulate different body parts mechanically or electrically. For example, different stimulators may stimulate the arm, abdomen, or wrist.

■ Tactile aids are cheaper than cochlear implants and do not involve surgery. However, a great deal of practice and training are needed to make optimal use of the tactile signals (Gelfand, 1997).

■ The *Tadoma Method*, a manual system for people who are deaf and blind, involves them placing hands on the speaker's face to feel the vibrations of speech.

■ The listener feels the vibrations of the lips, cheeks, jaws, and vocal folds of the speaker. The listener also feels nasal and oral airflow. This method can be used to teach speech production to children who are deaf or deaf and blind.

Assistive Devices

■ New technologies have been created to support the communication needs of individuals who are deaf and hard of hearing. Some can be used alone, while others must be used in conjunction with interpreters, speech reading (discussed later in chapter), or other support systems.

■ *Safety alerting devices* help people with hearing impairments to gain information through flashing lights and/or vibrators on common devices. These devices help people know, for example, when the doorbell rings or a burglar alarm goes off.

■ *Closed captioning* on television provides subtitles on the screen to help people who are deaf know what is happening in a TV program.

■ *Telecommunication devices for the deaf* (TDDs) allow people who are deaf to use the telephone. The TDD is a portable terminal that both sends and receives typed messages via telephone (Gelfand, 1997).

✎ Concepts To Consider

There are a number of types of amplification available for people who are deaf. Describe two of these types of amplification (e.g., cochlear implants).

_____

_____

_____

_____

_____

_____

_____

_____

_____

Communication Training

General Guidelines

■ It is important to consider the impact of hearing loss on all aspects of a patient's life. Hearing loss often creates educational challenges for children and vocational challenges for adults (Schow & Nerbonne, 1996).

■ Acceptance of a hearing loss can vary from culture to culture. It is important to be sensitive to culturally determined reactions such as embarrassment or the belief that God has given a family a deaf child as a cross to bear (Nuru-Holm & Battle, 1998).

■ When working with children who have a hearing loss, it is important to begin speech and language training as early as possible. The family should be involved in speech and language training and stimulation activities.

■ The child must be under appropriate medical and audiological management, including being fitted with a customized hearing aid. The child and parents should be trained in proper care and use of the hearing aid.

- Clinicians who serve children should work closely with classroom teachers and with educators of the deaf. The development of auditory skills must be integrated into the child's educational and speech–language programs.

- Children must be placed in appropriate educational settings. Those settings exist along a continuum from full mainstreaming into the regular classroom to enrollment in a residential school for the deaf.

- For many adults, hearing problems account for a high level of psychosocial difficulty even after a hearing aid is acquired (Erdman & Demorest, 1998).

- Thus, when working with adults, clinicians frequently need to provide psychosocial counseling to help patients and their families deal with impacts of the hearing loss and attitudes toward aural rehabilitation.

- Older people with hearing losses may be served through clinics, senior citizen centers, and nursing homes and other long-term health care facilities. The patient's living setting must be carefully considered as aural rehabilitation efforts are carried out.

Auditory Training

- Auditory training is designed to teach a person with hearing impairment to listen to amplified sounds, recognize their meanings, and discriminate sounds from each other.

- Individuals who use hearing aids generally undergo a *hearing aid orientation*, which is provided by an audiologist or sometimes by a hearing aid dealer. The person is instructed in use and care of the hearing aid.

- *Desktop auditory trainers* are frequently more effective and powerful in amplifying speech than hearing aids. One reason is that hearing aids pick up all noise, including background, or *ambient*, noise, whereas auditory trainers pick up and amplify only the signal of interest (the speech of a speaker).

- When auditory trainers are used, the person with hearing impairment wears headphones. The clinician's or teacher's speech is fed to an amplifier through a microphone, and the amplified sound is fed to the earphones and the person's ear.

- Auditory trainers can be used with adults who are receiving articulation training. They are also used with children in educational and therapy settings; prelingually deaf children may especially benefit.

- An *FM auditory trainer* is a wireless system that can be used in group or individual treatment sessions. In a classroom, for example, the teacher and the child or children can move about within a certain range. The children and teacher both wear receiving and transmitting units so they can hear and talk with each other.

■ Ambient or extraneous noise in school classrooms is approximately 60 dB. The signal-to-noise ratio (S/N ratio), or the difference in dB between the stimulus of interest (usually the teacher's voice) and competing background noise, is often negative; that is, the teacher's voice cannot be adequately heard due to the background noise.

■ This negative S/N ratio is very detrimental to children with hearing impairments, and auditory trainers are extremely beneficial in such situations. The Acoustical Society of America is currently working toward recommendations and an action plan to reduce ambient noise and other acoustical barriers in classrooms (Soli, 1998).

■ Auditory training goals for children with hearing impairments include discrimination of environmental sounds, discrimination of speech sounds and word pairs, and discrimination of phrases and sentences. Use of a multimodal approach (e.g., mirrors, pictures, charts, and tactile cues such as feeling the throat and lips) is a necessary component of auditory training.

Speech Reading

■ Previously known as lipreading, *speech reading* involves deciphering speech by looking at the face of the speaker and using visual cues to understand what the speaker is saying.

■ In speech reading, the listener watches the movements of the lips, jaw, and tongue as well as the shape of the lips and mouth. The speaker's gestures, hand movements, and facial expressions are also observed to understand the total message being conveyed.

■ In English, only 30% of sounds are visible on the face. These include the labials /v/, /f/, /m/, /p/, and /b/. The labials are *homophenous*; that is, they look the same and may be confusing. Other sounds are less visible and very difficult to read. Ideally, speech reading should be supplemented with other means of communication.

Cued Speech

■ *Cued speech* is speech produced with manual cues that represent the sounds of speech. It may be used to supplement speech reading.

■ Cued speech differs from sign language because it is composed of eight signs or hand configurations for consonants and four signs for vowels.

■ People with hearing impairment do not use cued speech. Rather, those who are speaking to people with hearing impairment make hand gestures that correspond to the appropriate vowels and consonants.

■ The hand gestures that constitute cued speech are often helpful in assisting the person with hearing impairment to distinguish among homophenous sounds.

■ Research has demonstrated that people with hearing impairment benefit when the speaker uses cued speech. Nicholls and Ling (1982) showed that correct speech reading of syllables increased from 30% without cues to 84% with cues. A challenge in using cued speech is that speakers must be able to speak and cue simultaneously.

Oral Language Training: General Principles

■ The aforementioned communication methods help people who are deaf to understand speech that is spoken to them. To be fully successful communicators, however, these people benefit from learning to express themselves to others. Successful expression requires training.

■ Oral language training should begin as early as possible. Language stimulation programs are best carried out in both clinical and educational settings as well as the home. These programs should involve cooperative efforts of a team consisting of an audiologist, family members, a speech–language pathologist, and an educator of the deaf.

■ Parents of infants who are deaf should speak to their children as much as possible, talking about and labeling things in the environment. Caretakers can integrate visual with auditory stimulation by showing objects and naming them simultaneously as well as demonstrating actions when they are described.

■ Initially, it is best to select and teach functional words that children use in their daily environments. Subsequently, children can be taught phrase and sentence structures to express their individual ideas and needs more fully.

■ Clinicians should also focus on other structures and concepts that are especially difficult for children with hearing impairment. These include:

- grammatic morphemes such as past tense -*ed* and plural -*s*

- terms with dual meanings (e.g., *rock, pound*)

- antonyms (e.g., *up–down, light–dark*) and synonyms (e.g., *happy–joyful*)

- proverbs (e.g., "A penny saved is a penny earned")

- abstract terms (e.g., *lighthearted, flimsy*)

■ Children with hearing impairment have challenges with pragmatic skills. Clinicians must provide training in specific skills such as turn-taking, topic initiation, topic maintenance, and eye contact.

■ It is important to use visual cues in therapy sessions. These visual cues can include hand gestures, facial expressions, toys and other manipulatives, pictures, printed letters, books, and other visuals to supplement auditory input.

Speech, Rhythm, and Voice Training

- In teaching speech sound production, it is important to give many visual cues. Clinicians can use charts, pictures, and other visuals to assist children in correct sound production.

- Clinicians must pay special attention to affricates, fricatives, and stops. These sounds are especially difficult for children with hearing impairment.

- The voice-voiceless distinction is also critical for children with hearing impairment to learn. Clinicians can contrast the cognates /p/ and /b/, for example, through visual and tactile means.

- Clinicians must address any voice abnormalities such as hoarseness, harshness, high pitch, and monotone. Clients must learn to speak with proper volume, especially avoiding excessive loudness. Work with proper respiration—especially proper breath support—can be helpful.

- Resonance problems such as hypernasality and hyponasality must also be addressed. Clinicians may need to help clients balance oral-nasal resonance, and avoid cul-de-sac resonance (defined in Chapter 7).

- Goals in the area of prosody may include teaching normal intonation, smooth flow of speech, and modifying pauses that are placed inappropriately or are of inappropriate length.

- It is very helpful to use mechanical feedback devices such as the Visi-Pitch (described in Chapter 7) in working with voice and resonance problems.

Approaches to Training

Aural/Oral Method

- The aural/oral method is also called the *oral approach*, the *auditory-global approach*, and the *multisensory approach*. Users of the method attempt to use amplification methods such as hearing aids or cochlear implants to tap children's residual hearing.

- Children undergo intensive auditory training and speech reading instruction. It is expected that these children will eventually learn to speak and will fit into mainstream social, vocational, and educational settings (Martin, 1997; Stach, 1998).

Manual Approach

- Proponents of the manual approach believe that early in life, children who are deaf must be taught a comprehensive sign language system. The sooner the child learns this system, the better.

- The sign language system is viewed as part of the deaf culture and is the standard means of communication in the community of people who are deaf.

Therefore, children who are deaf learn not only a means of communication, but also a way of integrating into that community.

Total Communication

- Total communication, advocated by some experts, involves teaching both verbal and nonverbal means of communication. Signs and speech are used simultaneously. People who are deaf are taught speech and language along with a sign system. There is no attempt to tap residual hearing through amplification.

- Although critics believe that it is unrealistic to expect children to follow signs, read lips, and sign simultaneously, total communication is probably the most popular current teaching method for children with hearing losses in the profound-severe range (Martin, 1997).

 ## Concepts To Consider

What are the basic differences between speech reading, cued speech, and total communication? In what situations might each of these communication methods be appropriate?

_____

_____

_____

_____

_____

_____

_____

_____

Nonverbal Communication: Sign Language

American Sign Language

- American Sign Language, or ASL, is the best known of the sign language approaches. Because there are many variations of ASL, there is no single definition of it.

- ASL is widely used in the United States and Canada. It is not considered a manual version of English, but is rather viewed as a separate language.

- In ASL, signs are used to express ideas and concepts through complex hand and finger movements. Each sign expresses a different idea.

■ Different signs are made in quick succession, much like spoken words are put into sentences. However, the syntax of ASL differs from that of spoken Standard American English.

Seeing Essential English

■ Seeing Essential English (SEE 1) primarily employs ASL. It breaks down words into morphemes and uses written English word order.

■ SEE 1 uses some markers to help identify number and tense, and also uses specific signs for some verbs and articles (e.g., *the, an*).

Signing Exact English

■ Signing Exact English (SEE 2) is similar to SEE 1. However, it is used more widely than SEE 1 and is more flexible about precise word order in sentences.

■ SEE 2 breaks down words into morphemes that are words when they stand alone (e.g., *hot-dog*).

Fingerspelling

■ In fingerspelling, ideas are communicated through quick, precise movements made by the fingers.

■ Fingerspelling may be used alone or in conjunction with other methods such as ASL. Sometimes fingerspelling is used for unusual words that do not lend themselves to standard signs.

Rochester Method

■ The Rochester method uses a combination of oral speech and fingerspelling. Signs are not used in this method. The oral aspect of the Rochester method is traditional English.

Summary

☑ There are many approaches to the habilitation of people with hearing impairment. These people frequently have disorders of speech, language, voice, fluency, and resonance.

☑ People with hearing losses can be helped by amplification devices such as hearing aids, cochlear implants, tactile aids, and various assistive devices.

☑ These people may also receive communication training, which can consist of auditory training; speech reading; cued speech; oral language training; training in speech, rhythm, and voice; and various verbal and nonverbal approaches to communication.

CHAPTER HIGHLIGHTS

▶ Audiology is the study of hearing, its disorders, and the measurement and management of those disorders. Audiologists identify, evaluate, and rehabilitate people with hearing losses due to peripheral and/or central auditory impairments.

▶ The ear consists of three basic parts: the outer, middle, and inner ear. These parts must function normally in order for sound to be converted to electrical impulses within the cochlea and then sent to the brain via the auditory nervous system. Cranial nerve VIII, the acoustic nerve, sends sound impulses to the brain, where the sound is interpreted.

▶ Acoustics, a branch of physics, involves the study of sound as a physical event. The human ear perceives sound in terms of pitch or frequency, and loudness or intensity. Frequency is measured in Hertz, or cycles per second, while intensity is measured in decibels.

▶ Hearing is a miraculous ability that depends on the intricate, precise, and accurate workings of the auditory system. When the outer and/or middle ear malfunctions, a person may manifest conductive hearing losses. Sensorineural losses reflect malfunctioning of the inner ear, and mixed losses reflect both conductive and sensorineural components. People with central auditory and retrocochlear disorders manifest auditory nervous system impairments, which are challenging to assess.

▶ Assessment of hearing impairment depends upon the nature of the problem. Standard procedures in assessment include pure-tone and speech audiometry, which can be carried out through air- or bone-conduction testing. Acoustic immitance testing, involving tympanometry and/or acoustic reflex testing, is used to assess middle ear function.

▶ Electrophysiological audiometry and medical imaging are often employed when retrocochlear damage is suspected. This damage is usually caused by tumors, which can grow slowly and make diagnosis very challenging. New, sophisticated techniques such as electrocochleography and magnetic resonance imaging help teams of specialists assess possible pathology of the auditory mechanism.

▶ Hearing screenings quickly identify people with normal hearing and people who need more in-depth testing due to possible hearing losses. Infants and children who have hearing losses often need to be assessed with special techniques that allow for reflexive responses if necessary.

▶ People with hearing impairment manifest a range of communicative disorders. The severity of these disorders depends on the age of onset of the hearing loss as well as the degree of the loss. People with hearing losses may

(continues)

manifest problems in one or more of the areas of articulation, fluency, voice, resonance, and language.

▶ Aural rehabilitation involves an educational and clinical program implemented by teams to help people with hearing losses achieve their full potential. Aural rehabilitation usually includes several key components. Amplification, one component, can involve hearing aids, cochlear implants, tactile aids, and assistive devices.

▶ Communication training, a second component of aural rehabilitation, may involve one or more of several methods. These methods include auditory training; speech reading; cued speech; and training in oral language, speech, voice, fluency, and resonance. Various approaches to training may include a verbal emphasis (e.g., total communication and the aural/oral approach) or a nonverbal emphasis, which involves use of a form of sign language.

▶ Add your own chapter highlights here:

_____

_____

_____

_____

KEY TERMS

acoustic branch (of cranial nerve VIII)
acoustic immitance
acoustic neuroma
acoustic reflex
acoustics
acute otitis media
admittance
air conduction
ambient noise
American Sign Language (ASL)
amplifier
amplitude
analog hearing aid
analytic approach
aperiodic
attenuate

attenuator
audiogram
audiologist
audiology
audiometer
auditory brain stem response (ABR)
auditory branch (of cranial nerve VIII)
auditory-evoked potentials
auditory trainers
auditory training
aural atresia
aural/oral method
auricle
basilar membrane
bilateral

binaural
bone conduction
bone-conduction hearing aids
Carhart's notch
central auditory system
central electroauditory prosthesis (CEP)
cerebellopontine angle
cerumen
chronic otitis media
cilia
cochlea
cochlear implant
complex tone
compression
computerized axial tomography

conductive hearing loss
congenital hearing loss
contralateral pathways
cranial nerve VIII
cued speech
cycle
cytomegalovirus
deaf
decibel (dB)
decussate
dichotic listening
digital hearing aid
eardrum
electrocochleography
electrophysiological
  audiometry
endolymph
eustachian tube
external auditory canal
external auditory
  meatus
external otitis
fingerspelling
frequency
hard of hearing
hearing impairment
hearing level (HL)
hearing screening
herpes simplex
Hertz
homophenous sounds
impedance
impedance bridge/meter
incus
intensity
internal auditory
  meatus
interruptor switch
ipsilateral pathways
labyrinths
localization audiometry
logarithmic scale
loudness
magnetic resonance
  imaging
malleus
manual approach

masking
mediums
Meniere's disease
microphone
microtia
middle ear effusion
mixed hearing loss
monaural
myringoplasty
myringotomy
operant audiometry
organ of Corti
oscillator
ossicular chain
otitis media
otosclerosis
otoscope
otospongiosis
ototoxic drugs
oval window
pascals (pa)
perilymph
periodic
peripheral
pinna
pitch
postlingual deafness
prelingual deafness
presbycusis
pressure equalizing tube
programmable hearing
  aids
psychoacoustics
pure tone
rarefaction
receiver
recruitment
Reissner's membrane
retrocochlear
Rochester method
rubella
Seeing Essential
  English (SEE 1)
semicircular canals
sensorineural hearing
  loss

sensory substitution
  method
serous otitis media
signal-to-noise ratio
  (S/N ratio)
Signing Exact English
  (SEE 2)
simple harmonic motion
sound pressure
sound pressure level
  (SPL)
sound wave
speech audiometry
speech reading
speech reception thresh-
  old
spondee word
stapedectomy
stapedius muscle
stapes
stenosis
synthetic approach
syphilis
Tadoma method
telecommunication
  devices for the deaf
  (TDDs)
temporal bone
tensor palatini
tensor tympani
threshold
tinnitus
total communication
toxoplasmosis
transducer
tympanic membrane
tympanometry
unilateral
vestibular branch (of
  cranial nerve VIII)
vestibular system
von Recklinghausen
  disease
watts
word discrimination test
word recognition test

STUDY AND REVIEW QUESTIONS

Fill in the Blank

1. The three bones that constitute the ossicular chain are the
   malleus, _incus_, and _stapes_.

2. Key parts of the auditory nervous system include cranial nerve _VIII_,
   which has two branches: the _vestibular_ branch and the
   auditory/acoustic branch, which carries the electrical sound impulses
   from the cochlea to the brain.

3. A cycle consists of one instance of _compression_ and one instance
   of _rarefaction_ per second.

4. Stenosis, aural atresia, and otosclerosis all cause _congenital_
   hearing loss.

5. A person with otosclerosis will often have an audiogram reflecting
   Carhart's notch, a specific loss at 2,000 Hz as indicated by
   bone-conduction testing.

6. Sensorineural hearing loss can be caused by many things. _Presbycusis_,
   a hearing impairment in older people, results in a sloping, high-frequency
   loss. _Meniere's_ disease, which causes sensorineural hearing
   loss, is accompanied by vertigo and tinnitus.

7. People with _retrocochlear_ disorders usually have pathology involving
   cranial nerve VIII and/or the cerebellopontine angle. These disorders are
   most frequently caused by _acoustic neuroma_, which are often diagnosed by use of _auditory brain stem resp_, which helps in
   differential diagnosis.

8. Middle ear function is frequently assessed through use of acoustic
   immittance testing. An impedance meter, used for assessment, can allow one to carry out the procedures of _tympanometry_
   and _acoustic reflex_ testing, the two most common types of
   assessment of middle ear function.

9. People from different ethnic backgrounds have different incidence rates of
   hearing-related problems. Rates of _otitis media_ tend to be
   highest among Native Americans and Alaskan Eskimos, while rates of
   otosclerosis are highest among Whites.

10. The _tadoma_ method is a manual system, sometimes used to
    train people who are deaf and blind to feel the vibrations emanating from
    the speaker's face and laryngeal area.

Multiple Choice

11. A patient has her hearing tested, and the resulting audiogram has the configuration below.

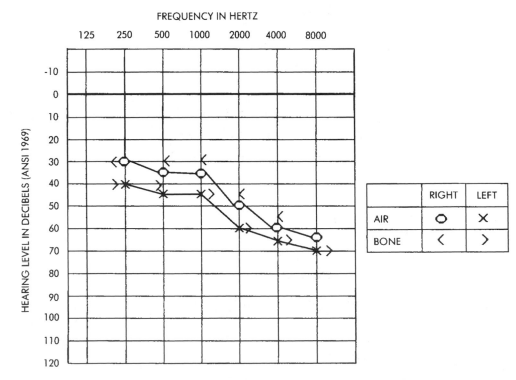

You can assume that this patient has:

A. a mixed hearing loss.

B. a conductive hearing loss.

C. sensorineural hearing loss.

D. noise-induced hearing loss.

E. a central auditory disorder.

12. A 65-year-old man with presbycusis comes to you complaining that when he is in social situations such as parties, people don't speak loudly enough. He says that the noise creates a problem for him in hearing what people are saying. This client has difficulty with:

A. signal-to-noise ratio.

B. auditory discrimination.

C. figure-ground discrimination.

D. pragmatic skills.

E. auditory memory.

13. Which one of the following is a homophenous pair?

   A. sheep–beep.

   B. man–ban.

   C. pan–fan.

   D. honey–money.

   E. list–gist

14. The muscle that exerts the pull that allows the eustachian tube to open during yawning and swallowing is the:

   A. tensor palatini.

   B. levator palatini.

   C. tensor tympani.

   D. stapedius muscle.

   E. levator veli palatini.

15. An infant with cleft palate will most likely have hearing problems because of:

   A. aural atresia.

   B. an incompletely formed cochlea.

   C. eustachian tube dysfunction.

   D. malformed ossicles.

   E. tympanic membrane dysfunction.

16. A sensorineural hearing loss is related to damage in which area?

   A. the external auditory meatus.

   B. the vestibular system.

   C. the tympanic membrane.

   D. hair cells of the cochlea.

   E. the ossicular chain.

17. Speech reception thresholds (SRTs) are:

   A. determined by the patient's response to a list of monosyllabic words presented at a low level of hearing.

B. determined by looking at the patient's pure-tone test results at the frequencies most important to speech.

C. the lowest level of hearing at which a person can understand 100% of the words presented.

D. the lowest level of hearing at which a person can understand 50% of the words presented.

E. the highest level of hearing at which a person can understand 50% of the words presented.

18. Popular forms of amplification today include hearing aids and cochlear implants. Which one of the following is NOT TRUE about these devices?

A. Cochlear implants may be used with children and also some adults who have sensorineural hearing loss.

B. Digital hearing aids provide a better signal-to-noise ratio than analog aids.

C. Cochlear implants can help prelingual children to make substantial progress through maximizing their potential.

D. A consideration in fitting clients with hearing aids is whether the clients are motivated to use and properly care for the aids.

E. Cochlear implants deliver amplified sound to the ear canal, while hearing aids deliver electrical impulses (converted from sound) directly to the auditory system.

19. A father comes to you regarding his daughter, who is 8 months old. The baby's hearing loss is bilateral, and she is profoundly deaf. The father states that he wishes for his daughter, as she grows older, to "fit in with children with normal hearing." He is interested in any possible amplification and says that he wants his daughter to lead a life that is "as normal as possible." Which training approach would best fit this father's wishes?

A. total communication

B. aural/oral method

C. manual approach

D. Rochester method

E. intensive training in American Sign Language and fingerspelling

20. Which of the following are likely to characterize the speech and language of people who are deaf?

     I. Omission of /s/ in almost all positions of words

    II. Consonant cluster reduction

   III. Occasional irrelevance of speech, including non sequiturs

   IV. Improper stress patterns, including excessive pitch inflections

    V. A voice that sounds strained and strangled

A. I, II, III, IV

B. I, III, V

C. I, II, IV, V

D. II, III, IV, V

E. I, II, III, V

REFERENCES AND RECOMMENDED READINGS

American Academy of Audiology. (1997). Audiology: Scope of practice. *Audiology Today, 9*(2), 12–13.

Bess, F. H., & Humes, L. E. (1995). *Audiology: The fundamentals* (2nd ed.). Baltimore, MD: Williams & Wilkins.

Cacace, A. T., & McFarland, D. J. (1998). Central auditory processing disorder in school-aged children: A critical review. *Journal of Speech–Language-Hearing Research, 41*(2), 355–373.

Erdman, S. A., & Demorest, M. E. (1998). Adjustment to hearing impairment I: Description of a heterogeneous clinical population. *Journal of Speech, Language, and Hearing Research, 41*(1), 107–122.

Flynn, M. C., Dowell, R. C., & Clark, G. M. (1998). Aided speech recognition abilities of adults with a severe or severe-to-profound hearing loss. *Journal of Speech, Language, and Hearing Research, 41*(2), 285–299.

Gelfand, S. A. (1997). *Essentials of audiology*. New York: Thieme Medical Publishers.

Helfer, K. S. (1998). In C. M. Seymour & E. H. Nober (Eds.), *Introduction to communication disorders: A multicultural approach* (pp. 277–305). Newton, MA: Butterworth-Heinemann.

Hood, L. J., & Berlin, C. I. (1996). Central auditory function and disorders. In J. Northern (Ed.), *Hearing disorders* (3rd ed.) (pp. 227–243). Needham Heights, MA: Allyn & Bacon.

Kelly, B. R., Davis, D., & Hegde, M. N. (1994). *Clinical methods and practicum in audiology*. San Diego, CA: Singular Publishing Group.

Martin, F. N. (1997). *Introduction to audiology* (6th ed.). Needham Heights, MA: Allyn & Bacon.

Mencher, G. T., Gerber, S. E., & McCombe, A. (1997). *Audiology and auditory dysfunction*. Needham Heights, MA: Allyn & Bacon.

Mueller, H. G., & Strouse, A. L. (1996). Amplification/assistive devices for the deaf and hard of hearing. In R. L. Schow & M. A. Nerbonne, *Introduction to audiologic rehabilitation* (3rd ed.) (pp. 27–55). Needham Heights, MA: Allyn & Bacon.

Nicholls, G. H., & Ling, D. (1982). Cued speech and the reception of spoken language. *Journal of Speech and Hearing Research, 25*, 262–269.

Nober, E. H. (1998). Hearing disorders. In C. M. Seymour & E. H. Nober (Eds.), *Introduction to communication disorders: A multicultural approach* (pp. 227–276). Newton, MA: Butterworth-Heinemann.

Northern, J. L. (1996). *Hearing disorders* (3rd ed.). Needham Heights, MA: Allyn & Bacon.

Nuru-Holm, N., & Battle, D. E. (1998). Multicultural aspects of deafness. In D. E. Battle (Ed.), *Communication disorders in multicultural populations* (2nd ed.), pp. 335–378. Newton, MA: Butterworth-Heinemann.

Roark, R., & Berman, S. (1996). Otitis media. In J. L. Northern (Ed.), *Hearing disorders* (3rd ed.), pp. 127–137. Needham Heights, MA: Allyn & Bacon.

Robinette, M. (1997). Top ten reasons universal newborn hearing screening should be the standard of care in the U.S. *Audiology Today, 9*(1), 21.

Schow, R. L., & Nerbonne, M. A. (1996). *Introduction to audiologic rehabilitation*. Needham Heights, MA: Allyn & Bacon.

Scott, D. M. (1998). Multicultural aspects of hearing disorders and audiology. In D. E. Battle (Ed.), *Communication disorders in multicultural populations* (2nd ed.), pp. 335–354. Newton, MA: Butterworth-Heinemann.

Soli, S. (1998). Classroom acoustics workshop. *Audiology Today, 10*(1), 27.

Stach, B. A. (1997). *Comprehensive dictionary of audiology*. Baltimore, MD: Williams & Wilkins.

Stach, B. A. (1998). *Clinical audiology: An introduction*. San Diego, CA: Singular Publishing Group.

Thedinger, B. S. (1996). Cochlear implants. In J. Northern (Ed.), *Hearing disorders* (3rd ed.) (pp. 291–298). Needham Heights, MA: Allyn & Bacon.

ANSWERS TO STUDY AND REVIEW QUESTIONS

1. Malleus, incus, stapes

2. VIII, vestibular, auditory/acoustic

3. Compression, rarefaction

4. Conductive

5. Carhart's notch

6. Presbycusis, Meniere's

7. Retrocochlear, acoustic neuroma, auditory brain stem response

8. Immitance, tympanometry, acoustic reflex

9. Otitis media, otosclerosis

10. Tadoma

11. C. A sensorineural loss is usually characterized by an audiogram reflecting a sloping, high-frequency loss.

12. A. People who have difficulty separating the signal of interest (speech) from background noise have difficulty with the signal-to-noise ratio.

13. B. *Homophenous pairs* are those words that look the same on the lips. *Man* and *ban* begin with bilabials, and thus the words look similar to listeners with hearing losses.

14. A. The muscle that exerts the pull that allows the eustachian tube to open during yawning and swallowing is the tensor palatini.

15. C. Infants with cleft palate frequently have eustachian tube dysfunction because of the oral-facial anomalies inherent within the cleft palate condition.

16. D. A sensorineural hearing loss is related to damage in the hair cells of the cochlea.

17. D. Speech reception thresholds (SRTs) are the lowest level of hearing at which a person can understand 50% of the words presented.

18. E. Hearing aids deliver amplified sound to the ear canal, while cochlear implants deliver electrical impulses (converted from sound) directly to the auditory system.

19. B. The aural/oral method emphasizes: (a) making use of residual hearing through amplification, and (b) helping people with hearing impairment learn to communicate so that they are comfortable in mainstream settings with hearing people.

20. A. People with hearing impairment do not typically have a strained-strangled voice quality unless there is a concomitant voice disorder.

CHAPTER 11

Assessment and Treatment: Foundational Principles and Procedures

PREVIEW OUTLINE

Assessment and treatment of clients with communicative disorders constitute the primary activities that speech–language pathologists engage in. In this chapter, we discuss foundational principles and procedures of assessment and treatment. The principles and procedures discussed are foundational, or standard, across most types of communication disorders. Specific information about assessment and treatment of various types of communication disorders can be found in chapters dealing with those specific disorders.

There is a difference between assessment and diagnosis. *Assessment* (also referred to as *evaluation*) refers to the process of arriving at a diagnosis. A *diagnosis* is an understanding of the problem, or the identification of a disorder by analysis of the symptoms presented and, in some cases, analysis of their underlying causes (Haynes & Pindzola, 1998; Nicolosi, Harryman, & Kresheck, 1996). In order to assess clients and arrive at a diagnosis, clinicians optimally use standard assessment procedures and a combination of standardized and nonstandardized assessment measures that are culturally and linguistically appropriate for individual clients.

Treatment in communicative disorders involves some common concepts and procedures. Although treatment is conceptualized in different ways, it essentially involves changing an existing, perhaps nonfunctional, pattern of communication. It requires working not only with clients, but also with people who routinely interact with them. And it requires sensitivity to relevant cultural and linguistic variables. Designing effective treatment procedures requires an accurate assessment of the client's problem. In this chapter, we summarize the basic principles, procedures, and concepts relative to assessment and treatment.

STANDARD ASSESSMENT PROCEDURES

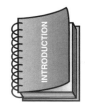

There are standard, or foundational, assessment procedures that are used across types of communication disorders. These procedures usually include a screening, obtaining a case history, a hearing screening, an oral-peripheral examination, an interview, a speech and language sampling, and obtaining related assessment data (Shipley & McAfee, 1998).

Screening

■ A screening is a brief procedure that helps determine whether a client should undergo further, more detailed assessment.

■ Clients who pass screening procedures are judged to have normal skills in the area tested, and thus are not assessed at length. Clients who fail screening procedures are scheduled for comprehensive assessments because they are judged to have potential communication disorders.

■ Screening procedures are used in many facilities, such as public schools, to determine who should receive full assessments and who should not.

Case History

Definition and Purpose

■ The case history yields detailed information that helps the clinician understand the client and his or her communication disorder and associated variables. The case history involves gathering information about the family, health, education, occupation, and other variables such as cultural and linguistic factors.

■ The emphasis of the case history depends upon the age of the client and the nature of the disorder. Relevant information is gathered through a printed case history form and interview of the client, family, or both.

■ The clinician should gather necessary identifying information (e.g., the client's name, date of birth, address and phone number) as well as other information summarized below (see Hegde, 1996a, for more detail).

Description of the Communication Disorder

Clinicians ask adult clients or parents of child clients the following questions:

■ What do you think is the problem?

■ When and under what circumstances did you first notice the problem?

■ What were the early signs of the problem?

■ How has the problem progressed? Has it changed over time or remained the same?

■ In your cultural community, is this issue viewed as a problem?

Prior Assessment and Treatment of the Disorder

Clinicians ask adult clients or parents of child clients the following questions:

- Have you seen any specialists before this evaluation?
- What did these specialists recommend? Did you follow up on their recommendations?
- Did you (or the child) receive treatment?
- If so, what were the results of treatment?

Family Constellation and Communication

Clinicians ask adult clients or parents of child clients the following questions:

- Is there any family history of communication disorders?
- Who currently lives in the home? What is their relationship to you (your child)?
- How many sisters and brothers do you (does the child) have?
- Does the child communicate with other family members?
- Does the child play with other children? How does the child play with others? How does the child communicate with peers?
- What language(s) do you speak at home? What is your (your child's) first or primary language? Do you (does your child) fluently speak, read, and/or write in the primary language and English?

Prenatal, Birth, and Developmental History

These questions are usually asked if the client is a child:

- How was the mother's health during the pregnancy? Did she have any major accidents or illnesses? Did she take any drugs?
- What were the birth condition and birth weight of the child?
- Was the child premature or full term? Were there any complications at birth? What type of delivery occurred (feet first, head first, breech, Cesarean)?
- Did the child have any feeding or nursing problems?
- How would you describe your child's physical development? If it seemed normal, what were the specific problems?
- Have you ever noticed any signs of hearing loss? If so, what were those signs?
- How would you describe your child's speech and language development?
- Were you ever concerned about your child's speech and language development? If so, why?

Medical History

Clinicians can ask adult clients or parents of child clients the following questions:

■ During the early childhood years, did the child (did you) have any illnesses? What kinds of illnesses?

■ Did the child (did you) have any major traumas or accidents of any kind?

■ What kinds of surgical and medical treatment did you (your child) have?

■ Are you (is your child) currently taking any medications? What medications are they? How long have you been taking them?

Educational History

Clinicians can ask adult clients or parents of child clients the following questions:

■ What level of education have you completed?

■ What grade is the child in? Has the child been held back or advanced a grade?

■ Has the child received any special education services? What kinds of services has he or she received?

Occupational History

Clinicians can ask adult clients the following questions:

■ What is your current occupation? What types of tasks do you do on your job? Does your communication problem negatively affect your job performance?

■ How is your relationship with your colleagues and supervisors? How do they react to your communication problem? Are you concerned about their reactions?

■ Do you think you are unable to get a job or receive a promotion because of your communication problem? Why do you think so?

■ What is your occupational goal in seeking treatment at this time?

Prognosis

■ Frequently, clients and their families wish to know the prognosis for improvement of a communication disorder. A *prognosis* is a professional judgment made about the future course of a disorder or disease. It is a predictive statement about what might happen under various future circumstances.

■ For example, a clinician might predict what might happen if a disorder of fluency remains untreated in a 4-year-old child versus what might happen if the child receives treatment. Or a clinician might predict whether a client who has sustained a stroke will possibly be able to return to his or her previous job.

■ Clinicians must be extremely careful in making statements of prognosis. The "Code of Ethics" in Appendix A delineates the parameters of what is considered ethical in making prognostic statements to clients.

■ Factors influencing the prognosis for a client include:

– the severity of the disorder;

– the client's general health;

– the physiological course of an underlying disease;

– the time of intervention (e.g., whether therapy occurred after a child had been stuttering for 2 years, or when the child first began to stutter);

– the quality and intensity of treatment offered;

– the consistency with which treatment is received;

– family support for the client and participation in the treatment process;

– the client's motivation to work hard in treatment and outside the treatment setting;

– social reinforcement for maintaining gains made in treatment; and

– the client and family's religious and cultural beliefs about the necessity for and efficacy of treatment.

Hearing Screening

■ A hearing screening is a quick procedure to determine whether a client can be assumed to have normal hearing or needs to be more thoroughly evaluated by an audiologist.

■ Clinicians should:

– screen the hearing of all clients whom they assess;

– use a screening procedure adopted at their clinical sites;

– make sure the ambient noise in the screening situation does not compromise validity and reliability of screening results;

– generally, screen hearing at 20 or 25 dB HL for 500, 1,000, 2,000, and 4,000 Hz; screen at 25 dB HL for 500 Hz;

— screen younger children at 15 dB HL for 500, 1,000, 2,000, 4,000, and 8,000 Hz; and

— refer the client who fails the screening test to an audiologist for a comprehensive hearing evaluation.

Oral-Peripheral Examination

■ This involves an examination of the oral and facial structures to evaluate their structural and functional integrity from the standpoint of speech production.

■ The oral-peripheral examination helps identify or rule out obvious structural abnormalities that may require medical attention.

■ The oral-peripheral examination is an important standard and common assessment procedure that is used with a variety of clients, including children and adults with articulatory-phonological disorders, cleft palate, neurological problems, and others that affect speech production. (For more detailed information on the components of an oral-peripheral examination, see Shipley & McAfee, 1998.)

✎ Concepts To Consider

Standard components of any assessment include a case history, hearing screening, and oral-peripheral examination. What are two important facets of each of these components?

_____

_____

_____

_____

_____

_____

_____

_____

_____

Interview

■ An interview involves a face-to-face exchange with the client, family members, or both to obtain additional information and to clarify and expand upon the information given on the printed case history form.

■ There are three basic purposes of interviewing (Haynes & Pindzola, 1998; Shipley, 1997):

- to obtain data or gather information

- to convey information

- to provide release and support

■ An important component of the interview is the clinician's establishing rapport with the client and any family members present. Rapport involves respect, trust, and a harmonious relationship between the clinician and the family.

■ Establishing trust between the clinician and the family involves (Peterson & Marquardt, 1994; Shipley & Wood, 1996):

- orienting the interviewees to the nature of the interview

- explaining why certain information is requested

- not making the client feel rushed

- listening

- using appropriate verbal and nonverbal communication

- assuring the client of (and maintaining) confidentiality

■ Maintaining rapport and establishing trust also involve recognizing and accounting for cultural and linguistic variables that might influence the interview. For example, the family might need an interpreter present to assist in the process. Or the family might come from a culture where it is considered inappropriate to reveal personal details. Clinicians must be sensitive to these issues (Roseberry-McKibbin, 1997).

■ During the interview process, it is important to occasionally reflect or report to clients and family members what they have been saying. In this way, clinicians can make sure that they are recording accurate information (Shipley, 1997).

Speech and Language Sample

Nature and Purposes

■ The speech and language sample is the primary means of assessing a client's speech and language production. Many clinicians record the sample on audiotape for further listening, and some clinicians may videotape the sample.

■ Generally, a speech and language sample is more naturalistic than standardized tests. Many clinicians use speech and language samples to supplement the results of standardized tests.

■ The goal of speech and language sampling is to obtain a representative sample of the client's speech–language production in naturalistic contexts that reflect the client's everyday speech and language usage.

■ Speech and language samples can be gathered during conversation between the client and the clinician, or between the client and a caregiver or other interlocutors. It is best to gather speech and language samples that reflect the client's interactions with several different interlocutors.

■ Clinicians can allow the sample to be completely unstructured, or they can manipulate contexts and materials to varying extents to evoke specific productions from clients.

■ Speech and language samples can be used when analyzing a client's articulatory-phonological skills, language skills, or both. With both adults and children, sometimes clinicians want to obtain information about production of speech sounds in naturalistic conversational contexts. Other times, clinicians want information about the client's language skills in the areas of syntax, morphology, pragmatics, and semantics.

Procedures for Gathering the Sample

■ Procedures for gathering language samples may vary from clinician to clinician and from setting to setting. However, in most settings, the following procedures are recommended for the optimal gathering of a representative speech and language sample (Hegde, 1996a; Shipley & McAfee, 1998):

■ Tape-record the entire sample in stereo for an optimal dynamic range. Be sure that the presence of the tape recorder does not cause the client to be self-conscious, thus interfering with the naturalness of the sample obtained.

■ Obtain 50–100 utterances. This may take at least 30 minutes.

■ Observe carefully and take notes on the context of the utterances that may not be clear from the audiotaped sample. For example, when working with a 3-year-old child, the clinician might want to take notes on what books, toys, and other manipulatives are being used at certain times during the gathering of the sample.

■ Use a quiet room and avoid noisy stimulus materials. Some clinicians, when using toys, cover the table with a soft cloth to prevent additional noise on the audiotape.

■ Carefully select stimuli that are appropriate for the client's cultural-linguistic background, educational level, occupation, and age.

▨ In the case of most adults, use objects and pictures only when necessary. In most cases, clinicians can converse with adults about relevant topics specific to the individual client. However, when evaluating adults with neurogenic disorders, clinicians may need to use pictures and objects.

▨ In the case of children, use procedures appropriate to the child's age. For most young children, it is best to have parents bring several favorite books and toys from home. Many young children will react best to interesting, attractive games, toys, and books that are appropriate to their age level.

▨ Use age-appropriate conversational topics (e.g., movies, sports) with older children. If necessary, the clinician may need to use pictures with older children who are reluctant to converse.

▨ When appropriate, especially with young children, begin by having the child interact with one or more family members such as a parent or sibling. As the child's comfort level increases, the clinician may interact alone with the child.

▨ Do not bombard a child or adult client with multiple questions. Let the client initiate the conversation sometimes, and allow enough periods of silence to encourage the client to initiate speech.

▨ With an unintelligible client (especially a child) who is being audiotaped, repeat what the client says so that the utterance can be understood on the audiotape.

▨ Ask as few yes–no questions as possible. Ask primarily open-ended questions; this usually involves wh-questions such as "What is...?" or "Why do...?"

▨ Obtain a home language sample if the family is willing to tape-record the client at home. This home sample would supplement the sample collected in the clinic and can give the clinician additional information about the client's speech–language skills in different settings.

▨ Clinicians can analyze language samples informally or formally. Some clinicians use formalized analysis methods; others calculate mean length of utterance and otherwise conduct an informal analysis of sample results. Clinicians are increasingly turning to computerized language-sample analysis methods because they yield very specific information in an efficient time period.

Obtaining Related Assessment Data

▨ Many times, it is important for clinicians to obtain assessment data in areas related to the communication disorder. While speech and language assessment data are of greatest concern to speech–language pathologists, assessment data in related areas contributes to an overall understanding of the client as a whole person.

■ When working with children, clinicians may want to obtain related assessment data in the form of results of:

- hearing evaluations

- behavioral evaluations

- medical evaluations

- educational psychological evaluations

- reports from regular and special educators (e.g., teachers, resource specialists)

- reports about current medications and their side effects

■ When working with adults in medical settings, clinicians may want to obtain assessment data related to:

- the patient's current medical-neurological diagnosis

- the patient's medical prognosis

- medical personnel's current and future medical treatment plans for the patient

- the patient's current medications and their side effects

- brain imaging and radiologic data that might be related to diagnosis of the communication disorder

- audiologic findings that might be related to or integrated with the communication assessment

- physical rehabilitation plans that might affect treatment of the communication disorder

■ Clinicians may work on teams with other professionals. Westby, Stevens-Dominguez, and Oetter (1996) have described three kinds of teams:

- *Multidisciplinary teams*: Team members represent multiple disciplines, but each member conducts his or her individual evaluation, writes a separate report, and has little interaction with other team members.

- *Transdisciplinary teams*: Multiple disciplines work together in the initial assessment, but service is provided by one or two team members.

- *Interdisciplinary teams*: Team members from multiple disciplines interact and use each other's suggestions and information in interpreting data. The team collaboratively writes the evaluation report and intervention plan.

Summary

☑ Most clinicians use standard, common assessment procedures when working with clients who represent a wide range of communication disorders.

☑ These common procedures include screening, gathering a case history, conducting a hearing screening and oral-peripheral examination, conducting an interview, gathering a speech and language sample, and obtaining available related assessment data.

☑ After these standard assessment procedures are completed, most clinicians then administer standardized tests as the next step of the evaluation process.

PRINCIPLES OF STANDARDIZED ASSESSMENT

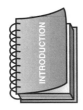

INTRODUCTION

Standardized, norm-referenced assessment is very popular in speech–language pathology. It offers a number of advantages to clinicians: ease of test administration, ease of test scoring, and some assurance of reliability or stability when the test is readministered. For clinicians in the public schools, standardized test scores comply with legal requirements for determining children's eligibility for treatment. Standardized tests yield quantitative scores and can be judged according to their validity and reliability as measures of appropriateness for use with specific populations.

Nature and Purposes of Standardized Assessment

◼ A *standardized test* is one that is *systematic*. Standardized tests have explicit directions and strict controls about what the examiner must say and do; specific stimuli are used, and there are explicit rules for scoring the test (Klein & Moses, 1999; Tomblin, 1994).

◼ The goal of having such explicit rules in standardized testing is that the behaviors being measured not be influenced by the examiner's personal or subjective biases. In addition, the creators of standardized tests hope to guarantee that the measurement process will be uniform across examiners (Tomblin, 1994).

◼ The results of standardized tests yield quantitative information, resulting in scores (numbers). These scores (explained more later) allow the client's performance to be compared to the performance of peers.

■ A standardized test is not the same as a *norm-referenced test*. A test can be standardized without being norm-referenced; however, many tests are frequently norm-referenced as well as standardized.

■ In creating norm-referenced tests, the authors select tasks that they believe are valid in measuring certain behaviors and administer those tasks to groups of subjects who are thought to be representative of the population. The performance of the large sample is calculated, resulting in normative data (Haynes & Pindzola, 1998). Thus, *norms* represent the average performance of a typical group of people on a test in its process of standardization.

■ The primary purpose of norm-referenced tests is to compare the individual client's score to the average score of the norming group. In that comparison, the clinician determines: (a) if the client has a problem, (b) if the problem is clinically significant, and (c) whether the problem warrants intervention.

■ Ideally, the client is represented in the norming sample. For example, if a White, middle-class, 8-year-old girl is being tested, other White, middle-class, 8-year-old girls should be included in the norming sample.

■ As discussed in Chapter 12, clients tested are often not represented in the norming sample. This is a major problem when clinicians attempt to assess culturally and linguistically diverse children.

■ A recent survey of public school clinicians in Oregon, for example, showed that 42% of them viewed standardized testing with culturally and linguistically diverse children as problematic (Huang, Hopkins, & Nippold, 1997).

■ Use of standardized tests with these diverse children is problematic because, for example, a test might have been normed on middle-class, monolingual, English-speaking, White children in Utah, Arizona, and Illinois. Such a test would be invalid for use with a bilingual, Spanish-speaking child who immigrated from Cuba at age 5 years and lives in Louisiana.

■ Unfortunately, many clinicians do not carefully examine the norming samples of tests they use, and thus norm-referenced tests are used inappropriately (Roseberry-McKibbin, 1995).

■ Ideally, standardized, norm-referenced tests (hereafter referred to as *formal tests*) should be representative of the clients who are tested. They should be representative in the areas of:

  – cultural and linguistic background

  – socioeconomic status

  – gender

  – age

  – geographic region

■ However, many formal tests are not diverse in the above-listed areas. In addition, many of these tests have small sample sizes. According to Haynes and

Pindzola (1998), most experts state that if a test has subgroups, there should be at least 100 subjects per group. This is frequently not the case.

■ Another disadvantage of formal tests is that, although administration and scoring procedures are fairly similar across examiners and are thus repeatable or replicable, tasks are so highly structured that they are usually not representative of the client's behavior in natural environments. And standardized tests rarely give information about how clients arrived at answers or the strategies they used to complete the activities (Westby et al., 1996).

■ In addition to these problems, many formal tests have a limited sampling of behaviors, which helps keep the length of the test manageable. For example, in a test of child language, there may be only two or three items that sample the child's production of plural -s.

■ A major problem in speech–language pathology testing is that many clinicians use the results of formal tests to create treatment goals. These treatment goals are based on a very limited sampling of specific behaviors, and thus the goals have a poor foundation.

■ Because the goal of formal testing is to sample a broad range of behaviors, clinicians should take the items that the client answered incorrectly on the formal test and create informal probe measures that sample the behaviors of interest in much greater depth.

■ Formal tests do not give clinicians specific guidance for planning treatment or evaluating treatment progress. It is critical for clinicians not to use formal tests for those purposes.

■ Unfortunately, the use of formal tests to create treatment goals and measure treatment progress is common nationwide. This is highly inappropriate, and experts urge clinicians to create treatment goals and assess treatment progress not on the basis of formal test results, but on that of informal measures.

■ Thus, the optimal use of formal tests is as follows:

1. Administer a formal test (e.g., *The Orangevale Child Language Test*).

2. Examine incorrect items and record them. For example, "The child missed 3/4 items assessing the use of *is-verbing*, and 2/4 items assessing the use of regular past tense *-ed*."

3. Use informal probe tasks to assess these forms in more depth. For example, use conversational speech and structured tasks with word cards to assess the child's production of *is-verbing* and regular past tense *-ed*.

4. Document the accuracy of production of the forms on the informal tasks. For example, "The child was 40% accurate for production of *is-verbing* in response to looking at pictures and being asked 'What is _____ doing?'" and "The child was 20% accurate for production of plurals during a board game when she was asked 'What are these?'"

5. Create treatment goals based upon these informal probe measures. For example, "The child will produce *is-verbing* with 80% accuracy when shown action pictures and asked 'What is _____ doing?'"

6. Measure treatment progress by assessing accuracy of the child's production of the target forms using tasks similar to the informal probe tasks (see "Treatment of Communication Disorders" later in chapter for more details).

This is an appropriate and valid use of formal test results for creating treatment goals and assessing treatment progress. Again, use of formal tests and their resulting scores for creation of treatment goals and assessment of treatment progress is inappropriate and invalid. Formal test results should always be supplemented with the results of informal assessment.

 Concepts To Consider

Describe why the use of formal (standardized, norm-referenced) tests for creation of treatment goals and assessment of treatment progress is inappropriate and should be avoided.

_____

_____

_____

_____

_____

_____

_____

_____

_____

Types of Scores in Standardized Assessment

■ As stated earlier, the goal of formal testing is to yield scores or quantitative measures that compare the client's performance to that of a normative group—a group in which the client is represented.

■ First, the clinician calculates the client's *raw score*. Raw scores are the actual scores earned on a test. For example, on an aphasia test, a patient might receive a raw score of 55, indicating that he or she answered 55 items correctly. The raw score is then converted so it can be viewed on a distribution.

- To successfully compare the client's performance to that of a normative group, test makers use *distributions*. Distributions yield measures of the client's performance as compared to the performance of the norming sample.

- An important component of a distribution is the *mean*. The mean is the arithmetic average of the scores of the norming sample. Another important component of a distribution is the standard deviation.

- The *standard deviation* is the extent to which scores deviate from the mean or average score. It reflects the variability of all the measures or scores of the norming sample. The larger the standard deviation, the more variable the scores. The smaller the standard deviation, the less variable the scores.

- Among scores that have a normal distribution, 34.13% will fall within one standard deviation above the mean and 34.13% will fall within one standard deviation below the mean (Tomblin, 1994). In other words, if scores are normally distributed in a bell-shaped curve, 68% of the sample will have scores between 85 and 115 (assuming 100 is the average score). The standard deviation is 15 points.

- A client's score enables the clinician to see where the client performs in relation to the mean. The client's score(s) may be expressed in terms of its standard deviation from the mean. Scores may also be expressed in terms of percentile ranks.

- *Percentile ranks* are converted scores that show the percentage of subjects who scored at or below a specific raw score. Percentile ranks use percentile points to express a client's score relative to the norming sample. For example, if a child's score is at the 25th percentile, 75% of children will do better on the test than that child did.

- The 50th percentile is equivalent to the mean and *median*. The median is the score in the exact middle of the distribution; it divides the distribution into two parts so that an equal number of scores fall to the right and to the left of it.

- Usually, clients whose scores place them one standard deviation below the mean will score slightly below the 16th percentile. People whose scores are two standard deviations below the mean score close to the second percentile (Tomblin, 1994).

- Formal tests often yield age equivalency and grade equivalency scores. Scores indicating *age equivalency* show the chronological age for which a raw score is the mean or average score in the standardization sample. Scores indicating *grade equivalency* show the grade placement for which a raw score is the mean or average score.

- Thus, for example, a 6-year-old's score on a test might be typical of the score of a 4-year-old in the norming sample. Or a fifth grader's score might be typical of the average score of the third-grade children in the norming sample.

■ Because age- and grade-equivalency scores are easier for parents and clients to understand than percentile ranks and standard deviations, many clinicians use them to explain test performance. However, experts do not recommend this practice (see Haynes & Pindzola, 1998, and Tomblin, 1994, for further discussion of this issue).

Foundations of Measurement: Evaluating Psychometric Properties of Formal Tests

When clinicians select formal tests to use with certain populations, they can evaluate those formal tests according to the broad parameters of validity and reliability.

■ Recent research indicates that many clinicians express a low level of concern with these psychometric characteristics of tests (Huang et al., 1997); thus it becomes even more important to understand and apply the concepts of validity and reliability to the evaluation of tests.

Validity

■ Validity refers to the degree to which a measuring instrument or test measures what it purports to measure. For example, for many years, the *Peabody Picture Vocabulary Test–Revised* (PPVT–R) purported to measure intelligence. This was not valid, because the PPVT–R measured only a single skill: that of receptive vocabulary. Receptive vocabulary is one very small part of the broad construct of intelligence. Thus, the PPVT–R came to be viewed as *invalid* for measuring intelligence.

■ However, the PPVT–R did measure receptive one-word vocabulary skills; thus, it was and is considered to be a *valid* measure of receptive one-word vocabulary skills (Tomblin, 1994).

■ There are several kinds of validity that clinicians can look for when selecting tests and evaluating their appropriateness for use with given populations. These kinds of validity include *concurrent*, *construct*, *content*, and *predictive* validity.

Concurrent Validity

■ This refers to the degree to which a new test correlates with an established test of known validity. For example, many new intelligence tests are evaluated against the well-known, trusted, and established *Stanford-Binet Intelligence Test*. If the new intelligence test correlates highly with the *Stanford-Binet*, then concurrent validity is established for the new test (Tomblin, 1994).

■ Too high a correlation suggests that the new test may be as valid as the old one and that the two tests are too similar, raising the question of the need for the new test. Thus, concurrent validity can be challenging to establish.

Construct Validity

■ This refers to the degree to which test scores are consistent with theoretical constructs or concepts. Construct validity includes any qualitative or quantitative information that supports the test maker's theory or model underlying the test (Hutchinson, 1996).

■ For example, a language test that shows higher scores for older children compared to younger children is consistent with the theoretical construct that language changes (improves) with age.

■ Construct validity is challenging to establish because it requires that measurements be based on a theory. The test must then be developed in a way that is consistent with the theory. Next, the test creator(s) must demonstrate through supporting research that the test indeed conforms to the predictions of the theory (Tomblin, 1994).

Content Validity

■ This is a measure of validity of a test based on a thorough examination of all test items to determine if the items are relevant to measuring what the test purports to measure, *and* whether the items adequately sample the full range of the skill being measured.

■ For example, a test of articulation should include all speech sounds in all word positions and in phrases and sentences. Omission of sounds or inclusion of items not relevant to measuring articulation would reduce the content validity of the test.

Predictive Validity

■ This refers to the accuracy with which a test predicts future performance on a related task. For example, a test of language competence may be shown to predict academic performance. Many universities use *Graduate Record Examination* (GRE) scores as a criterion for admission into their master's degree programs. This practice is based on the belief that GRE scores have predictive validity—that the scores predict how well students will perform academically in the graduate program.

■ Predictive validity is also known as *criterion-related validity* because future performance is the criterion used to evaluate the validity.

Reliability

■ Reliability means the *consistency* or *stability* with which the same event is repeatedly measured. Scores are *reliable* if they are consistent across repeated testing or measurement. The best way to increase reliability of any measurement is to repeat the measurement a number of times. The more measurements are taken, the more stable or reliable the overall measure will be.

■ In assessment, reliability of the test is influenced by several factors (Silverman, 1998; Tomblin, 1994):

– fluctuations in examinee's behavior—the examinee may behave differently during various parts of a test due to factors like fatigue, attention span, the presence of medications in his or her system, and environmental distractions;

– examiner error—the examiner may be tired or distracted and thus misuse a test by not administering it according to the standardized procedures dictated in the manual; and

– instrumentation or equipment errors—equipment might not be calibrated, or might malfunction.

■ Most reliability measures are expressed in terms of a correlational coefficient. The *correlational coefficient* is a number or index that indicates the relationship between two or more independent measures. It is usually expressed through Pearson Product Moment r.

■ The highest possible positive value is $r = 1.00$; the lowest possible negative value is $r = -1.00$. An r value of 0.00 indicates that there is no relationship between the two measures. The higher the correlational coefficient, the greater the reliability of a test or measurement.

■ Different types of reliability are associated with measurement. These types of reliability are *interjudge reliability*, *intrajudge reliability*, *alternate form reliability*, *test-retest reliability*, and *split-half reliability*.

Interobserver or Interjudge Reliability

■ This refers to how similarly a subject's performance is independently rated by two or more raters or judges. The judges independently score the same set of behaviors, and then the judges' scores are calculated in terms of how well they relate.

■ The more similarly the judges independently rate the same subjects, the higher the *interjudge reliability coefficient*. Optimally, there will be interjudge reliability coefficients of .90 or above to show good agreement among the examiners. The closer the coefficient is to 1.0, the more reliable the scoring (Haynes & Pindzola, 1998).

Intraobserver or Intrajudge Reliability

■ This measures a client's performance over several different occasions as rated by the same rater or examiner. Put differently, one individual measures and records operationally defined target behaviors over a series of two or more trials.

■ Recorded measures or scores may then be compared to determine agreement. As with interjudge reliability measurement, the closer the scores are to one another, the higher the *intrajudge reliability coefficient*.

Alternate Form Reliability

■ This refers to the consistency of measures when two forms of the same test are administered to the same person. A test must have two versions, which sample the same behaviors, for a clinician to establish alternate form reliability.

■ Alternate form reliability is also known as *parallel form reliability*.

■ For example, the PPVT–R has two forms: A and B. One could use forms A and B of the PPVT–R with the same child and compare scores. If the scores are very similar, then the PPVT–R has established parallel form reliability.

Test-Retest Reliability

■ This refers to consistency of measures when the same test is administered to the same person twice. The results of the two test administrations are compared for consistency. Thus, for example, if a child is given a specific test and receives a score of 96, he or she should receive a similar score if the test is readministered.

■ Test-retest reliability suggests stability of scores over time.

Split-Half Reliability

■ This refers to a measure of the internal consistency of a test. One can determine split-half reliability by showing that the responses to the items on the first half of the test are correlated with responses given to the items on the second half of the test. Or one could compare answers on the even-numbered items of a test to answers on the odd-numbered items and see if those answers are correlated.

■ To derive split-half reliability, the first and the second half of a test should measure the same skill. Split-half reliability generally overestimates reliability, as it does not measure stability of scores over time.

Summary

☑ Many clinicians use formal (standardized, norm-referenced) tests to assess clients. There are advantages and disadvantages to using formal tests.

☑ Formal test results alone should never be used to establish treatment goals or measure treatment progress.

☑ Clinicians can analyze formal tests according to how reliable and valid the tests are, especially for the specific populations the clinician serves.

☑ Clinicians are increasingly using formal tests in conjunction with nonstandardized, informal tests in order to obtain the most complete profile of clients' abilities and skills.

PRINCIPLES OF NONSTANDARDIZED ASSESSMENT

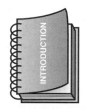

Because of some of the limitations inherent in formal assessment, many clinicians are supplementing formal test results with those of nonstandardized assessment measures. Nonstandardized, informal assessment measures have the advantage of being flexible, adaptable to individual clients, and valid as a basis for planning treatment (Klein & Moses, 1999). However, behaviors, qualities, or skills as measured informally may be poorly defined and subject to examiner bias. For example, the quality of vocal hoarseness may be subjectively defined differently by various examiners. The skill of cohesive adequacy in narratives is difficult to operationalize, thus making it subjective. A major challenge with informal assessment is to make it reliable and valid for optimal use with clients (Haynes & Pindzola, 1998). Clinicians have attempted to establish validity and reliability by using various types of nonstandardized or informal assessment measures including measurement scales, structured interviews or questionnaires, functional assessment, criterion-referenced testing, and dynamic assessment.

Measurement Scales

■ Sometimes clinicians use rating scales to document observations. These scales are typically *nominal* or *ordinal* in nature.

■ In a *nominal scale*, a category (e.g., hoarseness, hyponasality) is present or absent. Items or observations are classified into discrete groups (named groupings) that do not have a numerical relationship to one another. For example, a client might be rated as a *mild*, *moderate*, or *severe* stutterer. Or a questionnaire might ask a stutterer, for a particular item, to circle *always*, *sometimes*, or *rarely*.

■ An *ordinal scale* is a numerical scale that can be arranged according to rank orders or levels. For example, if a clinician is rating voice quality, an ordinal scale might look thus:

Breathiness	1	2	3	4	5	6
Harshness	1	2	3	4	5	6

Structured Interviews and Questionnaires

■ Questionnaires may be administered personally to clients or sent to clients, who fill them out and then bring them to the clinician. Clinicians who work with children often administer questionnaires to adults, such as parents and teachers, who are familiar with the child in question.

- Questionnaires are considered to be more valid with some populations than formal tests. For example, formal tests are generally inappropriate for use with culturally and linguistically diverse children and adults. Using questionnaires that account for linguistic and cultural background, clinicians can gather information that more validly reflects clients' actual skills and abilities in natural, daily life settings (e.g., Brice & Montgomery, 1996).

- Interviews may stand alone or be used in conjunction with questionnaires. Interviews are generally carried out for the purpose of gathering information about a particular client. Interviews have the advantage of being more personalized than questionnaires used alone.

- The use of questionnaires and interviews can yield quantitative data, qualitative data (verbal data expressed in words), or both. For example, a clinician working with an adult who stutters might ask the client to circle numbers on a scale reflecting attitudes toward stuttering, and also might record the client's verbal descriptions of his or her own attitudes toward stuttering.

Functional Assessment

The purpose of functional assessment is to assess a client's day-to-day communication skills in naturalistic, socially meaningful contexts.

- Speech–language pathology is increasingly turning to functional assessment because reimbursers and third-party payers are requiring documentation of functional outcomes of treatment.

- Many clinicians are targeting clients' functional communication skills during traditional assessments. Functional assessment requires the clinician to make targets, procedures, and settings of assessment as naturalistic and "real life" as possible.

To target a client's functional communication during an assessment, clinicians can use the following procedures (Hegde, 1996a):

- Observe the client's communication with family members and/or peers if appropriate.

- When assessing children, arrange a child-caretaker interaction that approximates their typical, everyday interaction. In this way, it is possible to observe naturalistic communication rather than artificial communication, which frequently results during testing.

- Whenever possible with children and adolescents, arrange for various peer interaction situations and observe communication patterns within those situations. Talk with two or three peers about how the client communicates in social contexts.

- Obtain several home speech and language samples. Tell the family to record natural, everyday communication interactions.

- In school (educational) settings, observe the child in the classroom, in the cafeteria, on the playground, and in other settings with peers.

- In school settings, obtain information from teachers and other professionals about the child's communication skills as observed in everyday settings such as the playground and classroom.

- In medical settings, observe the patient's interaction with health care providers and family members. Interview them as to when and how the patient communicates with them (e.g., How does the patient communicate with the physician? With the nurses? With the physical therapist?).

- When assessing adults, always interview at least one person with whom the client regularly interacts (e.g., colleague, significant other, friend).

- Place emphasis on conversational interaction. Do not make clinical judgments based solely on purely imitative or picture naming tasks (although use of those tasks, in conjunction with analysis of conversational interaction, may be necessary with some clients).

- Observe and record conversational speech in naturalistic situations outside the clinic room with various interlocutors.

- To the extent possible, create and structure assessment tasks that are meaningful to the individual client. This is especially important with linguistically and culturally diverse clients who do not relate well to the stimuli and pictures in standardized tests that are geared toward white, monolingual, English-speaking clients.

- When carrying out meaningful assessment tasks, use sentences that include names of family members, activities the client enjoys, interests that the client has, and so forth.

- Document variations in the disorder in natural settings. For example, in assessing the fluency of a person who stutters, document the person's degree of fluency in such naturalistic contexts as talking on the telephone, ordering in a restaurant, or purchasing items in a store.

- Instead of emphasizing the language structures the client produces in response to the administration of standardized tests, examine the effect the client produces when he or she attempts to communicate. For example, whether a patient with Alzheimer's dementia can successfully communicate his or her basic needs may be, at a certain stage, more important than the syntactic structure the patient uses to communicate those needs.

✎ **Concepts To Consider**

Why are more clinicians turning to nonstandardized, informal assessment measures? Summarize advantages and disadvantages of those measures.

_____

_____

_____

_____

_____

_____

_____

_____

_____

Criterion-Referenced Testing

■ Criterion-referenced testing is a form of assessment in which the examiner selects target behaviors to be assessed and uses stimulus materials that are effective for and individualized to the particular client.

■ Some level of performance is viewed as minimal for being deemed "acceptable." For example, when assessing swallowing, the clinician needs a standard defining unacceptable level of aspiration. Thus, criterion-referenced testing involves a qualitative evaluation of what is acceptable and what is unacceptable performance (Tomblin, 1994).

■ An example of criterion-referenced testing would be the clinician formulating specific questions and seeking answers to those questions. For example, the clinician might pose the question, "Does Susie use regular plural -s accurately in conversational speech?" Then the clinician might select 10 pictures with plurals in them and ask Susie, "What do you see here?" The clinician, using a predetermined passing criterion of 80% accuracy (for example), would judge whether Susie "passed" for correct production of regular plurals.

■ In standardized norm-referenced testing, a client's performance is explicitly evaluated against age-based norms. The purpose of norm-referenced testing is to rank individuals (McCauley, 1996). In criterion-referenced testing, the results are not compared against norms derived from the performance of a representative sample. Rather, skills are defined and individual performance is emphasized.

▪ Criterion-referenced measures may prove to be especially helpful when the norms of standardized tests do not apply to a particular client (e.g., a culturally and linguistically diverse client) or when the available standardized tests do not assess specific client skills of interest to the clinician (McCauley, 1996).

▪ Thus, criterion-referenced testing may assess aspects or skills that standardized tests do not include, and may assess those skills in greater depth than standardized tests do. Also, criterion-referenced testing is helpful in assessing a client's progress in treatment.

Dynamic Assessment

▪ Clinicians frequently use *static assessment*, or assessment that measures a client's abilities at one point in time. Static assessment accepts a client's current level of functioning as a predictor of how well the client will always function in the future.

▪ Because clients learn, change, and grow, static assessment is not optimal. Increasingly, clinicians are using dynamic assessment. *Dynamic assessment* (also referred to in Chapter 9) measures a client's ability to learn over time when provided with instruction (Roseberry-McKibbin, 1995).

▪ Dynamic assessment typically occurs in a test-teach-retest paradigm. The client (usually a child) is tested, and his or her skills are measured. Then the child is taught the skills that he or she did not manifest during testing. Finally, the child is retested to assess how quickly and well he or she learned the material presented. A unique feature of dynamic assessment, then, is the incorporation of intervention into the assessment process (Lidz & Peña, 1996).

▪ In dynamic assessment, the question asked is: What is the child's underlying language-learning *ability*? What is the child's ability to learn when provided with instruction or intervention?

▪ Because many children come from backgrounds where they are not exposed to the information assumed by formal tests, they score poorly on formal tests even if their language-learning ability is normal.

▪ Dynamic assessment controls for this mismatch between children's backgrounds and formal test assumptions. Again, the child's capability of learning and changing in response to intervention is evaluated as opposed to the child's knowledge of given areas at a particular point in time without intervention.

Summary

- ☑ Informal, nonstandardized measures include measurement scales, structured interviews and questionnaires, functional assessment measures, criterion-referenced measures, and dynamic assessment.

- ☑ These measures have many advantages for use with clients. Informal measures allow clinicians to tailor assessment to individual clients, create treatment goals, and monitor treatment progress.

- ☑ Clinicians must take precautions to ensure that informal assessment measures are reliable and valid.

TREATMENT OF COMMUNICATION DISORDERS: FOUNDATIONAL CONCEPTS

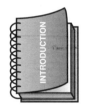

INTRODUCTION

Treatment, *remediation*, and *therapy* are all terms used to refer to ways of modifying communication disorders to achieve patterns of normal, functional, or socially more acceptable patterns of communication. Treatment follows a comprehensive assessment, which results in a diagnosis of a communicative disorder. Treatment procedures specific to given disorders are summarized in their respective chapters. In this section, a basic definition of treatment is given. Next, a treatment paradigm for communication disorders is described; this is followed by definitions of some basic treatment terms.

Treatment: Definition

- *Treatment* may be broadly defined as "teaching, training, any type of remedial or rehabilitative work, and all attempts at helping people by changing their behaviors or teaching new skills" (Hegde, 1998a, p. 12).

- A more strict definition of treatment is that it is a procedure in which contingent relations between antecedents, responses, and consequences (described later) are managed by a clinician to effect desirable changes in communication behaviors.

- Communication behaviors are considered disordered when they attract negative attention, create difficulty in interactions, and cause speakers to sound different than other people in their speech communities (Locke, 1998).

- Success in treatment of communication disorders depends upon how effectively the clinician is able to change the way speakers and their listeners react to each other (Hegde & Davis, 1995).

■ The clinician rearranges listener-speaker relations by first organizing his or her interaction with the client. Eventually, as the client learns new behaviors, the clinician must rearrange the communicative relations between the client and the client's family, friends, and other important people in the client's environment.

■ Historically, speech–language pathologists have focused upon the clinician-client relationship within the therapy room. Although clients have been successfully trained, in this manner, to produce appropriate communication behaviors, successful transfer to the environment has been limited. Today's clinicians are increasingly working to train clients in effective communication skills that can be transferred to clients' environments.

■ That goal can be accomplished in a number of ways. Clinicians can spend increased time working with the client in interactions with significant others as well as in situations outside the therapy room. In public schools, for example, clinicians can collaborate with classroom teachers and carry out therapy in classroom settings (Brice & Roseberry-McKibbin, 1999; Roth & Worthington, 1996).

A Treatment Paradigm for Communication Disorders

■ A *paradigm,* as used here, is an overall philosophy or perspective of treatment. Procedures and materials used in treatment are based upon the clinician's treatment paradigm.

■ Treatment paradigms vary greatly. A widely used paradigm holds that certain contingencies influence the behaviors treated by clinicians. A *contingency* is an interdependent relation between certain events, which are often called factors or variables. In this relation, events influence each other.

■ Communication behaviors manifested by clients are affected by two kinds of contingencies: (a) genetic and neurophysiological contingencies (which are generally not manipulable), and (b) environmental contingencies (which are generally manipulable).

■ *Environmental contingencies* can be defined as three sets of interdependent variables that correspond to:

  – antecedent events (used by clinicians to evoke target responses)

  – responses (of the client)

  – consequences (applied by the clinician) that follow the responses

■ Clinicians identify target behaviors for a client, arrange stimulus conditions for those behaviors, select materials and procedures to evoke responses, evoke the responses, and apply consequences to the responses. In this way, clinicians manipulate the environment to positively affect the client's behaviors.

- Clinicians' manipulation of the environment to positively affect clients' behaviors should be based on a particular scientific philosophy (Roth & Worthington, 1996; Hegde, 1998a). This philosophy states that all concepts and procedures used must be empirically validated; that is, procedures should be experimentally demonstrated to be effective.

- Unfortunately, many treatment concepts and procedures are not empirically validated. They are based upon speculation, anecdotal evidence, and/or opinions of "experts" who have not empirically tested their ideas. Many mistakes are made when clinicians "jump on a bandwagon" and vigorously use and promote treatment ideas that have never been subjected to scientific scrutiny.

- Ideally, treatment procedures should be objective, measurable, empirical, and reliable. Clinical procedures should include methods that help document the effectiveness of treatment.

- To help meet this need, the American Speech–Language-Hearing Association Task Force on Treatment Outcomes and Cost Effectiveness, created in 1993, has worked toward the goal of creating an outcomes database for speech–language pathology and audiology.

- This database is currently composed of data gathered by clinicians participating in various projects that reflect the ages and types of communication disorders manifested by clients. The data has been and will be used, in part, to create functional communication measures (FCMs) (ASHA, 1997).

- For example, FCMs for cognitive communication include seven levels. Level 1 is "No meaningful cognitive communication," and Level 2 is "Cognitive communication is limited to brief episodes of appropriateness with minimal cueing; client is unaware of deficits" (ASHA, 1997, p. 27). Level 7 is "Normal cognitive communication in all situations."

- Ideally, FCMs involve treatment procedures and measures that are empirically valid as well as effective in helping clients communicate to the best of their potential in their everyday living environments.

✎ Concepts To Consider

Define the term *treatment*. Summarize the above-described treatment paradigm for communicative disorders.

_____

_____

_____

_____

Basic Treatment Terms

There are some common terms that most clinicians use in describing treatment and its components. A list of these terms and their definitions follows:

■ *Antecedents* or *treatment stimuli*: Various objects, pictures, instructions, modeling, prompts, and other stimuli the clinician uses to evoke target responses.

■ *Aversive stimuli*: Events people tend to avoid; events people describe as unpleasant and hence work hard to avoid. For example, a person who stutters might try to avoid speaking on the telephone when possible.

■ *Avoidance*: An action that results in not coming in contact with an aversive event and hence is repeated in the future when such contact seems imminent (e.g., avoiding an aversive person by not going to a place at a time when he or she is likely to be there). Avoidance is a behavior exhibited by many clients (e.g., stutterers who avoid specific speaking situations). It is a behavior that needs to be reduced in some cases.

■ *Avoidance conditioning*: Teaching behaviors through negative reinforcement; teaching actions that help reduce or eliminate aversive events.

■ *Escape*: A behavior that reduces or terminates an aversive event after having come in contact with that event; a behavior that increases in frequency because it helped to reduce or terminate an aversive event (e.g., a stutterer's response of terminating a conversation with a hostile listener). Escape is a behavior to be reduced in some clients.

■ *Baselines*: Measured response rates in the absence of treatment; the natural rate of a response when nothing special is done to affect its frequency. Baselines are also known as the *operant level*; they help establish that the client did not produce the target behaviors and hence the treatment was necessary.

■ *Booster treatment*: Treatment given any time after the client was dismissed from the initial treatment. It is an important maintenance strategy and may involve the original or a new form of treatment.

■ *Constituent definitions*: Definitions of target behaviors in dictionary terms. This involves defining concepts with the help of other conceptual (not procedural) terms (e.g., *Language is* the mental capacity to communicate). Constituent definitions are not helpful in measuring the phenomenon being defined. They can be contrasted with operational definitions.

- *Operational definitions*: Definitions that describe how what is defined is measured (e.g., morphologic skills include production of plural morphemes in words, phrases, and sentences with 90% accuracy). Operational definitions, in contrast with constituent definitions, are helpful in quantitatively measuring changes in target behaviors during treatment.

- *Criteria*: Guidelines on making such clinical decisions as when to judge whether a response is trained, when to move on to another target, and when to dismiss the client from treatment.

- *Corrective feedback*: Information given to the client on incorrect or unacceptable responses with the effect of decreasing those responses (e.g., saying "No" or "Wrong" when an incorrect response is given).

- *Direct methods of response reduction*: Reducing behaviors by immediately providing a corrective feedback (e.g., reducing stuttering or asking inappropriate questions during treatment by saying "no"). Direct methods can be contrasted with indirect methods of response reduction.

- *Indirect methods of response reduction*: Reducing undesirable behaviors by positively reinforcing, and thus increasing, desirable behaviors. Nothing is done directly to decrease the undesirable behaviors.

- *Trial*: A structured and discrete opportunity to produce a response. A trial may involve showing various kinds of stimuli, asking questions, modeling, or prompting. The response given to each trial is scored separately.

- *Discrete trials*: Treatment methods in which each opportunity to produce a response (e.g., individual words in learning correct articulation; specific sentences) is counted separately. Each opportunity is clearly separated in time (e.g., by pausing for a few seconds after each attempt and scoring each response as correct or incorrect). Discrete trials are helpful in establishing target behaviors but are less efficient in promoting generalization to natural settings than spontaneous productions.

- *Evoked trial*: Clinical procedure in which modeling is not given; pictures, questions, and other stimuli are used to provoke a response (e.g., asking the client to name a picture or asking such questions as "Johnny, what is this?" while showing a picture or an object). Evoked trials follow modeled trials.

- *Modeled trial*: A discrete opportunity to imitate a response when the clinician models it. A modeled trial is typically preceded by a question (e.g., "What is this? Say . . .").

- *Modeling*: The clinician's production of the target response the client is expected to learn. Modeling is used to teach imitation and is effective in establishing target behaviors. It is used in the initial stages of treatment.

- *Exemplar*: A specific target response that illustrates a broader target behavior. Exemplars are individual items trained in therapy sessions (e.g., the word *soup* in teaching the /s/ or the phrase *two cups* in teaching the regular plural inflection).

■ *Extinction*: Simply withholding such reinforcers as attention to reduce a response. Extinction is appropriate in reducing such behaviors as crying and interfering questioning in treatment.

■ *Fading*: A treatment procedure in which the controlling power of a stimulus is gradually reduced while the response is maintained (e.g., making modeling less and less audible to the client until finally only an articulatory posture is modeled and then withdrawn).

■ *Follow-up*: An assessment procedure designed to find out if the clients have maintained their treatment gains. In most cases, follow-up involves recording a conversational speech sample to evaluate the continued use of clinically established communicative behaviors. Follow-up may involve a regular schedule (e.g., semi-annual or annual assessments following dismissal from treatment).

■ *Functional outcomes:* Effects of treatment that are generalized, broader, and socially and personally meaningful to clients, their families, caregivers, and others. Functional outcomes are qualitative effects (e.g., a treated stutterer's social communication) that go beyond quantitative changes in traditionally measured behaviors (e.g., reduction in the number of stuttering behaviors).

■ *Generality of treatment*: Presence of data that show that a treatment found effective in one situation, by one clinician, with some clients, is effective in other situations, when used by other clinicians, and with other clients. Generality is an important factor in judging treatment usefulness across situations.

■ *Generalized production*: Production of a clinically established behavior in natural settings with no particular or systematic reinforcement. Generalized production may be temporary unless reinforced.

■ *IEPs*: Individual Educational Plans for children with disabilities or special needs. IEPs are legally mandated in public school settings.

■ *IFSPs*: Individualized Family Service Plans are legally mandated for infants and toddlers with disabilities or special needs and their family members. The goal is to involve the family members in the treatment process.

■ *Imitation*: A process of learning in which the learner reproduces what is modeled by an instructor or clinician.

■ *Informative feedback*: Telling clients how well they are doing in treatment sessions; giving specific quantitative information on performance to motivate the client (e.g., telling the client, "During the last sessions, you were 70% correct; this time, you are 85% correct").

■ *Intermediate response*: A response that helps move toward the final target in a shaping procedure (e.g., vocalizing the /m/, opening the mouth while vocalizing, and closing the mouth in saying the word *mom*). An intermediate response is not stabilized by excessive reinforcement.

■ *Initial response*: The first, simplified component of a target response the client can imitate while shaping a target response (e.g., putting the lips together for production of the word *mom*).

■ *Maintenance strategy*: Various methods used to help maintain treatment gains in natural settings. These methods include training family members and others in evoking and reinforcing target behaviors and the client's self-monitoring of communicative skills.

■ *Manual guidance*: The use of physical guidance in a shaping process (e.g., moving a client's tongue with a tongue blade to a correct articulatory position; taking a child's hand and pointing to the correct picture).

■ *Mode of responses*: Manner or method of a response; typical modes include imitation, oral reading, and conversational speech.

■ *Peer training*: Training peers of clients to identify, prompt, evoke, reinforce, and record target behaviors in natural settings. Peer training is a response maintenance strategy.

■ *Physical setting generalization*: Production of clinically established responses in environments such as the home, school, and office, which are outside the therapy room.

■ *Physical stimulus generalization*: Production of clinically established responses to stimuli that were not used in training but are similar to stimuli that were used in training.

■ *Post-reinforcement pause*: Absence of responses following the delivery of a reinforcer. These pauses are more commonly observed under fixed-interval schedules of reinforcement.

■ *Pretests*: Procedures to measure target behaviors before starting treatment. Pretests are necessary to justify the need for treatment and to document changes under treatment. Pretests are compared with the results of posttests.

■ *Posttests*: Procedures designed to measure target behaviors after treatment to document changes from the pretests.

■ *Prompts*: Additional verbal (e.g., "The word starts with a *t*..." in teaching naming to aphasic patients) or nonverbal stimuli (showing an articulatory posture in the absence of voicing) that increase the probability of a target response. Prompts are useful with most clients.

■ *Probes*: Procedures to assess generalized production of responses without reinforcing them. Probes involve a criterion to be met before training is advanced to a more complex level or to another target behavior.

■ *Pure probes*: Procedures for assessing generalized production when only untrained stimulus items are presented.

■ *Intermixed probes*: Assessment of generalized production of trained responses by alternating trained and untrained stimulus items.

■ *Procedures of treatment*: Methods of treatment (e.g., modeling, instructions, verbal praise, prompting). Procedures are what the clinician does to teach target behaviors in clients.

■ *Punishment*: Procedures of reducing undesirable behaviors by response-contingent presentation or withdrawal of stimuli. Punishment includes corrective feedback, time-out, and response cost.

■ *Time-out*: A brief period of silence, inactivity, and lack of reinforcement imposed on a response to be reduced (e.g., a silent period of 5 seconds imposed on every instance of stuttering).

■ *Response cost*: A method of reducing responses by withdrawing reinforcers contingent on each response (e.g., taking a token away from the client for every incorrect production of a phoneme).

■ *Response generalization*: Production of new (untrained) responses that are functionally similar to those that have been trained.

■ *Response mode generalization*: Production of new (untrained) responses in a mode not involved in training (e.g., spontaneous production of untrained words after correct and reinforced imitation training).

■ *Stimulus generalization*: Evocation of established responses by stimuli not involved in training. For example, a child might have been trained to produce /s/ correctly in the words *see*, *sun*, and *saw*. If the clinician holds up a (untrained) picture of soup and says, "What's this?" and the child correctly says, "Soup," that is stimulus generalization.

■ *Self-control*: Deliberately maintaining, increasing, or decreasing specific behaviors of oneself. Self-control is useful in a response maintenance strategy and includes such procedures as self-monitoring correct responses and self-recording undesirable behaviors.

■ *Shaping*: A method of teaching nonexistent responses that are not even imitated. A target response is broken down into initial, intermediate, and terminal components and those are then taught in an ascending sequence. Shaping is also known as *successive approximation*.

■ *Targets of treatment*: Skills and behaviors a client is taught.

■ *Terminal response*: The final target behavior in a shaping procedure. For example, with a nonverbal child, the final target might be production of selected words in conversational speech the child produces in the home or other situations.

■ *Tokens*: Objects that are given for correct responses and later exchanged for backup reinforcers. Tokens require learning to be effective, and they are powerful because a variety of reinforcers can be used as backups. Tokens also help in resisting the satiation effect.

■ *Satiation*: An internal body state that renders primary reinforcers (such as food) temporarily ineffective. For example, a client might feel full and thus not desire the food reinforcers offered.

Reinforcers and Reinforcement: Basic Definitions

Clinicians shape and change clients' behavior through procedures such as reinforcement. Reinforcement is a key component of treatment programs and is used with clients who have a variety of communication disorders.

Reinforcement

Reinforcement is a method of selecting and strengthening behaviors of individuals by arranging immediate consequences under specific stimulus conditions. Types of reinforcement include those defined below:

- *Continuous reinforcement*: A method of reinforcing all correct responses in treatment sessions; this can be contrasted with intermittent reinforcement.

- *Intermittent reinforcement*: Reinforcement of only some responses or responses produced with some delay between reinforcers.

- *Differential reinforcement*: Teaching a client to give different responses to different stimuli (e.g., teaching the plural response to plural stimuli and the singular response to singular stimuli). Differential reinforcement involves reinforcing the correct response while ignoring the incorrect response to the same stimuli.

- *Differential reinforcement of alternative behaviors (DRA)*: Reinforcing a specified, desirable alternative to an undesirable behavior. DRA involves replacing undesirable behaviors with desirable behaviors that give the client access to the same effects or consequences (e.g., teaching a child to use words instead of whining to get attention).

- *Differential reinforcement of low rates of responding (DRL)*: Decreasing undesirable behaviors gradually by reinforcing progressively lower frequencies of that behavior (e.g., reinforcing a child for asking progressively fewer interfering questions during treatment until the frequency is reduced to zero or near zero).

- *Differential reinforcement of incompatible behaviors (DRI)*: Reinforcing a desirable behavior that cannot coexist with the undesirable behavior to be reduced (e.g., heavily reinforcing a child to sit quietly when the target is to reduce restless in-seat behavior or off-seat behavior during treatment).

- *Differential reinforcement of other behaviors (DRO)*: Specifying one behavior that will not be reinforced (e.g., leaving the chair in a group treatment session) while reinforcing many unspecified desirable behaviors (e.g., quiet sitting, coloring, reading, writing), any one of which is accepted.

- *Negative reinforcement*: Strengthening of behaviors by the termination of an aversive event. Negative reinforcement is involved in aversive conditioning (e.g., strengthening a stuttering person's avoidance of speaking situations because such avoidance also helps that person avoid or terminate aversive listener reactions).

■ *Reinforcement withdrawal*: Prompt removal of reinforcers to decrease a response; includes such procedures as extinction, time-out, and response cost.

✎ Concepts To Consider

What is reinforcement? Describe three types of reinforcement clinicians can use in treatment.

_____

_____

_____

_____

_____

_____

_____

_____

_____

Schedules of Reinforcement

Schedules of reinforcement are different patterns of reinforcement that generate different patterns of responses. Schedules of reinforcement include those described below:

■ *Fixed-interval (FI) schedule*: A schedule of reinforcement in which an invariable time duration separates opportunities to earn reinforcers. FI schedule is a form of intermittent reinforcement schedule based on time lapsed between two reinforcements (e.g., in an FI 2-minute schedule, correct responses given after a 2-minute lapse following the previously reinforced response are reinforced and any responses within the interval are ignored).

■ *Fixed-ratio (FR) schedule*: An intermittent schedule of reinforcement in which a certain number of responses are required to earn a reinforcer (e.g., reinforcing the fifth correct response during articulation training). The FR schedule helps fade or reduce reinforcement density.

■ *Variable-interval (VI) schedule*: A reinforcement schedule in which the time between reinforcers is varied around an average (e.g., reinforcing fluency on a VI 10 seconds means that the client is praised for fluent speech once in 10 seconds on the average, but from one instance of reinforcement to the other the duration will vary). The VI schedule is a form of intermittent reinforcement schedule; it generates a high and consistent response rate.

■ *Variable-ratio (VR) schedule*: A reinforcement schedule in which the number of responses needed to earn a reinforcer is varied around an average (e.g., reinforcing correct production of phonemes on a VR 10 means that an average of 10 correct responses is required before praising the client, but from one instance of reinforcement to the next, the number of correct responses will vary). The VR schedule is a form of intermittent reinforcement schedule that generates a high and consistent response rate.

Reinforcers

Reinforcers are events that follow behaviors and thereby increase the future probability of those behaviors. Reinforcers may be verbal or nonverbal and are essential to establish target behaviors. Descriptions of types of reinforcers follow:

■ *Automatic reinforcer*: Sensory consequences of a behavior that reinforce that behavior (e.g., the sensation associated with head banging that increases its frequency).

■ *Backup reinforcer*: Reinforcer given at the end of a treatment session in exchange for tokens the client earned in the treatment session. For example, if a child earns 10 happy face chips during the session, he or she might get a sticker at the end of the treatment session.

■ *Conditioned generalized reinforcer*: Reinforcer whose effect does not depend on a particular motivational state of the client. These reinforcers are effective in a wide range of situations and include tokens and money.

■ *Conditioned or secondary reinforcers*: Events such as praise, smiles, and approval that strengthen a person's response because of past experience.

■ *Negative reinforcers*: Events that are aversive and thus reinforce a response that terminates, avoids, or postpones them. For example, an aversive event (negative reinforcer) might be teasing endured by a boy who stutters. The teasing reinforces the boy's response of being silent because by being silent, the boy may avoid being teased.

■ *Positive reinforcers*: Events that follow a response and thereby strengthen them. Positive reinforcers are necessary in teaching any kind of skill to any client. They may be verbal (e.g., verbal praise) or nonverbal (e.g., the presentation of a token).

■ *Primary reinforcers*: Events whose reinforcing effects do not depend on past learning or conditioning. Primary reinforcers are biologically determined because of their survival value (e.g., food and water). They are useful for establishing target responses although not for promoting generalized productions. Primary reinforcers are also known as *unconditioned reinforcers*.

■ *Secondary reinforcers*: Social or conditioned reinforcers whose effects depend on past learning (e.g., social praise and tokens).

Summary

☑ Treatment involves teaching new skills to people who manifest disorders of communication. To teach those new skills, the clinician manages contingent relations between antecedents, responses, and consequences.

☑ Treatment should ideally be based upon a scientific philosophy that states that all procedures used should be experimentally demonstrated to be effective.

☑ Many terms are used in describing treatment. Some of these terms are used to describe reinforcement, various reinforcement schedules, and types of reinforcers.

AN OVERVIEW OF THE TREATMENT PROCESS

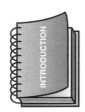

INTRODUCTION

There are various approaches to selecting treatment targets: the normative strategy, client-specific strategy, functional communication strategy, and integrated approach. When treatment targets have been selected, the clinician can consider various factors in deciding upon treatment sequence. Finally, the clinician can implement the procedures of follow-up and booster treatment.

Selection of Treatment Targets

There are different approaches to selecting treatment targets. It is possible to have an integrated approach to treatment selection. A few common approaches and an integrated approach are described as follows.

Normative Strategy

■ This strategy is based on the notion that especially for children, norms provide the best basis for selecting target behaviors. This approach is most frequently used in treating language and articulation disorders in children. Within this approach, age-based norms dictate the target behaviors.

■ For example, target responses for a 4-year-old child with language delay would be those language behaviors that are considered appropriate for a normally developing 4-year-old child. Similarly, phonemes selected for treatment in the case of a child with an articulation disorder will be age-appropriate sounds based on articulation norms.

Client-Specific Strategy

■ Within this strategy, behaviors that will improve the client's communication, that will help meet the social, academic, and other demands made on the client, will be selected. Some of these behaviors may be consistent with the normative strategy, but others may not be.

■ For example, in selecting language treatment targets for a 10-year-old developmentally disabled child, one might consider the special education class she attends and make an analysis of the educational terms she needs to learn. Those terms and their use in phrases and sentences might be the selected target instead of what might be appropriate for a normal 10-year-old.

■ The client-specific strategy is suitable for selecting target behaviors that are appropriate for clients of varied ethnocultural backgrounds. Because the approach emphasizes the individual's needs and uniqueness, it allows for a consideration of the particular cultural and linguistic background of the client in selecting target behaviors.

Functional Communication

■ This approach is very similar to the client-specific approach. In both approaches, what is most useful, what kinds of skills enhance communication, and what kinds of skills help meet the social and other demands made on the client are the main considerations in selecting target behaviors.

■ Within the functional approach, grammatical accuracy and speech production accuracy are less important than effective communication. For example, a clinician could choose one of two target behaviors for a client with aphasia. One target behavior might be the use of grammatically correct sentences, but another, more functional target behavior might be effective communication by means of phrases or sentences, gestures, signs, writing, or a combination of these and other means.

■ Functional communication targets help improve naturalistic communication. This approach is based on the assumption that any mode of response is appropriate, provided it results in effective communication.

Integrated Approach to Target Behavior Selection

■ Within this approach, treatment targets selected are appropriate for the client's age, ethnocultural background, individual uniqueness, and communication requirements. The targets selected should be functional and useful and should enhance natural communication in everyday situations.

■ As such, the approach places a greater emphasis on the client and effective communication and does not totally negate the importance of age-appropriate targets, especially for children.

✎ Concepts To Consider

Summarize the different approaches to selecting target behaviors. Which approach do you most favor? Why?

_____

_____

_____

_____

_____

_____

_____

_____

_____

Treatment Sequence

Treatment has a typical sequence although it is usually modified to suit an individual client. The sequence may be based on several factors: response complexity, degree of structure, response modes, multiple targets, training and maintenance, and shifts in treatment contingencies.

Response Complexity

■ Generally, treatment starts at a simple level and proceeds to more complex levels. At each level, a performance criterion must be met before the client is advanced to the next level of response complexity. Typical levels of response complexity include syllables, words, phrases, and sentences.

■ For example, a child with a w/r substitution who could produce the /r/ sound correctly in isolation might then progress to correct /r/ production in syllables, followed by words, phrases, and then sentences.

Degree of Structure

■ The sequence of treatment is partially based on the degree of treatment structure. Treatment is more structured in initial stages than in later stages. To establish the target behaviors, the clinician uses highly structured discrete trials in the initial stages of training and at the beginning of each new response topography.

■ As the client becomes more proficient in producing the target behaviors and the training is moved to more spontaneous kinds of productions, the treatment structure is loosened. The training environment becomes more similar to natural settings in which everyday communication takes place.

■ For example, an adult who stutters might initially work on producing fluent phrases with 80% accuracy in a one-one situation with the clinician in the therapy room. Eventually, after more training on longer utterances in different situations, the client might go with the clinician to a restaurant and practice ordering a meal using fluent speech.

Response Modes

■ Another factor influencing the sequence of treatment is the different response modes used in training. In most cases, the treatment starts with imitation. When the client reliably imitates target responses, modeling is withdrawn and evoked trials are introduced. Thus, imitation and spontaneous production are taught in that order.

■ Spontaneous productions may be more or less structured or controlled. This too, can create a sequence. Initial spontaneous productions may be more controlled and structured than the eventual naturalistic conversational speech. Reading, if it is a part of training, might introduce an additional sequence.

Multiple Targets

■ Most clients need to attain multiple targets in treatment. This influences the treatment sequence, as well. Clients with fluency disorders receiving fluency-shaping treatment, for example, are taught airflow management, gentle phonatory onset, and rate reduction by syllable prolongation roughly in that order, although those skills are all soon integrated and practiced.

■ Clients with language targets need to learn various language structures that must be sequenced. For instance, such pragmatic skills as conversational turn-taking and topic maintenance cannot be taught until the client is taught certain words, phrases, and sentences that make it possible for the client to talk on a topic.

■ When specific morphologic features are targets, they, too, must be sequenced. For instance, the child must master the present progressive *-ing* before mastering the auxiliary or copula *is*.

Training and Maintenance

■ A well-known sequence is based on initial training (establishment of target behaviors) and eventual maintenance of those behaviors in natural settings and over time. Although many maintenance strategies may be incorporated from the beginning of treatment, others are appropriately sequenced at later stages of treatment.

■ For example, while parents may be trained in identifying target behaviors from the beginning of treatment, prompting and reinforcing target behaviors produced in conversational speech at home and other natural settings will have to wait until treatment has progressed to that stage.

Shifts in Treatment Contingencies

■ *Treatment contingencies* refers to the pattern of reinforcement and corrective feedback given for correct and incorrect responses, respectively. Initially, the client is reinforced for every correct response. Soon, the reinforcement schedule is changed from continuous to intermittent.

■ For instance, the clinician may shift from a continuous reinforcement schedule to a schedule based on a fixed ratio of 2. In gradually sequenced steps the ratio may be stretched. This is important because in natural settings, the target behaviors may not be reinforced as heavily or as systematically as in clinical settings. When treatment is shifted to conversational speech, reinforcement may be sporadic, as it is in everyday communicative situations.

Follow-Up

■ Follow-up is a clinical procedure designed to find out if the client has maintained the target communicative skills and if he or she needs additional treatment. Follow-up involves assessment of communicative behaviors.

■ Typically, an extended conversational speech is recorded to analyze the continued production of communicative behaviors that were initially established. The need for treating additional targets may also be assessed. Follow-up in schedules may vary across clinics and may depend on the type of disorder; some may need more frequent assessments than others.

■ For example, successfully treated clients with fluency disorders need to be followed up for more than 2 years, whereas similarly treated children with articulation disorders may need to be followed up only for a year or less.

■ A general follow-up schedule is as follows:

- first follow-up assessment: 3 months post-dismissal

- second follow-up assessment: 6 months post-dismissal

- third follow-up assessment: 1 year post-dismissal

- subsequent assessments as necessary

Booster Treatment

■ Booster treatment is treatment offered anytime after the initial dismissal from services. Booster treatment is important for maintenance. Clients with certain disorders have a greater need for booster treatment than those with other kinds of disorders.

■ For example, successfully treated adults who stutter need more frequent booster treatments than similarly treated children with articulation disorders.

■ Booster treatment may be:

- identical to the original effective treatment

- a modified version of the original treatment

- a different form of treatment known to be more effective than the original

- much less extended than the original

Summary

☑ Clinicians may select treatment targets using the normative, client-specific, functional communication, or integrated approach.

☑ Treatment sequence is based on factors such as response complexity, degree of structure, response modes, multiple targets, training and maintenance, and shifts in treatment contingencies.

☑ Follow-up and booster treatment are implemented to ensure that clients have maintained skills taught in therapy and to assess whether they need additional treatment.

A GENERAL OUTLINE OF A TREATMENT PROGRAM

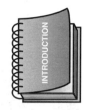

Successful treatment is based upon a thorough, individualized assessment of a client's communication skills. After the assessment, the clinician selects target behaviors for training, establishes baselines of those behaviors, and plans and implements a comprehensive treatment program. Finally, the clinician implements maintenance, follow-up, and booster treatment for the client.

General Outline

▶ **Step 1. Assess the client's communication behaviors**.

▶ **Step 2. Select target behaviors for training**.
Target behaviors are empirical response classes. When these response classes are taught or modified, they will reduce or eliminate the disorder.

Select short-term and long-term target behaviors. Make these target behaviors objective, measurable, and functional for each client.

▶ **Step 3. Establish baselines of target behaviors**.
Baselines are measured response rates in the absence of treatment. Baselines are usually gathered before treatment is initiated.

Establish baselines of all relevant response modes: conversational, modeled, and evoked speech, as well as oral reading if appropriate.

▶ **Step 4. Plan a comprehensive treatment program**.
A treatment program specifies what the client will be required to do, what the clinician will do, and how the two will interact.

Ideally, the program should be written after baselines are established and before treatment is started.

▶ **Step 5. Implement the treatment program**.
Careful management of behavioral contingencies is the most important aspect of a treatment program.

Manage two types of contingencies: those that will decrease undesirable responses and those that will increase desirable responses.

▶ **Step 6. Implement a maintenance program**.
Most clients need a maintenance program. Although some generalization of target behaviors may automatically take place, this generalization may not be maintained over time.

Select responses that are useful to the client and train the client and key people in the client's environment to use and reinforce those responses. Arrange for booster treatment.

▶ **Step 7. Follow up on the client's progress.**
Follow-up (previously described) is a procedure designed to assess response maintenance across time and in the natural environment. Responses are measured in the absence of treatment variables.

As previously stated, follow-up should be scheduled at regular time intervals to ensure that treatment gains are maintained.

▶ **Step 8. Arrange for booster treatment.**
Booster treatment (previously described), or treatment offered any time after initial dismissal from services, is very beneficial for many clients.

Conduct booster treatment sessions after a client has been dismissed from the program in order to help promote maintenance of target behaviors taught in treatment.

Summary

- ☑ Based on the results of an assessment, the clinician selects both short-term and long-term target behaviors for training. Before treatment is initiated, the clinician gathers baselines or measured response rates in the absence of treatment.

- ☑ After baselines are established, the clinician plans a comprehensive treatment program. This program is implemented through management of contingencies that will decrease undesirable responses and increase desirable responses.

- ☑ To help clients maintain target behaviors over time, the clinician implements a maintenance program. The clinician ideally follows up on the client's progress and, when necessary, arranges for booster treatment.

CULTURAL-LINGUISTIC CONSIDERATIONS IN ASSESSMENT AND TREATMENT

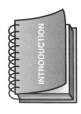

INTRODUCTION

Due to the increasing numbers of culturally and linguistically diverse (CLD) clients with communication disorders, clinicians need to be aware of special considerations that apply to CLD populations. Those considerations include prevalence and incidence of medical conditions and communicative disorders in various ethnocultural groups, potential sociocultural and linguistic barriers to service delivery, and the need for individualizing assessment and treatment.

Prevalence and Incidence Rates of Medical Conditions and Communication Disorders

■ Clinicians need to be aware that some CLD groups have higher prevalence and incidence rates of communication disorders or related medical conditions than others (Hegde, 1996a). (*Prevalence* refers to the current number of individuals; it is a head count. *Incidence* refers to the future occurrence of such an event in a population.)

■ Each client should always be treated as an individual. Clinicians must be careful not to stereotype clients from specific cultural-linguistic groups.

■ The presence of communication disorders and related medical conditions is related to a number of variables. These variables include, but are not limited to, lack of health insurance, low income, diet, and lack of access to medical services.

■ Hispanics tend, as a group, to have:

  – low prevalence of esophageal cancer

  – high prevalence of cardiovascular disease

  – higher prevalence of strokes and diabetes (especially adult-onset diabetes) than whites

  – overall low smoking rate

■ African Americans tend, as a group, to have:

  – high prevalence of traumatic brain injury, especially due to gunshot wounds in youth

  – high prevalence of strokes and hypertension

  – high prevalence of multi-infarct dementia

  – high prevalence of laryngeal, esophageal, and lung cancers

  – low incidence of cleft palate, especially cleft lip

  – overall low smoking rate

■ Asian Americans, as a group, tend to have:

  – high prevalence of cleft palate, especially in Japanese and Chinese Americans

  – high prevalence of nasopharyngeal cancer, especially in Chinese Americans

  – high prevalence of strokes

  – low prevalence of Alzheimer's disease, especially in Chinese Americans

  – overall low rates of alcoholism and smoking

■ Native Americans, as a group, tend to have:

- generally low prevalence of lung cancer

- high prevalence of cleft palate

- high prevalence of otitis media

- generally high rate of smoking

- high prevalence of alcoholism and fetal alcohol syndrome

■ Awareness of the above-listed tendencies can help clinicians be sensitive to the needs of clients from various ethnocultural groups, thus increasing the efficacy and thoroughness of the assessment and treatment processes.

Potential Sociocultural and Linguistic Barriers to Service Delivery

■ When working with CLD clients and their families, it is important to recognize any barriers to full utilization of clinical services. Such barriers might include:

- the overclassification of CLD children as needing special education services;

- client health care access problems (e.g., lack of health insurance), leading to underdiagnosis of problems such as middle ear infections;

- client presenting with more advanced states of communication disorders and related medical problems, caused by lack of health care and thus opportunities to prevent problems;

- client and family lack of facility with English, and, a lack of interpreters to serve as liaisons with the health care system;

- client and family lack of trust or belief in traditional, Western medicine and rehabilitation; and

- lack of transportation to and from health care facilities.

✎ Concepts To Consider

CLD clients often experience barriers that prevent them from receiving optimal services. How might clinicians help clients overcome these barriers?

_____

_____

_____

_____

_____

_____

_____

_____

_____

The Need for Individualizing Assessment and Treatment

While it is important to keep general ethnocultural and linguistic tendencies in mind, all clinicians are aware of individual factors that might affect service delivery to CLD clients and families. Clinicians must be careful to:

- explore to what extent a member of a cultural group is different from the majority of that group (e.g., an African American who does not speak African American Language or a southern rural white person who does);

- understand how refugee or immigrant status affects CLD people, and how CLD people born and raised in the United States differ from immigrants and refugees of the same cultural background (Roseberry-McKibbin, 1997);

- select standardized tests that have, in their standardization process, sampled the ethnocultural group to which the client belongs;

- avoid testing information about practices or events that may be culturally inappropriate (e.g., Christmas for Muslims);

- consider the client's home environment and past experiences (e.g., exposure to certain kinds of television shows, books, or toys) before selecting stimulus items to be used during assessment;

- consider the bilingual or multilingual status of the client, and select assessment tools that reflect that status;

- use trained interpreters to assess CLD clients who speak two or more languages;

- determine whether an underlying communication disorder exists that affects English, the primary language, or both;

- avoid diagnosing a communication disorder based solely on English production influenced by the primary language (e.g., labeling a Yugoslavian client who makes a d/th substitution in all word positions as having a disorder);

- be aware of the great heterogeneity of language patterns and dialects among members of the same general language group (e.g., the Hmong language includes the different dialects of Green Hmong, Blue Hmong, and White Hmong).

Summary

☑ The increasing numbers of CLD clients in our society make it very important for assessment and treatment to reflect sensitivity to the needs of those clients.

☑ Clinicians should be aware of the prevalence and incidence of medical conditions and communication disorders within certain groups. Clinicians must also recognize and help overcome potential sociocultural and linguistic barriers to service delivery.

☑ It is critical to individualize assessment and treatment for each client and family served.

CHAPTER HIGHLIGHTS

▶ When assessing clients who present a wide range of communication disorders, clinicians generally carry out a number of standard assessment procedures. These procedures include a general screening, gathering a case history, a hearing screening, an oral-peripheral examination, an interview, obtaining a speech and language sample, and obtaining of related assessment data.

▶ The vast majority of clinicians then use standardized, norm-referenced tests to assess the communication skills of their clients. Standardized tests have systematic procedures for administration and scoring. Norm-referenced tests allow the clinician to compare the client's score to the average score of the test's norming group, thus yielding information (scores) about how the client's performance compares with that of the norming group. Most standardized tests are also norm-referenced, and vice versa, and are frequently called formal tests.

▶ Formal tests can be evaluated according to their reliability and validity for use with specific client populations. Reliability refers to replicability, or a test's ability to yield scores that are consistent across repeated testing or measurement. Validity refers to the degree to which a test measures what it purports to measure. Even if they are both reliable and valid, formal tests should never be used to create treatment goals or assess treatment progress.

▶ Nonstandardized assessment measures are usually used to help create treatment goals, assess treatment progress, and provide functional descriptions of clients' communicative abilities in their daily environments. Commonly used nonstandardized, informal assessment measures include measurement scales, structured interviews and questionnaires, functional assessment tasks, criterion-referenced testing, and dynamic assessment.

(continues)

▶ Treatment involves changing a nonfunctional communication pattern of a client and requires systematic work with clients and their families. Although there are many approaches to treating communicative disorders, certain common concepts, principles, and procedures apply. A mastery of these concepts, principles, and procedures will help clinicians effectively treat clients with varied disorders of communication.

▶ Treatment targets may be selected on the basis of the normative strategy, the client-specific strategy, the functional communication approach, or an integrated approach. Within the normative strategy, targets are created from age-based norms. Within the client-specific strategy, targets are based on the individual uniqueness and needs of and the communicative demands placed on the client. The functional communication approach requires the selection of targets based on effective and useful communication in natural settings. An integrated approach requires that the targets be age appropriate and appropriate for the specific individual as well as functional.

▶ Treatment is sequenced based on response complexity, the degree of treatment structure, response modes, multiple targets, training and maintenance, and shifts in treatment contingencies. Based on these factors, various sequences are created: simpler responses are treated before complex responses, initial sessions are more structured than later sessions, imitation is used before spontaneous productions, certain targets are taught before certain other targets, certain maintenance procedures are implemented only in latter stages of training, and reinforcers are initially continuous and subsequently intermittent.

▶ Follow-up is an important procedure designed to assess maintenance of clinically established behaviors and the need for additional treatment. Typically a 3-, 6-, and 12-month follow-up schedule may be used; additional follow-up may be scheduled as necessary.

▶ Booster treatment is important to help maintain communicative skills when a client's performance deteriorates. The booster treatment may be the same as the original treatment, a modified version, or a different form of treatment. In any case, booster treatment is typically brief unless the deterioration in skills is substantial.

▶ When working with culturally and linguistically diverse (CLD) clients, clinicians must consider issues such as the prevalence and incidence of certain medical conditions and communication disorders within specific ethnocultural groups. Clinicians must also deal effectively with potential barriers to service delivery, such as lack of transportation and health insurance and possible differences in attitude toward rehabilitation. Finally, it is important to avoid stereotyping CLD clients; this can be managed by individualizing assessment and treatment for each client and his or her family.

(continues)

▶ Add your own chapter highlights here:

_____

_____

_____

_____

KEY TERMS

age equivalency scores
alternate form reliability
antecedent
assessment
automatic reinforcers
aversive stimuli
avoidance
avoidance conditioning
backup reinforcers
baselines
booster treatment
client-specific strategy
concurrent validity
conditioned generalized
    reinforcers
conditioned reinforcers
constituent definitions
construct validity
content validity
contingency
continuous rein-
    forcement
corrective feedback
correlational coefficient
criteria
criterion-referenced
    testing
diagnosis
differential reinforce-
    ment
differential reinforce-
    ment of alternative

behaviors (DRA)
differential reinforce-
    ment of incompatible
    behaviors (DRI)
differential reinforce-
    ment of low rates of
    responding (DRL)
differential reinforce-
    ment of other
    behaviors (DRO)
direct methods of
    response reduction
discrete trials
distribution
dynamic assessment
effectiveness of treat-
    ment
escape
ethnocultural generality
evaluation
evoked trial
exemplar
extinction
fading
fixed interval (FI)
    schedule
fixed ratio (FR) schedule
follow-up
functional communica-
    tion
functional outcomes
generality of treatment
generalized production

grade equivalency scores
high-probability
    behaviors
IEPs (individualized
    education plans)
IFSPs (individualized
    family service plans)
imitation
improvement
incidence
indirect methods of
    response reduction
informative feedback
initial response
integrated approach to
    target behavior
    selection
interdisciplinary team
interjudge reliability
interjudge reliability
    coefficient
intermediate response
intermittent reinforce-
    ment
intermixed probes
interobserver reliability
intrajudge reliability
intrajudge reliability
    coefficient
intraobserver reliability
maintenance strategy
manual guidance
mode of responses

modeled trial
modeling
multidisciplinary team
negative reinforcement
negative reinforcers
nominal scale of
  measurement
normative strategy
norm-referenced test
operational definitions
ordinal scale of
  measurement
paradigm
parallel form reliability
peer training
percentile rank
physical setting
  generalization
physical stimulus
  generalization
positive reinforcers
post-reinforcement
  pause

posttests
predictive validity
pretests
prevalence
primary reinforcers
probes
procedures of treatment
prognosis
prompts
punishment
pure probes
reinforcement
  withdrawal
reinforcers
reliability
response cost
response generalization
response mode general-
  ization
satiation
schedules of reinforce-
  ment
secondary reinforcers

self-control
shaping
split-half reliability
standard deviation
standardized test
stimulus generalization
target behaviors
targets of treatment
terminal response
test-retest reliability
time-out
tokens
topography
transdisciplinary team
treatment
trial
validity
variable interval (VI)
  schedule
variable ratio (VR)
  schedule

STUDY AND REVIEW QUESTIONS

Fill in the Blank

1. Standard assessment procedures for most communication disorders include
   __case history__, __screening__, and
   __oral peripheral__.

2. Most formal tests yield scores. The __raw__ score is the actual score the
   client earned on a test, while the __standard deviation__ shows how
   far the client's score deviated from the mean score of the norming sample.

3. A(n) __ordinal__ scale of measurement is a numerical scale that
   can be arranged according to rank orders or levels, while a(n) __numeri-
   cal__ scale classifies items or observations into named groupings or
   categories that do not have a numerical relationship to one another.

4. The purpose of __functional__ assessment is to assess a client's
   everyday communication skills in natural contexts, while __dynamic__
   assessment measures a client's ability to learn over time when provided
   with instruction.

5. A(n) _interdisciplinary_ team's members are from multiple disciplines, and they collaboratively write the evaluation report and intervention plan; a(n) _transdisciplinary_ team's members are from multiple disciplines, and though they work together in the initial assessment, treatment is provided by only one or two team members.

6. Measured response rates in the absence of treatment are called _baselines_; they are also known as the _operant_ level.

7. _probes_ are procedures to assess generalized production of responses without reinforcing them. _intermixed_ involve assessment of generalized production of trained responses by alternating trained and untrained stimulus items.

8. There are various types of reinforcers. _positive_ reinforcers are events that follow a response and thus strengthen it, and _secondary_ reinforcers are social or conditioned reinforcers whose effects depend on past learning (e.g., praise).

9. _intermittent_ reinforcement involves reinforcement of only some responses or responses produced with some delay between reinforcers. This is contrasted with _continuous_ reinforcement, in which all correct responses are reinforced.

10. When selecting treatment targets, a clinician may use the _normative_ strategy, which states that norms provide the best basis for selecting target behaviors. A clinician might also use the _functional communication_ strategy, in which communication targets help improve naturalistic communication.

Multiple Choice

11. If a test is being evaluated for internal consistency and whether responses to the items on the first half of the test correlate with responses to the items on the second half, then that test is being evaluated for:

    A. test-retest reliability.

    B. interjudge reliability.

    C. split-half reliability.

    D. parallel form reliability.

    E. predictive validity.

12. The concept of adequate *construct validity* means that:

    A. several judges have agreed that a test has been constructed appropriately and measures what it purports to measure.

    B. test items are relevant to measuring what the test purports to measure.

    C. the test accurately predicts future performance on a related task.

    D. test scores are consistent with theoretical concepts or constructs.

    E. if a test is new, it correlates highly with an established test of known validity.

13. Which one of the following is NOT a feature of norm-referenced, standardized tests?

    A. the provision of systematic procedures for administration and scoring of the test.

    B. the comparison of a client's score to that of a norming sample.

    C. ideally, the ensurance of consistency of administration and scoring across examiners.

    D. the provision of information that can be used to create treatment goals and assess treatment progress.

    E. ideally, the ensurance that the behaviors being measured are not influenced by the examiner's personal or subjective biases.

14. Which of the following are TRUE, and thus important for clinicians to remember, with regard to appropriate assessment for culturally and linguistically diverse clients?

    I. Some groups have tendencies toward certain conditions; for example, Hispanics tend to have a higher prevalence of adult-onset diabetes than whites.

    II. A potential barrier for CLD clients to take full advantage of service delivery is that CLD children tend to be underclassified as needing special education services.

    III. Some families may not believe in traditional Western concepts of medicine and rehabilitation.

    IV. A client who makes errors in English, due to the influence of a primary language or dialect other than English, should be diagnosed as having a communication disorder and consequently undergo remediation.

V. There can be great heterogeneity of language patterns and dialects among members of the same general language group.

A. I, III, V

B. I, II, III, V

C. II, III, IV

D. I, III, IV

E. III, V

15. You are seeing a 7-year-old child for language therapy and are working on the goals of accurately producing of the forms plural -*s* and regular past tense -*ed*. The best way to document the child's ongoing progress in attaining these goals would be to:

I. use the pre- and posttest results of a standardized test administered at the beginning and conclusion of treatment

II. use criterion-referenced measures

III. use conversational speech samples

IV. use informal probe measures specifically designed to assess production of these forms

V. ask the child how she thinks she is doing in production of the forms on the playground and at home

A. I, II, III, IV

B. III, IV, V

C. I, III, V

D. I, II, IV

E. II, III, IV

16. Baselines:

A. help establish the initial level of clients' behaviors.

B. help establish the need for treatment.

    C. help compare changes from the initial to the terminal phase of treatment.

    D. A, B

    E. A, B, C

17. Functional communicative behaviors are:

    A. age and norm based.

    B. useful only for adult clients.

    C. behaviors that promote communication in natural settings.

    D. useful only for clients with language disorders.

    E. behaviors that are displayed in the therapy setting but not in the client's natural environment.

18. Negative reinforcement:

    A. is involved in avoidance conditioning.

    B. is reinforcement that results from termination of aversive events.

    C. neither A nor B

    D. both A and B

    E. A only

19. The difference between modeling and imitation is that:

    A. modeling is clinician's behavior, and imitation is client's behavior.

    B. modeling is a treatment target, and imitation is a target behavior.

    C. imitation is usually superior to modeling as a treatment strategy.

    D. A, B

    E. A, B, C

20. IEPs and IFSPs differ in terms of:

    A. the emphasis placed on the family involvement in IFSPs.

    B. the need to write measurable treatment targets in IEPs.

    C. the need to make a thorough assessment of communicative behaviors in IFSPs.

    D. the need for IFSPs to be more highly individualized than IEPs.

    E. the need for IEPs to conform exactly to federal mandates.

REFERENCES AND RECOMMENDED READINGS

American Speech-Language-Hearing Association. (1997). Treatment outcomes data for adults in health care environments. *Asha, 39*(1), 26–31.

Brice, A., & Montgomery, J. (1996). Adolescent pragmatic skills: A comparison of Latino students in English as a second language and speech and language programs. *Language, Speech, and Hearing Services in Schools, 27*(1), 68–81.

Brice, A., & Roseberry-McKibbin, C. (1999). Turning frustration into success for English language learners. *Educational Leadership, 56*(7), 53–55.

Haynes, W. O., & Pindzola, R. H. (1998). *Diagnosis and evaluation in speech pathology* (5th ed.). Englewood Cliffs, NJ: Prentice-Hall.

Hegde, M. N. (1996a). *Pocketguide to assessment in speech–language pathology*. San Diego, CA: Singular Publishing Group.

Hegde, M. N. (1996b). *Pocketguide to treatment in communicative disorders*. San Diego, CA: Singular Publishing Group.

Hegde, M. N. (1998a). *Treatment procedures in communicative disorders* (3rd ed.). Austin, TX: PRO-ED.

Hegde, M. N. (1998b). *Treatment protocols in communicative disorders*. Austin, TX: PRO-ED.

Hegde, M. N., & Davis, D. (1995). *Clinical methods and practicum in speech–language pathology*. San Diego, CA: Singular Publishing Group.

Huang, R. J., Hopkins, J., & Nippold, M. (1997). Satisfaction with standardized language testing: A survey of speech–language pathologists. *Language, Speech, and Hearing Services in Schools, 28*(1), 12–29.

Hutchinson, T. A. (1996). What to look for in the technical manual: Twenty questions for users. *Language, Speech, and Hearing Services in Schools, 27*(2), 109–121.

Klein, H. B., & Moses, N. (1999). *Intervention planning for children with communication disorders: A guide for clinical practicum and professional practice* (2nd ed.). Needham Heights, MA: Allyn & Bacon.

Lidz, C. S., & Peña, E. D. (1996). Dynamic assessment: The model, its relevance as a nonbiased approach, and its application to Latino American preschool children. *Language, Speech, and Hearing Services in Schools, 27*(4), 367–372.

Locke, J. (1998). Where did all the gossip go? Casual conversation in the information age. *Asha, 40*(3), 26–31.

McCauley, R. (1996). Familiar strangers: Criterion-referenced measures in communication disorders. *Language, Speech, and Hearing Services in Schools, 27*(2), 122–131.

Nicolosi, L., Harryman, E., & Kresheck, J. (1996). *Terminology of communication disorders: Speech–language-hearing* (4th ed.). Baltimore, MD: Williams & Wilkins.

Peterson, H. A., & Marquardt, T. P. (1994). *Appraisal and diagnosis of speech and language disorders* (3rd ed.). Englewood Cliffs, NJ: Prentice-Hall.

Roseberry-McKibbin, C. (1995). *Multicultural students with special language needs: Practical strategies for assessment and intervention*. Oceanside, CA: Academic Communication Associates.

Roseberry-McKibbin, C. (1997). Interviewing and counseling with linguistically and culturally diverse clients. In K. G. Shipley (Ed.), *Interviewing and counseling in communicative disorders: Principles and procedures* (2nd ed.) (pp. 151–173). Needham Heights, MA: Allyn & Bacon.

Roth, F. P., & Worthington, C. K. (1996). *Treatment resource manual for speech language pathology.* San Diego, CA: Singular Publishing Group.

Shipley, K. G. (1997). *Interviewing and counseling in communicative disorders: Principles and procedures* (2nd ed.). Needham Heights, MA: Allyn & Bacon.

Shipley, K. G., & McAfee, J. G. (1998). *Assessment in speech–language pathology: A resource manual* (2nd ed.). San Diego, CA: Singular Publishing Group.

Shipley, K. G., & Wood, J. M. (1996). *The elements of interviewing.* San Diego, CA: Singular Publishing Group.

Silverman, F. H. (1998). *Research design and evaluation in speech–language pathology and audiology* (4th ed.). Needham Heights, MA: Allyn & Bacon.

Tomblin, J. B. (1994). Perspectives on diagnosis. In J. B. Tomblin, H. L. Morris, & D. C. Spriestersbach (Eds.), *Diagnosis in speech–language pathology* (pp. 1–28). San Diego, CA: Singular Publishing Group.

Westby, C. E., StevensDominguez, M., & Oetter, P. (1996). A performance/competence model of observational assessment. *Language, Speech, and Hearing Services in Schools, 27*(2), 144–156.

ANSWERS TO STUDY AND REVIEW QUESTIONS

1. Any three of these: a screening, obtaining a case history, a hearing screening, an oral-peripheral examination, an interview, obtaining a speech and language sample, obtaining related assessment data

2. Raw, standard deviation

3. Ordinal, nominal

4. Functional, dynamic

5. Interdisciplinary, transdisciplinary

6. Baselines, operant

7. Probes, intermixed probes

8. Positive, secondary

9. Intermittent, continuous

10. Normative, functional communication

11. C. If a test is being evaluated for internal consistency and whether responses to the items on the first half of the test correlate with responses to the items on the second half, then that test is being evaluated for split-half reliability.

12. D. The concept of adequate *construct validity* means that test scores are consistent with theoretical concepts or constructs.

13. D. Norm-referenced, standardized tests are NOT meant to provide information that can be used to create treatment goals and assess treatment progress. These tests are meant to provide systematic procedures for administration and scoring, an opportunity to compare a client's score to that of a norming sample, and, ideally, the ensurance of consistency of administration and scoring across examiners, as well as ensurance that the behaviors being measured are not influenced by the examiner's personal biases.

14. A. With regard to appropriate assessment for culturally and linguistically diverse clients, clinicians need to remember that some groups have tendencies toward certain conditions, some families may not believe in traditional Western concepts of medicine and rehabilitation, and that there can be great heterogeneity of language patterns and dialects in the same language group.

15. E. You are seeing a 7-year-old child for language therapy and are working on the goals of accurately producing the plural -*s* and regular past tense -*ed*. The best way to document the child's ongoing progress in attaining those goals would be to use criterion-referenced measures, conversational speech samples, and informal probe measures specifically designed to assess production of those forms.

16. E. Baselines help establish the initial level of clients' behaviors, help establish the need for treatment, and help compare changes from the initial to the terminal phase of treatment.

17. C. Functional communicative behaviors are behaviors that promote communication in natural setttings.

18. D. Negative reinforcement is involved in avoidance conditioning and is reinforcement that results from termination of aversive events.

19. D. Differences between modeling and imitation are that modeling is clinician's behavior, and imitation is client's behavior; and also that modeling is a treatment target, and imitation is a target behavior.

20. A. IEPs and IFSPs differ in terms of the emphasis placed on the family involvement in IFSPs.

CHAPTER 12

Research Design and Statistics: A Foundation for Clinical Science

PREVIEW OUTLINE

CHAPTER INTRODUCTION

Many speech–language pathologists in clinical practice believe that clinical science is irrelevant to "Monday morning" and the practical concerns of assessing and treating clients. Research and the statistics used in research are viewed as the province of scientists in "ivory towers" who are not interested in or concerned about practical applications to clients with communication disorders. And yet, practitioners regularly use, mostly unconsciously, scientific principles in their service to clients. Many clinicians gather statistics regularly to assess client progress. Clinicians who read scientific journals utilize their basic understanding of research design to understand journal articles and, perhaps, apply the knowledge gained to their clinical practice.

In this chapter, we discuss basic principles of research design and statistics as a foundation for clinical science. We assume that readers have had coursework that has given depth of knowledge in the areas covered; we seek to refresh readers' memories of some important concepts that have already been learned. We discuss the scientific method, characteristics of experimental and descriptive research, evaluation of research, and data organization and analysis (statistics). (A few of the ideas in this chapter are also covered in Chapter 11, on assessment and treatment. For the reader's convenience and ease of learning the material, the repeated ideas are worded almost exactly the same in both chapters.)

FOUNDATIONS OF THE SCIENTIFIC METHOD

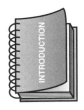

Scientists are people who use objective, experimental methods to systematically investigate questions. Research involves methods that scientists use as they carry out their investigations. These methods involve measurements, which must be valid and reliable in order to produce scientifically rigorous results.

The Philosophy of Science: Basic Precepts

■ Sometimes the terms *research* and *science* are used interchangeably. However, although their meanings overlap, they have different connotations. *Science* is a philosophy of events and nature that values evidence more than opinions. The scientist uses objective, experimental methods to systematically investigate research questions and produce valid and reliable results.

■ *Research* is what scientists do as they practice science. Research is the process of asking and answering questions; it includes steps scientists take as they search for uniformity and order in nature (Hegde, 1994; Silverman, 1998). Science is conceptual and philosophical; research is methodological. Basically, research is science in action.

■ The two philosophical hallmarks of science are empiricism and determinism. *Empiricism* is the philosophical position that statements must be supported by experimental or observational evidence.

■ According to the empiricist, sensory experience is the basis of knowledge. This sensory experience (the touching, seeing, tasting, smelling, and/or hearing of phenomena) must be objectively verifiable. In other words, events must be *observable* and *measurable*.

■ *Determinism* means that events do not happen randomly or haphazardly; they are caused by other events. Scientific activity based on determinism is a search for causes of events.

■ The goals of science are to:

　　— *describe* natural events or phenomena;

　　— *understand* and *explain* natural phenomena, especially in terms of cause-and-effect relationships;

　　— *predict* occurrences of events; and

　　— *control* natural phenomena by understanding the causes of events and predicting their occurrence.

■ Scientists frequently conduct research with the goal of explaining events and effects as stated above. An explanation of an event specifies its causes, and an event is scientifically explained when the scientist experimentally demonstrates its cause(s). As scientists attempt to explain events, they can use one of two approaches: the inductive method or the deductive method.

■ The *inductive method* is an experiment-first-and-explain-later approach. The researcher starts by conducting a series of experiments, and then he or she proposes a theory based on the results of those experiments.

■ In using the inductive method, a scientist would first observe events and later arrive at some general conclusions regarding the nature and causation of those events. In sum, a scientist who is using inductive reasoning first experiments and then proposes a theory based upon the results of the experiments.

■ The *deductive method* is an explain-first-and-verify-later approach. In this method, the investigator explains an event and then attempts to verify the explanation through the results of experiments.

■ In using the deductive method, a scientist would first make a series of proposals or statements without conducting any experiments or observations. Then the scientist would gather evidence to test those proposals. In sum, a scientist using deductive reasoning first proposes a theory and then verifies it.

■ Scientists use inductive and deductive reasoning to build theories. A *theory* is a systematic body of information concerning a phenomenon. A theory describes an event, explains why the event occurred, and specifies how it (the theory) can be verified. A theory specifies causal variables; a theory states that X causes Y.

■ While a theory is usually a comprehensive description and explanation of a total phenomenon, a *hypothesis* is concerned with a more specific prediction stemming from a theory. Hypotheses are testable propositions derived from a theory. As such, hypotheses are limited in scope as compared to theories.

■ For example, the *behaviorist theory* of language learning (see Chapter 3) explains the process of language learning in all children around the world. A *hypothesis* might address language learning in children with autism.

■ Hypotheses are usually formulated prior to an investigation and are predictive statements of cause-effect relationships between certain variables.

■ For example, a hypothesis might state, "When people who stutter are put in highly stressful speaking situations, their amount of stuttering will increase." In other words, the hypothesis is that stressful speaking situations will *cause* the *effect* of increased stuttering.

■ Hypotheses may be labeled either null or alternative hypotheses. The term *null* means zero, and a *null hypothesis* states that two variables are not related.

■ In the above example, the null hypothesis would be that stressful situations and stuttering are not related, that when people who stutter are placed in highly stressful speaking situations, the amount of stuttering does not increase.

■ The researcher hopes to *reject the null hypothesis* and *accept the alternative hypothesis*. The *alternative hypothesis* holds that there is a relationship between the variables specified.

■ In the above example, the alternative hypothesis is that there is indeed a cause-effect relationship between stressful situations and stuttering. That is, highly stressful speaking situations do cause people who stutter to become more disfluent.

■ As they test hypotheses, scientists gather data. *Data* are the result of systematic observation. Scientists observe events and record some measured values of those events. Scientific data are empirical; they are based upon actual events that resulted in some form of sensory contact.

■ *Qualitative data are verbal descriptions* of attributes of events, while *quantitative data are numerical descriptions* of attributes of events (Silverman, 1998). Qualitative data involve words; quantitative data involve numbers.

■ For example, a clinician might state, "The client has a severe articulation disorder characterized by multiple omissions of phonemes" (qualitative data). The clinician might further state, "In a 5-minute spontaneous speech sample, the client omitted word-final phonemes 75% of the time" (quantitative data).

■ When investigators gather data, they want the data to be both valid and reliable. *Validity* and *reliability* are critical aspects of any type of scientific measurement. Measures in speech–language pathology, whether they apply to research studies or clinical measurement of clients' skills, need to be valid and reliable.

✎ Concepts To Consider

Describe basic precepts of the philosophy of science. What are the goals of science? What methods do scientists use to arrive at conclusions?

_____

_____

_____

_____

_____

_____

_____

_____

_____

_____

Validity of Measurements

- *Validity* is the degree to which a measuring instrument measures what it purports to measure. For example, some child language tests purport to evaluate receptive language, but they actually evaluate auditory memory.

- There are different kinds of validity. *Predictive validity*, also called *criterion validity*, is the accuracy with which a test predicts future performance on a related task. For example, a graduate student's score on comprehensive examinations might predict whether or not he or she will be a competent clinician. Thus, future performance is the criterion used to evaluate the validity.

- *Concurrent validity*, considered a form of criterion-related validity, is the degree to which a new test correlates with an established test of known validity. For example, a new receptive vocabulary test might be correlated with the *Peabody Picture Vocabulary Test–Revised* (Dunn & Dunn, 1981) in order to establish concurrent validity. If the correlation is too high, however, there may be a question of the need for the new test.

- *Construct validity* is the degree to which test scores are consistent with theoretical constructs or concepts. Construct validity includes any information that supports the test maker's theory or model underlying the test.

- *Content validity* is a measure of test validity based on a complete examination of all test items to determine if the items adequately sample the full range of the skill being tested and if the items are relevant to measuring what the test purports to measure.

Reliability of Measurements

- *Reliability* refers to the *consistency* with which the same event is measured repeatedly. Scores are reliable if they are consistent across repeated testing or measurement.

- For example, a clinician, Susan Smith, measures a child's disfluencies on Monday, April 15, 2001. She states that the child is 35% disfluent in a 100-word sample. Susan becomes ill, and a substitute clinician named Donald Jones calculates the child's disfluencies on Wednesday, April 17, 2001. Donald states that the child, in a 100-word sample, is 37% disfluent. There is good reliability of these disfluency scores; they were consistent across repeated testing or measurement.

- Most measures of reliability are expressed in terms of a correlational coefficient. The *correlational coefficient* is a number or index that indicates the relationship between two or more independent measures. It is usually expressed through Pearson Product Moment r.

■ An *r* value of 0.00 indicates that there is no relationship between two measures. The highest possible positive value of *r* is 1.00; the lowest possible negative value of *r* is –1.00. The closer *r* is to 1.00, the greater the reliability of the test or measurement.

■ *Test-retest reliability* refers to consistency of measures when the same test is administered to the same people twice. The two sets of scores are correlated, suggesting stability of the scores over time.

■ *Alternate form reliability* (also known as *parallel form reliability*) means consistency of measures when two forms of the same tests are administered to the same people. For example, the *Test of Nonverbal Intelligence–Third Edition* (TONI–3; Brown, Sherbenou, & Johnson, 1997) includes Form A and Form B. If both those forms are administered to an adult client and the scores are very similar, then the TONI–3 has alternate form reliability.

■ *Split-half reliability* is a measure of internal consistency of a test. Split-half reliability is determined by showing that the responses to items on the first half of a test are correlated with responses given on the second half. Or the responses to even-numbered items should correlate with responses to odd-numbered items. Split-half reliability generally overestimates reliability because it does not measure stability of scores over time.

■ *Interobserver* or *interjudge reliability* refers to the extent to which two or more observers agree in measuring an event. For example, if three judges independently rate the fluency of a subject, there is high interjudge reliability if there is good agreement between judges. Optimally, good agreement results in an interjudge reliability coefficient of .90 or more.

■ *Intraobserver* or *intrajudge reliability* refers to the extent to which the same observer repeatedly measures the same event consistently. For example, if the same clinician rates a child's intelligibility over several sessions, those ratings should be consistent if there is good intraobserver reliability.

Summary

☑ Science, a philosophy valuing evidence and rigorous methods of investigating questions, is based upon empiricism and determinism.

☑ People who use the scientific method may use either inductive or deductive reasoning to create theories and test hypotheses.

☑ Validity and reliability of measurements are important hallmarks of good science.

EXPERIMENTAL RESEARCH

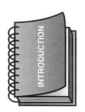

The hallmark of experimental research is the investigation of cause-effect relationships. Experimenters manipulate independent variables to assess the effect of these variables upon dependent variables. Group designs, the most popular type of experimental design in speech–language pathology, usually involve control and experimental groups. Single-subject designs, which usually involve 1–6 subjects, are experimental designs that help establish cause-effect relations based on individual performance as opposed to group averages.

Foundational Concepts

■ An *experiment* is a means of establishing *cause-effect* relationships. Experiments test *if-then* relationships. For example, *if* a person who stutters is put into a highly stressful situation, *then* will he or she stutter more? Does the highly stressful situation *cause* the *effect* of increased stuttering?

■ An experiment involves a controlled condition in which an independent variable is manipulated to produce changes in a dependent variable. An *independent variable* is directly manipulated by the experimenter. This manipulation causes changes in the dependent variable.

■ A *dependent variable* or *effect* is the variable that is affected by manipulation of the independent variable. Dependent variables must be defined very specifically so that they are measurable. Table 12.1 contains examples of independent and dependent variables.

TABLE 12.1

Examples of Independent and Dependent Variables

Independent Variable	Dependent Variable
Stressful situation	Amount of stuttering
Amount of noise in environment	Amount of difficulty hearing speech
Length and complexity of reading passage	Number of words a client with aphasia cannot read
Number of times client uses hard glottal attack	Amount of hoarseness present when client is speaking
Number of toys and games present in clinic room	Length of child's MLU as he or she interacts with the clinician

■ Good experiments involve conditions that are carefully controlled to eliminate *extraneous* or *confounding* variables. When establishing a cause-effect relationship, the experimenter must ensure that only the independent variable of interest is affecting the dependent variable.

■ Confounding variables are those that have an effect on the dependent variable; confounding variables should not have this effect, but they do. Confounding variables make it impossible for the experimenter to determine whether it was indeed the manipulation of the independent variable that caused a change in the dependent variable.

■ For example, an experimenter may want to find out if increased background noise (the independent, manipulated variable) causes subjects to speak more loudly (the dependent variable). The experimenter chooses a party situation and begins to play music louder and louder while measuring the loudness of the subjects' voices. As the music volume increases, the subjects simultaneously consume large quantities of alcohol.

■ The experimenter finds that the subjects are indeed speaking more loudly as the music is played more loudly. However, the increased loudness of the subjects' voices (dependent variable) may be due to the alcohol (confounding variable), the louder music (independent variable of interest), or both. Thus, the experimenter has not succeeded in determining whether the independent variable alone created the change in the dependent variable.

■ The types of experimental designs used in speech–language pathology can be placed in two broad categories: group designs and single-subject designs.

Group Designs

Basic Principles

■ In group designs, one or more groups of subjects are exposed to one or more levels of the independent variable. Then, the subjects' average performance on the dependent variable is analyzed to determine the nature of the relationship between the dependent variable and the independent variable (Schiavetti & Metz, 1997).

■ True experimental designs using groups rule out the influence of confounding variables through the use of experimental and control groups. An *experimental group* contains subjects who receive treatment and thus show changes in behaviors treated.

■ A *control group* contains subjects, matched with the experimental subjects on important variables such as age and disorder type, who do not receive treatment. The goal of having these two groups is to demonstrate that the experimental subjects improved and the control subjects did not, thus showing the efficacy of the treatment.

■ Researchers randomly draw a *sample*, or small number, of subjects needed for the study from the population. A *population* is a large, defined group (e.g., patients scheduled for laryngectomy surgery, people who stutter) identified for the purpose of a study.

■ *Random selection* is a method of selecting subjects to evaluate treatment effects or efficacy. To reduce experimenter bias in subject selection, each potential subject has an equal chance of being selected for the study.

■ The researcher identifies a large number of potential subjects, assigns each subject a number, and selects the number of subjects randomly (e.g., every 3rd, 6th, or 8th person). *Representativeness* is achieved when the subjects in this sample have the same characteristics as the population.

Pretest-Posttest Control Group Design

■ There are many kinds of group designs. Due to space limitations, this chapter discusses only the pretest-posttest control group design, which is considered a prototype of true experimental designs. Many other group designs are variations of this basic design.

■ In the *pretest-posttest control group design*, there are two groups: an experimental group and a control group. Each subject in each group undergoes a pretest and a posttest.

■ *Pretests* are measures of subjects' behaviors that are established before starting an experimental or routine teaching program.

■ Pretest measures are compared with *posttest* measures, which are measures of behaviors established after completing the program. Pre- and posttest measures, along with other control measures, help rule out the influence of confounding variables.

■ The pretest-posttest design is based on the logic that to assess the effects of an independent variable, the only difference between groups must be that variable. To isolate the effect of the independent variable, the two groups are, ideally, selected to be identical in all ways except that of the independent variable.

■ For example, an investigator might want to study the effects of enriched maternal speech on infant language development. She selects a control group and an experimental group of infant-mother pairs. The experimental group of mothers is taught specific strategies for enriching their infants' language; the control group of mothers is not taught those strategies. The vocalizations of babies in the experimental and control groups are measured before the experiment (pretest) and after the experiment (posttest).

■ To isolate enriched maternal speech as the independent variable of interest, the investigator must match the mothers on such characteristics as age, socioeconomic status, language background, and educational level.

■ If the mothers are not matched on socioeconomic status and educational background, for example, any increased vocalizations found in the experimental infants might be traceable to those variables rather than the mothers' use of language enrichment strategies.

■ Figure 12.1 illustrates the pretest-posttest control group design. Ideally, subjects are randomly selected from the population and randomly assigned to the two groups. The experimental group is exposed to the treatment variable (X, the independent variable), and the control group is not.

■ The dependent variable (0) is measured twice in each group: once before and once after the experimental group has received the treatment. This arrangement allows the investigator to evaluate the effect of the independent variable or treatment.

Advantages and Disadvantages of Group Experimental Designs

■ True experimental designs are the most powerful of the group design strategies. They are extremely useful in isolating cause-effect relationships between variables.

■ Well-conducted experimental group designs have strong internal validity (defined in greater detail later), in that extraneous or confounding variables are ruled out. Thus, the experimenter can be confident that it was indeed manipulation of the independent variable that caused the change in the dependent variable.

■ From a clinical standpoint, a major limitation of true group experimental designs is that it is not always possible to randomly draw subjects from specific clinical populations. To do this, one needs access to large populations of clients with specific disorders. Clinicians do not always have that access.

■ Another limitation of group experimental designs is that they may not allow extension of the study's results to individual clients. Most practitioners are interested in studies whose results will allow application to individual clients with whom they are working.

■ Group experimental designs thus yield helpful information for investigators and for the profession, but that information may have limited use for practitioners who seek application of results to individual clients. These practitioners may benefit from using single-subject designs.

Experimental group	01	x	02
Control group	01		02

Figure 12.1. The pretest-posttest control group design.

Single-Subject Designs

Basic Principles

■ Single-subject designs (SSDs) are experimental designs that have become increasingly popular in speech–language pathology research. These designs help establish cause-effect relations based on individual performances under different conditions of an experiment.

■ Group designs reliably allow the investigator to determine the average performance of the subjects in a group under the experimental condition(s) (Silverman, 1998). Single-subject designs allow extended and intensive study of individual subjects and do not involve comparisons based on group performances.

■ Instead of the pre- and posttests of group designs, SSDs measure the dependent variables continuously. Subjects are not necessarily randomly selected, and the results of SSDs are not always analyzed statistically.

■ Although SSDs may include only 1 subject, it is common for 4–6 subjects to be used. The data generated from each subject are not averaged as they are in group designs; rather, data based upon individual subjects' performances are recorded and displayed separately (usually in graphic form).

■ As stated, single-subject designs are *experimental* and must be distinguished from *case study designs* (explained later), which are *descriptive*. Case studies lack experimental control and frequently consist of descriptions of individual clients. Single-subject designs are experimental because they help establish cause-effect relationships.

■ The SSD strategy involves methods of demonstrating treatment effects by showing contrasts between conditions of no treatment, treatment, withdrawal of treatment, and other control procedures.

■ The two basic types of SSDs involve:

  – the ABAB design and its variations

  – multiple baseline designs and their variations

■ For purposes of space in this chapter, only basic prototypes of each type of design will be introduced.

✎ Concepts To Consider

Compare and contrast group and single-subject experimental designs. What are their similarities and differences? When would you use each type of design?

_____

_____

_____

_____

_____

_____

Types of ABAB Designs

- *ABAB designs* are used to evaluate treatment effects. In ABAB designs, the key terms *baseline* and *baserate* refer to data that show a client's pretreatment response rates. The term *baserate* also may refer to the action the investigator takes to achieve the baselines (Hegde & Davis, 1995).

- ABAB designs rely upon two conditions:

  - A phase: *no treatment phase*; target behavior is baserated with no treatment

  - B phase: *treatment phase*; target behavior is treated

- In the basic *ABA design*, the target behavior to be taught is baserated (A phase). The new treatment to be evaluated is then applied (B phase). When the subject's behavior increases, treatment is withdrawn (A phase). The researcher charts results to show that the results for the base rate and withdrawal conditions were similar but those for the treatment condition were different (see Figure 12.2).

- In the *ABAB design*, a target behavior is baserated (A phase), taught as the researcher applies the treatment (B phase), reduced by withdrawing or reversing the treatment (A phase), and then taught again by reinstating the treatment (B phase) to show that the treatment was effective. The researcher charts results to show that the no-treatment conditions (A phases) are convincingly different from the treatment conditions (B phases). Two variations on the ABAB design are *withdrawal* and *reversal*.

- In the *ABAB withdrawal design*, illustrated in Figure 12.3, a target behavior is base-rated (A phase), taught to the subject (B phase), reduced by withdrawing the treatment (A phase), and then taught again (B phase) to show that treatment was effective. For example:

  - A phase: baserate target behavior (e.g., fluency)

  - B phase: teach target behavior (e.g., increased fluency through technique of slowed rate of speech)

  - A phase: withdraw teaching (teaching of slowed rate of speech)

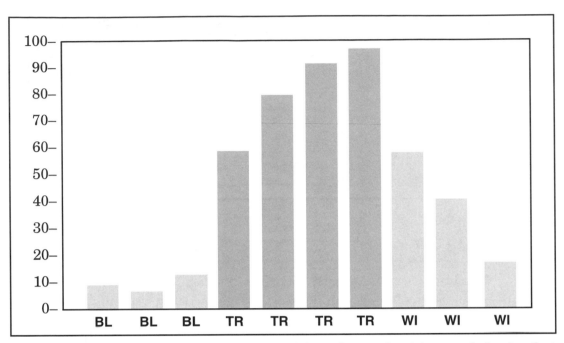

Figure 12.2. The controlling effects of the withdrawal procedure. A target behavior that is stable under baseline (BL) increases when treated (TR) and decreases when the treatment is withdrawn (WI). From *Clinical Research in Communicative Disorders: Principles and Strategies* (2nd ed.) (p. 230), by M.N. Hegde, 1994, Austin, TX: PRO-ED. Copyright 1994 by PRO-ED, Inc. Reprinted with permission.

- B phase: teach target behavior again (increased fluency through slowing rate of speech)

■ In the *ABAB reversal design*, a target behavior is baserated (A phase), taught to the subject (B phase), reduced by teaching its counterpart or an incompatible behavior (A phase), and then taught again (B phase) to show that the treatment was effective. For example:

- A phase: baserate target behavior (e.g., correct /r/ production for a subject who has a w/r substitution)

- B phase: teach target behavior to the subject (e.g., correct /r/ production)

- A phase: teach an incompatible behavior (e.g., production of a w/r substitution)

- B phase: again teach target behavior to subject (e.g., correct /r/ production)

■ Sometimes investigators do not wish to withdraw or reverse treatment as described above. In these cases, multiple baseline designs may be more appropriate.

Multiple Baseline Designs

■ As experimental designs, SSDs take various forms. The most basic is the *multiple baseline design*, in which the effects of treatment are demonstrated by

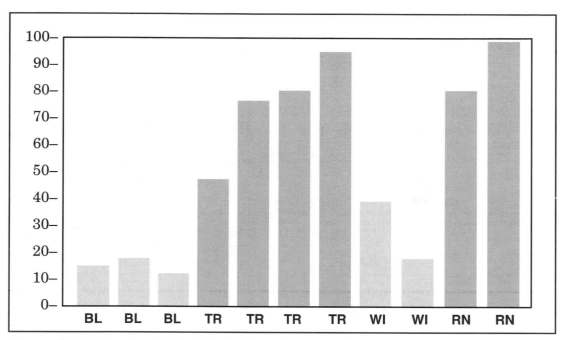

Figure 12.3. The controlling effects of a single withdrawal and reinstatement of treatment. A stable and low rate of a target behavior during the baseline (BL) increases during treatment (TR), decreases during withdrawal (WI), and increases again during reinstatement of treatment (RN). From *Clinical Research in Communicative Disorders: Principles and Strategies* (2nd ed.) (p. 234), by M.N. Hegde, 1994, Austin, TX: PRO-ED. Copyright 1994 by PRO-ED, Inc. Reprinted with permission.

showing that untreated baselines did not change and only the treated baselines did. The three variations of multiple baseline designs are across subjects, across settings, and across behaviors (Hegde, 1994; Hegde, 1996).

■ A *multiple-baseline-across-subjects design* involves several subjects who are taught a behavior sequentially to show that only treated subjects change and thus the treatment was effective. The researcher:

  – selects a target behavior to be taught to three or more subjects;

  – baserates the target behaviors in all subjects;

  – treats one of the subjects while repeating the baserates on the untreated subjects;

  – treats the second subject while repeating the baserates on the untreated subjects; and

  – alternates treatment and base rates until all subjects are trained.

■ A *multiple-baseline-across-settings design* involves a behavior being sequentially taught in different settings to demonstrate that the behavior changed only in a treated setting and thus treatment was effective. The researcher:

  – baserates a target behavior in three or more settings (e.g., the hospital room, hospital lobby, parking lot, and home);

- teaches the behavior in one setting;

- repeats the baserates in the remaining untreated settings;

- teaches the behavior in another setting; and

- continues to alternate baserates and teaching in different settings until the behavior is trained in all settings.

▪ A *multiple-baseline-across-behaviors design* involves several behaviors that are sequentially taught to show that only treated behaviors change and thus treatment was effective. The researcher:

- selects three or more target behaviors;

- establishes baserates on those target behaviors;

- trains the first behavior to a training criterion (e.g., 80% accuracy over three sessions);

- repeats the baserates on the remaining untreated behaviors;

- trains the second behavior while repeating baserates on the remaining untreated behaviors; and

- continues to alternate baserates and treatment until all the behaviors are trained.

Advantages and Disadvantages of Single-Subject Designs

▪ Single-subject designs are highly suitable for clinical research for many reasons (Hegde, 1994). First, clinicians can integrate research and clinical service by using the clients they serve as subjects in experiments that attempt to answer significant clinical questions. Clients who serve as subjects receive treatment; they are not denied treatment as clients in a control group might be if a group design is used.

▪ Another advantage of SSDs is that they help generalize from research studies to individual clients. Detailed descriptions of individual client characteristics and treatment effects can help establish generalizability of treatments across a wide variety of clients.

▪ Single-subject designs are much more easily replicated than group design studies. This is the case partially because clinicians do not need to seek unattainable random samples of clients. As stated, clinicians can use their own clients as subjects.

▪ A disadvantage of SSDs is that while statistical procedures for assessing the reliability of answers are available for group designs, they are not readily available for SSDs (Silverman, 1998).

Summary

✔ The goal of experimental research is to establish cause-effect relationships. In experiments, investigators inquire into whether certain variables have caused various effects.

✔ Investigators attempt to assess the effects of an independent variable on a dependent variable, and rule out confounding variables that might affect the dependent variable.

✔ Researchers may use group designs or single-subject designs to achieve that goal.

DESCRIPTIVE RESEARCH

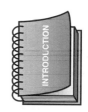

INTRODUCTION

While the goal of experimental research is to establish cause-effect relationships between variables, the goal of descriptive research is to describe phenomena. There is no manipulation of variables; descriptive research cannot demonstrate cause-effect relationships. Types of descriptive research include survey, case study, retrospective, comparative, and developmental research. Other research designs that are often considered descriptive in nature include ex post facto, correlational, and ethnographic designs.

Foundational Concepts

■ In *descriptive research*, the researcher is a passive observer who observes what is happening without interfering or manipulating. The researcher does not want his or her presence to interfere with the natural phenomena that are being observed (Schiavetti & Metz, 1997).

■ Unlike experimental research, descriptive research does not lead to cause-effect statements. This is the most important hallmark distinguishing descriptive from experimental research.

■ There are two types of variables in some kinds of descriptive research. The *classification variable* is analogous to the independent variable in experimental research, and the *criterion variable* is analogous to the dependent variable in experimental research.

■ For example, people with dementia might be compared to people without dementia on cognitive and linguistic measures. The classification variable would be group status (*dementia* as opposed to *without dementia*) and the criterion variable would be the performance on the cognitive and linguistic measures.

- Although descriptive research cannot lead to cause-effect statements, it is useful when it would be unethical to use experimental methods. For example, researchers would not tell one group of women to drink alcohol daily during pregnancy, tell a second group of women to not drink alcohol during pregnancy, and measure the language skills of babies of the two groups during the first 5 years of life. However, researchers can observe and measure the language skills of babies born to women who consumed notable quantities of alcohol during pregnancy and *describe* those language skills.

- Various types of descriptive research designs can be used to describe phenomena observed in an environment. Investigators choose the design that will be most efficacious in answering the research question(s) posed.

Ex Post Facto Research

- Ex post facto research does not fit comfortably under the rubric of either experimental or descriptive research. It is described in this section because, although it is not technically descriptive research, it is not purely experimental either.

- *Ex post facto research* is after-the-fact research. The investigator begins with the effect of independent variables that have occurred in the past. Thus, the investigator is making a retrospective search for causes of events.

- For example, the relationship between lung cancer and smoking is based exclusively on ex post facto research. Investigators have observed, using case studies, that smokers have a higher chance of developing lung cancer than nonsmokers. Most people with lung cancer report a history of smoking. On the basis of those observations, experts have concluded that there is a causal relationship between lung cancer and smoking.

- Although that conclusion makes sense, it is important to recognize the weaknesses as well as the strengths of ex post facto research. First, the *cause* of the observed effects cannot be experimentally manipulated. Second, confounding variables have not been ruled out. Because the investigator has no control over the independent variable or possible extraneous variables, a true cause-and-effect relationship cannot be established.

- In some situations, it is not possible to have control over independent variables—for example, researchers would not ask people to smoke and then observe over the years to see if they developed lung cancer. Thus, sometimes, ex post facto research is all that is available regarding certain observed phenomena.

- Consumers of research need to be aware of the limitations of this research, and take those limitations into consideration when making clinical decisions.

Ideally, ex post facto research should lead to a suggestion of variables that may be verified through other, stronger, more valid means of investigation.

Types of Descriptive Research Designs

Survey Research

■ Surveys assess some characteristics of a group of people or a particular society. Surveys attempt to discover how variables such as attitudes, opinions, or certain social practices are distributed in a population (Hegde, 1994). The purpose of survey research is to generate a detailed inspection of the prevalence of phenomena in an environment by asking people as opposed to direct observation (Schiavetti & Metz, 1997).

■ Because surveyors cannot assess an entire population, they attempt to survey a randomly selected, representative sample of that population. Each person in the sample is asked a set of questions designed to evoke answers of interest.

■ The two most common types of survey research tools are *questionnaires* and *interviews* (the two can also be combined). Many surveyors will use personal interviews when they want to obtain in-depth answers from survey participants. Questionnaires filled out by survey participants may yield a greater quantity of responses, but those responses may not contain the depth of those given in interviews.

■ An advantage of surveys is the wide range of data that can be obtained. For example, one can literally sample thousands of people through a survey. The problems of surveys are that (a) they cannot be used to illustrate cause-effect relationships, and (b) their samples are often biased because those who return surveys are more likely to be people who feel strongly about the issue surveyed.

Case Study Research

■ Case study research examines individuals in depth to illustrate important principles that might be overlooked in group studies (Schiavetti & Metz, 1997). As previously stated, case studies are *descriptive*, while single-subject designs are *experimental*.

■ Case studies are sometimes used to examine the characteristics of clients with rare disorders. For example, a child with Russell-Silver syndrome (a type of dwarfism) would be an ideal subject for a case study because the syndrome is rare and almost no literature exists that describes communication disorders in that population.

■ Case studies may help provide insight into the use of certain clinical techniques. For example, if a clinician is successfully using a specific computerized program with a voice client, a case study would be a useful tool for describing that treatment so that other clinicians and clients might benefit.

■ Case studies have two primary weaknesses. First, the researcher may be biased because of the excitement generated by a rare or unusual case. Second, the generalizability of case studies is extremely limited.

Retrospective Research

■ In retrospective research, the investigator examines data already on file. For example, administrators of a children's hospital might want to know how many of their patients in the past 5 years have had swallowing disorders. A search through the patient files would reveal the answer to that question.

■ A problem with retrospective research is that the data on file have usually been recorded by different people with varying levels of expertise. Thus, the data might or might not be valid and reliable.

Comparative Research

■ The purpose of *comparative research* is to measure the behaviors of two or more types of subjects at one point in time to draw conclusions about the similarities or differences between those subjects (Schiavetti & Metz, 1997). Subjects belong to certain categories or classifications by random chance, not experimental manipulation.

■ Comparative research might be used, for example, to compare people with head injury to people without head injury on tests of attention and memory. The results of those tests would enable the researchers to draw conclusions about similarities and differences of head-injured and non-head-injured subjects in the areas of attention and memory.

■ A difficulty with comparative research is that the similarities and differences found between groups of subjects might be due to variables other than the classification variable. For instance, in the above example, clients with head injury might perform differently than non-head-injured clients due to educational or socioeconomic differences, not head-injury status per se.

Developmental Research

■ The purpose of *developmental research* is to measure changes in subjects over time as the subjects age and mature. In developmental research, the independent variable is maturation. Developmental research has been used extensively to create developmental norms.

■ As an example, developmental research methods have been used in child phonology studies to study children's emerging phonological systems as the children get older. Developmental research has also been used to study the cognitive skills of older adults as they continue to age. There are three types of developmental research: longitudinal, cross-sectional, and semi-longitudinal.

■ In *longitudinal research*, the same subjects are studied over time. The investigator follows those subjects and observes the changes that occur *within* the subjects as they age or become more mature.

■ A major advantage of longitudinal research is that the investigator can directly observe changes in the behavior(s) of the same subjects as they age or mature. For example, investigators might observe the fluency of a group of 10 children between 18 months and 3 years of age. This yields valuable information about the development of fluency skills.

■ Disadvantages of longitudinal research are that it is (a) time consuming and (b) vulnerable to subject attrition. Thus, longitudinal studies often have small numbers of subjects, limiting the generalizability of the results.

■ Because of the disadvantages of longitudinal research, investigators often choose the cheaper, faster, and more popular *cross-sectional method*. In this method, researchers select subjects from various age levels and observe the behaviors or characteristics of the different groups.

■ For example, researchers might select a group of 3-year-olds, a group of 5-year-olds, and a group of 7-year-olds and observe the articulation characteristics of each group. The results of this observation could yield information about developmental norms, or characteristics of the articulation of normally developing children as they mature.

■ A problem with cross-sectional studies is that investigators make observations of differences *between* subjects of different ages in order to observe differences that occur *within* subjects as they mature (Schiavetti & Metz, 1997).

■ For example, in the above case, the three groups of children might be observed in the year 2000. It would be assumed that in the year 2002, the children who were 5 years old would perform like the group of 5-year-olds did in 2000. That might not be the case.

■ A plan that yields the best of both worlds, so to speak, is the *semilongitudinal* plan. In that plan, the total age span to be studied is divided into several overlapping age spans. The subjects selected are those who are at the lower end of each age span, and they are followed until they reach the upper end of their age span.

■ For example, researchers might select three groups of subjects and study the language development of those groups for 1 year (1999–2000). The groups might be as follows:

- 3-year-olds followed until the age of 4
- 4-year-olds followed until the age of 5
- 5-year-olds followed until the age of 6

■ In the year 2001, the researcher would have made observations both *between* and *within* subjects as time passed.

✎ Concepts To Consider

How does descriptive research differ from experimental research? What is the basic purpose of each type of design?

_____

_____

_____

_____

_____

_____

_____

_____

_____

Correlational Research

■ In *correlational research*, the researcher investigates *relationships or associations between variables*. A critical distinction between experimental design and correlational design is that experiments lead to cause-effect statements; correlational studies never do. Correlation does not imply causation.

■ An important distinction between experimental designs and correlational designs is that in a correlational design, the word *effect* would never be used. Rather, when correlations are described, the words *relationship* and *related to* are often used (Payne & Anderson, 1991).

■ A correlation is a statistical method of data analysis that suggests that two or more events are somehow associated or related. It suggests the *direction* (positive or negative) and the *strength* (high or low) of the relationship.

■ A *positive correlation* is found when high values of one variable predict high values of the other variable; when one event increases, the other event increases. For example, as the temperature rises on a hot July day, local grocery stores may sell increased quantities of ice.

■ A *negative correlation* is found when high values of one variable are associated with low values of the other variable. When one event increases, the other event decreases. For example, as a person who stutters experiences more pressure to communicate, her fluency decreases.

■ As previously stated, to express the strength and direction of correlational relationships, the Pearson product moment correlation coefficient is used. This is usually abbreviated *Pearson-r*. Pearson-r is a number ranging from -1.0 to +1.0 (see Figure 12.4).

■ The closer a number is to +1.0, the stronger and more positive the relationship. The closer a number is to -1.0, the stronger and more negative the relationship. The closer a number is to zero, the weaker the relationship.

■ Thus, if a researcher says that a strong relationship of $r = .35$ was found, the reader knows that the relationship is actually weak because .35 is closer to zero than to +1.0. Conversely, a relationship of $r = .95$ would be considered strong.

Ethnographic Research

■ Although not technically considered a type of descriptive research design, ethnographic research is not experimental. It involves observation and description of naturally occurring phenomena, and thus it is included under the aegis of descriptive research (albeit somewhat artificially).

■ *Ethnographic research* was originally designed by anthropologists as a means of conducting in-depth analytical descriptions of cultural scenes. The most common method of ethnographic research is for investigators to fully immerse themselves in the situation being studied. The investigators are attempting to fully understand naturally occurring phenomena in their own environment.

■ The investigators conduct detailed observations, making copious notes and sometimes video and audio recordings of phenomena and people being studied. The investigators do not formulate hypotheses, but rather take an inductive approach in which observations eventually lead to conclusions.

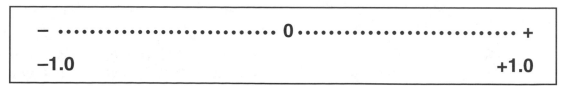

Figure 12.4. Positive and negative 1.0 in relation to zero.

■ Unlike experimental designs, in which the investigator approaches a situation with a hypothesis and then manipulates variables, ethnographic research designs are qualitative and rely on phenomenology. *Phenomenology* holds that to really understand people and situations, the investigator must get quite close to them and be actively involved.

■ In speech–language pathology, ethnographic research is advantageous for detailed study of clients, situations, and cultural groups when experimentation is not ideal or possible. Disadvantages of ethnographic research are that it is time consuming, it is often expensive, it yields data that are difficult to quantify, and it lacks the objectivity of experimental research. Ethnographic research is still relatively new in speech–language pathology.

Summary

☑ Descriptive research designs are used when investigators want to observe and describe phenomena that are naturally occurring in the environment. No cause-effect relationships can be inferred in descriptive research.

☑ Common descriptive research designs include ex post facto, survey, case study, retrospective, comparative, developmental, and correlational research. Ethnographic research is also descriptive in nature.

EVALUATION OF RESEARCH

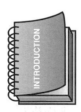

Research designs can be evaluated according to the parameters of internal and external validity. Internal validity asks, "Did the study demonstrate a cause–effect relationship?" External validity asks, "To which people and situations can these results be generalized?" Investigators must attempt to control for threats to both internal and external validity of a study.

Internal Validity

Definition

■ *Internal validity* is the degree to which data in a study reflect a true cause-effect relationship. A study with strong internal validity is one in which the dependent variable was affected only by manipulation of the independent variable. No confounding variables were present.

■ There are factors that can reduce the internal validity of a study. These *threats to internal validity* include instrumentation, history, statistical regression, maturation, attrition, testing, subject selection biases, and interaction of factors (Hegde, 1994; Schiavetti & Metz, 1997).

Instrumentation

■ Instrumentation refers to problems with measuring instruments that threaten internal validity. These measuring instruments include mechanical and electrical instruments, pencil-and-paper instruments such as questionnaires and tests, and human observers.

■ Mechanical and electrical problems may occur with instruments that need regular calibration or that are defective in some way; these problems affect validity.

■ For example, if subjects' hearing is tested at the beginning of a study, the audiometer is calibrated halfway through the study, and the subjects' hearing is posttested at the end of the study, the study's outcomes may reflect the midstudy audiometer calibration, not true changes in the subjects' hearing.

■ Instrumentation problems also occur when investigators use inadequate or inappropriate pencil-and-paper instruments. For example, an investigator might be attempting to distinguish language differences from disorders in Vietnamese refugee children who speak English as a second language. The use of standardized tests normed on monolingual, English-speaking, white children would be a serious threat to the internal validity of the study.

■ Behaviors are often rated by observers or judges with varying degrees of objectivity and expertise. Judges may reduce validity in several ways. They may become more experienced in measuring the variable of interest (e.g., glottal fry in subjects' voices) during the study and thus score more instances of the variable occurring during the posttest than during pretest observations, in which they missed some instances of glottal fry. Or they may become bored during the posttest and may not observe and score as vigilantly. Finally, criteria used by individual judges may become more or less stringent over the course of a study.

History

■ History includes the subjects' life events that may be partially or totally responsible for changes recorded in the dependent variable after the independent variable is introduced. In other words, history involves events that occur, in addition to the experimental variable, between the first and second (or more) measurements.

■ For example, the first author once treated a preschool girl with a moderately severe phonological delay. After 8–10 weeks, great improvement in intelligibility (the dependent variable) was noted as a result of the clearly superior treatment (the independent variable) the girl was receiving.

■ It was later discovered that during the 2nd week of treatment, the child had received pressure-equalizing tubes in her ears. Thus, the life event for this subject (the tubes) might have made some or most of the difference in her intelligibility—not the treatment.

■ Generally, the longer the time between measurements, the greater the chance of history having an effect on the study's results. Relevant events that occur outside the experimental setting, and thus outside the experimenter's control, have a greater chance of occurring in long-term studies (Schiavetti & Metz, 1997).

Statistical Regression

■ Statistical regression, also called *statistical regression to the mean*, refers to a behavior that goes from an extreme high or low point to an average level.

■ In clinical research, many clients seek treatment when their problem is at its worst. For example, clients who abuse their voices may seek treatment when they are the most hoarse after cheering at a ballgame. Thus, though the voice is very hoarse, it will not remain at that level of hoarseness. The voice will eventually (in most cases) sound less hoarse.

■ Subjects selected for a voice experiment that begins when they are at the peak of their voice problems (such as hoarseness) may begin to sound less hoarse as the experiment continues. The improvement in voice quality may be incorrectly attributed to the treatment.

Maturation

■ While history refers to events that occur outside the experimental setting, *maturation* refers to changes within subjects themselves; those changes can have an effect on the dependent variable.

■ Maturation refers to biological and other kinds of unidentified changes that take place in subjects simply as a result of the passage of time. The experimenter is not able to control those changes.

■ For example, an investigator may wish to study the effect of a language stimulation program on kindergarten children. The investigator measures the children's language skills in the fall of 2001, implements the program, and remeasures the language skills in May of 2002.

■ The children's skills have improved, and this improvement is attributed to the language stimulation program. Unfortunately, maturation, or getting older and thus more linguistically sophisticated, might be a partial explanation for the children's improvement.

Attrition

- Also called *mortality*, *attrition* refers to the problem of losing subjects as the experiment progresses. This has an effect on the final results as interpreted by the investigator.

- Group designs, which depend heavily on the analysis of results based on group averages, are very vulnerable to attrition. Attrition is a problem only when the investigator uses statistical analysis based on group means.

- Attrition is particularly problematic when it is *differential*. For example, if more severely affected subjects drop out of the experimental group and less severely affected subjects drop out of the control group, that would create great differences in the pre- and posttest scores of the two groups even if the treatment is ineffective.

- Attrition is not a threat in single-subject designs that have several subjects. Subjects who drop out of those studies can be replaced. Also, there are no groups of subjects to be statistically compared. A problem may be, though, that a single-subject design study with an N (number) of one will no longer exist if that subject withdraws from the study.

Testing

- *Testing* refers to a change that occurs in a dependent variable simply because it has been measured more than once. The dependent variable is affected because of the administration of pre- and posttests. In such cases, the investigator may incorrectly conclude that the treatment variable of interest was responsible for the change recorded.

- Some behaviors change when repeatedly measured or tested. *Reactive measures* are measures of behavior that change as a function of repeated testing.

- For example, attitude questionnaires filled out before and after treatment by clients who stutter are reactive. The clients may show significant attitude changes when they fill out the post-treatment questionnaire, even though their attitudes have not changed much.

- If possible, investigators should handle testing as a threat to internal validity by measuring behaviors directly, not by measures such as questionnaires.

Subject Selection Biases

- Subject selection biases are subjective factors that influence the selection of who participates in a study. A key feature of internally valid experiments is that differences found between experimental and control groups on posttests be attributable only to the treatment. However, if the two groups were different to begin with, differences in subjects themselves may produce the treatment effect.

■ To control for subject selection biases, it is best to use randomly selected and assigned groups. Another solution is to use groups that have very carefully matched subjects—that is, subjects who are similar on important variables.

Interaction of Factors

■ A study may be influenced by several of the above-described threats to internal validity. For example, a study involving the use of questionnaires to evaluate attitudes of spouses of people with aphasia might suffer from both testing and attrition.

■ Interpretation of data may especially be confounded by the interaction between subject selection and some other factor such as maturation (Schiavetti & Metz, 1997).

✎ Concepts To Consider

Briefly define internal validity and give two examples of threats to internal validity.

_____

_____

_____

_____

_____

_____

_____

_____

_____

External Validity

Definition

■ *External validity* refers to *generalizability*: to what settings, populations, treatment variables, and measurement variables this effect can be generalized (Campbell & Stanley, 1966). External validity is a matter of the extent to which the investigator can extend or generalize the study's results to other subjects and situations.

■ Threats to the internal validity of a study can ruin the study; the results may become meaningless and the investigator may not be able to form any valid conclusions about the relationships among the variables studied.

■ However, threats to *external* validity only *limit the degree* to which internally valid results can be generalized (Schiavetti & Metz, 1997). Most consumers of research do not expect that a single study can be generalized to a wide variety of settings and subjects.

■ External validity of a study can be threatened by several factors. These include the Hawthorne effect, subject selection, multiple treatment interference, and reactive or interactive effects of pretesting.

Hawthorne Effect

■ The *Hawthorne effect* is the extent to which the subjects' knowledge that they are participants in an experiment or that they are being treated differently than usual may affect the experiment's results.

■ For example, school-aged children who stutter might be taken from their classrooms, brought to a special room with an experimenter, and asked to read a story and interact in a game under a certain treatment condition. The children might react with increased or decreased fluency to the different setting, the change in routine, and/or the extra attention they are receiving, not the treatment itself.

Subject Selection

■ *Subject selection* is a threat to the external validity as well as the internal validity of a study. It is a threat to external validity when researchers and/or consumers of research try to extend and apply the study's results to subjects who differ from, or do not have pertinent characteristics in common with, the subjects in the study.

■ For example, a study might demonstrate that joint book reading was highly effective in increasing expressive language skills in preschoolers in that particular study. A reader might try, unsuccessfully, to use joint book reading to increase expressive language skills in preschoolers he or she was seeing.

■ The problem might be that the study was conducted with preschoolers of parents who had college educations and were of middle-class socioeconomic status, while the reader served children from homes where the parents were primarily high school graduates of low-income status.

■ If the reader had paid attention to the subject selection, he or she might not have tried to apply the study's results to a group of children with different characteristics than the subjects in the study.

Multiple Treatment Interference

- In most research studies, investigators assess the effects of a single independent variable. However, in some experiments, investigators assess the effects of multiple independent variables.

- *Multiple treatment interference* refers to the positive or negative effect of one treatment over another. This is likely when more than one experimental treatment is administered to the same subjects; it can also occur when treatment consists of a set of carefully sequenced steps (Schiavetti & Metz, 1997).

- For example, a clinician might be attempting to discover which method of reinforcement is most effective in increasing children's response rate during treatment: scratch-and-sniff stickers, verbal praise, or Fruit Loops. The three different methods of providing reinforcement would be the three treatment variables in the study.

- The overall effect observed in the subjects might be at least partially determined by the order in which the multiple treatments were applied. For example, if children's performance in the above study improved when they received Fruit Loops first, stickers second, and verbal praise third, then the study's results could be generalized only to children who were provided reinforcement in the same sequence.

- If the same treatments were applied in a different order, the same results might not be obtained. Generalizability of findings would then be affected because the results might be valid only in terms of the sequence in which the treatments were administered.

Reactive or Interactive Effects of Pretesting

- The dependent variable in a study might be assessed through a pretest that might sensitize the subjects to the treatment in such a way as to enhance the effect of the treatment variable. This is called *reactive or interactive effects of pretesting*.

- For example, people who regularly abused their voices through speaking loudly and using hard glottal attacks might fill out a questionnaire before treatment that assessed the frequency with which they used such abusive vocal habits.

- The subjects, thus sensitized to how often they abused their voices, might begin to modify their vocally abusive habits as a result of their increased awareness. At the end of treatment, the subjects' improved vocal quality might be attributed to the treatment, when in reality the subjects' increased awareness affected the improvement.

- In such cases, results of the study cannot be generalized to subjects who have not been given a similar pretest.

Summary

☑ Investigators who conduct studies must control for threats to the internal and external validity of those studies.

☑ Threats to internal validity can include instrumentation, history, statistical regression, maturation, attrition, testing, subject selection biases, and interaction of two or more of those factors.

☑ Threats to external validity include the Hawthorne effect, subject selection, multiple treatment interference, and reactive or interactive effects of pretesting.

DATA ORGANIZATION AND ANALYSIS: PRINCIPLES OF STATISTICS

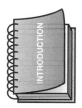

INTRODUCTION

Most studies conducted in speech–language pathology use statistics to help organize, summarize, and analyze data. There are dozens of statistical techniques available. Commonly used techniques include measures of variability and measures of central tendency. Measurement scales are often involved, as they are closely related to statistical scaling techniques.

Foundational Concepts

▨ Data organization and analysis techniques are statistical tools. These tools aid the investigator in drawing conclusions and making inferences from a study. Because descriptive and experimental studies use the same statistical techniques to analyze data, one cannot tell from the techniques used whether the study is experimental or descriptive (Schiavetti & Metz, 1997).

▨ When used in the singular form, *statistics* refers to the field of study involved with the art and science of data analysis. Statistics deals with *probability*, or the chance of something occurring. For example, if the probability of rain is 0.75, there is a 75% chance of rain.

▨ When used in the plural form, *statistics* refers to specific pieces of data that will be or have been gathered. For example, baseball statistics might include a baseball player's number of home runs and strikeouts (Grimmett, 1995).

▨ Kerlinger (1973) defines a statistic as a measure calculated from a sample. This differs from a *parameter*, which refers to a population value. Examples of statistics, or summaries of samples, include percentages, means, variances, standard deviations, and other measures calculated from samples.

■ According to Kerlinger (1973), there are several major purposes for statistics. The first purpose of statistics is to take large quantities of data and reduce them to manageable form. For example, if there are 100 individual scores on an examination, it is easier to calculate a mean and a standard deviation (defined later) than to look at and remember 100 individual scores.

■ The second major purpose of statistics is to aid the researcher in making inferences. An *inference* is a conclusion one arrives at through reasoning. Statistical inferences are frequently made from samples to populations. Researchers make observations on a sample, or small group of people, in order to make a decision about a larger group.

■ For example, investigators have studied the effects of exercise on cholesterol levels in samples of subjects. They have discovered that in those subjects, cholesterol levels were decreased when the subjects increased their exercise levels. Thus, the investigators *inferred* that people not in the study, the larger population of people with high cholesterol, might benefit from increased levels of exercise.

Statistical Techniques for Organizing Data

■ As stated earlier, data need to be organized and summarized. Statistics help the investigator do that organization and summarization. Silverman (1998) describes three foundational types of statistics used for data organization and summary: measures of central tendency, measures of variability, and measures of association.

■ Measures of association (also called measures of correlation) have been described already. Thus, measures of variability and measures of central tendency will be briefly discussed.

Measures of Variability

■ *Variability* refers to the dispersion or spread in a set of data. Common measures of variability include the range, interquartile range, semi-interquartile range, and standard deviation.

■ For example, if an instructor administers an examination to 50 students and the highest score is 100 and the lowest score is 40, there is great variability in that set of scores. But if the lowest grade is 90 and the highest grade is 100, there is very little variability in that set of scores.

■ The *range* is the difference between the highest and lowest scores in a distribution or set of scores. For example, a test on which the highest score is 100 points and the lowest score is 40 points, the range is 60 points. One hundred (highest score) minus 40 (lowest score) yields the *range* in that set of scores.

■ The range can be deceptive, because extremely high and low scores can make the range appear greater or more variable than it really is.

■ In the earlier example, let's say one student received a score of 40 on the examination. But the next highest score was 70, and 49 out of the 50 students received scores between 70 and 100. The one student scoring 40 caused the class to have a 60-point range in scores instead of a 30-point range.

■ To deal with this type of situation, the interquartile range and semi-interquartile range may be used. The *interquartile range* "cuts off" the highest and lowest 25% of the scores in a distribution. Thus, what is left is the middle 50% of the scores. The *semi-interquartile range* is the interquartile range divided by two.

■ For example, if 100 students take an examination and the 25 highest scores range from 75 to 100 and the 25 lowest scores range from 0 to 25, the interquartile range of those scores is 50 because the lowest 25 scores and the highest 25 scores are disregarded. The semi-interquartile range is 25: 50 (the interquartile range) divided by 2.

■ The *standard deviation* is the extent to which scores deviate from the mean or average score. The standard deviation reflects the variability of all measures or scores in a distribution. The larger the standard deviation, the more variable the scores. The smaller the standard deviation, the less variable the scores.

■ For example, if an instructor gives an examination to a class and the highest score is 100 and the lowest score is 50, that 50-point difference in the highest and lowest scores results in a large standard deviation.

■ If an instructor gives an examination on which the highest score is 100 and the lowest score is 85, that 15-point difference in the highest and lowest scores results in a relatively small standard deviation.

Measures of Central Tendency

■ The *central tendency* of a distribution or set of scores is an index indicating the *average* or *typical* score for that distribution. There are three measures of central tendency: mean, median, and mode.

■ The *mean* is the most commonly used measure of central tendency. To calculate a mean, the investigator adds up the scores and divides that total by the number of scores that were added together. For instance, $60 + 50 + 40 + 80 = 230$. Next, $230 \div 4 = 57.5$. Thus, the mean for this set of scores is 57.5.

■ The *median* is the score in the exact middle of the distribution. The median divides the distribution into two parts so that an equal number of scores fall to the right and to the left of it. The following illustrates a median score:

38   42   51   57   63   **69**   78   85   88   90   97

The median score is 69 because five scores fall below it, and five scores fall above it.

■ The *mode* is the most frequently occurring score in a distribution. This is illustrated as follows:

| 22 | 29 | 34 | 46 | 57 | **63** | **63** | **63** | 78 | 85 | 100 |

The mode is 63, because 63 is the most frequently occurring score in this distribution.

■ If distributions are relatively symmetrical, the three measures of central tendency should be the same. This would result in a *normal distribution* or *bell-shaped curve*.

✎ Concepts To Consider

Describe two measures of variability and two measures of central tendency.

_____

_____

_____

_____

_____

_____

_____

_____

Types of Measurement Scales

■ Psychological and social scientists typically describe what they term *levels of measurement*. Some of these levels of measurement are closely related to statistical scaling techniques. The four commonly used levels of measurement are represented by scales: nominal, ordinal, interval, and ratio scales.

■ In a *nominal scale*, a category is present or absent (e.g., hypernasality, hyponasality). Items or observations are classified into named groupings or discrete categories that do not have a numerical relationship to one another.

■ For example, in a survey of clinical practices, respondents might be asked if they "never," "sometimes," or "always" use a certain clinical practice. Or, a researcher might label diagnostic categories in a nominal way as "aphasia," "specific language impairment," "dementia," "dysphagia," and others.

■ An *ordinal scale* is a numerical scale that can be arranged according to rank orders or levels. Ordinal scales use relative concepts such as *greater than* and *less than*. The numbers in an ordinal scale and their corresponding categories do not have mathematical meaning. Also, the intervals between numbers of categories are unknown and probably not equal. Examples of ordinal scales of measurement are:

1 = strongly agree   2 = agree   3 = neutral   4 = disagree   5 = strongly disagree

1 = little hoarseness   3 = moderate hoarseness   5 = great hoarseness

■ An *interval scale* of measurement is a numerical scale that can be arranged according to rank orders or levels; the numbers on the scale must be assigned in such a way that the intervals between them are equal with regard to the attribute being scaled (Silverman, 1998). For example, in Figure 12.5, the attribute of distance is equal between one number and another.

■ A *ratio scale* has the same properties as an interval scale, but numerical values must be related to an *absolute zero point*. The *zero* suggests an absence of the property being measured. An example of a ratio scale is one that involves frequency counts in stuttering; it is possible to have zero instances of stuttering in a speech sample. Figure 12.6 below illustrates a ratio scale for the attribute of distance (Silverman, 1998).

Summary

☑ The use of statistical techniques enables investigators to organize, summarize, and analyze data in a useful way. These techniques include measures of variability and measures of central tendency.

☑ Measures of variability include the range, interquartile range, semi-interquartile range, and standard deviation from the mean.

☑ Measures of central tendency include the mean, median, and mode. Measurement scales used in studies include nominal, ordinal, interval, and ratio scales.

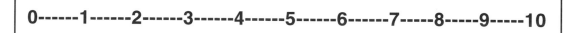

0------1------2------3------4------5------6------7-----8-----9-----10

Figure 12.5. Interval scale of measurement.

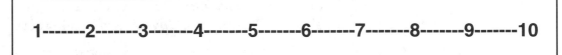

Figure 12.6. Ratio scale of measurement.

CHAPTER HIGHLIGHTS

▶ Science, a philosophy based on empiricism and determinism, uses objective experimental methods to systematically investigate research questions and produce valid and reliable results. Scientists may use either inductive or deductive reasoning to create theories and test hypotheses. Hypothesis testing is a major goal of science.

▶ A rigorous method of hypothesis testing is experimental research. An experiment is a means of establishing cause-effect relationships between variables. An independent variable is directly manipulated by the experimenter to cause changes in the dependent variable being studied. Ideally, confounding variables are ruled out as potential causes of changes in the dependent variable.

▶ There are many experimental group designs. In the basic experimental group design, there is at least one experimental group, which receives treatment, and one control group, which does not. These groups constitute the sample, a small number of subjects drawn from the population. The sample should be randomly selected and representative of the population.

▶ The pretest-posttest control group design is a prototype of experimental group designs. This design is based on the logic that the experimental and control groups are similar in every way except that of the independent variable of interest. Both groups are given a pretest, only the experimental group receives the treatment, and then both groups are given a posttest. This arrangement allows the researcher to evaluate the effect of the independent variable.

▶ Single-subject designs are experimental designs that demonstrate cause-effect relationships in small groups of subjects (usually 1–6 subjects) whose performance is recorded individually. ABAB designs and their variations are commonplace in single-subject design research. The A phase is the no-treatment phase, and the B phase is the treatment phase. Multiple baseline designs are another common type of single-subject research design.

(continues)

▶ Sometimes experimental research is not possible or desirable, so investigators use descriptive research strategies. In descriptive research, there is no demonstration of cause-effect relationships. Common types of descriptive research include ex post facto, survey, case study, retrospective, comparative, developmental, and correlational research. Ethnographic research is also considered descriptive in nature.

▶ Research can be evaluated in terms of its internal and external validity. The concept of internal validity means the degree to which data in a study reflect a true cause-effect relationship. External validity refers to the generalizability of a study's results.

▶ Possible threats to a study's internal validity include instrumentation, history, statistical regression, maturation, attrition, testing, subject selection bias, and interaction of two or more of those factors. Possible threats to external validity include the Hawthorne effect, subject selection, multiple treatment interference, and reactive or interactive effects of pretesting.

▶ Statistics can be defined as the field of study involved with data organization, summary, and analysis. Statistics involves probability. Two foundational types of statistical analysis used for data organization and summary include measures of variability and of central tendency.

▶ Levels of measurement used by scientists may be closely related to statistical scaling techniques. Four commonly used levels of measurement include nominal, ordinal, interval, and ratio scales.

▶ Add your own chapter highlights here:

_____

_____

_____

_____

KEY TERMS

A phase	alternative hypothesis	concurrent validity
B phase	attrition	confounding variable
ABA design	baserate	construct validity
ABAB design	baseline	content validity
ABAB reversal design	case study research	control group
ABAB withdrawal	central tendency	correlational coefficient
design	classification variable	correlational research
alternate form reliability	comparative research	criterion validity

criterion variable
cross-sectional research
data
deductive method
dependent variable
determinism
developmental research
empiricism
ethnographic research
ex post facto research
experiment
experimental group
external validity
extraneous variable
Hawthorne effect
history (as a threat to
   internal validity)
hypothesis
independent variable
inductive method
inference
instrumentation
internal validity
interobserver or inter-
   judge reliability
interquartile range
interval scale
intraobserver or intra-
   judge reliability
longitudinal research

maturation
mean
median
mode
multiple baseline design
multiple-baseline-
   across-behaviors
   design
multiple-baseline-
   across-settings design
multiple-baseline-
   across-subjects design
multiple treatment
   interference
nominal scale
null hypothesis
ordinal scale
parallel form reliability
Pearson product
   moment r
population
posttest
predictive validity
pretest
pretest-posttest control
   group design
probability
qualitative data
quantitative data
random sample

range
ratio scale
reactive or interactive
   effects of pretesting
reactive measures
reliability
representativeness
research
retrospective research
sample
science
semi-interquartile range
semilongitudinal
   research
single-subject design
split-half reliability
standard deviation
statistic
statistical regression
statistics
subject selection
subject selection biases
survey research
testing
test-retest reliability
theory
validity
variability

STUDY AND REVIEW QUESTIONS

Fill in the Blank

1. Researchers formulate and test hypotheses or predictive statements of cause-effect relationships between certain variables. The ___null___ hypothesis is a statement that two variables are not related, and the ___alternative___ hypothesis holds that there is actually a relationship between the variables specified.

2. A(n) ___confounding or extraneous___ variable has an impact on the dependent variable but shouldn't; this variable is what investigators hope to eliminate from their studies.

3. In group experimental designs, the _control_ group contains subjects who do not receive treatment, while the _experimental_ group contains subjects who do receive treatment.

4. In a(n) _ABAB w/drawl_, a target behavior is baserated, taught to a subject, reduced by withdrawing the treatment, and then taught again to show that treatment was effective.

5. _split half_ reliability is a measure of internal consistency of a test, and _test retest_ reliability means consistency of measures when two forms of the same test are administered to the same people.

6. In a(n) _multiple baseline across behaviors_ design, several behaviors are sequentially taught to show that only treated behaviors change in a subject, and thus treatment was effective.

7. The purpose of _comparative_ research is to measure the behaviors of two or more types of subjects at one point in time to draw conclusions about similarities or differences between those subjects.

8. In _ethnographic_ research, the investigator conducts detailed observations, immerses him- or herself in the environment being studied, and uses an inductive approach.

9. Threats to internal validity of a study can include _history_, or events in subjects' lives that may be partially or totally responsible for changes recorded in the dependent variable after the independent variable has been introduced. A possible threat to a study's external validity is the _Hawthorne effect_, in which subjects perform differently because they know they are participating in a study.

10. Measures of central tendency include the _median_, or exact midpoint of a distribution; the _mode_, or the most frequently occurring score; and the _mean_, or measure in which the investigator adds up scores and divides the total by the number of scores.

Multiple Choice

11. A measure of validity of the accuracy with which a test predicts future performance on a related task is called:

A. content validity.

B. concurrent validity.

C. construct validity.

D. predictive or criterion validity.

E. index validity.

12. *Reliability* means that a test or measure:

A. measures what it purports to measure.

B. has scores that are consistent across repeated testing or measurement.

C. has items that adequately sample the full range of the skill being tested.

D. correlates well with an established test of known validity.

E. is consistent with theoretical constructs or concepts.

13. An investigator carries out a study in which the effect of rate of speech upon stuttering during sibling interaction is being investigated. The investigator gathers conversational samples from children who stutter and their siblings. In the control group, siblings are asked to speak as they normally would at home. In the experimental group, siblings are asked to speak much more quickly than they would at home. The investigator wishes to measure the effect of rate of siblings' speech upon the amount of stuttering done by the children who stutter. In other words, the investigator is asking if increased rate of sibling speech causes children to stutter more. In the above study, the dependent variable is:

A. the amount of stuttering done by the children when they increase their rate of speech.

B. the rate of speech of the siblings in the experimental group.

C. the rate of speech of the siblings in the control group.

D. the combined amount of stuttering done by the children in both the experimental and the control groups.

E. B and C

14. An experimental design involving one or a few subjects would be called a:

A. case study design.

B. ex post facto design.

C. single-subject design.

D. single correlational design.

E. single-subject case study design.

15. In a single-subject design, the following are true:

     I. The A phase is the no-treatment or baseline phase.

     II. The B phase is the treatment phase.

     III. The A phase is the treatment phase.

     IV. The B phase is the no-treatment or baseline phase.

     V. There may be anywhere from 1 to 6 subjects.

  A. III, IV

  B. III, IV, V

  C. I, II

  D. I, II, V

16. A type of research in which independent variables have occurred in the past and the investigator is making a retrospective search for causes of events is called:

  A. retrospective research.

  B. ex post facto research.

  C. historical research.

  D. case study research.

  E. survey research.

17. A difficulty with cross-sectional studies is that:

  A. observations are made of differences *between* subjects of different ages in order to generalize about developmental changes that would occur *within* subjects as they mature.

  B. observations are made of differences *within* subject groups of different ages in order to generalize about developmental changes that would occur *between* subjects as they mature.

  C. the same subjects are studied over time, and this is expensive, time consuming, and difficult because subjects might drop out of the study.

  D. the total age span of children to be studied is divided into several over-lapping age spans, and it is difficult to follow subjects from the lower to the upper end of each age span.

  E. the investigator is examining data already on file to answer questions about children in various age groups, and that data might not be reliable.

18. A measure of variability denoting the extent to which scores deviate from the mean or average score is called the:

    A. deviant variability index.

    B. standard deviation.

    C. interquartile range.

    D. semi-interquartile range.

    E. standard variance squared.

19. A group of clinicians wishes to conduct research in a hospital setting. These clinicians work with clients who have voice disorders. Many of the clients are hoarse because they work in noisy factories where they shout a great deal during the work week. The clinicians devise a rating scale to evaluate the hoarseness of these clients during evaluation sessions. The scale looks like this:

1	2	3	4
almost no hoarseness	slight hoarseness	moderate hoarseness	great amount of hoarseness

    This type of scale would be called a:

    A. ratio scale.

    B. nominal scale.

    C. interval scale.

    D. logarithmic scale.

    E. ordinal scale.

20. The *range* in a distribution can be defined as:

    A. the difference between the highest and lowest scores in a distribution.

    B. the middle 50% of scores of a distribution.

    C. the middle 50% of scores in a distribution divided by 2.

    D. the variance plus the difference between the highest and lowest scores in a distribution.

    E. the lowest and highest 25% of a distribution.

REFERENCES AND RECOMMENDED READINGS

Brown, L., Sherbenou, R. J., & Johnson, S. K. (1997). *Test of nonverbal intelligence* (3rd ed.). Austin, TX: PRO-ED.

Campbell, D. T., & Stanley, J. C. (1966). *Experimental and quasi-experimental designs for research.* Chicago: Rand McNally.

Dunn, L. M., & Dunn, L. M. (1981). *Peabody picture vocabulary test–revised.* Circle Pines, MN: American Guidance Service.

Grimmett, D. R. (1995). *Statistics study cards.* Springfield, OH: Visual Education Association.

Hegde, M. N. (1994). *Clinical research in communicative disorders: Principles and strategies* (2nd ed.). Austin, TX: PRO-ED.

Hegde, M. N. (1996). *Pocketguide to treatment in speech–language pathology.* San Diego, CA: Singular Publishing Group.

Hegde, M. N., & Davis, D. (1995). *Clinical methods and practicum in speech–language pathology.* San Diego, CA: Singular Publishing Group.

Kerlinger, F. N. (1973). *Foundations of behavioral research.* New York: Holt, Rinehart, & Winston.

Payne, K. T., & Anderson, N. B. (1991). *How to prepare for the NESPA national examinations in speech pathology and audiology.* San Diego, CA: Singular Publishing Group.

Schiavetti, N., & Metz, D. E. (1997). *Evaluating research in communicative disorders* (3rd ed.). Needham Heights, MA: Allyn & Bacon.

Silverman, F. H. (1998). *Research design and evaluation in speech–language pathology and audiology* (4th ed.). Needham Heights, MA: Allyn & Bacon.

ANSWERS TO STUDY AND REVIEW QUESTIONS

1. Null, alternative

2. Confounding or extraneous

3. Control, experimental

4. ABAB withdrawal

5. Split-half, test-retest

6. Multiple-baseline-across-behaviors

7. Comparative

8. Ethnographic

9. History, Hawthorne effect

10. Median, mode, mean

11. D. A measure of validity of the accuracy with which a test *predicts* future performance on a related task is called *predictive* or criterion validity.

12. B. *Reliability* means that a test or measure has scores that are consistent across repeated testing or measurement. The other answers in this item relate to validity, not reliability.

13. A. The dependent variable is the amount of stuttering done by the children when they increase their rate of speech. The rate of speech of siblings in both groups is the independent variable, which is manipulated by the investigator.

14. C. Single-subject designs are *experimental* and may involve one or a few subjects. Case study designs are *descriptive*.

15. D. In a single-subject design, the A phase is the no-treatment or baseline phase, the B phase is the treatment phase, and there may be anywhere from 1 to 6 subjects.

16. B. A type of research in which independent variables have occurred in the past and the investigator is making a retrospective search for causes of events is called ex post facto research.

17. A. A difficulty with cross-sectional studies is that observations are made of differences *between* subjects of different ages in order to generalize about developmental changes that would occur *within* subjects as they mature

18. B. A measure of variability denoting the extent to which scores deviate from the mean or average score is called the standard deviation.

19. E. An ordinal scale of measurement would be represented by numbers that can be arranged according to rank orders or levels, but the intervals between the numerals are unknown and probably not equal.

20. A. The *range* in a distribution can be defined as the difference between the highest and lowest scores in a distribution.

CHAPTER 13

Special Topics in Speech–Language Pathology

PREVIEW OUTLINE

CHAPTER INTRODUCTION

At the beginning of the 20th century, there were no professionally trained speech–language pathologists or audiologists in the United States. There were no educational or professional training programs in the country. In Europe, the treatment of speech disorders was a domain of medicine. In the United States, it was the public schools that took a leading role in providing special teaching programs for children with communicative disabilities. By 1910 Chicago public schools began to hire specialists who worked with children with disorders of speech. These specialists were called speech correction teachers, and they worked mostly with children who stuttered or had disorders of articulation. Other disorders of communication began to be treated only later. In the early 1920s, the University of Wisconsin and the University of Iowa began to offer doctoral programs with an emphasis on speech disorders. Soon other universities across the country, such as Northwestern University, instituted degree programs in speech disorders.

Today, at the threshold of a new century, the profession of communicative sciences and disorders continues to undergo rapid changes and expansion. This expansion is due in large part to a phenomenal growth in the amount of research information concerning communication and its disorders. In this chapter, we discuss the following special topics: the nature of the ASHA and its professions of speech–language pathology and audiology, issues in certification and licensure, legislative issues in regulation of the professions, issues in counseling, basics of medical speech–language pathology, and craniofacial anomalies and genetic syndromes.

BACKGROUND AND NATURE OF ASHA AND THE PROFESSIONS

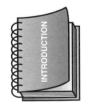

The American Speech–Language-Hearing Association (ASHA) is the national organization that fulfills many functions in research, legislation, and regulation of the profession. Most speech–language pathologists and audiologists are members of ASHA. Speech–language pathologists and audiologists are professionals who deal with normal development and disorders of communication, including language, speech, and hearing. ASHA and the professions of speech–language pathology and audiology are continually expanding to serve greater numbers of clients who need services relating to their communicative disorders. In this section, we discuss the ASHA organization, ASHA accreditation, and the professions of speech–language pathology and audiology.

The American Speech-Language-Hearing Association

■ The American Speech-Language-Hearing Association has undergone several name changes. In 1925, when it was established by a handful of people at the University of Iowa, it was called the American Academy of Speech Correction. In 1927 it was renamed the American Society for the Study of Speech Disorders. In 1934 the name was changed to the American Speech Correction Association.

■ In 1947, the organization was renamed the American Speech and Hearing Association (ASHA). The addition of "hearing" to the name was a significant event, recognizing the intertwined nature of speech–language pathology and audiology.

■ In 1978 the name was changed to the American Speech-Language-Hearing Association (the acronym is still ASHA) in order to reflect the field's deeper involvement in language and its disorders. This name stands today.

■ Although most members of ASHA are audiologists and speech–language pathologists in the United States, ASHA is not limited to U.S. citizens. Some ASHA members live in other countries such as Saudi Arabia, Canada, and Taiwan. ASHA represents the interests of 350 international affiliates in 65 countries.

■ ASHA has grown dramatically in recent decades. In 1935, the organization had fewer than 100 members; at the time of this publication, its membership exceeds 93,000 speech–language pathologists, audiologists, and speech-language and hearing scientists (ASHA, 1998). (In addition, there are approximately 40,000–50,000 speech–language pathologists, many of whom work in public schools, who are not members of ASHA.)

■ At the time of this writing, approximately 7.3% of ASHA members, international affiliates, and nonmember certificate holders are members of some ethnic or racial minority group. This percentage is far below the distribution of minorities in the general population.

■ Both the professional organization and the range of professional services are growing. At the time of this writing, 72% of audiologists are employed in health care facilities such as medical clinics, 23% in hospitals, and the rest in residential health care facilities (ASHA, 1998).

■ Currently, over 50% of speech–language pathologists work in school settings. Thirty-nine percent work in health care facilities, and 4% are employed in a college or university setting.

■ Eighty percent of ASHA members are certified speech–language pathologists. Thirteen percent are certified audiologists, and the rest of ASHA's membership comprises international affiliates, dually certified practitioners, those in the process of certification, and noncertified members.

■ ASHA is a national scientific and professional organization whose headquarters are located in the Washington, D.C., metropolitan area (in Rockville Pike, Maryland). As a scientific and professional organization, ASHA plays a major role in promoting awareness of communicative disorders in the public and the government.

■ ASHA has a number of goals. The most important of them include organized efforts to:

- ensure the quality of speech, language, and hearing services offered to the public;

- stimulate the development of speech, language, and hearing services to people who have communicative disorders;

- encourage scientific study and research into the basic processes of communication, disorders of communication, and the treatment of those disorders; and

- promote exchange of scientific and professional information through publications, conventions, and other continuing education activities.

■ ASHA publishes several scientific and professional journals and a number of publications that include scientific studies, clinical research, scholarly articles, and discussions of professional issues.

■ Currently, the basic requirement for membership in ASHA is a master's degree with a major emphasis in speech–language pathology or audiology. However, any member who also provides and/or supervises clinical services must meet or be in the process of meeting requirements for the association's clinical certification.

■ Those who do not provide or supervise clinical services may retain membership in ASHA without holding its clinical certificate. For example, research scientists who meet the academic requirement may be members of ASHA without possessing a clinical certificate.

■ Students who have declared their major as speech–language pathology or audiology may become members of the National Student Speech-Language-Hearing Association (NSSLHA), which is recognized by ASHA.

■ Benefits of membership in NSSLHA include reduced fees for conventions and scientific journals. Many colleges and universities have active local chapters of NSSLHA that sponsor professional and social events.

■ Within the last several years, ASHA has created a number of *special interest divisions* (SIDs) for members who wish to interact with other members who have similar interests. Any ASHA member may join one or more SID for a nominal annual fee.

■ At the time of this writing, there are more than 15 SIDs, and the number continues to expand. SIDs have been created in such diverse areas as Speech

Science and Orofacial Disorders, Aural Rehabilitation, and Communication Disorders and Sciences in Linguistically Diverse Populations.

Concepts To Consider

Summarize the nature and purpose of ASHA.

_____

_____

_____

_____

_____

_____

_____

_____

ASHA Accreditation

- ASHA has established standards of scientific and professional education in speech–language pathology and audiology. The standards include the kinds and variety of academic courses that must be offered and the amount and quality of clinical practice the student clinicians must have.

- Through its *Education Standards Board* (ESB), ASHA accredits those master's degree programs in speech–language pathology and audiology that meet its minimum standards.

- Through the *Professional Services Board* (PSB), ASHA evaluates clinical speech-language and hearing services offered by a speech and hearing clinic.

- Evaluations are conducted by ESB and PSB teams (specialists chosen by the respective boards), who analyze programs and services and decide whether certain minimum standards are met. The teams then make formal reports to their respective boards as to their findings.

- When selecting a college or university program in communicative disorders, students should make sure that the program is accredited by ASHA. ASHA accreditation means that the program meets the educational standards set by the national organization.

- Appropriate accreditation also means that the student, upon graduation with a master's degree in speech–language pathology or audiology, will be able to receive the national clinical certification from ASHA. A student who graduates from a university program that is not accredited by ASHA will not be certified.

The Professions of Speech–Language Pathology and Audiology

- Speech–language pathology is the scientific profession concerned with normal development and disorders of human communication (speech and language) and the assessment and treatment of those disorders. (For more information, see "Scope of Practice," Appendix B.)

- The term *speech–language pathologist* is preferred among members of the profession. However, some people use the terms *speech therapist* and *speech–language clinician*.

- *Audiologists* are specialists who are concerned with hearing, its disorders, and the assessment and rehabilitation of persons with hearing impairment. *Educational audiologists* may be found in educational settings such as public schools, and *industrial audiologists* are those who work in the industrial sector.

- Speech–language pathologists and audiologists work in a variety of professional settings such as hospitals, schools, private practices, rehabilitation clinics, skilled nursing facilities, and others.

- *Speech–language and hearing scientists* generally work in research laboratories and university departments. Their primary task is to generate new knowledge through research.

Summary

- ☑ ASHA, the national professional and scientific organization of communicative disorders professionals, has an interesting history, which includes phenomenal growth and change.

- ☑ With over 93,000 members, ASHA continually works to promote high ethical standards, pertinent legislation, and regulation of the professions of speech–language pathology and audiology.

- ☑ Students may join the ASHA-affiliated NSSLHA, the national student organization, which provides students with many benefits. Members of ASHA include speech–language pathologists and audiologists who work in a variety of professional settings to provide comprehensive services to individuals with disorders of language, speech, and hearing.

ISSUES IN CERTIFICATION AND LICENSURE

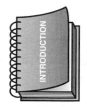

As mentioned earlier, a major function of ASHA is regulation of the professions of speech–language pathology and audiology. One way ASHA does this is through ASHA-administered certification, which helps ensure the quality of services provided (see Appendix C). Individual states also have licensing and certification requirements for their clinicians. The necessity of holding a state license, state certificate, ASHA certificate, or all three depends upon (a) the individual state, and (b) the professional setting in which the clinician works. Certification and requirements for supportive personnel are currently being discussed by ASHA and the states. In this section we discuss ASHA certification, state regulation of the professions, and issues regarding support personnel.

Certification

■ To ensure the quality of speech–language and hearing services offered to the public, ASHA has developed two clinical certificates that are issued to members who meet the academic and clinical standards of the association.

■ ASHA certifies speech–language pathologists and audiologists separately. The *Certificate of Clinical Competence in Speech–Language Pathology* (CCC-SLP) is issued to those individuals who have the master's degree or its equivalent in speech–language pathology and have fulfilled clinical practicum and fellowship requirements.

■ The clinical practicum requires a minimum of 25 hours of supervised observation of services and 350 clock hours of supervised clinical work with clients of all ages who have a variety of communicative disorders.

■ The clinical fellowship consists of additional, supervised clinical experience obtained after completing graduate education. This usually consists of 9 months of full-time, paid professional experience under the supervision of an ASHA-certified speech–language pathologist.

■ The *Certificate of Clinical Competence in Audiology* (CCC-A) has similar requirements, with the academic coursework, clinical practicum, and clinical fellowship completed in audiology. At the time of this writing, discussions are underway and steps are being taken to create and implement an Au.D., or clinical doctorate in audiology.

■ ASHA's certificates are not legal documents comparable to a state license. However, they are recognized by most employers, including hospitals, clinics, public school districts, and universities throughout the country. Many state licensure laws were modeled after the ASHA requirements.

■ Individuals who hold ASHA membership and clinical certification are committed to uphold the highest standards of clinical services. Treating people with communicative disorders is an ethical and socially responsible activity. Therefore, speech–language pathologists and audiologists who hold a certificate from ASHA are committed to its Code of Ethics (see Appendix A).

■ The Code of Ethics is an important document. It regulates all aspects of a professional's conduct. Violation of the code has serious consequences, including revocation of one's clinical certificate and cancellation of membership in ASHA.

State Regulation of the Profession

■ The state governments have laws and regulations that affect the work of speech–language pathologists and audiologists. Most states give *credentials* to their speech–language pathologists and audiologists working in the public schools.

■ A credential is typically issued by the state department of education or a related agency, depending on the individual state. Each credentialing agency has its own specifications, which affect the educational training and professional practice of speech–language pathologists and audiologists who work in the public schools.

■ Most of the coursework and clinical practicum experiences required by ASHA are also required from states' credentialing agencies. However, some state regulations may require coursework in education on the assumption that speech–language pathologists working in the schools must be familiar with certain educational methods and practices, including curriculum requirements.

■ A few states also combine a teaching credential with a credential in speech–language pathology. Such a credential requires more coursework in education, because the professional in this case is both a teacher and a speech–language pathologist.

■ Credentials issued by state agencies are specific to the particular state's public schools only. Those credentials may or may not transfer to another state's public schools. In other words, if a speech–language pathologist who works in California's public schools under California's credentials moves to Illinois, he or she may be required to satisfy additional requirements to work in Illinois public schools.

■ State public school credentials are specific to the public school setting only. They do not allow private practice, work in a hospital or clinic, or supervision of clinical practice in university speech and hearing centers.

■ A majority of states have passed licensure laws to regulate the professions of speech–language pathology and audiology. State licensure is not the same as state credentials, although they require similar coursework and clinic practicum.

■ Professional settings other than public schools (e.g., hospitals and private clinics) usually require either the ASHA Certificate of Clinical Competence, state licensure if it exists, or both. However, in many states, public school districts are also beginning to require or at least strongly encourage speech–language pathologists to possess state licensure and ASHA certification.

■ Most state licensure laws are based on the requirements specified by ASHA. Therefore, by meeting the ASHA requirements, graduates in most states will also meet the requirements for a license to practice speech–language pathology or audiology.

■ An important difference between a license and an ASHA certificate is that the ASHA certificate is issued by the professional organization. A license is issued by the individual state and carries the force of law. The state licensure is administered by a board or committee created by the state legislature.

■ There is state- and national-level discussion regarding the role of *supportive personnel* in rehabilitative settings, especially the public schools. Referred to also as *aides*, *assistants*, and *paraprofessionals*, these people are not currently mandated to possess certificates, credentials, or licenses in most states.

■ However, ASHA and many states are currently working toward developing a set of standards for support personnel. These standards will be used to regulate the *scope of services* provided by and the amount and type of *supervision* required of support personnel.

■ At the time of this writing, ASHA's guidelines for speech–language pathology assistants include the following:

  – completing a minimum of an associate's degree in an ASHA-approved speech–language pathology assistant training program (or equivalent course of study);

  – passing a uniform competency evaluation;

  – completing two field placements in different settings under the supervision of an ASHA-certified speech–language pathologist, and the requirement of competency assessments during field work.

■ ASHA's current strategic plan proposes a credentialing program for the registration of speech–language pathology assistants. This plan also proposes the registration and approval of technical training programs.

Summary

- ☑ ASHA regulates quality of service provision through ASHA certification, provided by the Certificate of Clinical Competence.

- ☑ States attempt to ensure quality of service provision by requiring a state license, a credential to work in the public schools, ASHA certification, or all three, depending upon the professional setting.

- ☑ Requirements for supportive personnel are underway to regulate scope of practice and supervision.

REGULATION OF THE PROFESSION: LEGISLATION AND ITS IMPLICATIONS IN SERVICE SETTINGS

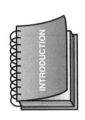

INTRODUCTION

A number of laws have been passed at both state and national levels that have impacted speech–language pathology and audiology. These laws have primarily mandated specific service provision requirements. In this section, we summarize some of the most key national laws, within the last two decades, that have impacted service provision in the public schools, employment, and health care settings.

Federal Legislation Impacting School Settings

Public Law 94-142

Enacted in 1975, the Education of the Handicapped Act (later retitled the Individuals with Disabilities Education Act) mandated free and appropriate education for disabled students from ages 3 to 21. Basic tenets of this law included the following:

- ■ Disabled children and youth from ages 3 to 21 years were guaranteed free and appropriate public education, in the "least restrictive environment," including special education and related services. (In some states, due to conflicts with state laws and court orders, children under age 5 and over age 18 were excluded.)

- ■ All students receiving special education services were to have individualized education plans (IEPs), determined by parents and professionals, that served as written records of commitments to meet students' goals.

■ Students and parents were guaranteed protection of their rights through due legal process, including the right to an impartial due process hearing and the right to examine all relevant records.

■ The federal government was to provide funds for local and state agencies to carry out prescribed programs and to monitor and evaluate those programs.

Public Law 99-457

■ These amendments to P.L. 94-142, enacted in 1986, were intended to provide early intervention that would reduce the number of children requiring special education services in later years.

■ P.L. 99-457 increased federal monetary support for states to provide services for disabled children between the ages of 3 and 6 years. It also created a new program that provided funds for service provision to infants and toddlers (up to 2 years) with disabilities.

■ An important tenet of P.L. 99-457 is that all school service providers must meet their state's highest requirements for their discipline (in many states, that meant a master's degree, which fulfilled the academic criteria for state licensing).

■ P.L. 99-457 established mandated development of individualized family service plans (IFSPs), requiring, among other things, information about:

– the child's present level of development

– the family's needs and strengths relating to the child's development

– the major goals for the child and family, and services to be provided

– a review of the plan at 6-month intervals or more frequently if needed

■ A major provision of P.L. 99-457 is multidisciplinary programming for infants and toddlers with disabilities and their families. This includes involvement of agencies outside the education setting (e.g., community programs).

■ Under P.L. 99-457, states were no longer required to report preschool children by disability category (e.g., hearing loss, mental retardation, learning disability). At-risk preschool children also became eligible for special education services, including those children who had experienced traumatic life events, depression, child abuse, and substance abuse.

Individuals with Disabilities Education Act (IDEA)

■ The IDEA (P.L. 101-476), enacted in 1990, reauthorized P.L. 94-142 and altered the language used in referring to its beneficiaries. Specifically, the term "disability" replaced the word "handicap."

■ The IDEA also expanded the number of categories of disabilities. Originally, P.L. 94-142 had 11 disability categories; the IDEA created 13 categories, newly including autism and traumatic brain injury.

■ The definition of special education was expanded to include instruction in all settings (not just the school), including training centers and workplaces.

■ The Amendments of 1997, Public Law 105-17, constitute the reauthorization of the IDEA. This reauthorization was signed into law by President Clinton on October 22, 1997. Foci of the reauthorization include (California Speech-Language-Hearing Association, 1997):

- increased, meaningful parental involvement in evaluations, including parental access to reports, test instruments, and other interpretative materials that contain personally identifiable information;

- improved educational results for children with disabilities;

- increased participation of special educators in the regular classroom setting, including involvement with curriculum;

- exploration of ways to increasingly serve children with learning problems in the regular classroom setting;

- prevention of inappropriate identification and mislabeling of children who are ethnically, linguistically, and racially diverse; and

- development of alternative assessments for children who cannot participate in regular assessments.

Federal Legislation Impacting Employment Settings

■ The Americans with Disabilities Act (ADA, Public Law 101-336), enacted in 1990, provides civil rights protection in the areas of employment, state and local government services, telecommunications, and public accommodations to all individuals with disabilities.

■ The ADA bars employment discrimination against qualified people with mental or physical disabilities, or disabilities that substantially limit one or more of the basic activities of life such as talking or walking.

■ The ADA requires that employers make "reasonable accommodations" for workers with disabilities. This includes making existing facilities such as public buildings and mass transportation accessible and arranging modified or part-time work schedules.

■ Employers must also provide special equipment for workers with disabilities. Examples include the provision of relay stations for users of telecommunication devices for the deaf (TDDs), auditory signals added to visual signs so that blind people can know when an elevator door is open, for example, and ramps for people in wheelchairs.

▤ According to the ADA, employers do not have to provide accommodations that impose an "undue hardship" on business operations. The meaning of the term "undue hardship" has been the subject of much discussion.

✎ Concepts To Consider

Describe one important point of each law: P.L. 99-457, IDEA, and ADA.

_____

_____

_____

_____

_____

_____

_____

Federal Legislation Impacting Health Care Settings

Health care legislation is under constant revision in the United States. One reason for this is that millions of Americans do not receive adequate health care. Statistics show that groups that are especially impacted are children, low-income people, and people from multicultural backgrounds.

▤ Several key pieces of health care legislation have been passed in preceding decades, but the entire health care system is still in flux at the beginning of a new century. This has service provision ramifications for the communicative disorders professions (Frattali, Curl, & Bevan, 1994).

Social Security Act (SSA)

▤ Passed in 1935, during the Great Depression, the SSA expanded the federal government's grant-in-aid assistance to the states. It was the federal government's first major step toward involvement in social insurance.

▤ The SSA provided the foundation for Medicaid and Medicare. It also provided for the general welfare of the public by establishing federal benefits for older people. The SSA also helped states provide more services for public health, maternal and child welfare, blind people, and dependent and disabled children.

■ Amendments to the SSA were made in 1965, 1967, 1972, and 1983. The amendments of 1983 had a real impact on speech–language pathology and audiology services. They offered incentive reimbursements for hospitals to provide more "efficient" and "cost-effective" treatment for patients.

■ Unfortunately, although inpatient rehabilitation units and rehabilitation hospitals were exempt from some of the flat-payment regulations imposed on other services, there were cost limits on services provided. This has resulted in the provision of fewer speech–language pathology and audiology services to patients.

U.S. Public Health Service Act

■ An important component of this act, passed in 1944, was the Health Maintenance Organization Act of 1973. This expanded the original U.S. Public Health Service Act to provide more basic medical services such as home health services, laboratory and X-ray services, and others.

■ Unfortunately, an effect of the Health Maintenance Organization Act was to limit speech–language pathology and audiology service provision. Health maintenance organizations interpreted part of the act to mean that 2 months, or 60 days, was a maximum for provision of speech–language pathology services in health care settings.

Balanced Budget Act of 1997

■ Signed into legislation by President Clinton, the Balanced Budget Act of 1997 is having a strong impact on Medicare.

■ A key provision of this act is that there is an annual cap of $1,500 per beneficiary for the disciplines of physical therapy and speech–language pathology outpatient rehabilitation services. Beginning in the year 2002, the cap will be updated annually based on the Medicare economic index.

■ The cap took effect on January 1, 1999. It does not apply to outpatient hospital services.

Future Trends

Sweeping changes lie ahead for health care reform in the United States. These changes, which will impact speech–language pathology and audiology, may include but not be limited to:

■ the increasing role of states in national health care;

- increasing accountability and the need for documentation of treatment effectiveness, including outcome measurements (see below);

- a greater need to prove that treatment has a documented positive impact on patients' activities of daily living; and

- increased professional collaboration—for example, the creation of interdisciplinary networks and teams to serve the needs of patients.

Speech–language pathologists and audiologists will increasingly have to prove the efficacy of their service in terms of functional gains and documentable outcomes. ASHA is currently developing a *National Outcome Measurement System* (NOMS). Professionals in all settings nationwide will collect treatment outcome data that will be put into a national outcomes database. Clinicians will be able to access that database and use the treatment efficacy data therein to provide support and documentation for the services they are recommending and providing.

Summary

☑ State and federal legislation has a major impact on speech–language pathology and audiology services provided in public school, employment, and health care settings. Such legislation can expand or limit the services provided to clients with communicative disorders.

☑ Future trends impacting health care settings include increased accountability for documenting functional gains and providing measurable outcomes of services provided.

COUNSELING

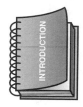

INTRODUCTION

Speech–language pathologists and audiologists frequently find themselves in a position where clients and families need help and support with emotional issues related to communicative disorders and their effects. This help and support can take place in the form of counseling. Counseling in the context of communicative disorders can be defined as creating an interpersonal, helping relationship whose goal is to support clients and families who experience emotional distress related to a communicative disorder. Families and clients who feel supported emotionally will frequently be more willing to cooperate with and carry out treatment recommendations. In many circumstances, speech–language

(continues)

pathologists and audiologists can successfully provide the support that clients and their families need.

However, speech–language pathologists and audiologists are not trained, qualified psychotherapists. It is imperative for professionals in communicative disorders to recognize their limitations and to be sensitive to when clients may need referrals to trained mental health professionals. Nevertheless, all speech–language pathologists and audiologists sometimes find themselves in situations where professionally appropriate counseling is needed as part of service provision. In this section, we discuss qualities needed to be effective in counseling activities, various counseling approaches, special issues in counseling, reactions and emotions related to communicative disorders, and potential defense mechanisms to be aware of when working with clients.

Qualities Necessary for Effective Counseling

- In order for speech–language pathologists and audiologists to be most effective in counseling activities, they should possess the following qualities (Shipley, 1997):

  - objectivity

  - competence and knowledge

  - honesty and openness

  - flexibility

  - empathy

  - trustworthiness

  - emotional stability

  - ability to motivate clients to take action

  - a nonjudgmental attitude

  - ability to be positive yet realistic

- While the adoption and application of all these qualities may seem like a tall order to many professionals, it must be remembered that acquiring these traits is a lifelong process. The most important thing is to be constantly aware of and continually working toward developing the qualities that make counseling and therefore treatment maximally effective for clients and their families.

Approaches to Counseling

There are different theories of counseling and providing help and support for others. Most speech–language pathologists and audiologists find the greatest success with directive, behavioral approaches to counseling, in which the focus is on the problem and action steps that can be taken to solve the problem. Nevertheless, it is important to be aware of other major approaches that have elements relevant to particular situations.

Psychodynamic Theory

- Based on psychoanalytic theory and created by Freud, this approach views behavior as the product of conflictual interaction between three systems: the id, ego, and superego. Anxiety is created when emotions arising from the conflicts among these three systems are repressed.

- Freud also discussed five psychosexual stages that develop from birth through adolescence. According to him, a healthy personality cannot develop without the successful resolution of each stage.

- Adults who have neuroses or problems can solve those problems through resolving difficulties that occurred during the development of one or more of the psychosexual stages.

- The purpose of psychoanalytic treatment is to make clients conscious of repressed issues and help them to resolve those issues so that the personality can be healthy and whole.

- The psychoanalytic approach to counseling is best undertaken by trained mental health professionals who understand it and believe in its efficacy. Use of the psychoanalytic approach is outside of the realm of communicative disorders professionals who are not specifically trained in its use and application.

Client-Centered Theory

- Also called the *person-centered theory*, this approach was created by Carl Rogers in the 1930s and 1940s. It was in large part a reaction to the rigidity of the psychoanalytic school of thought that predominated during those decades (Okun, 1992).

- According to this theory, clients need acceptance and positive unconditional regard in order to develop congruence between their self-concept and their behavior. The foundation of client-centered therapy is an empathic relationship between client and therapist that will allow the client to freely experience and express all his or her emotions in a completely accepting climate.

- In the nondirective client-centered approach, clients freely express their emotions while the clinician listens and responds to both the content and the feelings behind the words the client is saying. The clinician does not use specific techniques or recommend specific courses of action to change the client's behavior.

■ Proponents of the client-centered theory believe that the self-exploration and growth that occur in the nondirective, listening context make the client open to change. Eventually, the client is expected to take responsibility for determining goals and then to take action toward achieving those goals.

The process can be expressed thus:

▶ **Step 1**. The client is encouraged to freely express emotions. All these emotions are accepted and explored in a warm, empathetic climate of listening.

▶ **Step 2**. The clinician responds to both the content and the feelings of what the client expresses. Again, listening, not giving advice, is critical in this nondirective approach.

▶ **Step 3**. As a result of the warm, accepting relationship with the clinician, the client becomes open to change and self-growth.

▶ **Step 4**. This openness leads the client to take responsibility for determining goals and then to take action toward achieving those goals.

■ When confronted with emotional situations, many clinicians make the mistake of immediately trying to change clients' perceptions and behaviors by giving advice, information, and specific directions. But it is important for clinicians not to get clients back into a "cognitive role" prematurely (Fogle, 1998).

■ Instead, clinicians should first accept and acknowledge the feelings being expressed. For most clients, being understood and listened to is a critical, foundational first step, which precedes listening to advice and taking action to constructively change a situation (Luterman, 1996).

■ Many clinicians use elements of the client-centered theory in counseling clients with communicative disorders and their families. Elements of this approach can be helpful in the early stages of a clinician-client-family relationship, especially when the family is newly facing a major trauma with accompanying strong emotions such as shock and grief.

Behavioral Theory

■ A major influence in the development of behavioral theory was that scientists could not measure and document outcomes of the psychoanalytic and client-centered approaches to helping clients. Scientists wanted to measure the outcomes of helping approaches, based on quantifiable, objective, and observable behaviors (Okun, 1992).

■ Clinicians who use a behaviorist approach focus on what is observable, with an emphasis on environmental, external influences (Luterman, 1996). They believe that:

– all behavior is caused by environmental stimuli;

– human behavior is the product of external reinforcements;

- behavior is shaped and maintained by immediate consequences;

- reinforcement must be given immediately after a particular behavior has occurred; timing must be precise;

- positive reinforcement increases the chance that a behavior will reoccur;

- negative reinforcement, such as when a person's behavior causes an aversive stimulus to be removed, can also cause a behavior to reoccur;

- the reinforcement must be aversive enough or desirable enough to the client to cause a behavioral change; and

- behaviors that occur in the absence of reinforcement will be extinguished.

■ In the behavioral approach, clinicians focus on specific outcomes of counseling and interacting. Rather than discussing thoughts and feelings, clinicians emphasize clients' identifiable attitudes or behaviors and strive to make positive changes in those variables through the use of operant conditioning methods (reinforcement, punishment, and others).

■ Many speech–language pathologists and audiologists are comfortable with the behavioral approach because it:

- focuses specifically on areas that affect the client's communicative abilities;

- permits the creation of specific goals and objectives whose attainment can be objectively measured in a data-based manner;

- allows clinicians to measure the success of the counseling relationship; and

- allows for documentation of behavioral outcomes in a manner that is consistent with the demands of many of today's third-party payers, such as insurance companies.

■ Some experts believe that a strictly behavioral approach is limited in scope. According to Luterman (1996, p. 12) the behavioral approach leads to a "very narrow view of the clinician's role and responsibilities, reducing the clinical task to one of dispensing Fruit Loops."

■ Use of a behavioral approach may not be effective in the beginning of a client-clinician relationship, especially when there is an initial diagnosis of a communicative disorder, with accompanying strong emotions.

■ In such situations, a behavioral approach is most successful subsequent to a client-centered approach, which allows clients to express feelings first so that they may then focus on positive behavioral changes.

■ In all situations, it is the clinician's responsibility not only to listen empathetically but also to eventually provide specific guidance for behavioral changes that will make a measurable difference in clients' communication abilities.

Cognitive-Behavioral Theory

■ In this approach it is held that a client's *thoughts* are key to his or her feelings and actions. According to Albert Ellis, founder of the approach, the key variable is the *meaning* a person attributes to an event (Luterman, 1996).

■ The clinician helps the client focus on the problem, specifically identify the distorted thoughts or cognitions accompanying the problem, and replace the old distorted thoughts with newer, more rational thoughts that lead to behavioral changes. Clients are asked to assume responsibility for their behavior.

■ Proponents of the cognitive-behavioral theory believe that counseling is a three-step process:

 – Change the client's thinking ▶ change the belief system ▶ change the behavior

■ For example, a client with spasmodic dysphonia states that because of her voice, "Everyone looks down on me." She is resistant to therapy because of this belief, and is not making behavioral changes toward a better-sounding voice. Treatment is not succeeding. The clinician's job would be to:

 – *Help the client explore this thinking.* ("So you think that everyone looks down on you because of your voice. Does everyone look down on you, or just some people?")

 – *Challenge the client to test the validity of her old belief through experimentation.* ("When you go to the party tonight, observe people's reactions to you. Does everyone look down on you, or just some people?")

 – *Create a change in thinking through analyzing the data gathered through experimentation.* (Clinician: "What happened at the party?" Client: "Many people enjoyed talking to me at the party; several moved away and appeared uncomfortable.") Thus, after the party, the client and clinician would compare the client's old belief against the positive evidence gathered at the party.

 – *Create a change in behavior based on the new, positive evidence.* The clinician would use the positive evidence to motivate the client toward taking active steps to improve her voice through therapy techniques such as relaxation and easy onset.

■ The cognitive-behavioral approach thus explores discrepancies between a client's thoughts and reality, and helps the client to adopt a new set of thoughts or cognitions so that he or she can deal with the problem situation in a constructive way.

■ Many speech–language pathologists and audiologists are comfortable with the cognitive-behavioral approach and find it effective, because it deals with feelings and thoughts and helps the client change specific behaviors, which can then be directly measured and observed.

■ A limitation of the cognitive-behavioral approach is that it may, for certain clients, cut short the expression of legitimate strong emotions about a situation. Those emotions need expression and acknowledgment so that the counseling process can go forward (Luterman, 1996).

■ The cognitive-behavioral approach may be most helpful in dealing with adult clients who have such negative thoughts about their communicative disorder and its effects that treatment progress is hampered. If clinicians can help clients analyze, evaluate, and test their negative thoughts against reality, clients can move forward and take active steps to deal with their communicative disorder constructively.

Eclectic Approach

■ There are many other theories and approaches to counseling. However, most clinicians find that a combination of the client-centered, behavioral, and cognitive-behavioral approaches is most useful for providing help and support for clients.

■ Clients who are accepted and listened to nonjudgmentally, especially in the earliest stages of dealing with the impacts of a communicative disorder, become more ready to change their behaviors.

■ If feelings are accompanied by negative thoughts that are preventing progress, clinicians can deal with those thoughts openly and constructively through helping clients test the validity of the thoughts.

■ Finally, clinicians can recommend and help clients implement constructive behaviors that help them overcome the effects of the communicative disorder to the best of their potential. Those behaviors can be analyzed and measured so that both clients and clinicians can objectively, in a data-based manner, assess the progress being made.

Concepts To Consider

How do the client-centered, behavioral, and cognitive-behavioral theories of counseling differ from one another?

_____

_____

_____

_____

_____

_____

_____

_____

Special Issues in Counseling

Most speech–language pathologists and audiologists act in ways that are consistent with mainstream, Western beliefs. It is important, however, to be aware of the special, nonmainstream beliefs or practices that clients may bring to the counseling situation (Roseberry-McKibbin, 1997):

- *Gender* can influence a counseling relationship between a clinician and client. For example, in some cultural groups, a woman client may not be alone in a room with a male therapist. A male family member must be present at all times.

- *Age* is sometimes a factor in client-clinician relationships. Older people from some cultures might not respect a young clinician. Or, older patients might prefer to be referred to as "Mr." or "Mrs.," not by a first name as is common among younger Americans.

- *Culture* can influence counseling activities. In the United States, for example, open expression of emotion and directness of expression are encouraged. But indirectness is the norm in many cultures, and clients may be offended if a clinician is too frank or pushes them to be too emotive.

- *Time* can impact counseling with clients. In some cultures, being late is acceptable and common. In the United States, if clients are not prompt, professionals may be offended or angry. Clear communication about time expectations is needed.

- *Religion* can have an impact on the way families view services offered by communicative disorders professionals. Clients from some cultures, for example, believe in alternative methods of healing such as using herbs, massage, and religious rituals. Counseling clients to take advantage of therapy or rehabilitation opportunities might be unacceptable.

Reactions and Emotions Related to Communicative Disorders

Many clients and families experience strong emotions related to the communicative disorder and its effects, especially at the time of initial diagnosis. Clinicians should be able to recognize and deal with the following reactions:

■ *Shock and disbelief.* This is especially prevalent upon initial diagnosis of a communicative disorder. For example, a family who expected a healthy baby may undergo shock and disbelief when the doctor who delivers the baby reports that the infant has Down syndrome.

■ *Denial.* This can be seen when the client and/or family does not acknowledge the extent or implications of the communicative disorder—for example, when parents of a profoundly mentally retarded 5th grader continue to expect that he will be able to attend college someday. People who are in denial may become quite angry upon being confronted with reality. Clinicians must not take this personally, and must realize that acceptance is sometimes a long and multistage process.

■ *Anger.* This strong emotion can be composed of rage and hostility and actually be an attempt at self-protection. Clients and families may feel fear, powerlessness, and frustration; thus, anger ensues. This anger can be directed at the clinician and may even result in verbal abuse of the clinician.

■ *Grief.* This response involves sorrow and depression because of a loss, and it typically is experienced in stages. It is normal for clients and families to experience profound grief in response to diagnosis of a communicative disorder. Clinicians must allow clients to express their grief openly, for this will help clients move to a stage where they are ready to accept the situation and take constructive action.

■ *Guilt.* Sometimes clients and/or families believe that they have in some way caused or contributed to the communicative disorder; they blame themselves. They experience *personalization*, or the inappropriate assumption of responsibility for an event they did not cause. In addition, they may believe they are not "doing enough" to deal with the disorder. Clinicians need to gently and directly deal with guilt feelings expressed explicitly or implicitly, and allow open expression of those feelings. Giving information can be very helpful in alleviating feelings of guilt.

■ *Anxiety.* Clients may feel worry or apprehension because they are uncertain about a situation and its ramifications. Anxiety may be present throughout the therapeutic process and may arise in response to different situations (e.g., "How bad was my husband's stroke? The doctor didn't tell me anything." And later, "Will my husband be able to come home and go back to his job eventually?"). Clinicians can best deal with anxiety by encouraging open expression of questions and feelings, providing information and facts, and being willing to repeat information if it is not understood or heard the first time.

Defense Mechanisms

■ In order to deal with the strong emotions experienced in relation to communicative disorders, some clients and families may employ defense mechanisms.

■ Clients and/or their families who demonstrate prolonged use of one or more defense mechanism need to be served by professionals who are trained to deal with emotional issues. However, for many clients and family members, use of defense mechanisms is temporary and based upon the shock and trauma of dealing with a sudden blow, such as the diagnosis of a child with a severe disability or the profound changes brought about when a family member acquires a neurological problem.

■ Awareness of the defense mechanisms that clients and families may use can be most helpful to clinicians as they attempt to provide the most comprehensive and appropriate services possible. Common defense mechanisms include:

- *Rationalization.* In this form of resistance, the client provides a logical but untrue explanation of why something has occurred. For example, a client who stutters may explain away his lack of a social life by saying, "No one will talk to me because I stutter."

- *Reaction formation.* Clients who experience this have thoughts or emotions that are shocking and unacceptable to them; thus, they react with opposite emotions. For instance, the husband of an elderly Alzheimer's patient secretly wishes his wife would die. In reaction formation, he sacrifices all his own needs and wants to care for his wife, telling the clinician he loves his wife dearly and could not live without her.

- *Displacement.* The client takes his or her feelings of hostility or anger about a situation and transfers them to a safe object or person. For example, recently the first author was involved with parents who spent several hours blaming and castigating her for, among other things, stating in a report that their severely mentally retarded teenage daughter had "profound cognitive and linguistic delays."

- *Projection.* Clients attribute their own emotions, thoughts, or actions to someone else. For example, a mother told the first author that the school personnel who served her son never communicated with one another. The school personnel shared with the first author that this mother rarely communicated with school personnel, creating problems for everyone.

- *Repression.* Clients keep their thoughts and feelings under very strict control, out of view of others. Clients themselves are not aware of these thoughts and feelings, which are below the conscious level.

- *Suppression.* This is similar to repression. Clients keep their feelings and thoughts highly controlled, but they are consciously aware of those feelings. Suppression is the norm in some cultures. It should be viewed as a difference, not a defense mechanism, in those situations.

Summary

☑ Speech–language pathologists and audiologists sometimes have to deal with emotions that arise in response to communication disorders and their effects. Some situations require a referral to a trained mental health professional.

☑ In other situations, the clinician can successfully combine approaches to counseling to help clients and families take active steps to constructively deal with communicative disorders.

☑ Clinicians must be aware of phenomena that can impact counseling; these phenomena include special issues such as culture and gender, and clients' demonstration of emotional reactions and defense mechanisms. When clinicians are aware of and prepared for these phenomena, counseling and ultimately treatment efforts will prove much more successful.

MEDICAL SPEECH–LANGUAGE PATHOLOGY

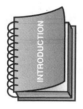

Thousands of speech–language pathologists work in a variety of medical settings. Those settings provide unique challenges and require a specific set of skills, which differ from those needed in other settings. As speech–language pathology becomes more and more specialized, clinicians need more in-depth knowledge about service to specific kinds of patients who are seen in medical settings. In this section, we discuss the scope of practice and responsibilities of clinicians in medical settings, medical team specialists and their roles, infectious disease control, patients with HIV and AIDS, and medical imaging techniques.

Practice and Responsibilities of Speech–Language Pathologists

In the majority of medical settings, speech–language pathologists carry out the following duties (Golper, 1997; Johnson & Jacobson, 1998):

■ *assessment and treatment of patients* in the areas of:

- mental or cognitive status (e.g., orientation, memory, attention)

- neurogenic speech and language disorders

- dysphagia

- voice disorders

- speech and resonance problems concomitant with or secondary to laryngeal, velopharyngeal, and/or oral surgery

- communication problems due to nonvocal, tracheostomized, and ventilator-dependent status

■ *participation on interdisciplinary teams*, including knowledge of the roles of each team member in the particular setting;

■ *staff education* (inservicing colleagues and other staff about various aspects of speech–language pathology);

■ *providing counseling and education* to families of patients, including facilitating interaction between the patient, family, and other team specialists;

■ *continuing education* (updating of one's own skills and competencies);

■ *participation in the medical facility's efforts to contain costs*;

■ *participation in the facility's internal and external reviews*, including providing a record of clinical activities and treatment efficacy;

■ *participation in quality management and quality assurance efforts* through monitoring and evaluating programs and resolving any problems in patient care, possibly including risk management, or identifying and reducing factors that put patients at risk in any way;

■ *securing reimbursements*, including documenting assessment findings and treatment progress for insurance companies as well as Medicaid and Medicare (Managed care companies, which provide health coverage at fixed costs, want to use facilities and providers that produce documented positive outcomes that directly impact patients' activities of daily living.);

■ *documentation of assessment and treatment activities*, often carried out through *SOAP notes*:

- S = *subjective* (observations such as the patient's complaint, what the examiner notices about the patient, e.g., patient says, "I'm always forgetful.")

- O = *objective* (examiner's objective findings, facts and data, e.g., "The patient was 90% accurate in defining 10 common words.")

- A = *assessment* (examiner's interpretation of findings, e.g., "Patient appears more oriented today.")

- P = *plan* (plans for treatment, steps taken or recommended, e.g., "Tomorrow we will begin left-right orientation.")

Medical Team Specialists and Their Roles

In every medical facility, the medical team specialists and their roles will be somewhat different. Speech–language pathologists tend to interact most with the following specialists, who usually perform the following services (Golper, 1997; Miller & Groher, 1990):

■ *Dieticians.* These nutrition specialists frequently interact with the medical team for patients with dysphagia. Clinicians consult often with dieticians about patients who need assistance with oral feeding.

■ *Infectious disease specialists.* These doctors are especially involved with patients who have AIDS and AIDS-related diseases; clinicians consult with them about patients who have speech, language, cognitive, and swallowing problems secondary to AIDS.

■ *Neurosurgeons.* These surgeons specialize in conducting surgery on the spinal cord, peripheral nerves, and brain; clinicians consult with them about speech-language disorders secondary to neurological problems.

■ *Nurses.* These specialists are directly involved in numerous aspects of patient care, and clinicians interact with them on almost a daily basis.

■ *Occupational therapists.* These specialists work with patients who need functional or adaptive restoration of upper-extremity disabilities. They may also help patients who have perceptual-motor and visual-perceptual disorders. Clinicians may work with them in providing assistance and adaptive devices for patients with dysphagia.

■ *Otolaryngologists or head and neck surgeons.* These doctors, who used to be called ear, nose, and throat (ENT) specialists, perform surgical services for patients with problems in the nasal, oral, laryngeal, pharyngeal, and esophageal structures. Clinicians consult with them about patients who have speech and swallowing problems.

■ *Pediatricians.* These physicians see children and youth (ages birth–21) who have medical diseases and developmental disorders. Pediatricians often refer to other specialists. Clinicians work with pediatricians regarding children who need early identification and treatment of communication disorders.

■ *Pharmacists.* These specialists dispense drugs. Clinicians work with pharmacists regarding patients whose medications may affect speech, language, cognition, and/or swallowing.

■ *Physical therapists.* These specialists carry out physical rehabilitation activities with patients who have physical disabilities due to disease or injury. Physical therapists help such patients to achieve adaptive and functional restoration of movement. Clinicians often work on rehabilitation teams with physical therapists.

■ *Plastic surgeons.* These surgeons provide reconstructive surgery to patients who have had parts or all of the mandible, maxilla, or tongue removed, for example, as well as patients who have velopharyngeal incompetence. Clinicians work with plastic surgeons in cases in which speech, resonance, or both are affected by the surgery.

■ *Prosthodontists*. These specialists construct prosthetic speech appliances for patients with such needs as obduration of clefts and fistulas and lifting of the velum for increased velopharyngeal closure, and patients who have had maxillary or mandibular surgery and need help in preserving their facial contours.

■ *Psychiatrists*. These doctors assess and treat patients with mental or emotional difficulties related to their medical problems. Treatment usually takes the form of psychotherapy, medication, or a combination of the two. Clinicians work with psychiatrists in cases in which patients have mental or emotional difficulties concurrent with a communication disorder.

■ *Pulmonary specialists*. These doctors manage patients with chronic and acute lung disorders. Clinicians may consult with them about patients who have speech, voice, and/or swallowing problems related to respiratory difficulties.

■ *Radiologists*. These doctors work with clinicians especially in dynamic evaluation of swallowing. Radiologists also carry out such diagnostic tests as magnetic resonance imaging (described later). Clinicians work with radiologists regarding patients who have swallowing problems and possible language and cognition problems secondary to diseases detectable through radiologic diagnostic tests.

■ *Social workers*. These professionals provide links between the hospital and the community, often helping meet patients' immediate social needs such as marital and psychological adjustments to disabilities, job placement, applying for benefits, obtaining family counseling, and others. Clinicians often work with social workers regarding patients and their families who have such social needs related to a communication disorder.

✎ Concepts To Consider

Summarize the role of speech–language pathologists in the medical setting. List four other medical team specialists that speech–language pathologists might interact with.

_____

_____

_____

_____

_____

_____

_____

Infectious Disease Control

Speech–language pathologists are increasingly serving in roles in which they come into contact with patients' bodily fluids: blood, saliva, mucous, and cerumen. Many clinicians have limited knowledge and use of appropriate procedures for avoiding infectious diseases. It is important for clinicians not to expose themselves—and thus others—to those diseases.

◼ Infections can have bacterial, viral, or fungal origins. Patients who may transmit infectious diseases to clinicians include but are not limited to those who:

  – are referred after head and neck surgeries;

  – are receiving dysphagia therapy;

  – have uncovered tracheostomies;

  – have HIV or AIDS;

  – are prone to bite clinicians (e.g., young children with behavior problems); and

  – are newborns who have infections acquired in utero or after birth.

◼ Medical facilities requiring the use of *universal precautions* require that all personnel who engage in patient contact must:

  – wear gowns if clothes are likely to become soiled;

  – wash hands before and after contact with patients;

  – put sharp instruments and disposable needles and syringes in a labeled "sharps" disposal container;

  – wear gloves if there is to be contact with broken skin, bodily fluids, or mucous membranes; and

  – protect the eyes and mouth if any splashes containing bodily fluid are likely.

◼ Hand washing should occur before and after patient contact, when coming on or off duty, after using the toilet, when the hands are dirty, and after wiping or blowing one's nose (Bleile, 1995). Hand washing should include the use of hot water, antibacterial soap, and paper towels. All areas of the hands and forearms should be washed for 1–2 minutes.

◼ Masks with clear plastic eye protectors should be worn when working with a patient who can transmit a disease through airborne means or through splashing; infections can enter through the eyes.

◼ Sterile gowns should be worn in surgery or when required by isolation precautions (those precautions are usually posted on the patient's door) (Golper, 1997).

■ Clinicians should use new gloves for each patient. Because latex and vinyl gloves are susceptible to tears and perforations, some clinicians wear two sets of gloves when working with especially high-risk patients.

■ Clinicians should take care to prevent bodily fluids (e.g., saliva) from contaminating things that cannot be disinfected (e.g., records, files).

■ It is wise to clean and disinfect all items and surfaces used if possible. This includes tables, equipment, toys, and other materials. Hospital supply stores often have powerful disinfectants that kill many microorganisms.

Working with HIV and AIDS Patients

■ Patients who are infected with the *human immunodeficiency virus* (HIV) experience depletions of *T lymphocytes*, a particular type of white blood cells. This eventually leads to extended, severe suppression of the immune system and consequent development of *acquired immune deficiency syndrome* (AIDS).

■ Patients may live for some years with a diagnosis of "HIV positive" before they develop AIDS. AIDS refers to the later stages of HIV infection. The immune system's failure predisposes the patient to the development of malignancies and severe, life-threatening infections (Vogel & Carter, 1995).

■ Many patients with AIDS experience their first symptoms in the head and neck (Benninger & Gardner, 1998). Patients with AIDS may have the following symptoms and communication problems (Benninger & Gardner, 1998; Golper, 1997; Hardman, Drew, & Egan, 1996; Vogel & Carter, 1995; Wallace, 1998):

  – AIDS dementia complex, with cognitive problems such as disorientation, confusion, loss of memory, loss of concentration

  – motor-speech impairment (e.g., dysarthria)

  – ataxia

  – dysphagia

  – articulation, swallowing, respiration, and voice problems due to candidiasis (yeast infections) that can occur in the mouth, esophagus, bronchial tubes, lungs, and trachea

  – apathy and social withdrawal

  – reduced verbal output

  – deterioration in handwriting

  – meningitis

  – encephalitis

- Kaposi's sarcoma (cancer that arises first in skin and then progressively affects other body sites, possibly including major organs)

- incontinence

- in children, hearing impairment secondary to middle ear disease

- in children, language delays, cognitive problems, and articulation disorders

■ Speech–language pathologists may serve patients with HIV or AIDS who have communication problems, swallowing problems, or both. Treatment may involve, among other things, the use of augmentative or alternative communication for patients who are deteriorating in speech, language, and/or cognitive function in the later stages of AIDS.

■ HIV has been found in certain human body tissues and in human excretions. When working with patients who are HIV positive or have AIDS, clinicians must be especially careful to observe universal precautions and to prevent transmission of the HIV virus.

Medical Imaging Techniques

While it is beyond the scope of this chapter to provide a detailed description of all available medical imaging techniques, we provide some basic definitions of imaging techniques that are commonly used with patients who have communication disorders. Speech–language pathologists who work in medical settings will encounter these techniques as used with patients, and should know the basics of what each involves (George, Vikingstad, & Cao, 1998; Golper, 1997; Nicolosi, Harryman, & Kresheck, 1996; Vogel & Carter, 1995):

■ *Tomography.* Also called *laminography*, this is a computerized radiographic method of taking pictures of different planes of body structures. It is used to scan brain structures, and is frequently used as a neurodiagnostic method for people with communication disorders such as aphasia secondary to stroke.

■ *Computerized axial tomography (CAT) scan* (also known as *CT scan* or *computed tomography*). In this radiographic imaging procedure, x- ray beams circle through segments of the brain and pass through tissue. A camera takes pictures of sections of the structure being scanned. The scanner detects density differences, and a computer analyzes the images generated by the scanning machine and produces pictures of the scanned structures. CAT scans can detect hemorrhages, lesions, tumors, and other pathologies. CAT scans are often used in the diagnosis of neuropathology associated with strokes.

■ *Electroencephalography (EEG).* This neurodiagnostic method records and measures electrical impulses of the brain through small surface electrodes attached to the scalp. EEG can show different kinds of brain waves associated with different kinds of activity (e.g., talking, listening, thinking). EEG indicates cerebral pathology by abnormal electrical activity and is often used to detect seizures.

■ *Magnetic resonance imaging (MRI)*. This neurodiagnostic imaging technique, in which the patient lies completely still in a cylinder container, is used to show fine detail in brain and spinal cord structure. MRI can also be used to provide images of the soft tissues, large blood vessels, and heart. The method is based on alignment and realignment of nuclei of atoms in the cell when a structure is placed in a strong magnetic field. Variations introduced in the amount of magnetic radiation will cause alignment and realignment of nuclei. Such changes produce electromagnetic signals, which a computer analyzes to produce images of the structure. MRI does not use x-rays and provides higher-resolution images than CAT scans, sometimes detecting lesions missed by CAT scans. However, MRI is expensive, and patients may have difficulty tolerating it.

■ *Positron emission tomography (PET)*. This neurodiagnostic procedure is a type of emission-computed tomography that allows imaging of metabolic activity through measurements of radioactivity in the section of the body being viewed (e.g., the brain). The patient is injected with a radioactive substance that spreads throughout the brain; the amount of radioactivity is then scanned, and observed differences in the amount of radioactivity suggest different rates of cerebral metabolism. Lower than normal metabolic rate suggests neuropathology. If the patient is suspected of having cerebral dysfunction secondary to a stroke, for example, PET scans can be helpful by evaluating the *function* of blood flow and brain metabolism (whereas CAT and MRI scans evaluate only *structure*).

■ *Single-photon emission computed tomography (SPECT)*. This neurodiagnostic procedure evaluates the amount of blood flowing through a structure. Also known as *regional cerebral bloodflow (rCBF)*, SPECT helps assess cerebral metabolism. The patient inhales xenon 133, a radioactive gas that immediately spreads throughout the cerebral hemispheres and enters the bloodstream. A scanner detects radiation uptake in cerebral blood, and a computer calculates the amount of blood flow in given regions and displays variations in blood flow with different colors. SPECT is helpful in diagnosing cerebral lesions associated with various neuropathologies causing communication disorders.

■ *Videofluoroscopy*. This is a radiologic method of examining movement of internal structures and recording the movement patterns for assessment and diagnosis. It is useful in assessing the functions of the velopharyngeal mechanism, vocal folds, swallowing, and respiratory movement. X-rays are transmitted through the tissue under observation; the soft tissue is coated with barium with the help of a nasal spray, and observers can have multiple views of the structures (e.g., frontal, lateral, base, and oblique views of the velopharyngeal mechanism) and their movements. The images are shown on a phosphorescent screen and recorded on a videotape for later examination and diagnosis.

Videofluoroscopy is often used to assess swallowing function in patients with confirmed or suspected dysphagia.

Summary

☑ Clinicians who work in medical settings have specific responsibilities related to assessment and treatment of patients, as well as participation in professional and institutional activities.

☑ Speech–language pathologists work on interdisciplinary teams whose members have specific roles, which differ slightly from setting to setting. As part of their jobs in medical settings, clinicians must rigorously practice infectious disease control measures, particularly when working with patients who are HIV positive or have AIDS.

☑ Some patients are assessed with specialized imaging techniques, and clinicians will often get medical reports that discuss findings of such procedures as CAT scans, videofluoroscopy, and others.

☑ When working with patients and with other medical professionals, clinicians should be familiar with imaging procedures as well as with their common abbreviations that are used in charts in medical settings.

CRANIOFACIAL ANOMALIES AND GENETIC SYNDROMES

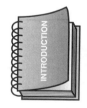

INTRODUCTION

Craniofacial anomalies, mostly due to genetic factors, create many clinical conditions and syndromes, some of which are associated with communicative disorders. In this section, major craniofacial anomalies including clefts of the lip and palate and some major genetic syndromes that are associated with communicative disorders are reviewed.

Craniofacial Anomalies

■ Craniofacial anomalies are abnormalities of the structures of the head and face. These abnormalities are congenital and in many cases due to genetic factors.

■ A variety of factors have been demonstrated or hypothesized to cause craniofacial anomalies. Clefts of the lip and the soft palate are better known to speech–language pathologists, but there are literally hundreds of genetic syndromes with craniofacial anomalies that are associated with communicative disorders (Bzoch, 1997; Jung, 1989; McWilliams, Morris, & Shelton, 1990; Shprintzen & Bardach, 1995; Shprintzen, 1997).

■ Selected syndromes with significant association with communicative disorders are summarized in a later section of this chapter.

Cleft Lip

■ A *cleft* is an opening in a normally closed structure. Cleft lip, therefore, is an opening in the lip, usually the upper lip. Lower lip clefting is very rare. Clefts of the lips alone are rare; they are usually associated with cleft of the palate.

■ However, clefts of the palate are often not associated with cleft lips. Clefting is a congenital disorder; it is present at the time of birth. A congenital disorder may or may not be inherited (Bzoch, 1997; Jung, 1989; McWilliams et al., 1990; Shprintzen & Bardach, 1995; Shprintzen, 1997).

■ Cleft lips are more often unilateral than bilateral, and they occur more frequently on the left side than on the right side. Rare bilateral lip clefts have an even greater tendency to coexist with palatal clefts than unilateral left lip clefts do.

■ Cleft lips alone rarely result in speech disorders and are less frequently associated with other genetic anomalies than palatal clefts (Shprintzen & Bardach, 1995).

Cleft Palate

General Facts

■ *Palatal clefts* are various congenital malformations resulting in an opening in the hard palate, the soft palate, or both. These malformations are due to disruptions of the embryonic growth processes resulting in a failure to fuse structures that are normally fused.

■ Cleft palates may be a part of a genetic syndrome with other anomalies. It is now believed that clefting of the lip and palate is etiologically different from clefting of the palate only (Shprintzen & Bardach, 1995).

■ The incidence of palatal clefts in different populations vary. In the U.S. population, about 1 in 600 to 750 live births may be diagnosed with clefting. The highest to the lowest incidence rates are found among Native Americans, Japanese, Chinese, Whites, and African Americans, in that order.

■ Generally, males tend to exhibit a higher frequency and greater severity of cleft lip (with or without cleft palate) than females, who tend to exhibit higher frequency of palatal clefts (without the cleft lip).

Overview of the Embryonic Growth of the Facial Structures

The most crucial period for genetic malformations is the embryonic period, which consists of the first 7 to 10 weeks of gestation. Most new organs emerge in the embryonic period. The 4th to the 6th week of pregnancy poses the greatest threat of embryonic disruptions, as it is the most sensitive period of growth. This period is characterized by:

■ Multiplication of embryonic cells during the first few weeks.

■ Development of three layers of cells from which different organs emerge.

■ Development of a marked bend in the top portion of the embryo, creating a bulge that becomes the primitive forebrain by the end of the 3rd week.

■ Development of a groove known as the *stomodeum*, which is the primitive mouth and nose.

■ Development of the *frontonasal process*, which develops into the nose, the central part of the upper lip, and the primary palate.

■ Development of two *maxillary processes*, which form most of the face, mouth, cheeks, and the sides of the upper lip; most of the hard palate; the alveolar ridge; and the soft palate.

■ Development of the *upper lip* and the *primary palate* (by the end of the 7th week). The upper lip does not develop as a single structure, hence it is prone to clefting. The nose and the midline of the upper lip are formed out of one structure, and the two sides of the lip are formed out of another structure. As a result, the cleft of the lip typically appears at either the right or the left side of the nose.

■ Development of the two *mandibular processes*, giving rise to the lower jaw (mandible), lower lip, and chin; these are formed and fused by the end of the 4th or 5th week.

■ Development of the mandible, which moves to a lower and more normal position.

■ Growth of the tongue, which initially lies higher, at the level of the nose; it drops down to its normal position when the jaw develops.

■ Growth of the hard and the soft palates; this growth is identifiable at the 5th week of gestation. The two shelves of the maxillary bone that form the hard palate remain in a vertical position, on either side of the high-placed embryonic tongue; when the tongue drops, the palatal shelves move in an upward and lateral manner and toward each other to form the roof of the mouth.

■ *Fusion* of the two shelves of the hard palate at the midline between the 8th and 9th weeks; this is a front-to-back fusion, a fact reflected in the clefting process. Also, fusion of the maxillary shelves with the triangular premaxillary bone (the primary palate) occurs, thus separating the mouth from the nose.

■ Growth of the muscles of the soft palate, initially as two separate halves. Palatal bones, as they move toward the midline, also bring the two halves of the soft palate together. By the 12th week, the muscle mass from the two sides fuses to form the soft palate.

✎ Concepts To Consider

Describe three critical anatomical structures that must develop intactly when a baby is in utero in order for the lip and palate to be normal. Which are the most critical weeks of gestation for the development of these structures?

_____

_____

_____

_____

_____

_____

_____

Etiology of Clefts

Clefts are related to a variety of genetic, chromosomal, environmental, and mechanical factors. Some of the more common factors are as follows.

Genetic Abnormalities

■ autosomal dominant inheritance in some syndromes (e.g., Apert syndrome, Stickler syndrome, van der Wude syndrome, Waardenburg syndrome, and Treacher Collins syndrome);

■ recessive genetic inheritance in some syndromes (e.g., orofacial-digital syndrome);

■ x-linked inheritance in some syndromes (e.g., oto-palatal-digital syndrome); and

■ chromosomal abnormalities (e.g., Trisomy 13).

Environmental Teratogenic Factors

The following are external factors that affect the genetic material:

■ fetal alcohol syndrome

■ illegal drug use

- side effects of certain prescription drugs (e.g., anticonvulsant drugs and thalidomide, a sedative)

- rubella

Mechanical Factors

- intrauterine crowding

- twinning

- uterine tumor

- amniotic ruptures

Classification of Clefts

- Clefts are classified in different ways. No system of classification captures the variations and combinations found in clefts. Therefore, none is universally accepted. Clefts vary in extent, often measured in thirds (⅓, ⅔, or ⅗) and widths.

- The major types of clefts include the following:

    - cleft lip (complete or incomplete, unilateral or bilateral);

    - cleft of alveolar process (unilateral, bilateral, median, or submucous);

    - cleft of prepalate (combination of previous types with or without prepalate protrusion or rotation);

    - cleft of the palate (of the soft palate, of the hard palate, or submucous);

    - cleft of prepalate and palate (any combination of clefts of the prepalate and palate); and

    - facial clefts other than prepalate and palate (e.g., such rare forms as horizontal clefts, lower mandibular clefts, lateral oro-ocular clefts, and naso-ocular clefts).

- Children might also manifest *microforms*, which are minimal expressions of clefts, including a hairline indentation of the lip or just a notch on the lip. Microforms are revealed only through laminographic examination.

- Microforms include *submucous clefts* (also called *occult cleft palate*), in which the surface tissues of the soft or hard palate fuse but the underlying muscle or bone tissues do not (Nicolosi et al., 1996).

Congenital Palatopharyngeal Incompetence

- Congenital palatopharyngeal incompetence (CPI) is not a form of cleft, but a related disorder. It refers to impaired velopharyngeal closing-valve functioning.

■ CPI is characterized by significant impairment of velopharyngeal functions as revealed by videofluoroscopy or endoscopy (inadequate velopharyngeal closure), although the laryngeal structures appear normal.

■ CPI may be caused by a short palate, reduced muscular mass of the soft palate, a deep or enlarged larynx, incorrect insertion of levator muscles (insertion to hard palate instead of the normal insertion to soft palate), or a combination of such factors.

■ People with CPI typically have hypernasal speech, which ranges in nature from mild to severe.

Communication Disorders Associated with Clefts

Hearing Loss

■ Children with clefts are prone to middle ear infections and hearing loss.

■ Eustachian tube dysfunction is also prevalent in children with clefts. This creates conditions conducive to conductive hearing loss especially.

Articulation Disorders

Articulation disorders are more significant if the palatal cleft is not repaired early or the repair is inadequate. Articulation disorders include errors such as those described below:

■ greater difficulty with unvoiced sounds than with voiced sounds, pressure consonants, audible or inaudible nasal air emission, and distortion of vowels; and

■ compensatory errors including various types of substitutions that help compensate for the inadequate closure of the velopharyngeal mechanism, such as substitutions of stops, fricatives, and affricates with unusual (often posterior) movements and posture of the tongue to stop the air or to produce friction noise (e.g., substitution of glottal stops for stop consonants, substitution of laryngeal fricatives for fricatives, and substitution of pharyngeal affricates for affricates).

Language Disorders

Language disorders may not be as significant as articulation disorders unless other conditions are associated; language may be normal in many cases. Common problems include:

■ initially delayed language development, with significant improvement as the child grows older; normal language possible by age 4 or so;

■ significant language disorders in children whose clefts are a part of genetic syndromes that include hearing loss, developmental disabilities, sensory problems, and so forth; and

■ relatively normal receptive language skills, with delays in expressive language.

Laryngeal and Phonatory Disorders

Children with palatal clefts tend to exhibit a higher prevalence of laryngeal and vocal disorders, which may include:

- vocal nodules;

- hypertrophy and edema of the vocal folds;

- vocal hoarseness, reduced vocal intensity, reduced pitch variations, and strangled voice; and

- Resonance disorders characterized by hypernasality, hyponasality, denasality, or a combination.

Assessment of Children with Clefts

Assessment of children with cleft palate includes all the standard procedures (e.g., case history, interview of the parents and the child if appropriate). The main concern is to assess speech sound production and velopharyngeal adequacy. It is also important to screen hearing and assess language.

Assessment of Velopharyngeal Incompetence

- The procedures include judgments about hypernasality and hyponasality, whose presence indicate velopharyngeal inadequacy.

- Objective assessment of the velopharyngeal mechanism includes an endoscopic examination of the velopharyngeal mechanism (*nasopharyngoscopy*). In naso-pharyngoscopy, the nasopharyngoscope is passed through the middle meatus and back to the area of velopharyngeal closure. The examiner can then observe the posterior and lateral pharyngeal walls, as well as the nasal aspect of the velum and the adenoid pad as the client produces sentences (Kummer & Marsh, 1998).

- Objective assessment also includes a videofluoroscopic examination of the velopharyngeal mechanism to observe the movements of the soft palate, the lateral pharyngeal wall, the posterior pharyngeal wall, and the tongue as the client produces consonant-vowel combinations, voiced and voiceless frica-tives, and selected phrases.

- Assessment includes an orofacial examination to take note of the clefts in the lip, the hard palate, and the soft palate as well as adequacy of the surgical repair of the cleft, facial abnormalities indicative of a genetic syndrome, and the velopharyngeal mechanism.

Assessment of Articulation Disorders

- Assessment of articulation and phonological disorders in children with clefts includes standard procedures used in assessing similar disorders in children without clefts.

■ However, special considerations are given to assess the kinds of errors and compensatory error patterns that are typical of children with cleft palates (e.g., pressure consonants).

■ Many clinicians administer the *Iowa Pressure Articulation Test* (a subtest of the *Templin Darley Test of Articulation*) as well as other standardized tests of articulation and phonological skills.

Assessment of Language Disorders

■ Assessing language disorders in children with clefts includes standard procedures used in assessing both language comprehension and production.

■ It is important to gather a comprehensive language sample to analyze the use of semantic, syntactic, morphologic, and pragmatic use of language.

Assessment of Phonatory Disorders

■ Assessing phonatory disorders in children with clefts includes standard procedures used in assessing voice disorders in children with no clefts.

■ The clinician makes clinical judgments about voice quality deviations (e.g., hoarseness, harshness, breathiness).

■ He or she also assesses vocally abusive behaviors, evaluates pitch and loudness of voice, and may conduct an instrumental assessment of voice disorders (e.g., with the use of Visi-Pitch or the Phonatory Function Analyzer).

Assessment of Resonance Disorders

■ This includes assessing hypernasality in conversational speech by making clinical judgments.

■ Rating of hypernasality in connected speech by two or more clinicians may also take place, and assessing hyponasality may be necessary.

Treatment of Children with Clefts

Treatment of children with clefts is a team effort involving several specialists including oral surgeons, pediatricians, orthodontists, otolaryngologists, psychologists, and speech–language pathologists. Often, the surgical repair of the palate is the major initial treatment implemented (Bzoch, 1997; Hegde, 1996b; McWilliams et al., 1990; Shprintzen & Bardach, 1995).

Surgical Management of the Clefts

■ *Primary surgery for the clefts* is the initial surgery, in which the clefts are closed.

■ *Secondary surgeries for clefts* are done to improve appearance and functioning, after the initial closure of the clefts.

■ *Lip surgery* is done to close unilateral or bilateral clefts of the lip; this is typically done when the baby is about 3 months old or weighs about 10 pounds.

■ *Palatal surgery* is done to close the cleft or clefts of the palate; this is typically done when the baby is between 9 and 24 months.

■ *V-Y Retroposition* or the *Veau-Wardill-Kilner* method of surgery is done to repair the cleft of the palate; single-based flaps of palatal mucoperiosteum are raised on either side of the cleft and brought together and pushed back to close the cleft; this push back (retropositioning of the flaps) lengthens the palate and improves chances of velopharyngeal approximation.

■ The *von Langenbeck surgical method* is performed to repair the cleft of the palate by raising two bipedicled (attached on both ends) flaps of mucoperiosteum, bringing them together and attaching them to close the cleft; this leaves denuded bone on either side and does not lengthen the palate.

■ *Delayed hard palate closure* is a surgical procedure in which the cleft of the soft palate is closed first, and the cleft of the hard palate is closed later.

■ *Pharyngeal flap* is a secondary palatal surgical procedure in which a muscular flap is cut from the posterior pharyngeal wall, raised, and attached to the velum; the openings on either side of the flap allow for nasal breathing, nasal drainage, and production of nasal speech sounds. The flap helps close the velopharyngeal port and thus reduce hypernasality.

■ *Pharyngoplasty* is another surgical procedure in which such substances as Teflon, silicone, dacron wool/silicone gel bag, and cartilage may be implanted or injected into the posterior pharyngeal wall to make it bulge and thus help close the velopharyngeal port.

Treatment of Articulation and Phonological Disorders

■ Treatment is sequenced from sounds, syllables, words, phrases, and sentences, in that order.

■ More visible sounds are taught before less visible sounds except for the linguadentals.

■ Stops and fricatives are taught before other classes of sounds.

■ Training on /k/ and /g/ may be inappropriate if the velopharyngeal functioning is inadequate.

■ If stimulable, fricatives, affricates, or both may be trained; in any case, they may be trained after stops are mastered.

■ Linguapalatal sounds, lingua-alveolars, and linguadentals should be taught, in that order.

■ Frequent presentation of auditory and visual cues and modeling may be helpful.

■ Compensatory articulatory positioning, where appropriate, may be taught.

■ The clinician may teach the child to avoid posterior articulatory placements and to articulate with less effort and facial grimacing.

■ Tactile cues and instruction to improve tongue positioning may be useful.

Treatment of Language Disorders

■ Early language stimulation by parents is needed in some cases.

■ When necessary, formal language treatment may be offered if language stimulation is not sufficient.

■ It may be especially important to stimulate expressive language, as it tends to be more delayed than receptive language.

Treatment for Resonance Disorders

■ Hypernasality due to velopharyngeal incompetence should not be treated until: (a) there are surgical or prosthetic efforts to improve the physiological functioning, and (b) the child is capable of velopharyngeal closure but is using previously established inappropriate compensatory articulation that can be modified.

■ Voice therapy techniques designed to reduce hypernasality can be used (e.g., increased loudness, discrimination training to distinguish oral and nasal resonance, lowered pitch, encouragement of increasing oral opening).

■ It is often helpful to teach the child to decrease intra-oral breath pressure on stop consonants and fricatives, while simultaneously using loose articulatory contacts.

■ Biofeedback instruments (e.g., Tonar II) to reduce hypernasality may also be useful.

✎ Concepts To Consider

Treatment for children with cleft palates can be surgical or traditional/therapy-based. Summarize two surgical and two traditional/therapy-based treatment methods.

_____

_____

_____

_____

_____

_____

Genetic Syndromes

- A *syndrome* is a constellation of signs and symptoms that are associated with a morbid process; a genetic syndrome is such a constellation with a known genetic basis.

- Many genetic syndromes are associated with communication disorders. Syndromes that involve the craniofacial complex and those that affect general intellectual functions tend to produce the most significant effects on communication (Jung, 1989; Shprintzen, 1997). Some of the most common syndromes that affect communication include the following (Hegde, 1996a):

Apert Syndrome

- This may be caused by spontaneous autosomal dominant mutations. Its transmission is limited because of low reproductive capacity of affected people.

- Its physical characteristics include syndactyly (digital fusion) involving the second, third, and fourth digits, cranial synostosis resulting in smaller anterior-posterior skull diameter, flat frontal and occipital bones and high forehead, increased intracranial pressure and compensatory growth in cranial structures.

- Other physical characteristics include midfacial hypoplasia (underdevelopment), an arched and grooved hard palate, conductive hearing loss in some individuals, class III malocclusion, irregularly placed teeth, thickened alveolar process, long or thickened soft palate, and cleft of the hard palate in 25–30% of cases.

- Communication problems include a tendency toward hyponasality, forward carriage of the tongue, and articulation disorders involving mostly alveolar consonants (e.g., /s/ and /z/) and labial dental sounds (e.g., /f/ and /v/). There may also be deficiency in language skills depending on the level of intellectual function and hearing.

Cri du Chat Syndrome

- This is caused by an absence of the short arm of the fifth chromosome (known as 5p). Its physical characteristics include a cry resembling that of a cat (hence the name) in the infant.

- Other physical characteristics include low-set ears, a narrow oral cavity, and laryngeal hypoplasia.

- Communication problems include articulation and language disorders typically associated with mental retardation.

Crouzon Syndrome

- This is caused by autosomal dominant inheritance, with varied expression in individuals. Its physical characteristics include *craniosynostosis* (fusion of the cranial suture, especially that of the coronal) and hypoplasia of the midface, maxilla, or both.

- Other physical characteristics include a small maxillary structure, sphenoethmoidal synchondroses, ocular *hypertelorism* (eyes that are far apart), a parrotlike nose, facial asymmetry and tall forehead, malocclusion Class III in some cases, a highly arched palate, shallow oropharynx, a long and thick soft palate, and *brachycephaly* (short head).

- Communication problems include conductive hearing loss in some individuals, articulation disorders associated with hearing loss and abnormalities of palatal oral cavity structures, hyponasality, and language disorders in the cases with hearing loss and cognitive deficits.

Down Syndrome

- This is caused by an extra whole number chromosome 21, resulting in 47, rather than the normal 46 chromosomes. Physical characteristics include generalized hypotonia; a flat facial profile; small ears, nose, and chin; and brachycephaly.

- Other physical characteristics include midface dysplasia, shortened oral and pharyngeal structures, a narrow and high arched palate, a relatively large and fissured tongue that tends to protrude, a short neck with excess skin on the back of it, hyperflexible joints, cardiac malformations in about 40% of cases, and short fingers.

- Communication problems include conductive loss in many cases and sensorineural loss in some. There may be language delays and disorders, especially deficient syntactic and morphologic features accompanied by relatively better vocabulary skills. Hypernasality and nasal emission, breathier voice, and articulation disorders may also be present.

Fragile X Syndrome

- This is caused by a fragile site on the long arm of the X chromosome. The syndrome is more severe in the male than in the female.

- Physical characteristics include a large, long, and poorly formed pinna, a big jaw, enlarged testes, and a high forehead.

■ Communication problems include jargon, perseveration, echolalia, inappropriate language or talking to oneself (more often in the male), lack of gestures and other nonverbal means of communication that normally accompany speech, voice problems, and articulation disorders.

Moebius Syndrome

■ This has a heterogeneous causation including agenesis or aplasia of the motor nuclei of the cranial nerves. There is sporadic, unpredictable occurrence in most cases and autosomal dominant inheritance in some cases.

■ Its physical characteristics include involvement of facial and hypoglossal nerves in most and of the trigeminal nerve in some cases.

■ There is also bilabial paresis and weak tongue control for lateralization, elevation, depression, and protrusion, unilateral or bilateral paralysis of the abductors of the eye, limited strength, range, and speed of movement of articulators, feeding problems in infancy, and a masklike face.

■ Communication problems include conductive hearing loss in only a few cases and delayed language in some cases, especially in children with frequent hospitalizations. There may also be articulation disorders ranging from mild to severe, with bilabial, linguadental, and lingua-alveolar sounds affected more than the others.

Pierre-Robin Syndrome

■ This is caused by autosomal recessive inheritance in most cases. In some cases, this syndrome may be a part of Stickler syndrome, in which case autosomal dominant inheritance may be the genetic basis.

■ Its physical characteristics include mandibular hypoplasia, *glossoptosis* (downward displacement of the tongue), a cleft of the soft palate (but typically not associated with cleft of the lips), velopharyngeal incompetence, a deformed pinna and low-set ears, and temporal bone and ossicular chain deformities.

■ Its communication problems include unilateral or bilateral conductive hearing loss associated with otitis media and cleft palate, delayed language and language disorders, hypernasality and nasal emission, articulation disorders, and hypercompensatory articulation.

Prader-Willi Syndrome

■ This is suspected to be caused by autosomal dominant inheritance and deletion in the region of the long arm of chromosome 15 (15q11-15q13) in some cases.

■ Its physical characteristics include low muscle tone, early feeding difficulties, failure to thrive initially, obesity after the first year, excessive eating, and underdeveloped genitals.

■ Communication problems include language disorders, mild to severe articulation problems, and nasal air emission.

✎ Concepts To Consider

Many syndromes are associated with speech-language problems. Describe two of these syndromes and their associated speech-language difficulties.

_____

_____

_____

_____

_____

_____

_____

Russell-Silver Syndrome

■ This is suspected to be caused by genetic factors, although information about etiology is very scarce. Babies with Russell-Silver syndrome have low birth weight, are small for their gestational age, and are considered to have dwarfism.

■ Physical characteristics include asymmetry of the arms and/or legs, a disproportionately large head, craniofacial disproportion, mandibular hypoplasia, a high, narrow palate, and *microdontia* (abnormal smallness of the teeth).

■ Communication problems often include hypernasality, feeding problems in infancy, articulation disorders, expressive and receptive language disorders, and an abnormally high-pitched voice (Buckholz & Roseberry-McKibbin, 1997).

Treacher Collins Syndrome

■ This is caused by autosomal dominant inheritance in most cases and spontaneous mutation in some. Its physical characteristics include underdeveloped facial bones including mandibular hypoplasia (small chin) and malar (cheek) hypoplasia, dental malocclusion and hypoplasia, and downwardly slanted palpebral fissures.

■ Other characteristics include *coloboma* (lesion or defect, usually a cleft) of the lower eyelid, stenosis or atresia of the external auditory canal, malformations of the pinna, and middle and inner ear malformations.

■ There is usually a high hard palate, a cleft palate in about 30% of the cases, a submucous cleft in some cases, a short or immobile soft palate, and sucking and swallowing problems in infancy.

■ Communication problems include congenital, bilateral, conductive hearing loss in many cases and sensorineural loss in some cases as well as language disorders typically associated with hearing impairment.

■ Other communication problems include hypernasality and nasal emission in cases with clefts and velopharyngeal incompetence, as well as articulation disorders consistent with hearing loss and gross oral structural deviations.

Turner Syndrome

■ This occurs only in the female and is caused by a missing or deformed X chromosome in most cases. A similar syndrome that occurs in both males and females is called *Noonan syndrome.*

■ Its physical characteristics include ovarian abnormality resulting in absence of menstruation and infertility, congenital swelling of the feet, neck, and hands, cardiac defects, webbing of the neck (excess skin over the neck), and a low posterior hairline.

■ Other physical characteristics include a broad chest with widely spaced nipples, *cubitus valgas* (elbows bent outward or away from the midline), pigmented skin lesions, a narrow maxilla and palate, and *micrognathia* (abnormally small lower jaw).

■ Further physical characteristics include anomalies of the auricle including low-set, elongated, and cup-shaped ears, thick earlobes, a high arched palate, a cleft palate in some cases, and evidence of right hemisphere dysfunction.

■ Communication problems include sensorineural loss in many cases (usually noticed after the 10th year); middle ear infections during infancy and early childhood; conductive loss in some cases; language and articulation disorders consistent with hearing impairment; and visual, spatial, and attentional problems.

Usher Syndrome

■ This is caused by autosomal recessive inheritance in most cases and is X-linked in rare cases. This syndrome may affect 50% of individuals who are deaf and blind.

■ Its physical characteristics include night blindness in early childhood, limited peripheral vision as visual problems worsen, eventual blindness, and cochlear abnormalities.

■ Communication problems include sensorineural loss, language and articulation disorders consistent with hearing impairment, and hypernasality and nasal emission.

Summary

☑ Craniofacial anomalies such as cleft lip and palate are due mostly to genetic factors, although environmental and mechanical factors may also play a role.

☑ People with clefts of the palate have communication disorders associated with those clefts; the disorders include hearing loss and disorders of language, articulation, resonance, and voice.

☑ When assessing children with clefts, it is important to assess velopharyngeal incompetence as well as articulation, language, phonatory, and resonance disorders.

☑ Treatment of children with clefts usually consists of surgical management combined with treatment of disorders of language, articulation, resonance, and voice.

☑ Many genetic syndromes are associated with communication disorders. Those syndromes often cause disorders of articulation, language, voice, and resonance.

CHAPTER HIGHLIGHTS

▶ The American-Speech-Language-Hearing Association (ASHA) is a national, professional and scientific organization that regulates quality of service provision, promotes relevant legislation, encourages research, and promotes exchange of information. Most speech–language pathologists and audiologists are members of ASHA.

▶ ASHA awards specific, national certification when its members meet certain requirements. Many states also have credentialing and licensing requirements that clinicians must meet, depending upon the professional setting.

▶ State and federal laws regulate service provision in public schools, employment settings, and health care settings. All communicative disorders professionals and clients are impacted by those laws, which are primarily influenced by the availability of funding.

(continues)

▶ Because of legislation and resulting budget cuts, provision of speech–language pathology and audiology services is often curtailed in many settings. Clinicians increasingly need to make the public aware of the communicative professions and the services offered. This can be done through marketing research and advertising. ASHA provides educational opportunities to teach its members about those areas.

▶ Clients and their families sometimes experience emotional reactions related to communicative disorders and their effects. Clinicians can make referrals to mental health professionals when it is warranted. In many cases, however, clinicians can provide the support and release families need.

▶ Various approaches to counseling (the client-centered, behavioral, and cognitive-behavioral approaches) can be combined to provide the most appropriate support for the stage that clients and families are currently in. Special issues can make counseling challenging. Those issues include culture, gender, and age of clients and clinicians. Clients may also demonstrate emotional reactions and defense mechanisms during counseling situations. Clinicians who are aware of and prepared for these special issues are generally successful in dealing with them.

▶ Speech–language pathologists sometimes work in medical settings, where they have a wide scope of professional responsibilities. They work on interdisciplinary teams that may consist of dieticians, infectious disease specialists, neurosurgeons, nurses, occupational therapists, otolaryngologists or head and neck surgeons, pediatricians, pharmacists, physical therapists, plastic surgeons, prosthodontists, psychiatrists, pulmonary specialists, radiologists, and social workers.

▶ Speech–language pathologists sometimes work with patients who may transmit infectious diseases through the bodily fluids of blood, cerumen, mucous, and saliva. It is important to take precautions when serving those patients, some of whom are HIV positive or have AIDS.

▶ Many medical settings use special imaging techniques to diagnose a variety of problems and diseases. Those techniques include computerized axial tomography, electroencephalography, fluoroscopy, magnetic resonance imaging, and positron emission tomography.

▶ Speech–language pathologists sometimes deal with clients who have craniofacial anomalies associated with clinical conditions and syndromes. Some clients have a cleft lip and/or palate. Others have a specific syndrome associated with disorders of language, articulation, voice, and/or resonance. Assessment and treatment may involve traditional methods as well as surgical intervention.

(continues)

▶ Add your own chapter highlights here:

_____

_____

_____

_____

KEY TERMS

acquired immune deficiency syndrome (AIDS)
Alport syndrome
American Speech-Language-Hearing Association
Americans with Disabilities Act
anger
anxiety
Apert syndrome
Au.D.
audiologist
behavioral theory
Certificate of Clinical Competence
cleft lip
cleft palate
client-centered theory
"Code of Ethics"
cognitive-behavioral theory
computerized axial tomography
congenital palatopharyngeal incompetence (CPI)
consumer
counseling
craniofacial anomalies
credential

cri du chat syndrome
Crouzon syndrome
delayed hard palate closure
denial
dieticians
displacement
Down syndrome
educational audiologist
Educational Standards Board (ESB)
electroencephalography (EEG)
fluoroscopy
fragile X syndrome
frontonasal process
grief
guilt
human immuno-deficiency virus (HIV)
Individuals with Disabilities Education Act
industrial audiologist
infectious disease specialist
laminography
magnetic resonance imaging (MRI)
mandibular processes
maxillary processes
microforms

Moebius syndrome
nasopharyngoscopy
National Outcome Measurement System (NOMS)
National Students' Speech-Language-Hearing Association
neurosurgeon
nurse
occupational therapist
otolaryngologist or head and neck surgeon
palatal clefts
pediatrician
personalization
person-centered theory
pharmacist
pharyngeal flap
pharyngoplasty
physical therapist
Pierre-Robin syndrome
plastic surgeon
positron emission tomography (PET)
Prader-Willi syndrome
Professional Services Board
projection
prosthodontist
psychiatrist
psychodynamic theory

Public Law 94-142
Public Law 99-457
pulmonary specialist
radiologist
rationalization
reaction formation
referral source
repression
Russell-Silver syndrome
shock
SOAP notes
Social Security Act
social worker
speech–language
 clinician

speech-language and
 hearing scientist
speech–language
 pathologist
speech–language
 pathology
speech therapist
stomodeum
submucous cleft palate
supportive personnel
suppression
syndrome
tomography
Treacher Collins
 syndrome

Turner syndrome
universal precautions
upper lip
U.S. Public Health
 Service Act
Usher syndrome
Veau-Wardill-Kilner
 surgery
von Langenbeck surgical
 method
V-Y retroposition
 surgery

STUDY AND REVIEW QUESTIONS

Fill in the Blank

1. In the medical setting, a(n) _pulmonary specialist_ manages patients with chronic and acute lung disorders, while a(n) _radiologist_ carries out diagnostic tests such as magnetic resonance imaging and participates in dynamic swallowing evaluations.

2. The _behavioral_ theory of counseling suggests that clinicians use operant conditioning methods and focus on specific outcomes of counseling and interacting with clients.

3. In the defense mechanism of _suppression_, the client keeps his or her feelings under control and is consciously aware of those feelings.

4. ASHA's _Professional Service_ Board evaluates clinical speech-language and hearing services offered by a speech and hearing clinic.

5. The _Americans c̄ disabilities Act_ is the law that requires that employers make "reasonable accommodations" in the workplace for employees with disabilities.

6. The IDEA created two new disability categories: _autism_ and _TBI_.

7. In medical settings, many clinicians use SOAP notes. SOAP is the acronym that stands for _subjective_, _objective_, _assessment_, _plan_.

8. Medical facilities requiring the use of _universal precautions_ _____ require that all personnel who engage in patient contact must, among other things, wash hands before and after contact with patients and wear gloves if there will be contact with bodily fluids, broken skin, or mucous membranes.

9. In the neurodiagnostic imaging method of _EEG electroencephalography_ electrical impulses of the brain are measured and recorded through small surface electrodes attached to the scalp.

10. Many genetic syndromes are associated with communication disorders. _downs_ syndrome is caused by an extra whole number chromosome 21, while _Moebius_ syndrome is caused by agenesis or aplasia of the motor nuclei of the cranial nerves.

Multiple Choice

11. A speech–language pathologist is conferencing with the family of a 16-year-old girl with severe language-learning disabilities. The girl reads at a 3rd-grade level and has been in special education placements since first grade. The speech–language pathologist tells the family, in a kind way, that their goal of their daughter attending medical school is unattainable. The family lashes out in anger against the speech–language pathologist, saying that he or she is wrong, pessimistic, and negative about their daughter and her abilities. In this situation, the family is utilizing the defense mechanism of:

    A. repression.

    B. reaction formation.

    C. displacement.

    D. suppression.

    E. projection.

12. It would be considered ethical for a speech–language pathologist to:

    A. guarantee the results of a treatment program to a worried patient.

    B. make a reasonable statement of prognosis when the spouse of a woman with aphasia asks about his wife's potential for improvement.

    C. make a diagnosis through the mail when he or she receives a letter from a friend in a distant state who is concerned about her son's articulation.

    D. allow an unsupervised assistant who is in the certification process to provide clinical services.

E. carry out a physician-recommended program of therapy with a head-injured patient even though the speech–language pathologist disagrees with the physician's recommendation.

13. Public Law 99-457:

A. increased federal support for services to disabled children 3–6 years of age and provided funding for infants and toddlers.

B. requires the development of individualized family service plans.

C. allows at-risk preschool children (not just those with documented disabilities) to be eligible for special education services.

D. A, B

E. A, B, C

14. A condition in which the surface tissues of the soft or hard palate fuse but the underlying muscle or bone tissues do not is called:

A. fusion disorder.

B. submucous or occult cleft palate.

C. class III palatal cleft.

D. submucosal cleft Class IV.

E. occult palate Class I.

15. In most states, to work in the public schools, speech–language pathologists and audiologists need:

A. a state license.

B. ASHA certification.

C. a state-issued credential from an agency such as the department of education.

D. A, B

E. A, B, C

16. Which one of the following is NOT TRUE?

A. Many state licensure laws are modeled after ASHA's requirements.

B. Violation of ASHA's Code of Ethics can have major consequences, including revocation of ASHA's clinical certificate and cancellation of ASHA membership.

C. A Certificate of Clinical Competence and state license are not necessarily required in order to practice in public school settings.

D. Some states require coursework in education or even a teaching credential for speech–language pathologists and audiologists who work in public school settings.

E. In order to receive a Certificate of Clinical Competence in speech–language pathology or audiology, a speech–language pathologists or audiologists needs only to have a state-granted credential to work in public schools.

17. A clinician who is using a client-centered approach to counseling a client with a communicative disorder will:

A. be very directive, making specific recommendations for behavioral changes.

B. help the client understand repressed conflicts between the id, ego, and superego.

C. help the client to overcome faulty thinking that is causing distress.

D. respond with acceptance and empathic listening to both the content and the feeling of what the client is saying.

E. give specific advice and look for measurable behavioral changes that occur as a result of the client implementing that advice.

18. P.L. 94-142, the Education of the Handicapped Act, was later reauthorized and retitled as:

A. the Americans with Disabilities Act.

B. the Education of Disabled Individuals Act.

C. the Handicapped Individuals Education Act.

D. the Individuals with Disabilities Education Act.

E. none of the above.

19. Speech–language pathologists working in medical settings frequently see patients who have been assessed with medical imaging techniques. A technique that uses x-ray beams that circle through segments of the brain and pass through the tissue is:

A. fluoroscopy.

B. MRI.

C. CAT scan.

D. EEG.

E. PET scan.

20. The surgical method of cleft palate repair that involves raising two bipedicled flaps of mucoperiosteum, bringing them together, and attaching them to close the cleft is called the:

A. von Langenbeck surgical method.

B. V-Y retroposition.

C. Veau-Wardill-Kilner method.

D. pharyngeal flap procedure.

E. pharyngoplasty.

REFERENCES AND RECOMMENDED READINGS

American Speech-Language-Hearing Association. (1998). ASHA membership grows to nearly 93,000, increases 5.9%. *Asha Leader, 3*(7), 5.

Benninger, M. S., & Gardner, G. M. (1998). Medical and surgical management in otolaryngology. In A. F. Johnson & B. H. Jacobson (Eds.), *Medical speech–language pathology: A practitioner's guide* (pp. 497–528). New York: Thieme Medical Publishers.

Bleile, K. (1995). *Manual of articulation and phonological disorders*. San Diego, CA: Singular Publishing Group.

Buckholz, P., & Roseberry-McKibbin, C. (1997). *A case study of a child with Russell-Silver syndrome*. Paper presented at the annual meeting of the American Speech-Language-Hearing Association, Boston, MA.

Bzoch, K. (Ed.). (1997). *Communicative disorders related to cleft lip and palate* (4th ed.). Austin, TX: PRO-ED.

California Speech-Language-Hearing Association. (1997). Substantive and subtle changes for federal IDEA. *CSHA Magazine, 26*(4), 14.

Dorland's illustrated medical dictionary. (1994, 28th ed.). Philadelphia: W.B. Saunders.

Fogle, P. (1998). Demystifying counseling. *ADVANCE for Speech–Language Pathologists & Audiologists, 8*(44), 24–26.

Frattali, C., Curl, B., & Bevan, M. (1994). Health care legislation: Implications for financing and service delivery. In R. Lubinski & C. Frattali (Eds.), *Professional issues in speech–language pathology and audiology: A textbook* (pp. 173–177). San Diego, CA: Singular Publishing Group.

George, K. P., Vikingstad, E. M., & Cao, Y. (1998). Brain imaging in neurocommunicative disorders. In A. F. Johnson & B. H. Jacobson (Eds.), *Medical speech–language pathology: A practitioner's guide* (pp. 285–336). New York: Thieme Medical Publishers.

Golper, L. A. C. (1997). *Sourcebook for medical speech pathology* (2nd ed.). San Diego, CA: Singular Publishing Group.

Hardman, M. L., Drew, C. J., & Egan, M. W. (1996). *Human exceptionality: Society, school, and family* (5th ed.). Needham Heights, MA: Allyn & Bacon.

Hegde, M. N. (1996a). *Pocketguide to assessment in speech–language pathology*. San Diego, CA: Singular Publishing Group.

Hegde, M. N. (1996b). *Pocketguide to treatment in speech–language pathology*. San Diego, CA: Singular Publishing Group.

Johnson, A. F., & Jacobson, B. H. (Eds.). (1998). *Medical speech–language pathology: A practitioner's guide*. New York: Thieme Medical Publishers.

Jung, J. H. (1989). *Genetic syndromes in communication disorders*. Austin, TX: PRO-ED.

Kummer, A. W., & Marsh, J. H. (1998). Pediatric voice and resonance disorders. In A. F. Johnson and B. H. Johnson (Eds.), *Medical speech–language pathology: A practitioner's guide* (pp. 613–633). New York: Thieme Medical Publishers.

Luterman, D. M. (1996). *Counseling the communicatively disordered and their families* (3rd ed.). Austin, TX: PRO-ED.

McWilliams, B. J., Morris, H. L., & Shelton, R. l. (1990). *Cleft palate speech*. Philadelphia: B.C. Decker.

Miller, R. M., & Groher, M. E. (1990). *Medical speech pathology*. Rockville, MD: Aspen Publishers.

Montgomery, J. B. (1994). Federal legislation affecting school settings. In R. Lubinski & C. Frattali (Eds.), *Professional issues in speech–language pathology and audiology: A textbook* (pp. 201–217). San Diego, CA: Singular Publishing Group.

Nicolosi, L., Harryman, E., & Kresheck, J. (1996). *Terminology of communication disorders: Speech-language-hearing* (4th ed.). Baltimore, MD: Williams & Wilkins.

Okun, B. F. (1992). *Effective helping: Interviewing and counseling techniques* (4th ed.). Pacific Grove, CA: Brooks/Cole.

Roseberry-McKibbin, C. (1997). Working with linguistically and culturally diverse clients. In K. G. Shipley (Ed.), *Interviewing and counseling in communicative disorders: Principles and procedures* (2nd ed.) (pp. 151–173). Needham Heights, MA: Allyn & Bacon.

Seikel, J. A., King, D. W., & Drumright, D. G. (1997). *Anatomy and physiology for speech, language, and hearing*. San Diego, CA: Singular Publishing Group.

Shipley, K. G. (1997). *Interviewing and counseling in communicative disorders: Principles and procedures* (2nd ed.). Needham Heights, MA: Allyn & Bacon.

Shprintzen, R. J. (1997). *Genetics, syndromes, and communication disorders*. San Diego, CA: Singular Publishing Group.

Shprintzen, R. J., & Bardach, J. (1995). *Cleft palate speech management: A multidisciplinary approach*. St. Louis, MO: Mosby.

Vogel, D., & Carter, J. E. (1995). *The effects of drugs on communication disorders*. San Diego, CA: Singular Publishing Group.

Wallace, G. J. (1998). Adult neurogenic disorders. In D. E. Battle (Ed.), *Communicative disorders in multicultural populations* (2nd ed.). Stoneham, MA: Andover Medical Publishers.

Zemlin, W. (1997). *Speech and hearing science: Anatomy and physiology* (4th ed.). Englewood Cliffs, NJ: Prentice-Hall.

ANSWERS TO STUDY AND REVIEW QUESTIONS

1. Pulmonary specialist, radiologist

2. Behavioral theory

3. Suppression

4. Professional Services

5. Americans with Disabilities Act

6. Autism, traumatic brain injury

7. Subjective, objective, assessment, plan

8. Universal precautions

9. EEG (electroencephalography)

10. Down, Moebius

11. C. In displacement, the client or family transfers their feelings of anger about a situation onto a safe object or person (frequently the clinician).

12. B. Principle of Ethics 1, Rule F, states that individuals may make a reasonable statement of prognosis. All other choices are forbidden by the rules in Principle of Ethics I, II, and IV.

13. E. P.L. 99-457 does all of the above, including mandating services for at-risk children.

14. B. A condition in which the surface tissues of the soft or hard palate fuse but the underlying muscle or bone tissues do not is called submucous or occult cleft palate.

15. C. In most states, public school systems require only a state-issued credential. Licensure and certification are required by many other settings such as hospitals and clinics.

16. E. In order to receive a Certificate of Clinical Competence in speech–language pathology or audiology, clinicians need a master's degree or its equivalent in speech–language pathology and must have fulfilled clinical practicum and fellowship requirements, as well

17. D. In the client-centered approach, the clinician does not give advice or specific recommendations for behavioral changes. Rather, he or she responds with acceptance and empathic listening to both the content and the feeling of what the client is saying, trusting that this will eventually lead to behavioral changes.

18. D. In 1990, the Individuals with Disabilities Education Act (IDEA) reauthorized and retitled P.L. 94-142 and made some changes in it.

19. C. A technique that uses x-ray beams that circle through segments of the brain and pass through the tissue is the CAT scan.

20. A. The surgical method of cleft palate repair that involves raising two bipedicled flaps of mucoperiosteum, bringing them together, and attaching them to close the cleft is called the von Langenbeck surgical method.

APPENDIX A

Code of Ethics of the American Speech-Language-Hearing Association
(Revised January 1, 1994)

The preservation of the highest standards of integrity and ethical principles is vital to the responsible discharge of obligations in the professions of speech–language pathology and audiology. This Code of Ethics sets forth the fundamental principles and rules considered essential to this purpose.

Every individual who is (a) a member of the ASHA, whether certified or not, (b) a nonmember holding the Certificate of Clinical Competence from the Association, (c) an applicant for membership or certification, or (d) a Clinical Fellow seeking to fulfill standards for certification shall abide by this Code of Ethics.

Any action that violates the spirit and purpose of this Code shall be considered unethical. Failure to specify any particular responsibility or practice in this Code of Ethics shall not be construed as denial of the existence of such responsibilities or practices.

The fundamentals of ethical conduct are described by Principles of Ethics and by Rules of Ethics as they relate to responsibility to persons served, to the public, and to the professions of speech–language pathology and audiology.

Principles of Ethics, aspirational and inspirational in nature, form the underlying moral basis for the Code of Ethics. Individuals shall observe these principles as affirmative obligations under all conditions of professional activity.

Rules of Ethics are specific statements of minimally acceptable professional conduct or of prohibitions and are applicable to all individuals.

PRINCIPLE OF ETHICS I

Individuals shall honor their responsibility to hold paramount the welfare of persons they serve professionally.

Rules of Ethics

A. Individuals shall provide all services competently.

B. Individuals shall use every resource, including referral when appropriate, to ensure that high-quality service is provided.

C. Individuals shall not discriminate in the delivery of professional services on the basis of race or ethnicity, gender, age, religion, national origin, sexual orientation, or disability.

D. Individuals shall fully inform the persons they serve of the nature and possible effects of services rendered and products dispensed.

E. Individuals shall evaluate the effectiveness of services rendered and of products dispensed and shall provide services or dispense products only when benefit can reasonably be expected.

F. Individuals shall not guarantee the results of any treatment or procedure, directly or by implication; however, they may make a reasonable statement of prognosis.

G. Individuals shall not evaluate or treat speech, language, or hearing disorders solely by correspondence.

H. Individuals shall maintain adequate records of professional services rendered and products dispensed and shall allow access to these records when appropriately authorized.

I. Individuals shall not reveal, without authorization, any professional or personal information about the person served professionally, unless required by law to do so, or unless doing so is necessary to protect the welfare of the person or of the community.

J. Individuals shall not charge for services not rendered, nor shall they mispresent. For purposes of this Code of Ethics, mispresentation includes any untrue statements or statements that are likely to mislead. Misrepresentation also includes the failure to state any information that is material and that ought, in fairness, to be considered, in any fashion, services rendered or products dispensed.

K. Individuals shall use persons in research or as subjects of teaching demonstrations only with their informed consent.

L. Individuals whose professional services are adversely affected by substance abuse or other health-related conditions shall seek professional assistance and, where appropriate, withdraw from the affected areas of practice.

PRINCIPLE OF ETHICS II

Individuals shall honor their responsibility to achieve and maintain the highest level of professional competence.

Rules of Ethics

A. Individuals shall engage in the provision of clinical services only when they hold the appropriate Certificate of Clinical Competence or when they are in the certification process and are supervised by an individual who holds the appropriate Certificate of Clinical Competence.

B. Individuals shall engage in only those aspects of the professions that are within the scope of their competence, considering their level of education, training, and experience.

C. Individuals shall continue their professional development throughout their careers.

D. Individuals shall delegate the provision of clinical services only to persons who are certified or to persons in the education or certification process who are appropriately supervised. The provision of support services may be delegated to persons who are neither certified nor in the certification process only when a certificate holder provides appropriate supervision.

E. Individuals shall prohibit any of their professional staff from providing services that exceed the staff member's competence, considering the staff member's level of education, training, and experience.

F. Individuals shall ensure that all equipment used in the provision of services is in proper working order and is properly calibrated.

PRINCIPLE OF ETHICS III

Individuals shall honor their responsibility to the public by promoting public understanding of the professions, by supporting the development of services designed to fulfill the unmet needs of the public, and by providing accurate information in all communications involving any aspect of the professions.

Rules of Ethics

    A. Individuals shall not misrepresent their credentials, competence, education, training, or experience.

    B. Individuals shall not participate in professional activities that constitute a conflict of interest.

    C. Individuals shall not misrepresent diagnostic information, services rendered, or products dispensed or engage in any scheme or artifice to defraud in connection with obtaining payment or reimbursement for such services or products.

    D. Individuals' statements to the public shall provide accurate information about the nature and management of communication disorders, about the professions, and about professional services.

    E. Individuals' statements to the public—advertising, announcing, and marketing their professional services, reporting research results, and promoting products—shall adhere to prevailing professional standards and shall not contain misrepresentations.

PRINCIPLE OF ETHICS IV

Individuals shall honor their responsibilities to the professions and their relationships with colleagues, students, and members of allied professions. Individuals shall uphold the dignity and autonomy of the professions, maintain harmonious interprofessional and intraprofessional relationships, and accept the professions' self-imposed standards.

Rules of Ethics

    A. Individuals shall prohibit anyone under their supervision from engaging in any practice that violates the Code of Ethics.

    B. Individuals shall not engage in dishonesty, fraud, deceit, mispresentation, or any form of conduct that adversely reflects on the professions or on the individual's fitness to serve persons professionally.

    C. Individuals shall assign credit only to those who have contributed to a publication, presentation, or product. Credit shall be assigned in proportion to the contribution and only with the contributor's consent.

    D. Individuals' statements to colleagues about professional services, research results, and products shall adhere to prevailing professional standards and shall contain no misrepresentations.

E. Individuals shall not provide professional services without exercising independent professional judgment, regardless of referral source or prescription.

F. Individuals shall not discriminate in their relationships with colleagues, students, and members of allied professions on the basis of race or ethnicity, gender, age, religion, national origin, sexual orientation, or disability.

G. Individuals who have reason to believe that the Code of Ethics has been violated shall inform the Ethical Practice Board.

Note. From "Code of Ethics," by American Speech-Language-Hearing Association, 1994, *Asha, 36* (March, Suppl. 13), pp. 1–2. Reprinted with permission.

APPENDIX B

Scope of Practice in Speech–Language Pathology

PREAMBLE

The purpose of this statement is to define the scope of practice of speech–language pathology and audiology in order to

(1) delineate areas of services and supports provided by ASHA members and certificate holders in accordance with the ASHA Code of Ethics. Services refer to clinical services for individuals with speech, voice, language, communication, and swallowing disorders, aimed at the amelioration of difficulties stemming from such disorders. Supports refer to environmental modifications, assistive technology, and guidance for communication partners to help persons with these disorders;

(2) educate health care, education, and other professionals, consumers, payers, regulators, and members of the general public about treatment and other services and supports offered by speech–language pathologists as qualified providers;

(3) assist members and certificate holders in their efforts to provide appropriate and high-quality services and supports to persons across the life span with speech, voice, language, communication, and swallowing disabilities;

(4) establish a reference for curriculum review of education programs in speech–language pathology.

The scope of practice defined here, and the areas specifically set forth are part of an effort to establish the broad range of services and supports offered within the profession. It is recognized, however, that levels of experience, skill, and proficiency with respect to the activities identified within this scope of practice vary among the individual providers. It may not be possible for speech–language pathologists to practice in all areas of the field. As the ASHA Code of Ethics specifies, individuals may only practice in areas where they are competent based on their education, training, and experience. However, nothing limits speech–language pathologists from expanding their current level of expertise. Certain clients or practice settings may necessitate that speech–language pathologists pursue additional education or training to expand their personal scope of practice. This scope of practice statement does not supersede existing state licensure laws or affect the interpretation or implementation of such laws. It may serve, however, as a model for the development or modification of licensure laws.

Finally, it is recognized that speech–language pathology is a dynamic and continuously developing practice area. Listing specific areas within this scope of practice does not necessarily exclude other, new, or emerging areas. Indeed, changes in service delivery systems, the increasing numbers of persons who need communication services, and technological and scientific advances have mandated that a scope of practice for the profession of speech–language pathology be a dynamic statement. For these reasons this document will undergo periodic review and possible revision.

STATEMENT

The goal of the profession of speech–language pathology and its members is provision of the highest-quality treatment and other services consistent with the fundamental right of those served to participate in decisions that affect their lives.

Speech–language pathologists hold the master's or doctoral degree, the Certificate of Clinical Competence of the American Speech-Language-Hearing Association, and state licensure where applicable.

These professionals serve individuals, families, groups, and the general public through their involvement in a broad range of professional activities. They work to prevent speech, voice, language, communication, swallowing, and related disabilities. They screen, identify, assess, diagnose, refer, and provide treatment and intervention, including consultation and follow-up services, to persons of all ages with, or at risk for, speech, voice, language, communication, swallowing, and related disabilities. They counsel individuals with these disorders, as well as their families, caregivers, and other service providers, related to the disorders and their management. Speech–language pathologists select, prescribe, dispense, and provide services supporting the effective use of augmentative and alternative communication devices and other communication prostheses and assistive devices.

Speech–language pathologists also teach, supervise, and manage clinical and educational programs, and engage in program development, program oversight, and research activities related to communication sciences and disorders, swallowing, and related areas.

They measure treatment outcomes, evaluate the effectiveness of their practices, modify services in relation to their evaluations, and disseminate these findings. They also serve as case managers and expert witnesses. As an integral part of their practice, speech–language pathologists work to increase public awareness and advocate for the people they serve.

Speech–language pathologists provide services in settings that are deemed appropriate, including but not limited to health care, educational, community, vocational, and home settings. Speech–language pathologists serve diverse populations. The client population includes persons of different race, age, gender, religion, national origin, and sexual orientation. Speech–language pathologists' caseloads include persons from diverse ethnic, cultural, or linguistic backgrounds, and persons with disabilities. Although speech–language pathologists are prohibited from discriminating in the provision of professional services based on these factors, in some cases such factors may be relevant to the development of an appropriate treatment plan. These factors may be considered in treatment plans only when firmly grounded in scientific and professional knowledge.

As primary care providers of communication treatment and other services, speech–language pathologists are autonomous professionals; that is, their services need not be prescribed by another. However, in most cases individuals are best served when speech–language pathologists work collaboratively with other professionals, individuals with disabilities, and their family members. Similarly, it is recognized that related fields and professions may have some knowledge, skills, and experience that could be applied to some areas within this scope of practice. Defining the scope of practice of speech–language pathologists is not meant to exclude members of other professions or related fields from rendering services in common practice areas.

The practice of speech–language pathology includes:

(1) Providing screening, identification, assessment, diagnosis, treatment, intervention (i.e., prevention, restoration, amelioration, compensation) and follow-up services for disorders of:

- speech: articulation, fluency, voice (including respiration, phonation, and resonance)

- language (involving the parameters of phonology, morphology, syntax, semantics, and pragmatics; and including disorders of receptive and expressive communication in oral, written, graphic, and manual modalities)

- oral, pharyngeal, cervical, esophageal, and related functions (e.g., dysphagia, including disorders of swallowing and oral function for feeding; orofacial myofunctional disorders)

- cognitive aspects of communication (including communication disability and other functional disabilities associated with cognitive impairment)

- social aspects of communication (including challenging behavior, ineffective social skills, lack of communication opportunities);

(2) Providing consultation and counseling, and making referrals when appropriate;

(3) Training and supporting family members and other communication partners of individuals with speech, voice, language, communication, and swallowing disabilities;

(4) Developing and establishing effective augmentative and alternative communication techniques and strategies, including selecting, prescribing, and dispensing of aids and devices and training individuals, their families, and other communication partners in their use;

(5) Selecting, fitting, and establishing effective use of appropriate prosthetic/adaptive devices for speaking and swallowing (e.g., tracheoesophageal valves, electrolarynges, speaking valves);

(6) Using instrumental technology to diagnose and treat disorders of communication and swallowing (e.g., videofluoroscopy, nasendoscopy, ultrasonography, stroboscopy);

(7) Providing aural rehabilitation and related counseling services to individuals with hearing loss and to their families;

(8) Collaborating in the assessment of central auditory processing disorders in cases in which there is evidence of speech, language, and/or other cognitive-communication disorders; providing intervention for individuals with central auditory processing disorders;

(9) Conducting pure-tone air-conduction hearing screening and screening tympanometry for the purpose of the initial identification and/or referral of individuals with other communication disorders or possible middle ear pathology;

(10) Enhancing speech and language proficiency and communication effectiveness, including but not limited to accent reduction, collaboration with teachers of English as a second language, and improvement of voice, performance, and singing;

(11) Training and supervising support personnel;

(12) Developing and managing academic and clinical programs in communication sciences and disorders;

(13) Conducting, disseminating, and applying research in communication sciences and disorders;

(14) Measuring outcomes of treatment and conducting continuous evaluation of the effectiveness of practices and programs to improve and maintain quality of services.

Note. From "Scope of Practice in Speech–Language Pathology," by American Speech-Language-Hearing Association, *Asha, 38* (Suppl 16). Reprinted with permission.

APPENDIX C

Standards for the Certificate of Clinical Competence of Practice in Speech–Language Pathology

The American Speech-Language-Hearing Association issues Certificates of Clinical Competence to individuals who present evidence of their ability to provide independent clinical services to persons who have disorders of communication. Individuals who meet the standards specified by the Association's Council on Professional Standards may be awarded a Certificate of Clinical Competence in Speech–Language Pathology (CCC-SLP) or a Certificate of Clinical Competence in Audiology (CCC-A). Individuals who meet the standards in both professional areas may be awarded both Certificates.

STANDARD I: DEGREE

Applicants for either Certificate must have a master's or doctoral degree.

Effective January 1, 1994, all graduate coursework and graduate clinical practicum required in the professional area for which the Certificate is sought must have been initiated and completed at an institution whose program was accredited by the Educational Standards Board of the American Speech-Language-Hearing Association in the area for which the Certificate is sought.

STANDARD II: ACADEMIC COURSEWORK

Applicants for either Certificate must have earned at least 75 semester (one quarter credit hour is equivalent to two-thirds of a semester credit hour) credit hours that reflect a well-integrated program of study dealing with (a) the biological/physical sciences and mathematics; (b) the behavioral and/or social sciences, including normal aspects of human behavior and communication, and (c) the nature, prevention, evaluation, and treatment of speech, language, hearing, and related disorders. Some coursework must address issues pertaining to normal and abnormal human development and behavior across the life span and to culturally diverse populations.

At least 27 of the 75 semester credit hours must be in Basic Scientific Coursework (see Standard II-A).

At least 36 of the 75 semester credit hours must be in Professional Coursework (see Standard II-B).

STANDARD II-A: BASIC SCIENCE COURSEWORK

Applicants for either Certificate must earn at least 27 semester credit hours in the basic sciences.

At least 6 semester credit hours must be in the biological/physical sciences and mathematics.

At least 6 semester credit hours must be in the behavioral and/or social sciences.

At least 15 semester credit hours must be in the basic human communication processes, to include coursework in each of the following three areas of speech, language, and hearing: the anatomic and physiologic bases; the physical and psychophysical bases; the linguistic and psycholingustic aspects. (The three broad categories of required education, and the examples of areas within these classifications, are not meant to be analogous to or imply specific course titles or to be exhaustive.)

STANDARD II-B: PROFESSIONAL COURSEWORK

Applicants for either Certificate must earn at least 36 semester credit hours in courses that concern the nature, prevention, evaluation, and treatment of speech, language, and hearing disorders. Those 36 semester credit hours must encompass courses in speech, language, and hearing that concern disorders primarily affecting children as well as disorders primarily affecting adults. At least 30 of the 36 semester credit hours must be in courses for which graduate credit was received, and at least 21 of those 30 must be in the professional area for which the Certificate is sought.

At least 30 of the 36 semester credit hours of professional coursework must be in speech–language pathology. At least 6 of the 30 must be in speech disorders, and at least 6 must be in language disorders.

At least 6 of the 36 semester credit hours of professional coursework must be in audiology. At least 3 of the 6 must be in hearing disorders and hearing evaluation, and at least 3 must be in habilitative/rehabilitative procedures with individuals who have hearing impairment.

A maximum of 6 academic semester credit hours associated with clinical practicum may be counted toward the minimum of 36 semester credit hours of professional coursework, but those hours may not be used to satisfy the minimum of 6 semester credit hours in speech disorders, 6 hours in language disorders, or 6 hours in audiology, or in the 21 credits in the professional area for which the Certificate is sought.

STANDARD III: SUPERVISED CLINICAL OBSERVATION AND CLINICAL PRACTICUM (375 CLOCK HOURS)

Applicants for either Certificate must complete the requisite number of clock hours of supervised clinical observation and supervised clinical practicum that are provided by the educational institution or by one of its cooperating programs.

The supervision must be provided by an individual who holds the Certificate of Clinical Competence in the appropriate area of practice.

STANDARD III-A: CLINICAL OBSERVATION

Applicants for either Certificate must complete at least 25 hours of supervised observation prior to beginning the initial clinical practicum.

Those 25 clock hours must concern the evaluation and treatment of children and adults with disorders of speech, language, or hearing.

STANDARD III-B: CLINICAL PRACTICUM

Applicants for either Certificate must complete at least 350 clock hours of supervised clinical practicum that concern the evaluation and treatment of children and adults with disorders of speech, language, and hearing. No more than 25 of the clock hours may be obtained from participation in staffings in which evaluation, treatment, and/or recommendations are discussed or formulated, with or without the client present.

At least 250 of the 350 clock hours must be completed in the professional area for which the Certificate is sought while the applicant is engaged in graduate study.

At least 50 supervised clock hours must be completed in each of three types of clinical settings.

The applicant must have experience in the evaluation and treatment of children and adults, and with a variety of types and severities of disorders of speech, language, and hearing. At least 250 of the 350 supervised clock hours must be in speech–language pathology. At least 20 of those 250 clock hours must be completed in each of the eight categories listed below.

1. Evaluation: Speech disorders in children

2. Evaluation: Speech disorders in adults

3. Evaluation: Language disorders in children

4. Evaluation: Language disorders in adults

5. Treatment: Speech disorders in children

6. Treatment: Speech disorders in adults

7. Treatment: Language disorders in children

8. Treatment: Language disorders in adults

Up to 20 clock hours in the major professional area may be in related disorders.

At least 35 of the 350 clock hours must be in audiology. At least 15 of those 35 clock hours must involve the evaluation or screening of individuals with hearing disorders, and at least 15 must involve habilitation/rehabilitation of individuals who have hearing impairment.

STANDARD IV: NATIONAL EXAMINATION IN SPEECH–LANGUAGE PATHOLOGY

Applicants must pass the national examination in the area for which the Certificate is sought.

STANDARD V: THE CLINICAL FELLOWSHIP

After completion of academic coursework (Standard II) and clinical practicum (Standard III), the applicant then must successfully complete a Clinical Fellowship.

The Fellowship will consist of at least 36 weeks of full-time professional experience or its part-time equivalent.

The Fellowship must be completed under the supervision of an individual who holds the Certificate of Clinical Competence in the area for which certification is sought.

The professional experience shall involve primarily clinical activities.

The Supervisor periodically shall conduct a formal evaluation of the applicant's progress in the development of professional skills.

Note. Adapted with permission from the American Speech-Language-Hearing Association, *Standards and Implementations for the Certificate of Clinical Competence of Practice in Speech–Language Pathology*. The standards are listed here; implementation procedures are not. Those procedures can be found in the source document, available from ASHA.

APPENDIX D

Study and Test-Taking Tips for the NESPA

Many readers of this book are preparing for the National Examination in Speech Pathology and Audiology (NESPA). This purpose of this appendix is to provide readers with a brief orientation to the NESPA and to give study and test-taking tips to help readers pass the NESPA. (*Note*: Some of these suggestions may also be applied to studying for and passing comprehensive examinations in graduate programs; readers may apply the information to their individual programs as needed.)

NATURE AND PURPOSE OF THE NESPA

■ The NESPA is "designed to measure examinees' academic preparation in and knowledge of the field" (*A Guide to the NTE: Speech Language Pathology Specialty Area Test*, Princeton, NJ: Educational Testing Service, 1995, p. 9). Essentially, the purpose of the NESPA is to ask questions in all areas of speech–language pathology to assess whether or not examinees are prepared to competently serve as speech–language pathologists in a variety of clinical settings.

■ The NESPA has 150 multiple-choice questions, which are to be answered within 2 hours' time. These questions assess examinees' knowledge of:

- the evaluation process (29%)

- remediation (how to plan and implement treatment) (66%)

- administration (5%)

■ Questions on the NESPA are gathered from courses in undergraduate and graduate programs in speech–language pathology. The questions cover all age levels from newborns to geriatric patients (Educational Testing Service, 1995).

■ Passing the NESPA is one of the requirements for obtaining a Certificate of Clinical Competence issued by the American Speech-Language-Hearing Association. Some individual states may use the NESPA as part of their licensing requirements. Some individual graduate programs may use the NESPA as part of the requirements to obtain a master's degree.

■ It is necessary to obtain a score of 600 to pass the NESPA. An examinee may score 600 by answering approximately 60–65% of the questions correctly.

STUDY TIPS FOR PREPARING FOR THE NESPA

■ Many test takers, being human, attempt to memorize a great deal of information right before the examination. Research indicates that ideal learning does not occur under those conditions.

■ It is best to start studying at least several months before the NESPA is taken. Ideally, you should try to study a little bit each day. Many examinees attempt to study for several hours only on weekends. It is optimal to study a little bit daily rather than try to "cram in" studying on weekends only.

■ If you studied 15 minutes a day 6 days a week, that would equal 1.5 hours of study a week. If that was done for 3 months, you would have studied for 18 hours total.

■ When it comes to studying, more is usually better. However, reality dictates that 15 minutes of studying a day for several months is the most many people can manage. When you do a little studying each day, you learn more than if studying was crammed into large blocks of time right before the examination.

■ Many adults learn best in a multimodal fashion. That is, they retain information best if they read it, write it, say it aloud, and discuss it with others, as opposed to just passively reading it. Thus, it is ideal to study both alone and with other people if possible. You should try to form study groups that meet once or twice a week. Many adults learn best in a study group format.

■ It is very helpful, in trying to retain information, to write the information down. You might make flash cards with pertinent information. These flash cards can be carried in a purse or pocket and pulled out during "dead time," when you are waiting in line at the supermarket or at a red light, for example. It is surprising how much dead time most of us have that we are not aware of.

■ It is extremely helpful to take a practice NESPA examination. Several are available and are listed at the end of this appendix. It is best to set aside 2 hours and take a practice examination with no interruptions. While it is challenging for many busy people to find a 2-hour uninterrupted time block, we have found that this is the very best situation for preparing to actually take the NESPA.

■ Many NESPA workshop attendees have told us, after taking the examination, that they ran out of time at the end because they worked too slowly. They had never before been required to answer 150 multiple-choice questions in 2 hours. Thus, taking a practice examination in an uninterrupted 2-hour time block is the very best way for you to be prepared for the actual situation ahead.

■ Many examinees stay up late the night before an examination. They spend those late hours "cramming" for the examination the next day. For many people, this does not work well when taking the NESPA. The NESPA questions (unlike some essay and fill-in-the-blank questions) do not necessarily require rote, pre-memorized answers. Rather, many questions require a great deal of reading, careful thought, and subjective judgment decisions.

■ Such higher-level thought questions are usually best and most accurately answered if you have had a good night's sleep before the examination. In our opinion, the night before the NESPA is best spent sleeping and attempting to wake up refreshed to answer challenging questions the next day.

TIPS FOR TAKING THE NESPA

■ Right before the examination is taken, it is best to go to the bathroom. While you may find this tip humorous, laughter quickly fades when you discover that if you take 10 minutes during the NESPA to go to the bathroom, that is 10 minutes lost during the examination.

■ In other words, if the NESPA is administered from 8:00 to 10:00 in the morning, you do not get to take 10 minutes in the bathroom during the examination and then continue taking the test until 10:10. Time spent in the bathroom is time lost in test-taking!

■ It is best to wear loose, comfortable clothing during the examination. Bring a sweater or wrap, even if the weather outside is warm. We have found that room temperatures may be too hot or cold for everyone's comfort and may distract from thinking and doing your best.

■ Many examinees feel very nervous. Deep breathing is an excellent way to deal with feelings of nervousness. Deep breathing also enhances concentration by providing increased oxygen to the brain.

■ Bring a watch to have out on your desk during the examination. We have found that some testing rooms do not have clocks (which can be very distressing for those not wearing watches).

■ Be constantly mindful of time. You have approximately 48 seconds to answer each question. As stated earlier, we have found that many, many examinees' greatest problem was that they ran out of time at the end. It is quite upsetting to have 10 minutes left with 25 questions still to answer. *Keep moving along*, even if you are unsure of each answer. At the end of the first hour of the test, you should be on #75.

■ Occasionally, you will encounter a question that seems deceptively simple and quick (as in the following example). There are a few of these on the NESPA. Answer them as best you can, and use the time you saved on those questions to answer the questions requiring more reading.

> ▶ Which is the primary cranial nerve involved in innervation of the muscles of the larynx?

> A. cranial nerve VIII

> B. cranial nerve IX

> C. cranial nerve II

> D. cranial nerve X

> E. cranial nerve XII

> The answer is D, cranial nerve X.

■ Many NESPA questions require a great deal of reading. Those questions involve cases in which a clinical decision is necessary. Examinees have shared with us that they were unhappily surprised by the sheer number of these complicated questions. Knowing that such questions exist is very helpful. An example follows:

> ▶ A 6-year-old child with a repaired posterior cleft palate has been referred to you by her teacher. The child's speech is hypernasal with numerous articulatory errors, including glottal stops, distortions of sibilants, and substitutions of w/r and j/l. The cleft palate team, consisting of an orthodontist, plastic surgeon, pediodontist, and oromaxillofacial surgeon, is involved in consulting with you in this case. During phonation of /u/, a palatopharyngeal gap exceeding 15 millimeters is observed. The parents are eager for their child to get as much assistance as possible and have indicated their willingness to provide as much support as is necessary. Given this information, which of the following will be your *first* priority in clinical management of this case?

> A. Therapy beginning with the easy initiation /u/ blended with stop consonants to lower tongue position, reduce nasality, and eliminate glottal stops

> B. Blowing exercises to strengthen velopharyngeal valving

> C. Therapy to remediate the w/r and j/l substitutions

> D. Ear training to identify distortion of sibilants

E. Referral to the appropriate specialists to determine physical management of the palatopharyngeal gap

The answer is E.

■ Read all choices before you decide on the best answer. Reading all choices increases the chances of answering the question accurately.

■ Never leave any questions blank. Always answer each question. You are never penalized for guessing incorrectly, but you are always penalized for leaving items blank and unanswered in that you have no chance to get an unanswered question right.

■ If you do not know the answer to a question, guess. Your first guess is usually the right one. We have heard dozens of times over the years that examinees changed their answers, only to find later that the first guess was actually the right one.

■ If you are unsure of your answer on an item, answer it as best you can, circle that item in the test booklet (not on the answer sheet) and, if time permits, come back to that item after you have completed the examination. In this way, you keep moving forward.

■ Constantly check your answer sheet to make sure you are filling in the right bubble for the item you think you are on. It is horrifying to come to question #130 and find that you are one item "off" because you accidentally skipped a question on the Scantron answer sheet. Keep checking!

■ If you erase an answer, erase very thoroughly. The Scantron machines that score the examinations are quite sensitive, and may pick up and score your erasure rather than your actual answer. Some examinees find it helpful to fill in the bubbles adequately but not so firmly that erasure is almost impossible.

■ Bring three or four sharpened pencils with good erasers to the examination. Do not assume that the NESPA proctor has extra pencils or a pencil sharpener.

■ Try to relax as much as possible. This is easier said than done. The more relaxed you are, the higher your likelihood of passing the examination. Remember that if you should fail the NESPA, you can take it again. (*Note*: Policies about the number of retakes change occasionally, so check into the latest available information about this.)

PRACTICE NESPA EXAMINATIONS

A Guide to the NTE Speech–Language Pathology Specialty Area Test, Princeton, NJ: Educational Testing Service, 1995. This book contains a complete 150-question actual NESPA examination (with answers), practice sample questions, and test-taking strategies. It can be ordered when you fill out the application form for taking the NESPA. It may also be available at local bookstores; phone first to check. The book may be ordered directly from:

Educational Testing Service
The Praxis Series
Princeton, New Jersey 08541-6000

How to Prepare for the NESPA National Examinations in Speech Pathology and Audiology, K. T. Payne & N. B. Anderson, San Diego, CA: Singular Publishing Group, Inc. 1991. This book contains suggestions for preparing for the NESPA as well as a complete 150-question NESPA examination with answers at the back of the book. The book may be ordered directly from:

Singular Publishing Group, Inc.
401 West A Street, Suite 325
San Diego, Ca 92101-7904
(619) 238-6777

INDEX

Page numbers in italics refer to illustrations.

ABOUT THE AUTHORS

Celeste Roseberry-McKibbin received her Ph.D. from Northwestern University. She is an associate professor of speech pathology and audiology at California State University, Sacramento. She also currently serves as a part-time itinerant speech–language pathologist in the Elk Grove Unified School District, where she provides direct services to elementary school students. She has worked in educational and medical settings with a wide variety of clients ranging from preschool-aged children through geriatric patients. She has copre-sented a number of workshops on taking and passing the National Examination in Speech Pathology and Audiology.

Dr. Roseberry-McKibbin's research interests are in the areas of bilingualism and second-language acquisition, multiculturalism, and assessment and treatment of multicultural students with communicative disorders. She has written over 25 publications and has made over 100 presentations at the local, state, and national levels. She lived in the Philippines from the age of 6 to the age of 17, when she came to live in the United States permanently.

M. N. (Giri) Hegde is a professor of communicative sciences and disorders at California State University, Fresno. He holds a master's degree in experimental psychology from the University of Mysore, India, and a post-master's diploma in medical psychology from Bangalore University, India. His doctoral degree in speech–language pathology is from Southern Illinois University in Carbondale, Illinois.

Dr. Hegde is a specialist in research methods, fluency disorders, language, and treatment procedures in communicative disorders. He has made many pro-fessional and scientific presentations to national and international audiences on a wide variety of topics in communicative disorders. He has published many research articles and over 18 books on a wide range of subjects in speech–language pathology. He has received numerous state and national professional accolades and honors, including the ASHA Fellow Award.